The Psychodynamic Treatment of Women

The Psychodynamic Treatment of Women

Anne E. Bernstein, M.D.
Clinical Professor of Psychiatry
College of Physicians and Surgeons
of Columbia University;
Attending Psychiatrist, Presbyterian Hospital
New York, New York

Sharyn A. Lenhart, M.D.
Associate Attending Psychiatrist
McLean Hospital
Belmont, Massachusetts

American Psychiatric Press, Inc.

Washington, DC
London, England

Note: The authors have worked to ensure that all information in this book concerning drug dosages, schedules, and routes of administration is accurate as of the time of publication and consistent with standards set by the U.S. Food and Drug Administration and the general medical community. As medical research and practice advance, however, therapeutic standards may change. For this reason and because human and mechanical errors sometimes occur, we recommend that readers follow the advice of a physician who is directly involved in their care or the care of a member of their family.

Manufactured in the United States of America on acid-free paper
96 95 94 93 4 3 2 1
First Edition
American Psychiatric Press, Inc.
1400 K Street, N.W., Washington, DC 20005

Library of Congress Cataloging-in-Publication Data
Bernstein, Anne E.
The Psychodynamic Treatment of Women / Anne E. Bernstein, Sharyn A. Lenhart
p. cm.
Includes bibliographical references and index.
ISBN 0-88048-368-7
1. Women—Mental health. 2. Psychodynamic psychotherapy. I. Lenhart, Sharyn A., 1948– . II. Title.
[DNLM: 1. Psychoanalytic Therapy. 2. Women—psychology.
WM 460.5.W6 B531p]
RC451.4.W6B469 1993
616.89'0082—dc20
DNLM/DLC 92-48733
for Library of Congress CIP

British Library Cataloguing in Publication Data
A CIP record is available from the British Library.

For everything there is a time. A time to be born
and a time to die—a time to tear down
and a time to build . . .

Ecclesiastes

Dedicated to those valuable family and friends, both living and dead, who inspired our decision to build this book together.

Contents

Preface

Our initial mandate from the American Psychiatric Press was a broad one: to write about the psychodynamic treatment of women. This meant that we were obligated to discuss and provide examples of major issues for women whose diagnoses spanned categories from high functioning, classically analyzable conditions to behaviors and cognitive and perceptual deficits that sometimes required prolonged institutional care.

The major categories of issues were clear and have, from the beginning, been reflected in our chapter titles. In reviewing the initial proposal, Dr. Carol Nadelson suggested that pulling things together might best be accomplished by a genetic format, which turned out to be a most helpful and organizing principle. Although a problem like self-esteem dysregulation may begin in children or surface anywhere in the life cycle, we elected to discuss it at the stage in which it appears most prevalent (i.e., in the middle years of adulthood) but also to mention it when it arises in childhood and maximally in adolescence, and again when widowhood and illness bring it to primacy in the later years.

The psychodynamic treatment of women began with Freud and his early "classical psychoanalytic" colleagues. Most important contributions came from women analysts. The fallacy lay in taking the male model as the norm, in denying the prevalence of sexual abuse in childhood, and in trying to deduce problems and solutions for women from this phallocentric point of view.

During the last 15 years, women writers, psychiatrists, psychologists, and analysts discovered that not only do women differ from men anatomically, but in the facets of their ego and superego functioning women sees themselves primarily in relation. Their valuing of relationships above other goals often seems to have an instinctual basis, a drive quality much like sexuality or aggression. Closer inspection reveals that women have been carefully taught these values. A great deal of conflict stems from the contrary messages that women have received in a male-dominated society. The definition of self in relation to others will be a pivotal concept essential to the understanding of women's conflicts and the recollection of these conflicts throughout the life cycle.

As we patiently tackled our chapters, one by one, we recognized the magnitude and complexity of psychodynamic issues specific to women and the need to unify them in one definitive work. No work on female psychodynamics could be complete without discussing issues like infertility, abortion, adoption, divorce, widowhood, and grandmotherhood, to name a few. Nor could we fail to acknowledge the importance of AIDS, alternate life-styles, or committed partnerships. There is no way to illustrate the importance of self-esteem issues without reference to the plastic surgery and cosmetic industries or to the growing addiction of women to alcohol, tobacco, and prescription and over-the-counter drugs. The project became a massive one because of issues begging to be discussed—for example, incest, sexual harassment, rape, and battering—that cause such frequent and profound psychiatric morbidity. Each of our chapters threatened to demand a book of its own. What we have done is to try to provide a brief but in-depth study of many issues and the psychodynamic treatment involved. For those who would care to look further—to read, and even write, more—we have provided an extensive and comprehensive list of references. Our hope is to have set our readers firmly on the path of further exploration of the multitude of psychodynamic problems specific to women.

Anne E. Bernstein, M.D.
Sharyn A. Lenhart, M.D.

Acknowledgments

The American Medical Women's Association (AMWA) is an organization that promotes networking among women physicians and encourages them to work together on projects that make their expertise available to others. It was through the AMWA that the present authors met, presented collaborative workshops, and validated their mutual respect for collegial relationships between women. We are grateful to the AMWA for setting the scene for what has been a personally enriching collaboration.

Our families have been gracious to us both during our working visits. We are especially grateful to our husbands, Drs. Richard K. Bernstein and Lloyd F. Price, for their patience and encouragement. The friendship of our daughters, Lili Bernstein and Allison and Heather Price, has been a special pleasure.

We are grateful to our colleagues who shared patient material with us and who are acknowledged by name in the text, and also to our legal experts, who have been cited.

We are indebted to our patients, who furnished the laboratory for observation and whose responses in treatment have helped confirm our hypotheses about the specific and special nature of women and their psychology. In some instances, we have obtained consent to publish their material at length; in other instances, we have, in the interest of protecting privacy and confidentiality, disguised the material and presented briefer vignettes.

Mostly, we are grateful to each other for the patience, forbearance, and humor it took to hammer out the organization and style of the book, and for the integrity of meeting agreed-upon deadlines and furnishing information uniquely available to one or the other of us. We appreciate the meticulous care given the manuscript by our editor, Greg Kuny. His standards of excellence forced a precision that we might not have otherwise exercised.

Each of us wishes to thank some special people who have been inspirational and supportive or technically helpful to us individually:

For Dr. Bernstein: The idea of selecting a coauthor was governed by the experience of having written two prior books with Gloria Marmor

Warner, M.D. We had been dear friends, spending working vacations together with our husbands and children. We laughed a lot and never argued. We envisioned a lifetime of collaboration and shared enjoyment of grandchildren. Life was shattered by "Dr. Gloria's" premature death at the age of 50. Collaboration with another woman represented my conscious hope of softening the pain of that loss. I dedicated the book to "Dr. Gloria" before the first word of the text was written. However, in the spirit of equality, the generic dedication represents the new collaboration. I would like to acknowledge the competent technical assistance of Susan Congdon; photocopier Jeanine Fredrick; and Pat Gian, whose organizational help was invaluable. Laura Bernstein assisted with the references, as did the librarians at both Columbia University College of Physicians and Surgeons and the New York State Psychiatric Institute.

For Dr. Lenhart: Warm appreciation and respect are extended to Rosanne Labree, Lyn Dietrich, Debbie Pennino, and Pam Hastings of the McLean Mental Health Sciences Library for graciously providing invaluable research assistance; to Ann Montague for preparing this manuscript with professionalism and calm good humor; and to Marian Bodeman for extending support and assistance in cutting through an innumerable amount of red tape. Thanks to colleagues Maria Smith, Eileen Kahan, Clyde Evans, Freade Klein, and Connie Cutter for generously contributing their clinical and theoretical expertise.

Greatest appreciation is extended to my family, who generously supported me through this lengthy project. I thank Mildred and Sidney Price and Al and Betty Winograd for providing an important boost when it was crucially needed. I thank my daughters, Allison and Heather Price, for helping with the housework, for allowing me to take time away from our time together, and for being curious, enthusiastic, and appreciative of my work. Most of all, I thank my husband, Dr. Lloyd Price, who helped me both professionally and personally, providing encouragement, perspective, companionship, criticism that was both intelligent and sensitive, careful proofreading under exhausting circumstances, and a consistent and calming sense of respect and caring for me and for this project.

Introduction

Women seek psychodynamic treatment twice as frequently as men, and they manifest unique problems. In this volume, we present an overview of the general problems experienced by women and detail methods of treatment that we have utilized with positive outcomes. Our material has come from patients with a wide range of diagnoses—from high-functioning patients (candidates for psychoanalysis) to patients whose behavioral, cognitive, and perceptual difficulties have sometimes required prolonged institutional care. These patients were treated using psychodynamic psychotherapy as well as medication and a multidimensional treatment team approach when necessary. Although intensive, prolonged inpatient care has been virtually eliminated because of the constraints in funding, we do not consider this development to be good psychiatric medicine. We present and discuss patients who did respond to brief, intensive psychodynamic psychotherapy. We differentiate between psychoanalysis and psychodynamic psychotherapy.

Our material is organized in terms of the life cycle. We discuss each issue at length at the genetic phase at which it is most prevalent, referring to each issue briefly as it occurs in other developmental phases. We include discussion on a range of anxiety, depressive, and personality disorders that are responsive to psychodynamic intervention. For our purposes we have confined ourselves to insight-oriented and ego-supportive therapies, rather than behavior or cognitive therapies. This focus does not reflect a prejudice against other therapies but a desire to explicate psychodynamic treatment.

We discuss treatment paradigms for women and strategies that have been worked out by nonphysician therapists. It is apparent that there are issues around anxiety, depression, and anger that are specific to women. Secondarily, the attempt by women to relieve these often unbearable affects leads to other problems such as sexual promiscuity, child battering, and/or abuse of alcohol, street drugs, and tranquilizers. We cite and illustrate the way in which we utilize this new information and these new conceptualizations.

Our point of view encompasses so-called classical analytic concepts as applied in a dyadic relationship between therapist and patient. We also discuss concepts drawn from object-relations psychology, interpersonal psychology, self psychology, and cognitive psychology. In addition, we mention biochemical, behavioral, and group techniques when appropriate. As physicians we present recent contributions from neurology, neurobiology, chemistry, and pharmacology in the appendixes.

We have chosen several topics that deal with either problems specific to women or problems for which women increasingly present themselves for treatment. Women come with anxiety disorder, generalized anxiety, somatization, panic attacks, and multiple personality disorder. All of these are more common in women than in men. We are seeing more female patients with posttraumatic stress disorder secondary to specific assaults occurring because of their sex. Depressive disorders, dysthymia, and major depression are more prevalent in women. The rate of suicide and homicide is also increasing in women. We are seeing increasing drug abuse with physician-prescribed tranquilizers and energizers, illegal drugs, and legal drugs and alcohol. More women than men are smoking. We see masochism and passivity as well as rage and note when it is nonproductive.

Adolescent girls in search of identity often become victims of bulimic symptoms, bulimia nervosa, and anorexia nervosa. These last two disorders are often life threatening and require medical, behavioral, and psychodynamic management. Out-of-wedlock pregnancy, drug abuse, and acquired immunodeficiency syndrome (AIDS) are at epidemic proportions in the adolescent population.

Premenstrual syndrome and/or late luteal phase dysphoric disorder (proposed in the upcoming DSM-IV as depressive disorder not otherwise specified) are being contested as diagnostic entities by some feminists who are fearful of the scapegoating of women. Yet we have seen these disorders, and we must treat them both medically and psychiatrically if indicated. If premenstrual syndrome is not a psychiatric diagnosis, patients who could feel better with psychodynamic therapy or psychotropic medication will not have insurance coverage for treatment.

Women have enormous, even if not exclusive, problems with self-esteem regulation. The quest for youth, beauty, and tranquility (or tranquilization) is a major problem for women, even if men are not exempt in these areas or manifest them differently. Currently, women find themselves having to handle the problems of career and motherhood, combining these two worlds and networking for self-esteem regulation at this stressful period. Problems of infertility and the quest for a baby are shared by spouses, but women often present these problems as if they bear the guilt or the responsibility, or both. Often it is women who require the invasive diagnostic and therapeutic procedures, as well as hormonal and other treatments for infertility.

Sexual harassment, rape, and battering are most frequently but not exclusively the problems of women.

Women for the most part are themselves responsible for love relationships. They worry more and assume more responsibility for finding a partner and for establishing a committed relationship. This occurs among heterosexual, bisexual, and gay women. Until recently, single women by far outnumbered single men. Therefore these women have had to resolve the issue of "settling" if they wanted security, a home, and family, rather than waiting to fall in love.

Women have special problems in relation to their hormonal cycles and reproductive organs. Genital surgery occurs in both men and women, but its psychiatric morbidity in women is clearly demonstrable. It is not difficult to understand that mastectomy, with its resultant visible physical mutilation, would by problematic. Yet the greatest psychiatric morbidity results from hysterectomy, even when this surgery is performed for a benign condition.

There may be a male menopause or involution, but more women require treatment, both medical and psychiatric, at this phase of life for reasons that are complex and multidimensional.

Yet another phenomenon for women has been called the "sandwich generation." Women still are primarily responsible for the care of children and increasingly almost solely responsible for the care of elderly parents, parents-in-law, grandparents, and other relatives.

Grandmotherhood may be either a liability or a phase in development that promotes growth and resolution of previously unresolved conflicts. Widowhood is becoming an increasingly common and prolonged period in the life cycle of women, bringing opportunities for growth as well as problems requiring a variety of treatment interventions.

We share with the reader our ideas as well as the input of other investigators and thinkers. We would hope to focus and sharpen both awareness of and psychodynamic treatment for the problems of women.

No work on female psychodynamics could be complete without discussing issues like abortion, adoption, divorce, and infanticide, to name a few. Nor could we fail to acknowledge the importance of AIDS, alternate life-styles, or committed partnerships. There is no way to illustrate the importance of self-esteem issues without reference to the plastic surgery and cosmetic industries or to the growing addiction of women to alcohol, tobacco, and prescription and over-the-counter drugs. The project became a massive one because of the need to discuss issues such as incest, sexual harassment, rape, and battering, which cause such frequent and profound psychiatric morbidity.

Each topic has required a different approach. In the cases of harassment, rape, and battering, to cite some examples, the psychiatric literature is replete with sources, which we have quoted and referenced. The material on incest is complicated because Freud changed his mind about its reality and because incest has become the "in" topic of the decade. These factors require that we use our own clinical experience to sift the wheat from the chaff. In the case of infertility, there are only one or two references in the psychiatric literature, mostly from abroad. The bulk of the information is found in the obstetrical and gynecological literature, in which the psychological problems of depression and stress in the marital relationship have been given some attention. Having successfully treated a number of women who came for depression because of infertility, we learned about the gynecological diagnostic and treatment procedures and the often profound effect of these on life-style, self-esteem, anxiety, and depression. We also learned that the process caused conflict that had once been resolved to reemerge because of the symbolism of the process or because of the guilt that often manifested itself. In the case of infanticide we have treated only two patients. Because children are murdered every day, our approach has been to turn to the limited psychiatric literature and to detailed case reports by investigative journalists. In several instances—formulations about self-esteem, for example—our work was informed by the writing and thinking of psychologists, social workers, sociologists, and "feminist" writers.

It is difficult to say which portion of our task was most daunting—reading and citing hundreds of articles and abstracting them in a meaningful way with the addition of our own clinical experience, or examining in depth our clinical experience in an attempt to formulate psychodynamic issues and to generate new hypotheses.

Each of our chapters threatened to demand a book of its own. What we have done is to try to provide a brief but in-depth study of many issues and the concomitant psychodynamic treatment. For those readers who would care to look further, we have provided an extensive and comprehensive list of references. Our hope is to have set our readers firmly on the path of further exploration of the multitude of psychodynamic problems specific to women.

To illustrate the treatment of women with various psychodynamic issues we have chosen patient material from two treatment modalities. The first type of material is gleaned from *classical psychoanalysis*, alternately called *reconstructive treatment*. In psychoanalytic treatment the patient is seen four or five times a week and uses the psychoanalytic couch to decrease social interaction and encourage free association aloud by the patient and silently by the analyst. This process leads to the understanding of the unconscious. The analyst adopts a neutral stance that is nonadversarial and nonjudgmental, in the context of which a regressive transference neurosis develops and is analyzed. By this we mean that the patient repeats with the analyst relationships with parents and siblings, revealing the conflicts therein and the defenses, symptoms, characterological traits, and adaptation that have been determined by these conflicts. Through interpretation, the patient learns about these motivations for attitude and behavior and becomes free to adapt in ways that cause less pain to herself and others and that bring more successful functioning. Candidates for psychoanalysis are those patients who can be depended upon to tolerate anxiety, depression, and anger that may be generated in the process while remaining functional and not endangering themselves or others.

Psychodynamic psychotherapy (also known as *reparative treatment*), on the other hand, is done face to face and may take place at a frequency of two to five times a week. The patient is not encouraged to develop a regressive transference neurosis. Transferences do occur and are interpreted in order to help the patient resolve conflicts in a way that is less painful to herself and others and improves her ability to function. Ideally, interpretations are made to help the patient contain and cope with anxiety, panic, depression and suicidality, and rage. Growth also occurs in the context of the psychotherapeutic relationship itself. Patients who are more ill require advice, support, cognitive explorations, and prohibition of harmful behaviors either by contract between therapist and patient or through the use of periodic partial or full hospitalization.

In this introduction we have outlined problems that are important in the lives of women, and defined the two modalities of treatment that we will predominantly discuss.

Chapter 1

Female Psychology: A Historical Overview

The most valid contributions to female psychology have been made by women, and in recent years. This has for the most part been a result of listening to women and female child patients. Listening does not occur in a vacuum. Most therapists have been schooled in Freudian theory. They began to realize, however, that their female patients were not validating that theory but were providing information and therapeutic response to new hypotheses.

The psychodynamic treatment of women, however, began with Freud and his colleagues,† who, despite their accomplishments, made two significant errors. First, they assumed that the model for psychodynamic treatment of men, with its phallocentric point of view, could be used to deduce problems and solutions in the treatment of women. Second, these early investigators denied the prevalence of sexual abuse in childhood and its importance in disrupting normal development.

During the last 15 years, women writers, psychiatrists, psychologists, and analysts have discovered that women differ from men not only anatomically but in their ego and superego functioning. A woman sees herself primarily in relation (to other persons, things, etc.). This valuing of relationships above other goals often seems to have an instinctual basis, a drive quality much like sexuality or aggression. Closer inspection, however, reveals that women have been carefully taught these values in the context of important early relationships (Bernstein and Warner 1984,[86] pp. 1–52). A great deal of conflict stems from the contrary messages they received growing up in a male-dominated society.

†Very important early contributions, in fact, came from women analysts.

The definition of self in relation to others will be a pivotal concept essential to the understanding of women's conflicts and their recollection throughout the life cycle.

Although Freud's work regarding women was largely incorrect, he was the first psychodynamic theorist to formulate ideas about what he considered to be nonpsychotic psychiatric disorders. If nothing more, his work was heuristic; it gave other analysts a starting point for investigation and correction.

Freud's Views on Female Psychology

Freud acknowledged that his exploration of female psychology was insufficient (Freud 1925[1]). Although much of his work was with female patients, he wrote, "We know less about the sexual life of little girls than of boys. But we need not feel ashamed of this distinction; after all, the sexual life of adult women is a 'dark continent' for psychology" (Freud 1926b,[2] p. 243). Freud further recognized that the definitive work on female sexuality would have to be done by female analysts (Freud 1933[3]).[†]

As noted above, Freud's earliest work was with female patients (Breuer and Freud 1892[4]), and many of his most important early psychoanalytic discoveries derived from this work (Freud 1905a[1901],[5] 1905b,[6] 1915[1914][7]). After formulating an entire theory of female psychology (Freud 1920a,[8] 1920b,[9] 1923a,[10] 1923b,[11] 1924a,[12] 1924b,[13] 1925,[14] 1931,[15] 1933[1932][16]) and knowing the intimate fantasies of women and details of their sexual lives, Freud still found women to be a mystery.

There are several reasons for Freud's puzzlement. The first is that Freud constructed a theory of infantile sexuality (Freud 1905b,[6]

[†]We would have to amend this view to add that the psychology of women is determined by more than their sexuality. Thus, in the present volume we discuss the work of women who are not psychoanalysts who have made major contributions not only to female psychology in general but to the study of female sexuality in specific.

1923b,[11]) based on a male model. He began with the idea that all children have sexual drives that center around mucocutaneous junctions and proceed from one primary zone to the next. In the first year of life, the mouth is the organ of pleasure. In the second year, sexual excitement focuses on the anus and the activities of holding on and letting go of fecal contents. In the third year, he believed that the leading erogenous zone was the penis for boys and the clitoris, the equivalent (in Freud's view) of a little penis, for girls (Freud 1923b,[11] 1924a,[12] 1924b[13]). In addition, Freud hypothesized that the oedipal phase, or the phase of a triadic relationship with the parents, overlays the phallic phase. Therefore, for Freud (1905b[6]), sexuality for both sexes was essentially phallic. Later, Freud (1925[14]) hypothesized that the oedipal conflict was related to the child's discovery of the anatomical differences between the sexes. The boy in love with his mother, perceiving his father as a rival, would develop the fantasy that if there was a human without a penis, he might lose his. Thus, the fear of castration would lead him to give up the love of his mother and identify with his father. All the paternal injunctions, perceived or fantasied, would coalesce in the superego. Freud regarded castration anxiety as the major motivation for superego formation.

Freud postulated that when a little girl discovered the anatomical differences between the sexes, she would feel a sense of genital inferiority and would be envious of the penis. Because of her castrated state, she would angrily blame and reject her mother (1924b[13]) and turn to her father, wishing to have his penis or a penis equivalent (i.e., his baby). Another possible outcome to the feeling of genital inadequacy would be identification with the father and homosexuality.

Freud stressed that a normal outcome for a little girl would be to change the sex of her object choice. She must, he thought, give up masturbation with her inferior organ, the clitoris, and switch to the vagina as her major erogenous zone. In fact, for Freud the sine qua non for achieving normal female adult sexuality was that the female gave up clitoral (i.e., masculine) orgasms in a shift to the vagina as her primary erogenous zone and achieved vaginal (i.e., feminine) orgasms. He also postulated that the little girl must relinquish her aggressiveness

(1933[1932][16]) and become passive and masochistic. Freud believed that because a girl considers herself castrated (1925[14]), she lacks castration anxiety and, therefore, one motivation to form a strong superego (i.e., one that is autonomous, impersonal, and not swayed by emotion). He stated that women necessarily lack a sense of justice, are less ready to submit to the necessities of life, and are influenced in their judgment by the emotions. Yet another inferiority of mental structuralization would be in the capacity to form an ego ideal. The female child's rejection of her mother for not having given her a penis, Freud reasoned, would interfere with the child's ability to introduce the maternal ego ideal (1925,[14], 1926a[17]).

Freud was not aware of early primary femininity arising out of a preoedipal identification between daughter and mother, despite the fact that there is a long pregenital relationship between mother and child (see Chodorow 1978[84]; Stoller 1968[75]). He did not address himself to gender identity and its formation. Despite his belief in the overdetermination of fantasies and conflicts, Freud did not explore what early pregenital factors might contribute to making penis envy such a decisive influence on sexuality and on the structuralization of the mind. Throughout his writings, Freud viewed himself as the father in the transference. He wrote very little, however, about his patient's maternal transferences.

Freud recognized countertransference as the analyst's unconscious response to the patient's productions based on the analyst's own unresolved infantile conflicts. These infantile conflicts span all stages of development. Because Freud was his own analyst, he could not have achieved a deep enough level of regression to understand conflicts of the oral stages of development.

Many times he acted out his own maternal countertransference feelings by giving food to his patients. Also, we know that he required continued oral gratification, smoking (i.e., sucking) even when he realized that he had cancer of the mouth.

Freud's analysis of his oedipal conflicts was conducted through transference relationships with male colleagues and friends as well as with patients. Those women with whom he worked, such as Helen Deutsch and Princess Marie Bonaparte, were women who were identified with their fathers, as was his daughter, Anna.

In Freud's time there was no infant or child observation. He could not have known of phenomena such as orgasm in infant girls or that girl children often insert objects into the vagina before beginning clitoral masturbation. He did not realize that masturbation continues throughout latency in normal girls. He prematurely abandoned the seduction theory (Freud 1909b[18]). He never reversed himself again in that area despite statements that "phantasies of being seduced are of particular interest, because often they are not phantasies but real memories" (Freud 1917[1916–1917],[19] p. 370). He noted that "actual seduction . . . is common enough" (1933[3]) and that "the girl who was made the object of sexual seduction in her early childhood may direct her later sexual life so as constantly to provoke similar acts" (1939[1934–1938][20] pp. 75–76). The insistence, nevertheless, that seduction was an oedipal fantasy and not a real occurrence helped keep us blinded to what we now realize is a shockingly high incidence of father/daughter incest and abuse.

Further Views of Female Psychology

As noted above, Freud predicted that the definitive work on female sexuality would be done by female analysts (1933[1932][16]), and, in fact, some of his female colleagues attempted such work. Deutsch postulated that the detachment of girls from their mothers is a gradual process rather than the sudden hateful rejection that Freud thought would necessarily be the outcome of penis envy and consequent devaluation of women (Deutsch 1944[21]). Whereas Freud attributed female masochism, passivity, and narcissism to penis envy, Deutsch felt that masochism was a normal component necessary to motherhood. She also noted that women seemed more inner directed, intuitive, and empathic than men (Deutsch 1930[22]).

Deutsch disagreed with Freud's idea that mothers prefer their sons as a way of having a penis; she realized instead that mothers wish to perpetuate themselves and their own maternal relationships through intense relationships with their daughters (Deutsch 1945[23]). Deutsch also reported that there are two sexual organs in the woman, the clitoris for the origin of pleasurable sensations, and the vagina and internal organs for reproduction. She surmised that sexual excitement flows from the clitoris to the vagina and disagreed that a girl must give up her clitoris as the primary organ of pleasure, in favor of the vagina. Deutsch (1925[24]) realized that female sexuality was the product of both the pregenital and the genital phases of development. She did agree with Freud, however, that first a woman wants a penis, and then a baby (Deutsch 1944[21]).

Princess Marie Bonaparte (1935[25]) described primary vaginal sensations in female children. However, she, too, remained committed to Freud's basic theories about female sexuality.

Karen Horney (1926/1967[26]) was the first to challenge Freud's views about female sexuality. She interpreted these views as the wishful fantasies of men, due to masculine narcissism, which places the penis at the center of sexuality. Horney thought that men overvalue their penis because of the fear of castration. She also contended that men cling to their infantile fantasies to compensate for breast and reproductive envy (Horney 1932[27]).

Horney's most popular formulations (1933a,[28] 1933b[29]) had to do with the role of an aggressive male-oriented society in generating female inferiority and psychopathology. In taking the position that society influences the intrapsychic world, Horney came into an important metapsychological conflict with Freud, who had insisted that culture reflects the external projection of intrapsychic structures (Freud 1930[1929][30]). As an example, Freud (1912b[1912–1913][31]) used the incest taboo to illustrate the projection of superego injunctions onto cultural mores.

Later, Clara Thompson (1942[32]), reaching the same basic conclusions as Horney, explained penis envy and masochism in women on the basis of socioeconomic restrictions and forced dependency, and of the cultural sanctions imposed on women relevant to the expression of their sexuality.

Freud had one male colleague who interested himself in female psychology. Jones (1927[33]) recognized that girl children recognize their gender even prior to awareness of the presence or absence of a penis. He believed that basic femininity developed instinctually (Jones 1935[34]).

Melanie Klein (1928,[35] 1932[36]) was the first to acknowledge and then make supraordinate the influence of the preoedipal mother and the oral phase of development.† Central to Klein's thesis was the hypothesis that infants are capable of fantasy formation that allows the female infant to be consciously aware that she has a vagina and her father has a penis. This implies an early cognitive awareness that other investigators and infant observers have been unable to validate. We depend on observers of infants and animals to validate hypotheses drawn from adult female studies.

In the experimental observation of monkeys, Harlow demonstrated that separation of mother and infant primate, even when needs for food, warmth, and clinging were satisfied, led to failure of these infants to assume appropriate sexual roles later on (Harlow and Harlow 1962,[39] 1966[40]).

Phyllis Greenacre (1948[41]) agreed with Freud about the vicissitudes of the Oedipus complex. She hypothesized that women, feeling hurt by the discovery of the anatomical difference between the sexes, may well anticipate new injury and seem generally more worrisome and fearful than male peers. Greenacre pointed out the unconscious fantasy of castration as a punishment for masturbation and the unconscious fantasy of an illusory penis. She observed that the illusory phallus might be placed, in fantasy, in the oral, anal, or genital apparatus. She postulated two causes for this seemingly odd finding. First, she noted the poor somatic differentiation of vagina, urethra, and anus. Second, she noted the coexistence of vaginal sensation with oral sucking behavior.

Greenacre (1952b,[42] 1953a/1971,[43] 1953b/1971[44]) pointed out that the fear of loss of love seemed more important in female development than castration anxiety. She recognized and described two pregenital

---

†Lampl de Groot (1928[37]) and Brunswick (1940[38]) also acknowledged the role of the preoedipal mother. However, these two investigators still insisted on the dominant influence of the oedipal father in determining the sexuality of his daughter.

phases. In the first phase the recognition of genital differences was more meaningful in terms of self-worth and in attempts at differentiation from the maternal figure. That is, Greenacre focused on the meaning of the first pregenital phase for self and object representations and for narcissistic issues. In the second pregenital stage the issues were, according to Greenacre, oedipal and would be conceptualized by the female child in sexual terms.

Greenacre was the first to notice a positive consequence of female anatomy. She postulated that the female, failing to adequately compete anatomically with the male, would experience compensatory growth in intellectual sublimation and a turning to a creative fantasy life. Later creative aims might become procreational. On the negative side, Greenacre noted that vague female genital awareness might be associated with vagueness in ambition. She also thought that problems in abstract and analytical thinking were predicated on an incomplete body image. Keiser (1956[45]) confirmed the hypothesis about the influence of body image on ego styles.

It was not until much later that Lerner (1974a,[46] 1974b[47]) understood that the mislabeling or failure to name female genitalia contributed to both penis envy and learning failure in girls. The tactile access and genital naming that boys experience allow them to more easily incorporate a picture of their genitalia into their internal self representations. In addition, boys are taught early by both mothers and fathers to positively invest their motoric system and motor activities. Girls invest the motor system only when they picture themselves as graceful, delicate, and cuddly (Green 1976[48]; Korner 1973[49]; Murphy 1962[50]).

Judith Kestenberg (1956a,[51] 1956b,[52] 1975[53]) also took for granted that the oedipal wish for the father was the prime impetus in women's sexual development. Kestenberg was interested in other sources of femininity as well. Both she (1968[54]) and Erikson (1968b[55]) explored the meaning and ramifications of the existence of an inner genital space. Kestenberg developmentally placed the wish to fill that space with a baby before the oedipal period and before full separation from the mother had been achieved. Pondering the importance of the mother/daughter relationship in terms of similarities in rhythms of movement and a shared internal space, Kestenberg wondered if the girl baby might have difficulty distinguishing her inner space from an inner space shared with the mother. Kestenberg conceptualized that one of the primary developmental tasks of the girl was separation of her genital space from her mother's and from her own alimentary and excretory spaces. She also related female masochism to the adult female's later capacity for the pain of childbirth and the self-sacrifices a mother must make. Kestenberg was among the first to notice the male's wish to carry and bear a baby; she therefore did not see the wish for a baby as a consolation prize for castration, because this wish was present in both sexes. She related this wish in both sexes to the desire to restore the early blissful symbiotic relationship with the mother.

Female analysts had indeed heeded Freud's admonition to turn to their own experience to know more about femininity (Jones 1955,[56] p. 421). What they were beginning to contribute was a recognition of the importance of the early relationship of the female child and her mother.

Margaret Mahler and colleagues, in many papers (Mahler 1963,[57] 1967[58]; Mahler and Furer 1963[59]; Mahler and La Perriere (1965[60]), provided, based on observation of children, the best understanding of the move from symbiosis to separation-individuation in both male and female children. Edith Jacobson (1950[61]) added to this understanding in terms of describing the vicissitudes of the processes of object relationships and identifications.

Contemporary Views of Female Psychology

Until the contemporary period, analytic investigators had all added to Freud's theories but kept the oedipal conflict as central to development and focused great importance on penis envy and the dominant role of the father in determining the sexuality and psychology of women. The first major challenge to Freudian sexual psychology came from the laboratory observations of nonanalysts. Masters and Johnson (1966[62]) established forever the primacy of the clitoris as the erotic focus for female sexual stimulation. In discussing Masters and Johnson's findings,

Sherffy (1966,[63] 1973[64]) dissolved the myth of any difference between so-called clitoral and vaginal orgasms. She pointed out that Freud was wrong in thinking that a major maturational task of women was to change their leading erogenous zone from the clitoris to the vagina. In keeping the clitoris as the primary erogenous organ, women were not, as Freud thought, failing to give up their inferior organ for a psychological reason. They were responding to the "hard wiring" of the cluster of nerve endings that causes orgasm in women, which is located in the clitoris and not in the vagina. Women who are orgasmic in response to vaginal thrusting alone are being stimulated by friction or traction on the clitoris. Furthermore, women are able to achieve multiple orgasms without a refractory period.

Many analysts were willing to accept that Freud made one error, but still clung tenaciously to the rest of his theory. These included child observers such as Roiphe, Galenson, and Parens, among others (Galenson 1971[65]; Galenson and Roiphe 1971[66]; Galenson et al. 1975,[67] 1976[68]; Parens 1971[69]; Roiphe 1968[70]; Roiphe and Galenson 1972,[71] 1973[72]).

Among analysts it was Stoller (1964,[73] 1965,[74] 1968[75]), working on gender identity, who introduced a new concept that he called "core gender identity." The sense of one's sex and gender role, Stoller contends, were determined by labeling at birth and by habitual patterns of differential handling of boy and girl children. He believes that there is a primary femininity—that the little girl is happy to be female, holds herself differently from the little boy, and daydreams, plays, wears clothes, and uses a different vocabulary than he does. In the course of normal development, this occurs by the age of 2 years. Stoller argues that these developments precede the recognition of the anatomical differences between the sexes and, furthermore, that this core gender identity is fixed by age 2 years and cannot be changed.

Mayer (1985[76]) reported on several women patients who felt that men lacked something crucial: the so-called feminine capacities of empathy and emotional receptivity. These women felt that they had these capacities and feared to lose them. In analysis with these patients, Mayer found that this formulation rested on a fantasy that the woman is genitally open, a capacity that can be endangered and lost, and indeed has been lost, by the male sex. Women, Mayer noted, have a state of primary femininity resulting in part from the pleasure obtained from the touchable aspects of the female genitalia: the mons pubis, labia, clitoris, and the parting between the labia and the introitus. The notion of an opening and a potential inner space develops concomitantly with and prior to the appreciation of the anatomical differences between the sexes. Young girls at the period of discovery of the anatomical differences develop the fear that what they have could be lost or sealed over and that, in fact, boys have lost access to their inner genital and its sensations and receptivity. This fear may exist side by side with penis envy and the sense of having been castrated, that is, having lost a penis.

Horney (1926/1967,[26] p. 66) first referred to "female genital anxiety, like the castration dread of boys." She pointed out that wishing for a penis may serve as a defensive function against worrying about losing what one already has (i.e., the female genitalia).

Applegarth (1976[77]) suggested that superego content is different in girls than in boys, though women do not lack a superego. If indeed, as Freud (1905b[6]) suggested, the presence of castration anxiety motivates superego formation, the girl's superego formation may also rest on castration anxiety (i.e., loss of the genital she already has).

Money and Erhardt (1972[78]) studied hormonally and genetically aberrant children whose sex was designated by the physician at birth based on a guess after observation of the external genitalia. Genetic studies often revealed those guesses to be wrong, but at 2 years the children's gender identity nevertheless corresponded to the gender that they were assumed to be during their rearing. Kleeman's (1971,[79] 1975[80]) observations of children lent support to the role of cognitive functioning for core gender identity formation. He noted the importance that parental expectations play in how the child will enter the oedipal conflict. Kohlberg (1966[81]) found that even boys reared by single mothers but labeled as boys override the exclusive contact with a woman.

Karme (1981[82]) studied women with severe penis envy and hypothesized that their envy is based on a variety of fantasies:

> (1) the penis as umbilical cord, a means of attachment to mother; (2) the penis as baby, a means of completing mother and/or . . . self; (3) the penis as an object that can unite with and separate from mother with pleasure to both and without damage to either; (4) the penis as the undamaged, and undamageable, external version of the womb; (5) the penis as breast; (6) the penis as a defense against murderous rage; (7) the penis as a weapon of competition for mother with father and brothers . . . ; (8) penis envy as a means of blocking the wish for sexual expression for fear of losing mother by inhibiting sexual responsiveness and pleasure; (9) penis envy as part of general feeling of envy of both men and women. (p 443)

Schafer (1974[83]), an analytic investigator, challenged Freud's formulations about female psychology from a metapsychological point of view. Specifically, Schafer dealt with what he regarded as Freud's misconceptions about the morality and objectivity of women, his neglect of their preoedipal development, and the problem of pejorative labeling. Yet it fell to writers outside of the fields of psychoanalytic psychology and psychiatric medicine to focus on the role of the mother and the mother/daughter relationship as pivotal in determining the vicissitudes of female psychology and sexuality (Chodorow 1978[84]; Friday 1973[85]).

Bernstein and Warner have reviewed the literature concerning female psychology and sexuality. They have also reviewed the histories of their patients and the patients of some of their colleagues. Out of this work came the book *Women Treating Women* (Bernstein and Warner 1984b[86]), in which the authors propose alternate viewpoints based on the primacy of the relationship of mother and daughter. Among the findings is the recognition of the ubiquitous occurrence of a transient period of penis envy. This transient phase is also transitional in separating mother and child. Boys often use their penis as a transitional object, whereas girls may use the fantasy of an illusory penis to serve the same function. The persistence of penis envy or of the illusion of a phallus with accompanying castration anxiety is a reparative phenomenon—that is, this wish or fantasy repairs preoedipal damage. The baggage of the failure of one stage of development is carried into the next. Much of the damage is done when mothers tend to perpetuate the symbiosis of infancy with their daughters.

Pathogenic mothers experience their daughters as extensions of themselves both physically and emotionally. The physical concerns of the mothers are often projected onto the daughters. There may be a reversal of parental roles in which the daughter prematurely becomes mother to her mother. Sometimes the daughter is even offered, consciously or unconsciously, by the mother to the father as love or sex object.

In addition, the daughter is regarded as a narcissistic object and is called upon to meet her mother's narcissistic needs, both conscious and unconscious. The mother's demand may be to be perfect and beautiful, and to perform excellently in all or selective endeavors. Sometimes there is a double message. The conscious one is to be better than mother; the unconscious one is not to compete. Very often masochism, depression, unstable self-esteem regulation, and difficulties with independence and independent relationships are the legacy.

The fantasies, identifications, and self and object representations that derive from the mother/daughter relationship are primarily responsible for some women's otherwise unintelligible reactions to surgery, the menopause, the problems of being in the "sandwich generation" (see Chapter 4), and the positive and negative aspects of grandparenting (see Chapter 7), to list just a few examples. The original mother/daughter relationship and its subsequent evolution bear significantly on each developmental stage and its concomitant psychopathology.

In recent years there have been many other authors from the disciplines of medicine, psychology, anthropology, and the social sciences who have contributed a great deal to the understanding of several discrete issues relevant to the psychodynamic understanding and treatment of women. Specifically, Gilligan (1982[87]), abandoning the male model, has contributed to our understanding of moral development in women. Her premise is that rather than having rigid standards of fairness, women have the tendency to take a broader view in terms of the consequences for many of the individuals with whom they have relationships. Her second premise is that women consider loyalties and the well-being of a group, or the value of a concept or project, and that this does not reflect masochism but altruism.

The Stone Center theorists (Surrey 1983[88]; Jordan et al. 1983[89]) have elucidated a parallel theory for female development based on the importance of relationships. The authors focus attention on the close relationship of a mother to her children, especially daughters. In these relationships children are encouraged to grow in the context of an evolving relationship. The children are neither forced to separate nor maintained as narcissistic extensions of the mother. Mother and child both grow together, and this evolving relationship helps in the growth and maintenance of self-esteem for both members of the dyad. Women, Surrey and colleagues note, also attend to the issue of the development of a collaborative flexible work style that is neither selfish nor masochistic. In this kind of relationship, empathy evolves (Jordan et al. 1983[89]).

This view of female development has consequences for the psychodynamic treatment of women, in which women get well in a setting of an evolving, growth-producing, empathic relationship. Women who have not had the benefit of such a relationship get depressed. They also become depressed when a relationship is not working because they tend to hold themselves individually responsible for the failure of that relationship. The depression is not the result of dependency but rather the result of an overvaluation of the relationship and a sense of responsibility for its well-being.

Jean Baker Miller (1976[90]) has emphasized that women are forced to live in a male-dominated culture, which is contrary to their own psychology of nondominance and submission. Women are defined by a culture that does not understand, support, respect, or value their unique capabilities and style. Some of the realities with which women have to cope in a male-dominated culture are 1) abuse in childhood, 2) exclusion from certain vocations and opportunities, 3) unequal distribution, 4) less pay for equal work, 5) sexual harassment, and 6) rape.

Good psychological health can offer women the ability to cope without internalizing the deprecation. Implementing cultural change is a larger, more complicated task. Coming full circle, some women are raising children of both sexes and continue to raise sons who deprecate them. These women do this because they have internalized negative values about themselves.

The explosion of data about the real external limitations and impediments that women experience can help both women and their therapists to find a balance between what is internal and what is external. Nancy Friday (1973[85]), from a literary point of view, and Nancy Chodorow (1978[84]), as a scientist, were the earliest women to write about the profound consequences for female development that arise from the early mother/child relationship. Chodorow concentrates particularly on the issues of parenting. The major contribution of both authors relevant to the psychodynamic treatment of women revolves around the issue of the female child being treated as the narcissistic extension of the mother. Both Friday and Chodorow understood the consequences of such an extension for self-esteem development and the inability to express anger.

The Stone Center theorists (Surrey 1983[88]; Jordan et al. 1983[89]) and other individuals (Lerner 1985[91]) have more fully elucidated the tendency of women to express their anger against introjected selfobjects. In other words, the self and object representations remain merged, and the anger is directed not only against an introjected object representation but against the merged selfobject representation. We think that mobilization of anger directed against a developmentally primitive selfobject is more difficult because the patient must first separate her self and object representations. Therefore the problem of separation-individuation must initially be resolved, which is easier with an 18-month-old child than with an adolescent or adult woman. This dynamic is especially operative in women who have been abused early in their development, before separation-individuation is consolidated.

Very frequently there is a polarization in the literature and in its clinical integration between those investigators with a primarily "intrapsychic" focus and those with an "environmental" focus. There is also a polarization between lay workers in the field of female psychology, analysts, psychiatrists, psychologists, and other mental health professionals. We find these theoretical polarizations counterproductive for women in life, work, practice, and theory building.

Women who have been trained as medical professionals have initially been pressured to identify with masculine standards of competition and "work first." These women then have to integrate the female characteristics of altruism, generativity, and nurturing. This often produces conflict or reactive overidentification with male standards and a sense of alienation from female professionals in order to be accepted or to prove themselves worthy. These women may also receive negative comments from female professionals who are displacing their anger at male professionals. The better outcome would be integration of the positive aspects of all competing psychologies.

Because we are physicians, we must keep in mind the contributions that have recently come from neurology, neurobiology, chemistry, and psychopharmacology. For information on gender differences in the brain, see Appendix A.

We have surveyed the most prominent theories of female psychology. Our work illustrates a synthesis of the work of most theorists but excludes Freud's erroneous hypotheses about female sexual development.

Notes

1. Freud S: Some psychical consequences of the anatomical distinction between the sexes (1925), in The Standard Edition of the Complete Psychological Works of Sigmund Freud, Vol 19. Translated and edited by Strachey J. London, Hogarth Press, 1961, pp 241–258
2. Freud S: The question of lay analysis: conversations with an impartial person (1926b), in The Standard Edition of the Complete Psychological Works of Sigmund Freud, Vol 20. Translated and edited by Strachey J. London, Hogarth Press, 1959, pp 177–258
3. Freud S: Femininity (1933), in The Standard Edition of the Complete Psychological Works of Sigmund Freud, Vol 22. Translated and edited by Strachey J. London, Hogarth Press, 1964, pp 112–135
4. Breuer J, Freud S: Studies on hysteria (1892), in The Standard Edition of the Complete Psychological Works of Sigmund Freud, Vol 2. Translated and edited by Strachey J. London, Hogarth Press, 1966, pp 1–319
5. Freud S: Fragment of an anal analysis of a case of hysteria (1905a[1901]), in The Standard Edition of the Complete Psychological Works of Sigmund Freud, Vol 7. Translated and edited by Strachey J. London, Hogarth Press, 1953, pp 1–122

6. Freud S: Three essays on the theory of sexuality (1905b), in The Standard Edition of the Complete Psychological Works of Sigmund Freud, Vol 7. Translated and edited by Strachey J. London, Hogarth Press, 1953, pp 123–245
7. Freud S: Observations on transference-love (further recommendations on the technique of psychoanalysis) (1915[1914]), in The Standard Edition of the Complete Psychological Works of Sigmund Freud, Vol 12. Translated and edited by Strachey J. London, Hogarth Press, 1958, pp 157–173
8. Freud S: Beyond the pleasure principle (1920a), in The Standard Edition of the Complete Psychological Works of Sigmund Freud, Vol 18. Translated and edited by Strachey J. London, Hogarth Press, 1955, pp 1–64
9. Freud S: The psychogenesis of a case of homosexuality in a woman (1920b), in The Standard Edition of the Complete Psychological Works of Sigmund Freud, Vol 18. Translated and edited by Strachey J. London, Hogarth Press, 1955, pp 145–172
10. Freud S: The ego and the id (1923a), in The Standard Edition of the Complete Psychological Works of Sigmund Freud, Vol 19. Translated and edited by Strachey J. London, Hogarth Press, 1961, pp 1–66
11. Freud S: The infantile genital organization: an interpolation in the theory of sexuality (1923b), in The Standard Edition of the Complete Psychological Works of Sigmund Freud, Vol 19. Translated and edited by Strachey J. London, Hogarth Press, 1961, pp 139–145
12. Freud S: The dissolution of the oedipus complex (1924a), in The Standard Edition of the Complete Psychological Works of Sigmund Freud, Vol 19. Translated and edited by Strachey J. London, Hogarth Press, 1961, pp 171–179
13. Freud S: The economic problem of masochism (1924b), in The Standard Edition of the Complete Psychological Works of Sigmund Freud, Vol 19. Translated and edited by Strachey J. London, Hogarth Press, 1961, pp 155–170
14. Freud S: Some psychical consequences of the anatomical distinction between the sexes (1925), in The Standard Edition of the Complete Psychological Works of Sigmund Freud, Vol 19. Translated and edited by Strachey J. London, Hogarth Press, 1961, pp 241–258
15. Freud S: Female sexuality (1931), in The Standard Edition of the Complete Psychological Works of Sigmund Freud, Vol 21. Translated and edited by Strachey J. London, Hogarth Press, 1961, pp 221–243
16. Freud S: New introductory lectures on psycho-analysis: femininity (1933[1932]), in The Standard Edition of the Complete Psychological Works of Sigmund Freud, Vol 22. Translated and edited by Strachey J. London, Hogarth Press, 1964, pp 112–135

17. Freud S: Inhibitions, symptoms and anxiety (1926a), in The Standard Edition of the Complete Psychological Works of Sigmund Freud, Vol 20. Translated and edited by Strachey J. London, Hogarth Press, 1959, pp 75–175
18. Freud S: Notes upon a case of obsessional neurosis (1909b), in The Standard Edition of the Complete Psychological Works of Sigmund Freud, Vol 10. Translated and edited by Strachey J. London, Hogarth Press, 1955, pp 151–320
19. Freud S: Introductory lectures on psycho-analysis, Part III: general theory of the neuroses (1917[1916–1917]), in The Standard Edition of the Complete Psychological Works of Sigmund Freud, Vol 16. Translated and edited by Strachey J. London, Hogarth Press, 1963, pp 241–476
20. Freud S: Moses and monotheism (1939[1934–1938]), in The Standard Edition of the Complete Psychological Works of Sigmund Freud, Vol 23. Translated and edited by Strachey J. London, Hogarth Press, 1964, pp 1–137
21. Deutsch H: The Psychology of Women, a Psychoanalytic Interpretation, Vol 1. New York, Grune & Stratton, 1944
22. Deutsch H: The significance of masochism in the mental life of women. Int J Psychoanal 11:40–60, 1930
23. Deutsch H: The Psychology of Women, a Psychoanalytic Interpretation, Vol 2: Motherhood. New York, Grune & Stratton, 1945
24. Deutsch H: The psychology of women in relation to the functions of reproduction. Int J Psychoanal 6:405–418, 1925
25. Bonaparte M: Passivity, masochism and frigidity. Int J Psychoanal 16:325–333, 1935
26. Horney K: The flight from womanhood: the masculinity-complex in women as viewed by men and women (1926), in Feminine Psychology. Edited by Kelman H. New York, WW Norton, 1967, pp 54–70
27. Horney K: The dread of woman: observations on a specific difference in the dread felt by men and by women respectively for the opposite sex. Int J Psychoanal 13:348–360, 1932
28. Horney K: The denial of the vagina: a contribution to the problem of genital anxieties specific to women (1933a), in Feminine Psychology. Edited by Kelman H. New York, WW Norton, 1967, pp 147–161
29. Horney K: The problem of feminine masochism (1933b), in Feminine Psychology. Edited by Kelman H. New York, WW Norton, 1967, pp 214–233
30. Freud S: Civilization and its discontents (1930[1929]), in The Standard Edition of the Complete Psychological Works of Sigmund Freud, Vol 21. Translated and edited by Strachey J. London, Hogarth Press, 1961, pp 57–145

31. Freud S: Totem and taboo (1912b[1912–1913]), in The Standard Edition of the Complete Psychological Works of Sigmund Freud, Vol 13. Translated and edited by Strachey J. London, Hogarth Press, 1958, pp 1–162
32. Thompson C: Cultural pressures in the psychology of women. Psychiatry 5:331–339, 1942
33. Jones E: The early development of female sexuality. Int J Psychoanal 8:459–472, 1927
34. Jones E: Early female sexuality. Int J Psychoanal 16:263–273, 1935
35. Klein M: Early stages of the oedipus conflict. Int J Psychoanal 9:167–180, 1928
36. Klein M: The Psycho-analysis of Children. London, Hogarth Press, 1932
37. Lampl de Groot A: The evolution of the oedipus conflict in women. Int J Psychoanal 9:332–345, 1928
38. Brunswick K: The pre-oedipal phase of libido development. Psychoanal Q 9:293–319, 1940
39. Harlow HF, Harlow MK: The effect of rearing conditions on behavior. Bull Menninger Clin 26:213–224, 1962
40. Harlow HF, Harlow MK: Learning to love. American Scientist 54:244–247, 1966
41. Greenacre P: Human sexuality: research and treatment frontiers, in American Handbook of Psychiatry. Edited by Arieti S. New York, Basic Books, 1948, pp 665–691
42. Greenacre P: Some factors producing different types of genital and pregenital organization, in Trauma, Growth, and Personality. New York, International Universities Press, 1952b, pp 293–302
43. Greenacre P: Certain relationships between fetishism and the faulty development of the body image (1953a), in Emotional Growth: Psychoanalytic Studies of the Gifted and a Great Variety of Other Individuals, Vol 1. New York, International Universities Press, 1971, pp 9–30
44. Greenacre P: Penis awe and its relation to penis envy (1953b), in Emotional Growth: Psychoanalytic Studies of the Gifted and a Great Variety of Other Individuals, Vol 1. New York, International Universities Press, 1971, pp 31–49
45. Keiser S: Female sexuality. J Am Psychoanal Assoc 4:563–574, 1956
46. Lerner HE: Early origins of envy and devaluation of women: implications for sex role stereotypes. Bull Menninger Clin 38:538–553, 1974a
47. Lerner HE: The hysterical personality: a "woman's" disease. Compr Psychiatry 15:157–164, 1974b
48. Green R: Human sexuality: research and treatment frontiers, in American Handbook of Psychiatry, Vol 1. Edited by Arieti S. New York, Basic Books, 1976, pp 665–691

49. Korner AF: Sex differences in newborns with special reference to differences in the organization of oral behavior. J Child Psychol Psychiatry 14:19–29, 1973
50. Murphy L: The Widening Circle of Childhood. New York, Basic Books, 1962
51. Kestenberg JS: On the development of maternal feelings in early childhood: observations and reflections. Psychoanal Study Child 11:275–291, 1956a
52. Kestenberg JS: Vicissitudes of female sexuality. J Am Psychoanal Assoc 4:453–576, 1956b
53. Kestenberg JS: Children and Parents: Psychoanalytic Studies in Development. New York, Jason Aronson, 1975
54. Kestenberg JS: Outside and inside, male and female. J Am Psychoanal Assoc 16:457–520, 1968
55. Erikson E: Womanhood and the inner space, in Identity, Youth, and Crisis. New York, WW Norton, 1968b, pp 261–295
56. Jones E: The Life and Work of Sigmund Freud, Vols 1–3. New York, Basic Books, 1955
57. Mahler MS: Thoughts about development and individuation. Psychoanal Study Child 18:307–324, 1963
58. Mahler MS: On human symbiosis and the vicissitudes of individualism. J Am Psychoanal Assoc 15:740–763, 1967
59. Mahler MS, Furer M: Certain aspects of the separation-individuation phase. Psychoanal Q 32:1–14, 1963
60. Mahler MS, La Perriere K: Mother-child interaction during separation-individuation. Psychoanal Q 34:483–498, 1965
61. Jacobson E: Development of the wish for a child in boys. Psychoanal Study Child 5:139–152, 1950
62. Masters W, Johnson V: Human Sexual Response. Boston, Little, Brown, 1966
63. Sherffy M: The evolution and nature of female sexuality in relation to psychoanalytic theory. J Am Psychoanal Assoc 14:28–128, 1966
64. Sherffy M: The Nature and Evolution of Female Sexuality. New York, Random/Village, 1973
65. Galenson E: A consideration of the nature of thought in childhood play, in Separation-Individuation; Essays in Honor of Margaret S. Mahler. Edited by McDevitt JB, Settlage CF. New York, International Universities Press, 1971, pp 41–59
66. Galenson E, Roiphe H: The impact of early sexual discovery on mood, defensive organization, and symbolization. Psychoanal Study Child 26:195–216, 1971

67. Galenson E, Blau S, Vogel S: Disturbance in sexual identity beginning at eighteen months of age. International Review of Psychoanalysis 2:389–393, 1975
68. Galenson E, Miller R, Roiphe H: The choice of symbols. Journal of the American Academy of Child Psychiatry 15:83–96, 1976
69. Parens H: A contribution of separation-individuation to the development of psychic structure, in Separation-Individuation; Essays in Honor of Margaret S. Mahler. Edited by McDevitt JB, Settlage CF. New York, International Universities Press, 1971, pp 100–112
70. Roiphe H: On an early genital phase, with an addendum on Genesis. Psychoanal Study Child 23:348–365, 1968
71. Roiphe H, Galenson E: Early genital activity and the castration complex. Psychoanal Q 41:334–347, 1972
72. Roiphe H, Galenson E: Object loss and early sexual development. Psychoanal Q 42:73–90, 1973
73. Stoller RJ: A contribution to the study of gender identity. Int J Psychoanal 45:220–226, 1964
74. Stoller RJ: The sense of maleness. Psychoanal Q 34:207–218, 1965
75. Stoller RJ: The sense of femaleness. Psychoanal Q 37:42–55, 1968
76. Mayer EL: "Everybody must be just like me": observations on female castration anxiety. Int J Psychoanal 66:331–347, 1985
77. Applegarth A: Some observations on work inhibitions in women. J Am Psychoanal Assoc 24(suppl):251–268, 1976
78. Money J, Erhardt A: Man and Woman, Boy and Girl. Baltimore, MD, Johns Hopkins University Press, 1972
79. Kleeman J: The establishment of core gender identity in normal girls, introduction: development of ego capacity to differentiate. Arch Sex Behav 1:117–129, 1971
80. Kleeman J: Genital self-stimulation in infant and toddler girls, in From Infancy to Senescence. Edited by Marcus I, Francis JJ. New York, International Universities Press, 1975, pp 97–106
81. Kohlberg L: A cognitive-developmental analysis of children's sex role concepts and attitudes, in The Development of Sex Differences. Edited by Maccoby E. Stanford, CA, Stanford University Press, 1966, pp 82–173
82. Karme L: A clinical report of penis envy: its multiple meanings and defensive function. J Am Psychoanal Assoc 29:427–446, 1981
83. Schafer R: Problems in Freud's psychology of women. J Am Psychoanal Assoc 22:459–485, 1974
84. Chodorow N: The Reproduction of Mothering: Psychoanalysis and the Sociology of Gender. Berkeley, CA, University of California Press, 1978

85. Friday N: My Secret Garden: Women's Sexual Fantasies. New York, Pocket Books, 1973
86. Bernstein A, Warner G: Women Treating Women. New York, International Universities Press, 1984b
87. Gilligan C: In a Different Voice. Cambridge, MA, Harvard University Press, 1982
88. Surrey JL: Self in relation: a theory of women's development. Presentation at The Stone Center for Developmental Services and Studies Colloquium Series, Wellesley, MA, November 1983
89. Jordan J, Surrey J, Kaplan A: Women and empathy: implications for psychological development and psychotherapy. The Stone Center for Developmental Services and Studies, Work in Progress, Wellesley, MA, 1983, No 82
90. Miller JB: Toward a New Psychology of Women. Boston, MA, Beacon Press, 1976
91. Lerner HE: The Dance of Anger. New York, Harper & Row, 1985

Chapter 2

Adolescence

Upon cursory inspection, adolescence often looks more like a disease than like a stage in development, and this is more true now than it has been in the past. There has been research, however, that contradicts the view that adolescence is necessarily a period of turmoil and upheaval. Specifically, Offer and his colleagues (Offer 1969[1]; Offer and Offer 1968[2]; Offer et al. 1970[3]) studied large populations of adolescents in public high schools and found the incidence of turmoil and severe crises to be low. These studies were done in the late 1960s and early 1970s, and the adolescents came from traditional families and stable communities. Few adolescents grow up in that atmosphere today. In the best case, both parents work; in the worst case, we see the increasing prevalence of divorce, one-parent families, unemployment, and drug abuse by parents and within the community.

Felicity Barringer (1990[4]), in an article written for the *New York Times*, has amassed a group of impressive statistics on adolescence culled from various sources.[†] The National Center for Health Statistics tells us that as of 1988, 28% of 15-year-old women and 80% of 19-year-old women have had sexual intercourse at least once. As of 1989, according to the National Institute on Drug Abuse, 90% of youths are using alcohol and 48% marijuana, but the percentage of youths abusing cocaine

[†]The dilemma and conflict of our youth is portrayed in a cartoon by P.C. Vey with which the Barringer article begins. A woman is saying, "I know what you mean. My daughter doesn't know whether to get married, live alone, move in with somebody, all too frustrating; except for marijuana, or to become totally drug free or to quit drinking altogether, or have a child, or adopt or just ignore sex or become celibate and take more sedatives, or . . ." The turmoil we often see in adolescence is due in part to the many options faced by the adolescent.

has dropped to 10%. The Crime Control Institute tells us that the number of 10- to 18-year-olds arrested for homicide is 8.9 out of 100,000, a 65% increase from the period 1980 to 1989. The National Center for Health Statistics reports that the rate of suicide is still high: 16 out of 100,000 in the 20- to 24-year-old age group, and 10 out of 100,000 in the 15- to 19-year-old group.

Adolescent Development

Adolescence is ushered in by the physiology of puberty and sexual maturation. It is a period of intensified demand for adaptation, not only to intensification of sexual and aggressive drives but to the tasks of emerging adulthood and independence. Blos (1962[5]) has recognized adolescence as the terminal phase of the four stages of psychosexual development. By this he means that the genital phase, which has been partially interrupted by latency, is resumed. Thus, adolescence is a continuation of the progression from the oral through the anal, through the phallic, through the genital phases of infantile development. The genital phase of development needs completion without reliance on the structural organization of parents and usually with the help of a peer group. Ultimately, ties to the parents and other incestuous objects must be abandoned, and genital sexual impulses must become primary and directed toward nonincestuous objects (Bernstein and Warner 1981[6]).

Society impacts on self-esteem in women and particularly during adolescence. Gilligan (1990[7]) has observed that latency-age girls have a sense of authority but that by adolescence they have gotten society's message that it is better to keep quiet about themselves, their conflicts, and their relationships. They do this at the expense of their self-esteem. The vivacious and outspoken posture of latency turns to sullenness and silence during adolescence. (See Chapter 3 for discussion of women's self-esteem throughout the life cycle.)

The adolescent is in a vulnerable state, buffeted by endogenous and exogenous demands at the very time that major definitive tasks, both emotional and cognitive, must be accomplished. In the context of severe stressors, the adolescent must integrate a new body image as well as a new set of identifications. To accommodate these, old ideals and moral codes must be altered. In this process both the superego and the ego ideal must be disassembled, resculpted, and firmly internalized. Both Erikson (1956[8]) and Blos (1962[5]) emphasized the need for consolidation of the internal representation and further intrapsychic structuralization. Chused (1990[9]) has emphasized the role of action in the outside world and in terms of object relationships for self-definition. To this we add Ritvo's (1971[10]) observation that adolescence is the first time that an individual's sexual identification and sense of self as a sexual being is measured not just in terms of wishes but in terms of action. Rapaport (1967[11]) discussed the executive function of the ego in terms of activity and passivity relative to containing, restraining, and qualifying impulses. The development of the executive function of the ego is essential to the establishment of ego autonomy, which in turn impacts on the formation of the self representation. Chused's (1990[9]) emphasis on the importance of action will be illustrated in terms of its consequences for the adolescent, the family, and society, as well as the problems it presents in treatment.

In our view the processes cited above are rarely accomplished without anxiety, emotional lability, and regression to genetically more primitive modes of adaptation. This involves earlier modes of object relations, a revival of old struggles for autonomy, and old needs for dependency. The conflicts of earlier developmental phases may all be reactivated along with their concomitant defenses. Defenses more specific to adolescence include revolt to avoid dependency needs. This revolt may include contempt and derision of family and community standards along with identification and idealization of strange and different life-styles. These identifications and idealizations include religious cults, political causes, sexual mores, "alternate" life-styles, or exaggeration of involvement in some areas in which the rest of the community seems reasonably invested.

Hostility may be turned against the self, which accounts for accidents and suicide being the major causes of death during adolescence. Defensive withdrawal of investment in the self often results in hypochondriasis on the one hand and fantasies of grandiosity and entitlement on the other. Anna Freud (1936/1966[12]) recognized the defenses of asceticism and intellectualization. She pointed to the fact that in adolescence there is sometimes alternating with instinctual excess and eruptions (genital and aggressive) an antagonism to the instincts that reaches an intensity that far surpasses repressive capacity. Adolescents who exhibit ascetic behavior counter pressing instinctual desires with stringent prohibitions that often involve renunciation of all pleasure to the point of self-punishment. Freud also noted that, in general, the storms of instinct and affect (i.e., falling in love) bear an inverse relationship to the individual's intellectual capacity. In adolescence the reverse is the case. The greater the pressure of instinct and affect, the more the tendency to abstract and invest the intellect for the purpose of meditating on and attempting to resolve what are often esoteric or philosophical intellectual questions. This has some special implications for abuse victims during adolescence. The overinvestment of cognitive functioning often leads to a more functional adaptation. That is, these young women are able to become educated or job-oriented in contrast to their more promiscuous, self-destructive peers who often receive more clinical attention during adolescence and later life.

Any of these coping mechanisms can be transient. The seemingly sudden, almost meteoric changes in defenses make for turmoil and consternation in the family. We believe that rapidly changing coping mechanisms have to do with trial identifications. Erikson (1959[13]) conceptualized adolescence as a period of either solidification of *identity* as regards synthesis of new objects, sexual orientation, independent adulthood, and career choices, or *ego diffusion*. Adolescents seek or are brought to psychiatric attention because of profound lability or rigidity, severe enactment (commonly but incorrectly called "acting out"[†]), severe depression, or psychotic decompensation.

[†]*Acting out* is a technical term originating from psychoanalysis. It does not mean bad or dangerous behavior, which has become the common usage, but rather displacement of the analytic transference to the patient's life. Therefore, actions of adolescents not in treatment are not acting out but *enactment*.

In addition to the tasks, practical problems, and behaviors endemic to adolescence are the problems specific to young women. For young women the need to integrate a new body image includes an accommodation to increase in body size, the development of breasts, the enlargement of genitalia, and the development of genital, axillary, and other body hair. The most significant change is the onset of menstruation, which is a potent stimulator of the recurrence of anal-phase conflicts about messiness and control. It also stimulates castration anxiety in those women who have the unconscious defensive fantasy of possessing a penis. There is a fear of loss of control because the vagina is the single body orifice without a sphincter.

Problems Associated With Onset of Menstruation

Before discussing the intrapsychic meaning of menstruation, we now briefly discuss the real problems associated with the onset of the menstrual flow. Aside from premenstrual or late luteal phase disorders, which will be reviewed in greater detail in Chapter 5, there are problems more specific, but not confined to, adolescence.

The initial concern is the first menstrual period, which commonly occurs without warning. The young woman will have to learn how to control her menstrual flow. External pads often have the problem of visibility and of placing limitations on some activities such as swimming or sports that require short-shorts or skirts. For those women who prefer an internal tampon, the process of placing it properly, comfortably, and quickly requires a great deal of practice. (We will return to the anxiety that is often caused by the need to touch the genitalia.) Adolescent women are frequently concerned about doing internal damage. This concern occurs despite reassurance, and not always on an intrapsychic basis. A poorly placed tampon, or the placement of a tampon during sparse or intermittent flow when the vagina is dry, can be painful.

Early menstrual cycles may be irregular and unpredictable. The problem of cleaning stained underwear is not insignificant. Blood is soluble only in peroxide or other specific chemical formulas. Soap or detergent and water leave a residual stain. The first menstrual periods are frequently anovulatory and may or may not be more painful. This contributes to the fear that something may be physically wrong. These concerns and problems are intimate matters that the young woman often will not discuss with her mother or older sisters, and may feel hesitant to discuss with friends.

Although no limit need be placed on physical activities (because they do not add to the total amount of blood loss per cycle), some activities do precipitate an interval of brisker bleeding that may present an aesthetic problem and require specific care. Despite prior knowledge and reassurance, the worry about "bleeding to death" is not uncommon. A small amount of blood in the toilet bowl rapidly diffuses, which may exaggerate the perception of the extent of the blood loss, making menstruation more frightening. Water retention, emotional lability, and cramping, even if not severe and which may be acceptable and handled easily later on, are all new and frightening experiences. It is not without reason that menstruation is referred to as "the curse," "the red plague," and other negative labels, and that the women during menstruation is sometimes depicted as being "unwell." It is only in recent years (and in fact in one popular song) that menstruation is newly being referred to as "having my friend."

The occasional skipping of a menstrual period once the cycles have become more regular is a cause of worry about physical health in general, and about pregnancy in specific, in young women who are experimenting with various stages of heterosexual intimacy. Menstruation is the signal that pregnancy is now possible, and it is a realistic concern, as well as one that is involved with fantasy and intrapsychic processes.

Sexual Issues

Despite all the advertising about condoms as a protection against AIDS and unwanted pregnancy, most young women feel that the prevention of pregnancy is their problem, or at least their responsibility. This is not an irrational perception. Early forays into sexuality are often enacted and not verbalized, planned, or discussed. It takes a certain amount of maturation before women feel comfortable in verbalizing their needs for pregnancy or AIDS protection, or for gratifying sexual stimulation. Part of this hesitancy has to do with issues of entitlement or self-esteem. Until recently it also involved the preponderance of females over males in the general population. In the black and Hispanic communities, where accidental death, murder, suicide, and war still take a large toll of young men, women, as reported in one large study (Fullilove et al. 1990[14]), are forced to compete for the attention of available men, and they may hesitate to do anything that might "turn them off."

It is neither rare nor necessarily a signal of gender dysphoria for a young woman to wish that she was a guy, or even a little girl again. We will return to a discussion of the times that this is a response to intrapsychic conflict rather than to reality.

Intrapsychic Problems Specific to Adolescent Women

We now present a brief and broad review of the intrapsychic problems specific to female adolescents. We discuss specific problems that originate in this developmental stage and require treatment at that time, or in later years. We provide both brief illustrative vignettes and specific clinical case material to illustrate our psychodynamic approach to these problems.

Menstruation

As noted above, menstruation is a pivotal event. Intrapsychically it causes an increased narcissistic investment in the maturing woman's own body. When this investment is negative, it is because it gives rise to either conscious or unconscious feelings of damage, dirtiness, passivity, dyscontrol, shame, and disgust, all derivations from earlier developmental stages. Ritvo (1977[15]) has made a valuable contribution to the psychology of concealment. He believes that concealment is a widespread, if not universal, phenomenon having its roots in the repression of pregenital (particularly anal) strivings, as it may be a defense against early exhibitionistic wishes. If we look at the ego, rather than the instinctual determinants, concealment may be reflective of a lack of self-esteem, self-assurance, self-confidence, and pride in one's self.

Masturbation and the Establishment of an Adult Object Fantasy Life

In addition to anal instinctual and ego pressures associated with menstruation, there is the possibility that the required genital care and manipulation will mobilize more primitive masturbatory wishes and desires. The regression of these fantasies and wishes is further threatened by the surge of adolescent sexuality and the need for masturbatory release. Masturbation and the establishment of an adult object fantasy life are important preparation for the actuality of an intimate adult sexual relationship. Fearful avoidance of masturbation deters regression to infantile fantasies involving parental objects or to idealized, distancing latency-age sexual fantasies. Avoidance of masturbation does not constitute a positive step on the road to adult dyadic sexuality. One of the authors treated an adolescent who had been hospitalized for promiscuous sexual behavior that had resulted in physical injury to her. This high school student, from a middle-class family, was blatantly aggressively and defiantly seductive. She did not masturbate but rather enacted her sexual fantasies with a partner. She was actually compelled to pick up older men in public places. Her need to do this represented a way of protecting herself against overt incestuous wishes that became conscious in the course of treatment.

Maternal Introjects

We have treated patients who attempt to compensate for the loss of the mother by turning to a male as a substitute. Much of what masquerades as sexual desire in adolescence is participation in sex as a way of being held and comforted by the symbolic mother of earliest childhood. One of the present authors has reported on adolescent homosexual behavior as a search for the mother (Bernstein and Warner 1984b[16]).

The analysis of a female patient whose promiscuity was motivated by the repeated witnessing of the primal scene was also presented and discussed. The establishment of adult autonomy requires giving up archaic wishes for reunion with the mother along with oedipal wishes to replace her. What must be established is an ego ideal that contains both the wish to be cared for and the wish to be caring and nurturant. Some of the most serious psychopathology beginning in adolescence revolves around separation from the mother. Both anorexia nervosa and bulimia nervosa have elements of separation anxiety at their core. We will return to this at a later point.

The introjection of a bad mother with the failure of formation of an acceptable maternal ideal will also cause damage to the functioning of the superego. Blum (1976[17]) and Greenacre (1948/1952a[18]) pointed out the relationship of the female's fear of loss of her mother's love as a powerful force for superego integration. This contrasts with Freud's (1925[19]) formulation that castration anxiety was the force determining superego formation and that because girls were already "castrated" they would necessarily have a weak superego. We can agree with the many authors who believe that Freud confused different values in the superego with failure of structuralization. We believe that the identification of a woman with her mother's compassion and empathy tends to temper a stern (i.e., masculine) superego whose goal is talion punishment. We suggest that the willingness to negotiate, compromise, and forgive in order to avoid injury, death, starvation, and war represents an added affective component to the superego. Certainly the addition of this affective modulation requires more rather than less structuralization.† With respect to the problem of feminine masochism, we could pursue the same line of reasoning. Being sexually receptive or nurturant is a positive feminine ego adaptation and not equivalent to masochistic

†Some more recent documentation of these phenomena appeared in the *Sunday New York Times* (August 12, 1990) in the form of a telephone public opinion survey that revealed significant gender differences regarding the approach to military intervention in the Middle East.

submission. Maternal self-sacrifice represents an identification with an altruistic mother. This is a positive adaptation, not a form of punitive self-sacrifice.

Developmental Issues Related to Femininity

Femininity has its own biological line of development. Its representation in the ego ideal means that the superego will be an outcome of the normal resolution of the adolescent stage of development. The tasks of the adolescent female include the following:

1. Integration of pregenital impulses within the framework of adult genitality
2. The ability to be nurtured and to be nurturing
3. The ability to share in relationships as an autonomous, independent adult
4. The ability to actualize certain traditionally male strivings autonomously, or to actualize them vicariously, through a loving relationship
5. The ability to achieve sexual orgasm in which there is a fusion with a beloved partner, paralleling in both partners the very early blissful union with the mother, without fears of either engulfment or dissolution
6. The ability to share the desire for generativity and establish a nurturant relationship[†]
7. The ability to have a firm parental identification in the absence of one's birth parent(s)
8. The complex ability to be empathic and to have flexible self-object boundary in order to achieve empathic attunement to both one's own needs and the needs of others

---

[†]Erikson (1959[13]) adds to this "a nurturant atmosphere for children." We believe the wish to bear and nurture one's own biological child is not a requirement of the resolution of adolescent conflict. Women can be nurturant in other ways. Serving as mentor, teacher, surrogate, or adoptive or foster parent can be a successful sublimation of the need for one's own biological offspring.

Problems in Adaptation in Adolescence

Because adolescents so often get derailed from a satisfactory outcome of their adaptational tasks, we shall now address facets of their adaptation that may go wrong and the results of which may surface during adolescence or later in adulthood. We discuss the pathological entities with which adolescents present for treatment, keeping in mind that these may arise in later phases in the life cycle as well. We include the search for identity, anorexia and bulimia, and the abuse of chemical intoxicants, as well as the problem of depression and suicide. (Although the quest for eternal youth and beauty often begins in adolescence, it will be considered in Chapter 3.)

The Search for Identity

The search for identity—a process typified by the questions "Who am I?" and "What do I want?"—is quite overt during adolescence. These questions arise, in general, relative to life-style, religion, career choice, sexual identity, intimate relationships, motherhood, or any combination of the above.

Uncertainty and Identity

One of our patients said:

> *I was 16 and everyone was getting a driver's license, and I just was not ready. The worse year of my life was my senior year in high school when I was supposed to choose a college. I was not ready. I could not do my applications; I could not even complete my high school courses. I holed up in my room. I ate, I slept, I put my music on very loud to block out the world, to block out my mother's demand that I do my school work and finish my college applications. I was not ready. I had no idea who I was, where I wanted to be, or what I wanted to become. It was a study in avoidance and procrastination. I just was not ready, and there was no way I could get anyone to understand that. I pretended to be defiant and lazy but I was just stuck. I was not ready yet.*

Sexual Identity

One adolescent further along in her treatment said:

> *I didn't know where to go to college. I knew that I was smart and that I was expected to choose some elite and socially correct school. I know now that my mother, although she held a prestigious job, was unbalanced. She ran around looking feminine but efficient. No one had any idea of how crazy and disorganized she was at home. She beat the hell out of us because she felt bad. My dad stayed away from it all, but he was calm and financially successful. I wanted to be like him. They [both parents] accused me of being a "dyke" because I would not dress up like Mom. That settled it. I applied to college and got in. That school had a reputation for homosexuality but it was top rate socially and academically. I knew it upset them. I did it for spite and I was glad. I had no inkling then that I was homosexual, but that must have been what really drove me. I wanted to be a man, calm and financially successful, and not a crazy intellectual, artsy person like my mother.*

* * *

Another women related:

> *My parents accused me of being a "dyke." I was the only girl among four brothers. I wore their hand-me-downs. My mother always dressed in a business suit. My father was a "fairy decorator." What did they expect. Yet I always have had boyfriends, and I want to get married and have children.*

Educational Choice

One adolescent patient made her adaptation by going to medical school because from the time she was a child she had wanted to be a physician. In medical school she suffered panic attacks during phlebotomies. She explained that her father had been a medical student who had switched to hospital administration because of a "blood phobia." She always knew that she was destined to do for him what he never could do for himself. Yet now she was experiencing her father's symptoms. The assessment that she was a talented, intellectually curious and happy student by those who taught her and know her led to the suggestion that she stay on in medical school and get psychiatric help.

She had been pressured to achieve in a counterphobic way. She was designated to do what her father could not. She shone academically and never rebelled but was enraged about not being allowed to be her own person. The rage led to a defensive identification with the hated parent and thus to her phobic response to blood letting.

She became asymptomatic, completed her training and chose a field of medicine unrelated to direct patient care, one in which she could use investigational and interpretive skills that she might have applied to another vocation if she could have made her own choice.

Religious Identity

One high school student was seen after her mother entered treatment. The mother, who was separated from her husband, was struggling as the single parent of three adolescents. She was working but she became depressed in the context of a difficult fight over a financial settlement during her divorce. Her most immediate concern was for her youngest child, a daughter, who had become active in a religious movement, removed from the family's background, that had the reputation for being a cult. The youngster was persuaded to see one of the present authors. She was a very angry young woman who insisted on her right to do whatever she pleased even if her parents did not approve. After all, she had not approved of their divorce. Why should she remain in a religion to which her father professed an allegiance while at the same time having a love affair outside of his marriage? She also felt, probably correctly, that her father had cheated in other areas of his life. Her mother was a "closet alcoholic," so how, the daughter wondered, had her religion helped her? Indeed the mother's alcoholism, confirmed by the other siblings, had gone undetected at work or in the community. The family's religious leader, with whom this young woman had tried to discuss the problem, contributed to the denial. Now she was determined to go to the cult's summer retreat where alcohol was forbidden, and neatness and discipline required, to get away from her home.

The mother was confronted and her denial was shallow enough that she agreed to go to Alcoholics Anonymous. Her daughter met her halfway and went to Alanon. Alanon was easy for the daughter, who had been seeking a structured system to put her life in order. Her mother was assigned a contact who was a coprofessional who helped in the period of alcohol withdrawal. Once clear of the drug she was able to put her household back to the state it had been for all her life before her alcoholism. Soon the house was cleaned up and the beer and wine bottles disposed of, and activities such as meals and doing laundry became a family effort and were done in a timely fashion. The young woman returned to the church in which she had been raised.[†] *Adolescents respond positively when a parent acknowledges a deficit and is seen to be actively struggling to improve.*

* * *

Another patient came to treatment because of her inability to get her daughter home, even for a visit, from Israel, to which the daughter had chosen to emigrate. The daughter was caught up in a movement designed to educate young people in orthodox Judaism. The movement provided a group home, hours of religious study, and the promise of an arranged marriage. Her family was Jewish in origin but atheist by persuasion. Her father worked dawn to midnight, Monday, Tuesday, and Wednesday, and quit at five on Thursday, at which time he and his wife drove to their vacation home, returning by midnight on Sunday. The mother's free time was spent in a vain attempt to help and influence a morbidly obese unemployed older sibling.

Encouraged to open a dialogue with her Israeli daughter, the mother found herself under the demand to "just once do something for me if you ever want me to come home even for a visit." The demand was a potentially onerous one, namely, that the mother establish a kitchen in strict conformity with Jewish dietary laws. When she did this, her daughter agreed to visit, and she invited friends that she had never had before. As the dialogue continued over several visits, the young woman began to think about remaining orthodox in

[†]There is a literature on cults and their insidious ability to interest and capture individuals who otherwise perceive themselves and are perceived by others as untroubled. In this case, the patient actively sought a cult affiliation as the answer to a chaotic home situation.

this country. She temporarily put off an arranged marriage, which she realized would have brought her an arranged and physically present family.

The young, newly orthodox woman stated quite clearly that she had never had an identity before. She insisted that her behavior was not rebellious. On the contrary, there was nothing to rebel against. She repeated softly, "There was nothing, nothing at all." What she did not realize was that her orthodoxy was the opposite of her parents' nonconformity.

Abandonment of religion or acquisition of one is often a way of separating from parents coping with the separation anxiety involved and establishing an individual identity. Before the so-called "yuppie" generation, there were the "hippies," rejecting any kind of orthodoxy in religion, sexual behavior, dress, schooling, career, home, or family building. The conformity, conservatism, and traditionalism of the 1950s was ripped asunder by the freedom and radicalism of the 1960s and early 1970s. The mid-1980s were characterized by a pendulum swing toward a 1950s mentality.

In each generation, adolescence and young adulthood have had their "markers" in terms of costumes, hair styles, food, and music preference. These are all attempts at establishing an identity separate from those of the parents but consensually valid in the peer group. On a rough sea of fluctuating wishes, tastes, and ambitions, and emotional lability, these givens become the ballast that allows the ship to continue safely in a single direction.

Adolescents who experience severe identity diffusion often isolate themselves from their peer group. They either reject the peer norms or adopt bizarre caricatures of these. Often they are not overtly angry or rebellious, and they sleep a lot and absent themselves from school and from functions within the family. Others are overtly sullen and diffusely and unreasonably angry. At the extremes, they may be profoundly depressed, actively suicidal, or psychotically decompensated.[†] They may

---

[†]Adolescents are at risk for both psychotic and major mood disorders, a finding that has been discussed widely in the literature. We find the contributions of Nicholi (1978[20]), Robins et al. (1959[21]), Barraclough et al. (1974[22]), Shaffer (1974[23]), and Pfeffer et al. (1984[24]) especially useful.

become prisoners of severe rituals that keep them from "falling apart" or of drugs that numb their senses or ameliorate their profound dysphoria. For some patients the illness itself and its treatment with medication may cause a narcissistic injury to the patient and his or her family and, therefore, once again exacerbate the illness. In addition, the illness or the refusal to take medication may be used to punish the family.

Suicide

Suicide is the leading cause of death in adolescents ages 15 to 24 (Pfeffer et al. 1983[25]). According to one report ("Most Youth Who Attempt Suicide" 1990[26]), 70% of all suicide attempts in youth are silent attempts. Blumenthal and Kupfer (1990[27]) feel that although most suicides involve the classical thread of helplessness, hopelessness, and isolation, more specific factors play a part in various stages of the life cycle. These authors point to anxiety disorders, homosexual orientation, and repeated failures due to learning disability. To these factors we would add broken families, youth unemployment, the decline in religious affiliation, access to firearms, medications prescribed for parents, and street drugs. (In one 16-year-old patient whom we have seen, the suggestion that her emotional pain was not real and that she should go take one her mother's prescription sleeping pills led to the impulsive, retaliatory consumption of the entire vial of phenobarbital.) Stanley and Barter (1978[28]) point to a nonproximate source of suicidal behavior: separation of a child before the age of 15 from his or her parents. In addition, the presence of low cerebrospinal fluid levels of 5-hydroxyindoleacetic acid (5-HIAA) has been noted by Van Praag (1984[29]) and Brown et al. (1982[30]), among others, to be associated with suicidal behavior.

The association of a family history of suicide and suicide was noted by Ranier (1984[31]). McIntire and Angle (1975[32]) correlated open hostility with family environment. These children had experienced home environments of indifference and low parental involvement. The authors also noted that overtly depressed adolescents often come from environments with high expectations for achievement and extreme parental control. The latter group, though few in number, had more lethal attempts. Green and Keown (1986[33]) found that increased arguments with parents, the breaking of seemingly important relationships, and geographic relocation were also important factors. Sack et al. (1985[34]) noted a correlation between adolescent suicide and intrapartum as well as perinatal conditions (e.g., perinatal hypoxia).

Sexual abuse is another factor linked to suicide in adolescents. Adams-Tucker (1982[35]) looked at the effects of sexual abuse in an outpatient sample and found the victims to be more depressed, withdrawn, and self-destructive than other patients. Briere and Pruntz (1986[36]) examined childhood sexual abuse and suicidality in 195 Canadian women treated at a community mental health center. Fifty-five percent of those women who were sexually abused as children were suicide attempters in childhood or adolescence in contrast to those women who were not abused (23%). Deykin et al. (1985[37]) described physically abused children and found a link between physical abuse and adolescent suicide.

There is also evidence that the presence of manifest psychopathology in parents, such as low self-esteem, depression, and alcohol abuse, as well as deficient parenting skills, increases the risk of adolescent suicide. Pfeffer (1986[38]) and McKenny et al. (1982[39]) have noted the role of maladaptive marriages and manipulative behaviors in relation to suicidality. Pfeffer (1986[38]) has put forth the theory of "the expendable child": one who is unconsciously no longer needed by the family and who senses this wish and sees suicide as a way out of this predicament. Pfeffer also describes rigid and unchanging family systems (in contrast to some of the more specific characteristics to which we have alluded) that leave the child no way out.

Recently there has been a rising occurrence and increasing interest in so-called cluster suicides—that is, a rash of suicides in response to one suicide in a community or the television media account of youthful suicide (Gould and Shaffer 1986[40]; Phillips and Carstensen 1986[41]). We are aware of, and support, the current trend toward discussions in the schools of violent and upsetting events, such as the explosion of the manned space mission Challenger 2 years ago. Discussion of accidental, homicidal, or suicidal death within peer groups offers the opportunity for ventilation of hostile and depressive feelings and mitigates isolation. It also gives knowledgeable teachers, counselors, and professional workers the opportunity to offer individual help to those young people who seem either unaffected or too profoundly affected.†

The authors have heard accounts of adolescents who were killed as a result of an accident, particularly a motor vehicle accident. Interestingly, none of these persons had a history of either expressed suicidal wishes or prior psychiatric treatment. None had a proximate cause in terms of loss, separation, violent or chaotic families, or the descent into psychosis. We know, however, from our experience with incest victims that when something is hidden or denied, other terrible things may also be happening. Another complicating factor is that impulsivity and grandiosity are often features of adolescence. Death may come as an unanticipated result.

We now present the histories of several adolescent patients who made serious suicide attempts for which they required hospitalization. Treatment is obviously not for the suicide attempt but for the underlying diagnosis. In addition, we discuss one patient whose submitted classwork caused a teacher to suspect suicidal ideation. One of the present authors confirmed that intervention was warranted. Indeed, the young woman was suicidal and was helped with her despair and the unsuspected realities of her life.

Attempted Suicide After Breaking Up With a Lover

The patient was 18 years old when she attempted to drive her car over an embankment abutting a river. Upon hospital admission, she was overtly depressed, agitated, and tearful, and remained actively suicidal. The patient refused to see family members, and, initially, she would not give a history.

---

†The authors wish to thank Ellen Klausner, Ph.D. candidate at Yeshiva University, for access to her paper on suicidal children.

The patient seemed to settle in with a peer group on a mixed adult and adolescent floor. Her initial depression abated without medication. She was seen every day and gave a history of an intact and functioning family but persisted in her contention that they would not understand her and her wish not to see them. Her mental status was otherwise unremarkable. At the end of a week, when the patient was urged to do her laundry, she had a panic attack. Her clothing had to be laundered separately. Insisting that her clothes were a part of her and that she could not let them out of her sight, the patient had to sit in the room until the washing and drying process was complete. She responded to persistent interpretations about her separation anxiety by revealing that separation was the reason for her suicide attempt. It seemed to her female therapist that, in order for the patient to cope with separation anxiety, the transference was becoming eroticized. She judged this from the patient's glances, her undressing gaze, and finally her flirtatious manner in terms of grooming herself for sessions and literally batting her eyes. When this was interpreted, the patient revealed that she had been involved in a lesbian relationship from which her lover had been moving away for weeks. The more eagerly the patient waited on her lover or tried to curry her favor, the worse the siutation became. Her lover finally broke it off entirely on the day preceding the suicide attempt. The more the patient realized that she had been used, abused, and discarded, the angrier and, therefore, less suicidal she became. She revealed that she always carried a pocket knife, ostensibly to protect her lover. However, she had smuggled it into the hospital, secretly planning that she could use it to cut her throat. She surrendered it voluntarily on one condition: that the therapist take it home and keep it for her rather than putting it in a locked drawer on the unit. The patient's fantasy, which later became conscious, was that she had merged with her therapist and was therefore not separated from her knife or the therapist. She was as merged with the therapist as she had once been with her clothing.

The staff experienced the patient as needful of and resistant to nurturing. After finally attaining the patient's permission to meet her parents, the therapist found the mother masculine, aloof, and businesslike. The father, on the other hand, was very histrionic, concerned, and tearful. When the patient asked about the meeting, the therapist shared her thoughts about it. Relative to her mother, the patient replied, offhandedly, "Yeah, she [the mother] has ice in her tits." Of her father, she said, "He wears the skirts in the family." The patient went on to discuss her brothers. The older one, who was in a prestigious profession, had sexually abused her when she was a child. Her adaptation had been to tough it out. If that is what the guys do, she thought, she would do it too. Her youngest brother was simply dismissed as a baby who never had a mother and did not know which end was up. Her one role model was a grandmother whose death anniversary coincided with the patient's attempts at suicide. The patient denied having been aware of this at the time.

The one visitor that the patient would accept was a man from her school whom she had been dating on and off. He was a very nurturing and supportive figure. When he observed that she could not part with her clothes, he offered to go out and buy her a duplicate set, and she accepted. She went out on pass with this young man and things went well.

Upon discharge from the hospital the patient continued in outpatient therapy with the same therapist. She began interviewing for jobs but returned home to live temporarily. When the therapist took a vacation, the patient gave her a small gold wishbone and instructed her to bring it back with her. The fear and then the underlying wish that the therapist would be killed was analyzed in the transference. Although the patient continued to feel that she was more attracted to women than men, she was no longer involved in the gay community. She continued to see the same young man, and the two were engaged. On the occasion of her marriage, she gave the therapist permission to dispose of her knife, the one that she had given to the therapist upon entering the hospital. She continued to work and went to college part time.

The patient had previously eschewed pregnancy but began to find motherhood more and more attractive. This shift represented an identification with the therapist, who had been pregnant and given birth twice during the course of her treatment (i.e., 5 years). She successfully terminated treatment but contacted the therapist in a panic a couple of weeks before she was scheduled to deliver her first child. Her demand was that the therapist intervene to see that she would not be put to sleep during delivery or ever be separated from her child prior to leaving the hospital. She was afraid that she would take the wrong baby home. This was unanalyzable. The therapist intervened to guarantee no anesthesia or medication that would cause unconsciousness, and to arrange rooming in. The patient, who gave birth to a daughter, chose a foreign-language name that indicated her "ownership" of the child.

Three years later, pregnant again, the patient called with the same requests about labor and delivery and the postpartum period. She came with her husband for an appointment. She was evidently a good mother: her daughter was thriving and well adapted to a prenursery program. The patient was seen one more time, later, when her two children were away from home and she felt panicky. She was helped to identify the separation anxiety, and she wished to confront it without using any medication.

Multiple Suicide Attempts and Self-Mutilation

Another patient, an 18-year-old woman, was admitted to the hospital after a third attempt at wrist slashing. Estranged from both parents, the patient was at school and was being supported by her grandparents. Angry about being in the hospital, she remained mute in her sessions but spoke occasionally to staff and other patients. Her father lived in another city; her mother, dependent on both alcohol and prescription drugs, was unreliable in visiting or coming to see the social worker assigned as an adjunct to the daughter's treatment. Her grandparents agreed to support a prolonged hospitalization.

An experimental music therapy program was instituted, and she wanted a guitar, which her grandparents readily supplied. The patient was amazingly talented at her new instrument, picked up a variety of popular and folk songs, and entertained patients, staff, and visitors. She began to bring her guitar to session and mutely strum it.

Invited to play tunes, she readily agreed. The ones she chose were usually nostalgic and sad. Coaxed little by little to come out of her shell, she began to verbalize in snatches. For a while the therapist was empathic enough to verbalize her feelings correctly. After the first break in empathy, the patient stole a razor blade and cut her thigh. After a recurrence in which she lacerated her breast, it was agreed that she would no longer be taken to the emergency room for suturing but that her therapist would be called around the clock to suture her wounds. The rationale was that this behavior was a communication meant for a transference object. Therefore, the therapist had to separate from the psychotic maternal acting out by establishing her reality as a physician. It was felt that this reality testing would avoid transference reenactment and would not lead the patient to increased dependency, regression, or enactment in order to gain attention from the psychotic maternal transference object. This plan was based on the observation that the self-mutilation was an autistic mechanism of rage release rather than an hysterical bid for attention and escalating interaction with the therapist. The patient was apprised of the plan for her surgical management of her wounds if she cut herself again.

Quite suddenly she began to talk in session. She gave a history of neglect by her mother and physical abuse by her father. At times when she had tried to escape his belt or fists, he had broken down her door. Her grandparents knew about this but encouraged her not to antagonize her father. She was initially enraged with them, but they were the most dependable figures in her life. She recognized her mother's illness but was furious that her mother was not "in tune" enough with her to realize that she was being, or about to be, brutalized, and to step in. Later, in a minor dispute between patients on her floor, in a rage the patient again cut her thigh open. In accordance with the plan, the therapist came to the hospital and attended to the wound. For the first time the patient cried. She became able to talk about the self-mutilating behavior. It happened when she felt numb and in danger of disappearing (her defense against murderous rage). Although when "in her right mind" she could not figure a way to get possession of a "sharp" (i.e., a cutting instrument), in her numb (and raging) state, she zoomed in on how to either get into the utility room or steal from a patient who was not on "razor precautions."

On the next occasion when her rage was out of control, she collected a bunch of large safety pins and pinned the curtains around her bed together. (This was when there were curtains around all beds, even in psychiatry, for the purpose of medical examinations and procedures.) Quite correctly, the staff called the therapist to the floor. When asked what she was doing, the patient replied very calmly, "Trying not to cut myself." She could not contain the rage, but now her skin was no longer the barrier—the bed curtains were. She let the therapist in behind the curtains and then discussed the precipitating episode and related it to her father's behavior. For the first time the patient revealed that she had at times felt physically capable of snatching the belt and beating her father to death. She would have used the buckle that often cut her to cut him up "like chopped meat." Interpretations dealt with her real ability to intervene with other persons before she got so mad that she felt like killling them. As a result she began to be angry with those persons whom she experienced as unempathic or impinging on her rights.

To her surprise, the staff encouraged her more normal adolescent behavior. She requested and got her hair styled. Her grandparents took her out for clothing and allowed her to "do her thing" with her purchases even though they were a very staid, proper old New England couple.

When the patient confronted her grandparents with their failure to protect her, they were frank in their answer. Her mother was sick and seemed to need this man, and they had been unaware that the patient had been abused. They also told her that they knew that her mother was physically abused but that they could not seem to get her to leave the situation. In addition, they mentioned that they had left their entire multimillion-dollar estate to her, their granddaughter, because they considered their daughter, her mother, unreliable, and thus depended on the patient to care for her mother. This helped the patient to soften her attitude toward her mother, whom she phoned and invited to visit. During all of these visits her mother looked so put together and her behavior was so impeccable that the staff began to wonder if the patient was delusional. When she was confronted with this, she became angry and said, "Of course that is what's so crazy. She looks fine and then she behaves crazy and in an irresponsible way." This explanation seemed more credible when the mother's visits became unreliable. The patient would become enraged on these occasions, slam her pillows, and scream at the therapist. She had not hurt herself in 6 months.

The patient's grandparents told the therapist that their daughter had deceived the "best psychiatrists" in the world, and they all felt that a social worker should see the patient's mother as part of the patient's treatment. Her mother agreed to a detoxification program.

The patient was the featured artist in a final concert given by the musical therapy program. The mother attended and brought the patient an appropriate gift. Her mother had never bought her anything before in her life; her grandparents had supplied all her needs. The patient began to leave the hospital on pass. She shopped and went to museums, and returned in good spirits. Once she met her mother for lunch.

She and her mother requested an overnight pass for her to stay at her mother's apartment. She returned to the hospital late that night. She seemed fine and told the staff simply that she did not feel safe to be out of the hospital at night. Everyone was delighted that she was able to recognize her need to return. The next morning she was unarousable. Even before the toxicology reports it was clear that she had overdosed. Her therapist passed the nasogastric tube and did the lavage. She was furious with the patient and shouted at her, "How could you do this!" Apparently the patient's mother had had a boyfriend over who was drunk and invited the mother to leave. The mother assented to the boyfriend's request. The patient also assented, but took a handful of her mother's pills.

The therapist was upset about her countertransference outburst and thought that a very difficult year had been lost. To her surprise the patient responded favorably and lovingly. She said, "You got mad; you gave a damn. I let you down, don't make excuses for me. I will never do any of this stuff again. I know that you really love me." The psychotic transference resolved because the therapist, unlike the mother, cared. Once out of the psychotic transference, all of the patient's prior behavior was open for analysis. The patient subsequently left the hospital to attend college, got married, and now has a very successful career in which she is constantly involved in violence, as a bystander and a recorder. Her career represents a successful sublimation of lingering pain and rage. Real trauma cannot be analyzed away, but patients can channel their affects in productive, rather than destructive, ways.

Potential Suicide Noted by a Teacher

A patient was diagnosed and brought into treatment because of a creative writing assignment given to a high school class, which was shown to one of the present authors. Excerpts are as follows:

> *Joan's eyes flit from window to window, along the roadway. Eyes, meanwhile alert, ready to investigate any noise, curtains slide across windowsills. Ladies smooth satin sashes, teasing Joan with occasional coy peeks at the warm black hole inside—warm wombs, the rooms, meanwhile Joan feels innumerable eyes staring from every dark area. Judgmental eyes that tell Joan to go home. Home to dark amorphous blankets and pillows. Outside daylight cold staring eyes, unwelcome trespassers. Home to a place that reeks of age of regressive states of social disconnection and removal. . . .*

> *Joan's surroundings yield a cold barren wasteland, devoid of the mysterious bonds existing between humans. Joan feels her place is a place of disregard by the world. . . .*
>
> *Joan sees daddy driving, Joan's backseat baggage, determined eyes disregard him in the mirror. . . . old man, pile of rags . . . old man stops, a stream stagnant clogged. Joan chokes all responses slowly from within, drags a stick roadside, sits. . . . The old man starts, jerking deathlike dance past Joan. . . . Joan hears discordant buzzes feels the earth bowels shifting into first gear and she sidles home fading quickly into the light of day.*

The teacher, sensing something ominous and suicidal in the writing, brought it in for evaluation. She said that Joan would come to class in a black raincoat that she never removed, sit silently in an otherwise participatory group, and then slink off.

Joan was invited to her grade advisor's office for a general chat. She seemed "somber and downhearted," which led to some direct questioning. Joan revealed that her parents had "put her out" and that she had been living for weeks with the clothes on her back moving from the home of one friend to another. No one knew that her parents had put her out. Her parents were contacted and confirmed her story but were unwilling to discuss the matter further. Joan had just turned 18. They no longer felt responsible for her. She had been accepted, with a scholarship, into one of the finest colleges in the country. They had no intention of helping her to pay her way or otherwise support her. They were unwilling to meet to discuss this decision. Joan, they said, could come home and collect her belongings.

With nowhere to go, her bright future obliterated, Joan admitted to being suicidal. Indeed, she had a plan for violent suicide. Her counselor made a fast decision: to contact the referring teacher and find another teacher who would be willing to take Joan home temporarily to live with his or her family, and not to call the police or take her to a treatment facility. Within days one of Joan's teachers, the father of daughters in elementary school, welcomed Joan to their household in exchange for chores and baby sitting. Joan thus became an independent minor eligible for additional tuition support. She lived with her new "family" for the last 3 months of high school and through the summer, *during which she worked at her usual summer job. Her new "family" took her off to college and made it known that she was welcome to come "home" on school breaks, holidays, and for the summer if she wished.*

She had a brilliant first year at college, and when she visited the high school she was dressed in blue jeans and a bright colored shirt. She was cheerful, and it seemed that she had actually grown in height, or maybe she was no longer slouched over. No one, including Joan, seemed able to understand why her parents rejected her. She believed that it was because she was "too bright and too weird" (i.e., creative) for her blue-collar parents. They refused any further contact with her. She went on to a stellar career.

This last patient would seem to fit Pfeffer's (1986[38]) description of an "expendable child."

Other Conditions That Place the Adolescent at Risk

In addition to adolescents who are overtly suicidal or have suicidal ideation, there is a group of youngsters whose behavior or compulsions put them at risk for serious physical illness or even death. Such adolescents may be at risk due to many factors, including anorexia, bulimia, violent delinquent behavior, drug abuse, or pregnancy.

Anorexia and Bulimia

Anorexia nervosa is defined in DSM-III-R (American Psychiatric Association 1987[42]) as refusal to maintain body weight over minimal norms (i.e., weight more than 15% below these norms), intense fear of gaining weight or of becoming fat, and, in women, the absence of at least three consecutive expected menstrual cycles. *Bulimia nervosa* is defined in DSM-III-R as episodes of binge eating at least twice a week for 3 months, a feeling of lack of control over eating behavior during bingeing episodes, a persistent overconcern with body weight and shape, and the use of self-induced vomiting, laxative (i.e., purging) diuretics, dieting, or vigorous exercise to prevent weight gain. These two disorders can be diagnosed separately but are often found to overlap. Anorexic persons who limit food intake may have episodes of binge eating as well as purging, vigorous exercise, and the use of diuretics.

These disorders have both psychological and biochemical determinants. We have found that sometimes the most seriously ill patients have been abused as children. Biochemical changes may precede, accompany, or follow behavioral changes, making it difficult to make judgments about cause and effect. (For material about biochemical changes, see Appendix B.)

Sours (1980[43]), in his book *Starving to Death in a Sea of Objects*, begins:

> There is no disturbance in human development more enigmatic to clinicians and alarming to parents than anorexia nervosa. Typically adolescent girls, anorectics become morbidly fascinated with anything to do with eating—food, cooking, restaurants—to the extent of insisting that everybody, except themselves, eat heartily, while at the same time they remain deeply involved in a grim struggle to lose weight, beyond the expectation of any ordinary dieter. Usually of average weight, the dieting anorectic decides to lose ten to fifteen pounds initially but often goes on to drop 50% of her body weight and sometimes dies. (p. 3)

To this preliminary description we would only add that often an anorexic person begins as a slightly overweight adolescent who wishes to lose a few pounds and to tone up her muscles by exercise. At some point a too thin or even starved adolescent sees her body as fat. The bulk of the literature indicates that distorted body image leads to the syndrome of anorexia.[†]

Bruch (1979[45]), who contributed much to the literature on anorexia nervosa, points out that the illness was named "anorexia nervosa" over

---

[†]One of the authors (Bernstein and Warner 1983[44]) reported three patients for whom distortion of body image was the trigger for anorexic behavior. These patients had used the bulky Milwaukee brace for a prolonged period for the correction of scoliosis.

100 years ago by Sir William Gull in England. There are references to still earlier observations in a work by Morton (1689[46]), who reported a "nervous consumption" and described a patient as "a skeleton only clad with skin."

Between the time of Morton's observations and the 1970s, anorexia nervosa was a rare disease. It could not be treated, and little attempt was made to understand the psychodynamics. It was not until it became an epidemic disease in the 1970s that it was studied.

By 1979 data were accumulated revealing that the disease has a 10:1 to 20:1 female-to-male ratio and that middle- and upper-class children seem to be at highest risk. Typically, the anorexic person will have had a premorbid history of compliance and perfectionism.[†]

The anorexic person's mother is typically "perfectionistic, domineering, overwhelming and overcaring" (Sours 1980,[43] p. 6). Bernstein and Warner (1984[16]), on the basis of their experience in treating anorexic patients, have taken this description one step further, indicating that the mother is intrusive and invasive and does not allow separation, and the father is often distant and uninvolved and does not help his daughter separate from her mother. Bruch (1973[48]) points out that the introjected mother is the person whom the adolescent is starving and trying to control and punish. Some concomitants of this struggle with the mother include the wish never to have a baby and the wish not to menstruate and not to be like the unconsciously hated mother.

One of the tasks of adolescence is the establishment of an identity. We have found that conflicts often arise between the need for intimacy and interpersonal relations and the pressure for independence, achievement, and autonomy. Devlin and Walsh (1989[49]) have discussed the relationship between depression and eating disorders. One point of view (Keys et al. 1950[50]) attributes depression, irritability, low energy, and concentration to the effects of semistarvation. Another point of view (Altshuler and Weiner 1985[51]) maintains that eating disorders are a

[†]Levenkron (1978[47]), in his book aptly titled *The Best Little Girl in the World*, provides an excellent description of the anorexic woman and her world.

masked form of depression. Several recent reviews summarize in detail the complicated relationship between eating disorders and depression (Swift et al. 1986[52]; Hudson and Pope 1987[53]; Strober and Katz 1988[54]).

Certainly anorexia and bulimia have many psychodynamic determinants. The relative weight of separation from mother, the need to establish an identity in the face of conflicting demands, body-image issues (part of the problem of establishing an identity), and depression must be assessed for each patient.

No disagreement exists now on the fact that what is required is a comprehensive medical psychological approach, which may involve the use of antidepressant medication. Weight must either be maintained or gained to the point at which the patient is no longer in danger of cardiovascular collapse and death. Because antidepressant medication is used in conjunction with other treatment modalities, it is difficult to assess its effectiveness. We have seen an improvement in the binge-purge behavior of anorexic patients when treated with antidepressent medication. We have also seen agitated patients with insomnia improve after treatment with antidepressant medication.

Some anorexic patients must be hospitalized and re-fed via a variety of invasive enteric means, either intravenous, nasogastric tube, or major vein cannulation. Other patients can be managed in the hospital by both positive and negative reinforcers (Agras 1987[55]). Inpatient behavioral programs, strict or lenient, and hospital milieu care have reported success in treatment of anorexic and bulimic patients (Eckert et al. 1979[56]; Pillay and Crisp 1981[57]; Touyz et al. 1984[58]). Russell et al. (1987[59]) compared family and individual outpatient psychotherapies for anorexic and bulimic patients after hospital discharge and found that family therapy produced greater improvement. It is our experience that anorexic patients resist treatment, resist having the therapist involved with the family, and refuse to be seen with the family. To compound this, the family, especially the mother, resists recognizing the disorder, resists obtaining psychodynamic treatment for the daughter, and resists involving herself or other family members in treatment.

A general rule for the psychodynamic treatment of the anorexic adolescent on an outpatient basis is that the subject of her weight and eating patterns should not become the subject of discussion or of a power struggle within the treatment. Rather the patients are required to have an internist or family practitioner who deals with nutrition, weight maintenance, or weight gain. A contract is established that guarantees physical health so that psychodynamic treatment can deal with emotions, conflict, and ego functioning.

A Persistently Intrusive Mother

A patient recently seen had moved from another city to do a college internship. The worst of her anorexia was over, but sensitive liver enzyme tests had not yet returned to normal levels. The patient painted a very benign picture of her family, as she had done persistently with her former therapist. Yet she seemed very sad when discussing them and was preoccupied with their health in a clear reaction formation. As her response to her family was analyzed, she became conscious of her anger at her "managed life." She was looking well and was obviously happy in her work, where she had made several friends. Also, she had begun to date one particular man. Her parents came to visit. She anticipated showing off the city and herself. She found herself not complimented by her mother but criticized about not eating enough, being too thin, and a variety of other things. Her boyfriend's family came to town and invited her to dinner, and she spent the entire weekend with them. Upon returning, she contrasted them with her own family in terms of their flexibility. The patient began to view her mother as anxious, punctual, and prearranged. She made summer plans only to find that her mother had already arranged her summer.

Anorexia and Obsessive-Compulsive Disorder

A patient who had had a history of severe anorexia in adolescence came for treatment in her last year of graduate school. She felt depressed and was obsessive about her health and her grades. The patient was very angry in her demeanor toward the therapist. She at first refused to look at the therapist. Chopped, disconnected sentences alternated with periods of silence. When questioned about her behavior, she revealed that during her treatment for anorexia she had often spent many hours in silence. The therapist inquired as to whether that was not very uncomfortable for her. For the first time she looked at the therapist and replied that of course it was. She said that it was often difficult to talk to "get out of her head." She acknowledged that she would like some help with that problem.

Early in the course of the patient's treatment, a dream signaled the emergence of murderous rage toward the mother-therapist. The patient began to feel fat, started a diet, and became obsessed with her exercise. Her diet consisted of vast quantities of caffeinated beverages and sugar snacks. Her mother put an article in the community publication about her daughter's graduation and began to insist on a graduation party. The patient became enraged at her mother's narcissistic use of her success. Meanwhile, therapist and patient were working on other issues in her life, her need for friendships, her shyness, and her criticism of others that revealed an identification with her mother. The patient made a friend, an achievement to which she, but not her mother, had aspired. She was invited to various graduation parties. In anticipation of a break before continuing her studies, she became bulimic. She went to a donut store and bought two of each kind. She tasted a bit of each, and then, not trusting herself, she threw the rest into the garbage. However, no attention was paid in the treatment to the eating disorder behavior.

The patient reported a conversation with her mother during which the patient expressed a feeling of boredom. In reality the preparation for comprehensive examinations was boring for this bright woman. Her mother replied, "You should use the time to make some friends." The patient became furious and hung up the telephone. When asked why this response from her mother generated such rage, whereas the therapist's attempt to encourage her friendships seemed to be well accepted, the patient replied, "She eats me up!" She was incredibly startled by this primitive response from her unconscious; its meaning in terms of her disordered eating behavior was not lost on her. Without interpretation her eating and exercise behavior have returned to normal. Therapy directed toward her longing for and making of relationships continues. It is clear, however, that the dynamics of this patient's anorexia, perfectionism, and episodic bulimia are far from being resolved. Indeed, it seems that apart from these compulsive episodes of enactment or acting out, her depression is not yet solved.

The following case, in which the mother was seen in psychotherapy and the daughter took psychotropic medication and was followed by her physician, is an exception to the family's usual reluctance to enter treatment of their anorexic or bulimic daughter.

Treatment of the Mother

One young patient resisted psychodynamic treatment but agreed to medical management and antidepressant medication under the very real threat that otherwise she would have to be hospitalized. The patient's mother asked for treatment for herself to help her daughter. First, she recognized her inability to deal with her daughter's anorexic and reclusive behavior, and, second, she was open to the possibility that her own behavior might have precipitated her daughter's illness. Indeed, she was a compulsive perfectionist who exercised avidly and kept her own weight below normal but not in a dangerous or unaesthetic way. Her daughter's chronic medical illness kept the mother overprotective and overinvolved. Her husband was often out of town on business, and she substituted involvement with her daughter as a source of emotional intimacy and gratification.

Soon she became more engaged and began to disengage from her daughter. When the family participated in activities not centered around their daughter, who was not invited to family meals, the daughter became more curious and less reclusive. One day she appeared at the dinner table and asked, "Can I have something to eat?" Her mother replied, "Sure, grab a plate, meat's in the oven, vegetables are on the stove, and dessert is in the refrigerator." As the dinnertime conversation continued, the mother never looked at what her daughter ate. Gradually the daughter began to eat and even request food, and she gained weight. The mother's concern about her daughter's condition led to an understanding of the mother's history of binge eating during her own adolescence.[†]

[†]We have treated several adult bulimic patients, male and female, who were overweight as children, and others who were anorexic, cachectic, skinny, or puny as children and/or adolescents. One patient said, "I would never eat for my mother, and now I will not stop eating because my mother wants me to."

Delinquent Behavior

Another maladaptation to the stress of adolescence is delinquent behavior. This type of behavior constitutes a spectrum disorder that at the most pathological end is not amenable to the psychodynamic therapy that we have discussed and will discuss relevant to the treatment of other disorders of female psychology. Juvenile delinquency is defined in legal terms as usually applicable to youth below the age of 18 who exhibit behavior that is punishable by law. These offenses range from murder, burglary, assault, robbery, and rape, to truancy, sexual activity including peeping and acts involving minors, and "incorrigibility" (Conger and Petersen 1984[60]).

Because of the increasing incidence of heinous crime, murder, assault, and rape, youngsters from the age of 14 are in some locales classified as adults, tried, and penalized under adult statutes. Fewer girls than boys are involved in such crimes, but girls are frequently detained for prostitution. Delinquency among disadvantaged groups has always been noted. We are beginning to notice that significant social class differences in official delinquency records may be due to discrimination against youths from lower classes (Braithwaite 1981[61]). At least one careful study has revealed that predatory crimes against persons occur three times as often and predatory crimes against property twice as often among youths from the lower socioeconomic class than among youths from other socioeconomic classes. However, no difference in the rate of victimless crimes, such as drug abuse or drunkenness, can be found between youths of different socioeconomic classes (Elliot and Ageton 1980[62]).

Several recent changes in the patterns of delinquency too new to have been documented in the psychiatric literature but known to us through our newspapers and other media reports are 1) a sharp upsurge in racially motivated crime; 2) an upsurge of heinous crime committed by youngsters of middle- and upper-class parents; and 3) a strong relationship between drug abuse and serious crime—for example, deliberate murder, accidental murder (in which the weapon is a motor vehicle), and "wilding rampages," involving personal assault, rape, and murder. Often these crimes are connected with drug abuse.

Drug Abuse

Drug abuse may be determined in part by depression and anxiety. The authors do not have firsthand experience with either sociopathy or drug abuse by disenfranchised youth, because these adolescents do not get into the health care system. They have no insurance, and their families do not apply for Medicaid. The links between poverty, socioeconomic despair, and drug abuse are understood and discussed in the media without any attempt at psychodynamic understanding. Some adolescents observe the gold chains, big cars, and sexy women associated with the drug bosses. Even adolescents in intact families with both parents working, sometimes at multiple jobs, see an easier way. We recognize the need to understand and treat those economically advantaged adolescents who are involved in alcohol or drug abuse. This care should be available to disadvantaged adolescents as well. Some of the drug abuse occurs in economically comfortable families in which there is no history of drug abuse or family turmoil (Elliot and Ageton 1980[62]). Kalogerakis (1973[63]) reported on emotionally troubled adolescents and their families from the family physician's viewpoint.

The problem for the psychodynamic psychotherapist is to ascertain the meaning of the need for the drug and then work out appropriate steps to eliminate the need. This may require a period of preliminary inpatient care. The reason for drug abuse may be involved with acting out against the parents or therapist, or the need to fill an inner emptiness. (See Appendix C for data on specific drug addictions.)

Cocaine Addiction

The patient, a 19-year old college dropout, was admitted for inpatient detoxification for severe and persistent cocaine abuse and a recent drug overdose. Her father was an ambitious man from a disadvantaged family who had achieved phenomenal financial success as an investment broker. Her mother, a housewife, and somewhat depressed, had devoted her life to her children. The patient's older sister, a successful businesswoman, was living in another city, and her younger sister lived at home with her parents.

The patient requested a therapist because "I need to talk, too." During her initial sessions, she discussed a long-standing history of cocaine addiction and promiscuity involving a series of live-in boyfriends, all of whom were addicts and somewhat devaluing of her. Her initial pressure to talk with a therapist remained unclear until after discharge to a drug halfway house, where she began to explore the possibility that her sexual provocativeness and life-threatening addictions always resulted in parental intervention. She noted, "It's the only time I exist for them, I guess."

She then went on to reveal the family secret—her younger sister was mentally retarded and blind. The parents had experienced this defective child as a punishment for their eloping against their families' wishes. So intense had been their guilt and denial that the sister was kept at home and continually cared for by the patient's mother, despite the sister's being 17 years of age and a severe management problem. The patient and her sister had been seen as fine, beautiful children with no problems, and they were either ignored completely or the focus of anxious and overcontrolling attention lest something "spoil them." During her growing up, the patient often stole food and money as a means of getting some supplies from her parents, and she continued an alternating passive-dependent, passive-aggressive stance, accepting financial supplies on a continued basis from her parents and often using the money to purchase high-status material goods or to buy drugs.

During the next 2 years, the patient made significant progress in her therapy. She was able to move to an apartment, obtain a job as a department manager, maintain her drug abstinence, and develop an intimate, stable relationship with a man. Eventually she convinced her parents to enter family therapy, where they ultimately dealt with their sadness and guilt regarding her sister's deficits. The family also addressed separation issues that permitted the family to place the sister in a residential home and to assist the patient in preparing for her wedding.

Cocaine Abuse

A young woman who was the daughter of a "blue blood" New England family attended a prestigious northeastern college. She seemed unsure of herself and scattered in her academic pursuits, and began forays into what her family considered an alternate life-style—that is, she became interested in theatre and production as an offshoot of her traditional English major. She began to see a therapist because of the open disapproval of her family and the lethargy and depression that was troubling her.

The patient experienced the therapist as being on the side of a liberal arts education and became overtly angry at her parents. She began to experiment with available on-campus drugs, such as "pot" and some alcohol (i.e., beer). She flaunted this to her parents in her midwinter break, and they threatened to withdraw her from school. She placated them and returned to school only to begin to experiment with snorting cocaine. Her academic performance began to fail. Nevertheless, she continued this behavior despite her therapist's efforts to point out that her defiance was in her fantasy defeating her parents but in reality defeating herself. It was only the death of another student from adulterated cocaine that brought the patient back to reality testing. With the cessation of drug use, she was able to begin to analyze her rage at her parents. She remembered that she had been a physically abused child. She showed the therapist a scar hidden by her hair, the evidence of a laceration that had required 50 sutures to close. The injury was the result of her mother's having thrown a vase at her head. The patient came to recognize that her masochistic behavior was the result of her identification of herself as someone who must deserve abuse.

Secret Drug Abuse and Depression

One of the authors saw a young woman who had a postgraduate degree from a respected professional school. Her major complaint was depression, which she felt was the result of her husband's long hours on the fast track in a prestigious investment banking corporation, and of his steady abuse of cocaine to keep him going. She had gone deeply into her trust fund to support his habit and was now at the end of her rope. She and her husband met with the therapist, at which time he acknowledged his problem and his desire for detoxification. (This was just before his company was going to discharge him.) A paternalistic organization made a 3-month hospitalization possible for him.

In the context of the husband's inpatient treatment it came to light that the patient chronically and secretly abused drugs herself. She had felt very empty for many years and had been sustained through graduate school only because of her husband's constant physical presence and support. When he went to work and had to be away from her, she began using drugs and in fact introduced him to drug use. Her history was of being the "poor little rich girl" whose family gave her nannies and everything she named in the way of clothes, toys, and pets. Her parents were seldom around physically; they traveled abroad for long intervals most of the patient's life. Her father seemed to appreciate his daughter's intellectual gifts. The daughter was successful in an attempt to please him and gain his love. Meanwhile, she had met her husband in college. Coming from an old but not affluent family, he met the parents' standards and was clearly intellectually gifted. The two were married as college students and supported by her family. He experienced this financial support as validation. His own family did not value his intellect or financial ambitions, but her family did. Two very empty young people were in different ways mutually supportive until reality severed what had been a blissful symbiotic relationship.

The husband recovered in treatment and wanted the freedom to return to the fast lane. Unable to handle her husband's wish and not willing to be treated for her addiction, the woman separated from him and returned to her parents' home.

Smoking

Cigarette smoking is the largest preventable cause of death in the United States. Smoking tends to begin in adolescence, and the use of tobacco has risen dramatically in young girls. Surveys show that this is not because of ignorance of the health hazards. A majority of teenagers believe that smoke can harm their health. They are aware that smoking is habit forming, that it is better not to start, and that it has been proven to cause heart disease (Evans et al. 1979[64]). Despite decreases in peer pressure, in parental smoking, and in smoking in men of all ages, adolescent girls continue to smoke at increasing rates.

It has not been possible to pinpoint specific personality traits that are predictive of smoking behavior. It has been suggested that women's liberation (women and men having equal rights) as depicted in popular culture, such as in the Virginia Slims advertisement "You've come a long way, Baby," is the culprit. Thus smoking has become an equal-opportunity killer. If this hypothesis is correct, it would mean that culture influences intrapsychic processes and not the other way around. There is, however, a vast literature which postulates that culture is the external manifestation of intrapsychic needs. The intrapsychic changes in women have produced the feminist movement and raised the consciousness of women. It did not give them anything new. We have another hypothesis that stems from our work with adolescent girls. These girls are under more performance pressure than prior generations. For disadvantaged women the sign of adulthood is early sexuality and pregnancy. One young black woman seen in an outpatient clinical setting pointed out that academic distinction or economic reward was a less likely and more distant source of gratification than sexuality and the prospect of motherhood. Motherhood, the fantasy of a baby that would love her, seemed a more easily attainable goal. For young women who have the opportunity of a career and motherhood or who face the perceived obligation of work, outside the home as well as in motherhood, the future does not look carefree and promising. It is a source of anxiety. Smoking may be started to allay that anxiety. It has been shown that smoking is causally related to anxiety. The more a person smokes, the more anxiety he or she experiences (Thomas 1973[65]) and the more the person smokes in order to handle the anxiety. The anxiolytic properties are, however, short lived. The anxiety then reemerges, which is why some individuals chain-smoke.

In a 1990 issue of the *Journal of the American Medical Association*, two studies pointed to the relationship between smoking and depression (Anda et al. 1990[66]; Glassman et al. 1990[67]) Other data (Enscobedo et al. 1990[68]) illustrate the relationship between initiation of smoking, usually in adolescence, and degree of education in people of both sexes and all racial and ethnic backgrounds but of low socioeconomic groups. We know that helplessness and hopelessness are characteristic of early school dropouts in our inner cities.

Pregnancy

Another maladaptation to the stresses and conflicts of adolescence has been the epidemic of adolescent pregnancy. There were approximately

500,000 adolescent pregnancies in 1984 (Hofferth 1987[69]).[†] There are several determinants. First, premarital intercourse seems to have become a more socially approved pattern since the 1960s (Conger 1984[70]). Second, contraceptives are often not used because of either ignorance or typical adolescent risk-taking behavior and denial (Chilmon 1978[71]). Some adolescents are willing to accept pregnancy or even seek it out because of factors such as gaining acceptance as an adult, holding a boyfriend, getting attention from peers, escaping from school, having someone to love, or seeking a change in an unrewarding existence (Planned Parenthood Foundation 1976[72]). Also, the refusal to use birth control in American culture is probably related to women's culturally determined habitual sexual subservience to men. Third, pregnancy itself may be valued as a source of self-esteem when other avenues seem blocked. Black adolescents growing up in matriarchal families often have their mothers' support for unwed pregnancy. (Lest this sound like a biased view, we refer the readers to the bibliography, which cites the work of authors who represent this culture.) Lastly, there has been a rise in pregnancy in relation to substance abuse (Zuckerman et al. 1987[73]). We discuss later the case of a young woman pressured to premature sexuality by her mother's unconscious wishes.

The consequences of this unprotected sexual behavior are

1. Abortion[††]
2. Endangerment of physical health of gestational and postpartum mother and her child (Task Panel on Mental Health and American

---

[†]Adolescent pregnancy has leveled off, perhaps because of an awareness of AIDS and increased use of condoms.

[††]Outcome morbidity studies are conflicting. Cates et al. (1983[74]) found lower rates of morbidity and mortality in adolescents than in adult mothers. Higher rates of morbidity have been found by Waldhera and Nair (1980[75]). McAnarney et al. (1988[76]) found that psychological outcomes are unclear. Our in-depth psychodynamic studies of women reveal that there is psychological trauma that may resurface at several junctures. These junctures will be discussed in subsequent chapters as they relate to experiences later in the life cycle.

Families 1978[77]), especially low birth weight in infants (McCormick et al. 1984[78])
3. Abandonment, neglect, and higher risk of child abuse
4. Negative psychosocial outcome—both educational (Cord and Wise 1978[79]) and economic—for adolescent mothers
5. Repeated pregnancy (Wetzel 1987[80])
6. Sexually transmitted disease (Hardy 1988[81])

There is a complex interrelationship between promiscuity, intravenous drug abuse, unprotected sex with persons who abuse intravenous drugs, and acquired immunodeficiency syndrome (AIDS). AIDS becomes related to sexuality and drug abuse in late adolescence and early adulthood. When AIDS is the result of sexual transmission, some of the psychodynamic problems are similar to those of other sexually transmitted diseases, especially herpes. AIDS is unique because of its, at present, inevitably fatal outcome. Because it is most frequently transmitted to women and their fetuses as a result of sexual practices, we will discuss it in Chapter 5.

Because most teenage pregnant females or teenage mothers are not available for in-depth psychodynamic treatment, we can only give some vignettes that shed light on the psychodynamic determinants. In Chapter 5 we discuss the psychodynamic determinants of the wish to abort and the consequences of abortion throughout the life cycle.

Pressure to Enact a Mother's Unconscious Wishes

The patient, a 14-year-old adolescent from a highly functional upper-class intact family, was brought by her mother because of a downturn in her school grades and because she seemed to be depressed. Reluctant to talk at first, she gradually revealed that her mother was very restrictive about her social engagements, which included situations that seemed quite unremarkable to the therapist. In particular, the patient's mother had been enraged with her for coming home from a party 30 minutes late and had accused her of being a whore. Prior to this her mother had questioned her intensively about her "boyfriends" and had insisted on imparting a lot of intimate sexual information before her daughter was ready to hear it or to become sexually or romantically involved. The patient began to withdraw from her friends, disengage from her interest in school activities, and have unwanted sexual fantasies. Afraid to act out and angry at her mother, she became depressed.

As therapist and patient began to discuss her anger at her mother's intrusiveness, the patient became more active academically and socially. She began to dress and behave seductively. On the one hand her mother seemed eager to assist in the purchase of suggestive clothing, and on the other hand she berated her daughter when she saw her dressed to go out. The patient verbalized very directly that she was getting a double message, felt tormented, and considered running away from home. She was encouraged to share these feelings with her mother. When she did this, her mother called to request a private appointment with the therapist, to which the daughter agreed. With much tearfulness and difficulty, her mother revealed that at age 16 she had been caught up romantically with a classmate. She had been drawn into a very intensive and active sexual relationship and had become pregnant. Her boyfriend abandoned her, after which she sought and obtained an abortion. She determined never to fall in love again and eventually married a good, productive, caring, and successful businessman by whom she dutifully had two daughters. (The patient's sister was younger by 6 years.) The mother, when confronted, was able to recognize her own ambivalence and also her heretofore unconscious attempt to push her daughter into repeating her experience.

The mother was seen several times supportively. She was unable to reveal her secret to her daughter but was willing for the therapist to do so. The patient was strong enough to forgive and to learn, and began to feel clear about ambivalent messages and free to pursue her own life.

Transference Acting Out

A 21-year-old woman—but still an adolescent patient in terms of her dependency on her family, her failure to set individual goals, and her inability to come to terms with her own sexuality—came to treatment amid the crisis of career choice. She was a very gifted and advanced college graduate who had taken a community social welfare job because she was undecided on a future direction. Her father, a successful physician, had brought his children up on a vast country estate. Her mother had served as homemaker and was frequently depressed. Her two oldest brothers were in various stages of medical education.

In analysis it became apparent that the patient was stongly identified with a helpless, depressed, somatizing mother and had been discouraged by both parents from seeking an appropriate career. The patient decided on social work and entered graduate school. She became identified with her image of her analyst, who, unknown to the patient, was well into pregnancy. She began social, then sexual, relationships with men. She was able, for the first time, to masturbate and discover how to be orgasmic. The patient was living in her own city apartment.

The patient denied the analyst's pregnancy, being the only one of all the analyst's patients to take that path. The unconscious reasons for the denial were her envy of the analyst's sexuality and of her ability to have a child (and, by extension, the husband that the analyst had) and her wish to fill her own sense of emptiness. Then she herself became accidently pregnant by a casual sexual partner and decided on an abortion. The resultant conscious perception of her feelings of emptiness led to an analysis of the transference identification and of the void in her life caused by her mother's depression. This patient's case illustrates both the pressure of the unconscious feelings of emptiness and the denial of these feelings along with the attempt to identify with the transference mother-analyst, who was perceived to have the things that the patient wanted, that is, sexuality without conflict and a family.

As we have attempted to illustrate, adolescence is a stormy stage of development. In its most normal presentations, it often looks like a disease rather than a developmental phase. The adolescent is confronted by a series of developmental tasks. These must be accomplished despite the strong and often tempting pull of regression and the forceful physiological, intrapsychic, and social thrusts toward adulthood.

An adolescent often looks like a small sailboat on a fast-changing sea: sometimes becalmed, sometimes carried too quickly by the current, often struggling unsuccessfully to master both rudder and sail, and sometimes rudderless entirely. In the worst case, the adolescent adrift sets a course that jeopardizes health and life and may end in destruction for the adolescent or anomie in the family, in the community, or in society at large. The vicissitudes, the volatility, the rapidity of change, and the tendency toward action frequently make the adolescent difficult to treat and too often impossible to rescue. Some of our most ill adolescents are fortunate enough to get help. The stories of these young persons' journeys are often the most gratifying and should press us to widen the scope of prevention and intervention.

Notes

1. Offer D: The Psychological World of the Teenager: A Study of Normal Adolescent Boys. New York, Basic Books, 1969
2. Offer D, Offer JL: Profiles of normal adolescent girls. Arch Gen Psychiatry 19:513–522, 1968
3. Offer D, Marcus D, Offer JL: A longitudinal study of normal adolescent boys. Am J Psychiatry 126:914–924, 1970
4. Barringer F: What are youth coming to? New York Times, August 19, 1990, pp 1, 5
5. Blos P: On Adolescence. New York, Free Press, 1962
6. Bernstein AE, Warner GM: Introduction to Contemporary Psychoanalysis. New York, Jason Aronson, 1981
7. Gilligan C: Making Connections: The Relational Worlds of Adolescent Girls at Emma Willard School. Cambridge, MA, Harvard University Press, 1990
8. Erikson EH: The problem of ego identity. J Am Psychoanal Assoc 4:56–121, 1956
9. Chused JF: Neutrality in the analysis of action-prone adolescents. J Am Psychoanal Assoc 38:679–704, 1990
10. Ritvo S: Late adolescence: developmental and clinical considerations. Psychoanal Study Child 26:241–263, 1971
11. Rapaport D: The theory of ego autonomy, in Collected Papers. Edited by Gill MM. New York, Basic Books, 1967, pp 722–744
12. Freud A: The ego and the mechanisms of defense (1936) [revised edition], in The Writings of Anna Freud, Vol 2. New York, International Universities Press, 1966
13. Erikson EH: Identity and the Life Cycle. New York, International Universities Press, 1959

14. Fullilove MT, Fullilove RE, Haynes K, et al: Black women and AIDS prevention: a view towards understanding the gender roles. Journal of Sex Research 27:47–64, 1990
15. Ritvo S: Adolescent to woman, in Female Psychology: Contemporary Psychoanalytic Views. Edited by Blum HP. New York, International Universities Press, 1977, pp 127–137
16. Bernstein AE, Warner GM: Women Treating Women. New York, International Universities Press, 1984b
17. Blum H: Masochism, the ego ideal, and the psychology of women. J Am Psychoanal Assoc 24(suppl):157–191, 1976
18. Greenacre P: Anatomical structure and superego development (1948), in Trauma, Growth, and Personality. New York, International Universities Press, 1952a, pp 149–164
19. Freud S: Some psychical consequences of the anatomical destination between the sexes (1925), in The Standard Edition of the Complete Psychological Works of Sigmund Freud, Vol 19. Translated and edited by Strachey J. London, Hogarth Press, 1961, pp 241–258
20. Nicholi AM Jr: The adolescent, in The Harvard Guide to Modern Psychiatry. Edited by Nicholi AM Jr. Cambridge, MA, Belknap Press/Harvard University Press, 1978, pp 519–540
21. Robins E, Gassner S, Kayes J, et al: The communication of suicidal intent: a study of 134 consecutive cases of successful (completed) suicide. Am J Psychiatry 115:724–733, 1959
22. Barraclough B, Bunch J, Nelson B, et al: A hundred cases of suicide: clinical aspects. Br J Psychiatry 125:355–373, 1974
23. Shaffer D: Suicide in children and early adolescence. J Child Psychol Psychiatry 15:275–291, 1974
24. Pfeffer CR, Zuckerman S, Plutchik R, et al: Suicidal behavior in normal school children: a comparison with child psychiatric inpatients. Journal of the American Academy of Child Psychiatry 23:416–423, 1984
25. Pfeffer CR, Plutchik R, Mizruchi MS: Suicidal and assaultive behavior in children: classification, measurement, and interrelations. Am J Psychiatry 140:154–157, 1983
26. Most youth who attempt suicide go unidentified, unhelped. Psychiatric News, Vol 26, May 18, 1990
27. Blumenthal SJ, Kupfer DJ: Suicide Over the Life Cycle: Risk Factors, Assessment, and Treatment of Suicidal Patients. Washington, DC, American Psychiatric Press, 1990
28. Stanley EJ, Barter J: Adolescent suicidal behavior. Am J Orthopsychiatry 83:180–185, 1978

29. Van Praag HM: Depression, suicide and serotonin metabolism, in The Neuro-Biology of Manic Depressive Illness. Edited by Post IM, Ballinger JC. Baltimore, MD, Williams & Wilkins, 1984, pp 601–618
30. Brown GL, Ebert MH, Goyer PF, et al: Aggression, suicide, and serotonin: relationships to CSF amine metabolites. Am J Psychiatry 139:741–746, 1982
31. Ranier JD: Genetic factors in depression and suicide. Am J Psychother 38:329–340, 1984
32. McIntire MS, Angle CK: Evaluation of suicidal risk in adolescents. J Fam Pract 2:339–341, 1975
33. Green JW, Keown M: Depression and suicide in children and adolescents. Compr Ther 12:38–43, 1986
34. Sack L, Sturner W, Lipsitt L, et al: Relationship of maternal and perinatal conditions to eventual adolescent suicide. Lancet 1:624–627, 1985
35. Adams-Tucker C: Proximate effects of sexual abuse in childhood. Am J Psychiatry 139:1252–1256, 1982
36. Briere J, Pruntz M: Suicidal thoughts and behaviors in former sexual abuse victims. Canadian Journal of Behavioural Sciences 18:413–423, 1986
37. Deykin EY, Alpert JJ, McNamarra JJ: A pilot study of the effect of exposure to child abuse or neglect on adolescent suicidal behavior. Am J Psychiatry 142:1299–1303, 1985
38. Pfeffer CR: The Suicidal Child. New York, Guilford, 1986
39. McKenny P, Tishler C, Keeley C: Adolescent suicide: a comparison of attempters and non-attempters in an emergency room population. Clin Pediatr (Phila) 21:266–270, 1982
40. Gould MS, Shaffer D: The impact of suicide in television movies: evidence of imitation. N Engl J Med 315:690–694, 1986
41. Phillips DP, Carstensen LL: Clustering of teenage suicides after television news stories about suicide. N Engl J Med 315:685–689, 1986
42. American Psychiatric Association: Diagnostic and Statistical Manual of Mental Disorders, 3rd Edition, Revised. Washington, DC, American Psychiatric Association, 1987
43. Sours JA: Starving to Death in a Sea of Objects: The Anorexia Nervosa Syndrome. New York, Jason Aronson, 1980
44. Bernstein AE, Warner GM: Onset of anorexia nervosa after prolonged use of the Milwaukee brace. Psychosomatics 24:1033–1034, 1983
45. Bruch H: The Golden Cage: The Enigma of Anorexia Nervosa. New York, Vintage Books, 1979
46. Morton R: Phthisiologia: On a Treatise of Consumption. London, S Smith and B Walford, 1689

47. Levenkron S: The Best Little Girl in the World. New York, Warner, 1978
48. Bruch H: Eating Disorders: Obesity, Anorexia Nervosa, and the Person Within. New York, Basic Books, 1973
49. Devlin MJ, Walsh BT: Eating disorders and depression. Psychiatric Annals 19:473–476, 1989
50. Keys A, Brozek J, Henshel A, et al: The Biology of Human Starvation. Minneapolis, MN, University of Minnesota Press, 1950
51. Altshuler KZ, Weiner MF: Anorexia nervosa and depression: a dissenting view. Am J Psychiatry 142:328–332, 1985
52. Swift WJ, Andrews D, Barklage NE: The relationship between affective disorder and eating disorders: a review of the literature. Am J Psychiatry 143:290–299, 1986
53. Hudson JI, Pope HG Jr: Depression and eating disorders, in Presentations of Depression: Depression in Medical and Other Psychiatric Disorders. Edited by Cameron OG. New York, Wiley, 1987, pp 33–66
54. Strober M, Katz IL: Depression in the eating disorders: a review and analysis of descriptive, family, and biological findings, in Diagnostic Issues in Anorexia Nervosa and Bulimia Nervosa. Edited by Garner DM, Garfinkel PE. New York, Brunner/Mazel, 1988, pp 80–111
55. Agras WS: Eating Disorders: Management of Obesity, Bulimia and Anorexia Nervosa. Elmsford, NY, Pergamon, 1987
56. Eckert ED, Goldberg SC, Halmi KA, et al: Behaviour therapy in anorexia nervosa. Br J Psychiatry 134:55–59, 1979
57. Pillay M, Crisp AH: The impact of social skills training within an established in-patient treatment programme for anorexia nervosa. Br J Psychiatry 139:533–539, 1981
58. Touyz SW, Beumont PJV, Glaun D, et al: A comparison of lenient and strict operant conditioning programmes in refeeding patients with anorexia nervosa. Br J Psychiatry 144:517–520, 1984
59. Russell GFM, Szmukler GI, Dare C, et al: An evaluation of family therapy in anorexia nervosa and bulimia nervosa. Arch Gen Psychiatry 44:1047–1056, 1987
60. Conger JJ, Petersen AF (eds): Adolescence and Youth: Psychological Development in a Changing World, 3rd Edition. New York, Harper & Row, 1984; see p 616
61. Braithwaite J: The myth of social class and criminality reconsidered. American Sociological Review 46:36–57, 1981
62. Elliot DS, Ageton SS: Reconciling of race and class differences in self-reported and official estimates of delinquency. American Sociological Review 45:95–110, 1980

63. Kalogerakis MG: The Emotionally Troubled Adolescent and the Family Physician. Springfield, IL, Charles C Thomas, 1973
64. Evans R, Henderson A, Hill P, et al: Smoking in children and adolescents: psychosocial determinants and prevention strategies, in Smoking and Health: A Report of the Surgeon General, Vol 17 (DHEW Publ No [PHS]-79-50066). Washington, DC, U.S. Department of Health, Education and Welfare, U.S. Government Printing Office (No 017-000-00218-0), 1979, pp 1–30
65. Thomas CB: The relationship of smoking and habits of nervous tension, in Smoking Behavior: Motives and Incentives. Edited by Dunn WL Jr. Washington, DC, Winston, 1973, pp 157–170
66. Anda R, Williamson D, Escobed AL, et al: Depression and the dynamics of smoking. JAMA 264:1541–1545, 1990
67. Glassman A, Helzer J, Coveny L, et al: Smoking, smoking cessation and major depression. JAMA 264:1546–1549, 1990
68. Enscobedo L, Anda R, Smith P, et al: Sociodemographic characteristics of cigarette smoking initiation in the United States. JAMA 264:1550–1555, 1990
69. Hofferth SL: Teenage pregnancy and its resolution, in Risking the Future. Edited by Hofferth SL, Hayes CD. Washington, DC, National Academy Press, 1987, pp 78–92
70. Conger JJ: Adolescent sexuality, in Adolescence and Youth: Psychological Development in a Changing World, 3rd Edition. Edited by Conger JJ, Peterson AF. New York, Harper & Row, 1984, p 277
71. Chilmon ES: Adolescent Sexuality in a Changing American Society: Social and Psychological Perspectives. Washington, DC, U.S. Government Printing Office, 1978
72. Planned Parenthood Foundation: Eleven million teenagers: what can be done about the epidemic of adolescent pregnancies in the United States? New York, Planned Parenthood Foundation of America, 1976
73. Zuckerman BS, Amaro H, Beardstein W: Mental health of adolescent mothers: the implications of depression and drug use. J Dev Behav Pediatr 8:111–116, 1987
74. Cates W, Schulz KF, Grimes DA: The risks associated with teenage abortion. N Engl J Med 309:621–624, 1983
75. Waldhera A, Nair C: Legal abortions among teenagers in Canada, 1974 through 1978. Can Med Assoc J 122:1386–1388, 1980
76. McAnarney R, McAnarney MD; Hendee WR: Adolescent pregnancy and its consequences. JAMA 262:76, 1988
77. Task Panel on Mental Health and American Families: Report of the Sub-Task Panel on General Issues and Adult Years, President's Commis-

sion on Mental Health. Washington, DC, U.S. Government Printing Office, 1978, p 3

78. McCormick MC, Shapiro S, Starfield B: High risk mothers: infant mortality and morbidity in four areas in the United States, 1973–78. Am J Public Health 79:18–23, 1984
79. Cord J, Wise L: Teenage mothers and teenage fathers: the impact of early childbearing on parents' personal and professional lives. Fam Plann Perspect 10:199–205, 1978
80. Wetzel JR: American Youth: A Statistical Snapshot. New York, William T Grand Foundation, 1987, pp 11–13
81. Hardy JB: Premature sexual activity, pregnancy, and sexually transmitted diseases: the pediatrician's role as counselor. Pediatr Rev 10:69–76, 1988

Chapter 3

Problems of Self-Esteem Regulation

The term *self-esteem* is defined in *Webster's Collegiate Dictionary* as "a confidence and satisfaction in oneself." Most women, at least in Western culture, do not have this sense of satisfaction. Even when not depressed, they often have highs and lows, and the highs tend to be ephemeral and not sustained. These mood swings do not always indicate affective illness or premenstrual syndrome, even though it has become fashionable to report any mood lability as "premenstrual syndrome." Men complain less of self-esteem problems and are less aware of feelings of low self-esteem. When aware of them, men often handle them differently through action, aggression, or sadistic control.

In this chapter we provide a historical overview of the literature relevant to self-esteem, including 1) classical psychoanalytic concepts; 2) current theories, which elaborate separate and parallel lines of female development; 3) issues of gender-related socialization; 4) the dominant culture's support of the subordinate role of women; 5) recent literature documenting the high prevalence of incest and sexual abuse of women, with its disastrous psychological consequences; and 6) integration of relevant theoretical models of developmental lines that affect self-esteem.

Dysregulation of self-esteem will be viewed as a spectrum disorder of varying severity. In attempting to understand self-esteem dysregulation, we find that we are dealing with a kind of Möbius strip in which very important internal dynamics are projected onto environmental situations and cultural norms are reintrojected and integrated. We will demonstrate the vicissitudes of self-esteem regulation by presenting cases of patients who illustrate the influence of various psychodynamics.

The relationship between self-esteem and alcohol/drug abuse, eating disorders, and excesses in the use of cosmetics and cosmetic surgery is addressed.

Classical Psychoanalytic Concepts in the Regulation of Self-Esteem

Freud (1925[1]) thought that women, when noticing the anatomical differences between the sexes, necessarily felt envious and inferior. To this, Horney (1967[2]) added that it is not the organ difference itself that causes women to be envious, but the fact that the phallus confers power and privilege. To accept this formulation would mean accepting that culture determines all psychodynamics rather than that culture is also a reflection of psychodynamics. Accepting classical psychodynamic formulations also requires that we believe that there is an obligatory confusion between the presence of the phallus and power and privilege. The answer to the problem of self-esteem regulation in women must come from other than narrow classical formulations about the psychology of women. However, classical psychodynamics are still relevant in understanding the importance of early issues of separation and individuation.

Freud (1914a[3]), in his paper on narcissism, wrote about *self-regard*, a term synonymous with self-esteem. The infant, he tells us, is born at the center of his or her world—the narcissist par excellence. Initially, all needs are met instantly. Inevitably there must be a certain amount of frustration. Slowly there is a dawning reality in the infant: that he or she is dependent on others. In a situation that Winnicott (1960[4]) has described as "good enough mothering," the infant will be mostly gratified but frustrated at times. The child will develop internal representations of the parents (i.e., parental object representations) and a picture in his or her mind of himself or herself (i.e., a self representation). Under optimal conditions each of these representations will be mostly good and only partly bad or frustrating. However, as Annie Reich (1960[5]) pointed out, if the infant has to strive against major trauma or threats to his or her bodily integrity, the infant may compensate by altering his or her self representation. That is, the infant's image of himself or herself may become artificially inflated. This mechanism involves a magical denial of helplessness and substitution of the fantasy of greatness and power. This denial and the concomitant fantasy substitution often alternate with a state of severe deflation of the self representation accompanied by depression. The extreme case was described by Renée Spitz in 1946 (Spitz and Wolf 1946a[6]). He observed chronically hospitalized, neglected infants with no primary caretaker who developed apathy, failure to thrive, and marasmus, and who eventually died.

The establishment of basic trust is intrinsic to self-esteem regulation. Erikson (1950[7]) conceptualized the development of basic trust as the normal outcome of the first year of life. To trust that one will be cared for is to trust that one will be positively regarded. Abused children often position themselves for repeated abuse in accordance with Freud's (1914b[8]) theory of repetition compulsion. The sometimes conscious but often unconscious narcissistic fantasy is to emerge the victor so as to achieve a better intrapsychic outcome.

If childhood sexual abuse occurs prior to clear self-object differentiation, the child will introject a sadistic devaluating self or a fused sadistic self-object image. Abuse that occurs later, when self and object representations have been better delineated, may cause the child either to identify the self with the sadism of the abuser or to develop a self representation that is denigrated (i.e., perceived as deserving of abuse). In addition, there may be superego deformations. A pathological superego may be critical, punitive, and demanding. This superego says in effect, "You haven't done or been good enough," or "You made a crucial mistake and have to do better, give more, etc." Alternatively, there may be superego lacunae that allow sociopathic behavior.

If a child is fortunate and things go relatively well, anxiety is minimized. The ego's function will differentiate, and a primitive superego, the embodiment of parental injunctions, will emerge. Simultaneously, there will be the development of an ego ideal, the representation of what the individual would like to be. At first it will be the precipitate of the old pictures of the parents. It will reflect the expression of adoration for the perfection the small child once attributed to his or her parents.

The problem of not living up to the ego ideal is the fear of loss of love. If the ego ideal remains falsely inflated, the individual will have set standards beyond hope of achievement and self-esteem regulation will necessarily suffer. Optimally, the ego ideal, the self representation, and the object representations will be equally invested. This will result in a firm and realistic sense of self-esteem, one that accurately mirrors the individual's characteristics, potentialities, and abilities (Jacobson 1964[9]).

As noted earlier, Freud makes this a virtually impossible outcome for a female because of her "anatomical inferiority." Annie Reich (1953[10]), accepting Freud's formulation, tells us that a woman often finds a solution in taking a male object in the place of her ego ideal. The overvaluing of the male object is meant to counteract envious aggression. The result she posits is a love-hate relationship between women and men, whom women envy and wish to be. Other psychodynamics are involved in self-esteem regulation as it evolves in the father-daughter relationship.

The answers to the problem of self-esteem in women have to come from other sources than narrowly Freudian formulations about the psychology of women. We believe that a psychology of women that emphasizes the mother-daughter relationship and women's valuing of relationships and of a moral responsibility toward others will explain many problems relating to self-esteem regulation, masochism, and depression.[†]

Current Theories of Self-Esteem Regulation

Bernstein and Warner (1984b[11]) focused on the importance of the preoedipal relationship with the mother to the development of self-esteem. Simultaneously and since then, supporting data have come from many

[†]We are noticing parallel but opposite problems in men involving increasing narcissistic entitlement, rage, and sadism. Although it is not our purpose to discuss these issues, perhaps the same factors that are, on the one hand, acting to worsen women's lot are, on the other hand, acting to worsen men's lot.

sources. Chodorow (1978[12]) and Friday (1978[13]) documented that women maintain long-lasting intimate bonds with their mothers. Some problems of depression and self-esteem dysregulation may arise from the experience of the mother as being overinvolved and both self-critical and critical of her daughter. In this situation, the mother experiences her daughter as a small replica of herself. The mother keeps her female baby physically closer, and the closeness continues for a longer period of time. The female baby is experienced as more vulnerable, and, as a rule, her mother delays and interferes with her child's attempts at separation and autonomy. The result is that this female child (and, later, adult woman) is more anxious and doubtful about her decision making and even her ability to care for and protect herself.

In addition, mothers may project their own feelings onto their daughters instead of regarding them as separate persons with separate needs and desires. For example, an adolescent female patient responded to the question "Tell me something about your mother?" by replying, "Want to know what kind of mother I have? The kind who says, 'Go put a sweater on, I'm cold.'" Mothers who tend to perceive their daughters as extensions of themselves give messages both subtle and overt, insisting that their daughters be the persons that they, the mothers, wanted to be or that they want their daughters to be. If a little girl gets angry, cries, is dirty, or is slow at training and learning, the mother feels and acts as if the daughter shamed her personally. "How could you do this to me?" the mother asks. These mothers perceive their daughters' success or failure as reflecting directly on their own self representation. Even the attempt to separate is often perceived by these mothers as a loss of part of themselves. It is not unusual for adult daughters of well-functioning mothers to call them every day.

In addition, these mothers give their daughters mixed messages. The daughter may be urged, on the one hand, to succeed and excel and yet, on the other hand, not to surpass the mother. A narcissistic mother does not want her daughter to fail, but neither does she want her daughter to outdo her. The self-esteem of the narcissistic mother is too low for her to tolerate her daughter's being prettier, smarter, more talented, or more organized. Her praise for her daughter will always be tainted with spoken or implied reservations. For example, the mother of one of our successful patients waxed ecstatic to her daughter about how handsome one of our daughter's husband and son looked at a family occasion, overlooking her daughter's new dress that others had especially admired.

The daughter of a pathologically narcissistic mother treads a thin line. She is exquisitely sensitive to her mother because the two are so identified with each other. Dr. Mia Friedland points out something that is both classic and correct: "A little girl knows her mother's feelings as well as she knows the insides of her own pockets." Unconsciously, the little girl lives with fear of the loss of her mother's approval and love. Carried into adolescence this problem may result in sexual acting out that is not intended to spite the mother, which is the common formulation. Rather the sexual acting out may be an unconscious attempt to carry out the mother's unconscious wishes. Mothers who treat their daughters as narcissistic extensions of themselves produce daughters who are functionally damaged in terms of depression and self-esteem regulation. Abelin (1971[14]) has pointed out that this effect can be muted by the presence of a father who is involved with his daughter. In this situation, the father's most important role in his daughter's psychology may be in disrupting this type of symbiotic tie between daughter and mother.

Another outcome occurs for the many women who have had a good relationship with a mother who was nonintrusive and who did not engulf them out of her own narcissistic needs. These daughters will identify with a developmental model that emphasizes the importance of relationships, mutuality, and responsibility toward others.

Whereas Freud conceptualized relationships as secondary to or deriving from the satisfaction of primary drives, Melanie Klein placed object relations at the center of her psychology. She contended that love and gratitude arise spontaneously in the infant in response to the love and care of its mother (Klein 1953[15]). Klein stated that out of this gratitude the infant will attempt to save his or her love object and gratify, restore, and repair it. Attempts that fail will result in depression and loss of self-esteem.

A series of current theorists have elaborated a different way of understanding the primary importance of affiliative relationships for women. Surrey (1985[16]) writes that women grow in the context of mutually empathic relationships beginning with the all important mother-daughter relationship. Women's development does not involve, as in men's development, sequential separation from important relationships but rather the maintenance and valuing of these relationships that change to accommodate each developmental stage. The growth of these relationships, as Jordan (1986[17]) observes, involves an interest in and attunement and responsiveness to the experience of the other at both a cognitive and intuitive level. Gilligan (1982[18]) has elaborated a theory of a women's moral development in which responsibility to others is stressed rather than adherence to a fixed set of ethical values.

Tannen (qtd. in Rose 1990[19]), discussing the differences in conversation between men and women, notes that men and women have different hierarchies of priority:

> My husband was simply engaging the world in a way that many men do: as an individual in a hierarchical social order in which he was either one-up or one-down. In this world, conversations are negotiations in which people try to achieve and maintain the upper hand if they can, and protect themselves from others' attempts to put them down and push them around. Life, then, is a contest, a struggle to preserve independence and avoid failure.
>
> I, on the other hand, was approaching the world as many women do: as an individual in a network of commerce. In this world conversations are negotiations for closeness in which people try to seek and give confirmation and support and to reach consensus. They try to protect themselves from others' attempts to push them away. Life, then, is a community, a struggle to preserve intimacy and avoid isolation. Though there are hierarchies in this world too, they are hierarchies more of friendship than of power and accomplishment.

Problems may occur for relationally oriented women when their attempts to value and maintain a relationship are not reciprocated; when they are misinterpreted and mislabeled as pathological dependency; or when the relationship fails. Because their self-esteem is invested in the success of the relationship, these women may assume full responsibility for its outcome and become depressed, even when the quality of the relationship is less than optimal (Stiver 1984[20]).

Dominant, Male Culture and Women's Roles

Beginning in childhood, girls may begin to observe that their values and orientation are not the dominant ones (Miller 1976[21]). Furthermore, they may also observe the denigration of the mother, to whom they have become so deeply attached, by the father (Stiver 1984[20]). Women, early in development, incorporate this denigrated perception into their own intrapsychic representations. Growing up, females often observe their father's empowered role both within the family and in the community. In most families, the father is less frequently available than the mother, and therefore daughters work harder at trying to obtain his attention. Many fathers value so-called feminine characteristics in their daughters. They encourage coyness, flirtatiousness, and even seductivity. They may even turn to their daughters for the kind of adoring, romantic relationship that their wives, overburdened in other areas, may not provide. In the least traumatic case this results in competition between mother and daughter or even anger of the mother toward her daughter. In the most traumatic case this can result in the daughter's taking the mother's place with father in a sexual relationship and may also involve becoming the parent/caretaker for a dysfunctional mother. Abused girls tend to be daughters of psychotic, depressed, detached, alcoholic, or drug-addicted mothers. Later in this chapter we will discuss the relationship between depression, the addictions, and poor self-esteem regulation.

Another more benign but nevertheless pathogenic scenario occurs due to the tendency of men to play more rough-and-tumble games with their sons and not with their daughters. The message to the daughters is that they are to be excluded from these more stimulating and exhilarating activities. This exclusion leads to a feeling of loss and devaluation. Fathers teach their sons earlier on how to take a punch and to punch back. Even when adult women venture into more adventurous and competitive arenas, they often withdraw from aggression. They accept the punch as punishment and penalty for their daring.

Societal norms are evidenced outside of the family in the playground, day care, or nursery school. Self-assertion by females is devalued. Healthy displays of anger are inhibited and seen as destructive and pathological (Miller 1983[22]). Females' emotional concerns and displays of affect are both encouraged and disparaged. Girls are expected to cry and cling, but boys are not. Although women are expected to cry and cling, this behavior is narrowly limited in a way that surpasses the cognitive capacity of the little girl to comprehend or the ability of the ego to modulate affect (e.g., she may cry but only a little).

For the woman, even if the earliest pitfalls are negotiated, problems still lie ahead. In a study of clinicians' attitudes, Broverman et al. (1970[23]) found that clinicians believed that for a woman to have a healthy adjustment she must accept the norms for her sex even though she may recognize that these are considered subordinate and valued less. Thus women must struggle to behave in a way that will not call their femininity into question, and yet not in such a "feminine" way that their judgment, maturity, or seriousness of purpose will be questioned. When anger results from the stress of this conflict, it is often viewed by clinicians as pathological. When anger is displaced and outbursts occur without proximate provocation, women are criticized or criticize themselves and lose self-esteem (Miller 1983[22]). When the anger is turned inward, the result is depression or loss of self-esteem and self-devaluation.

Nadelson et al. (1978[24]) have pointed out that "self-actualization, the pursuit of independent goals, and risk taking have not been seen by our society as consistent with 'feminity'" (p. 1092). Women are often conflicted about activities that are regarded as aggressive or competitive because of fear of loss of approval, rejection, and isolation from valued relationships if established norms are violated (Miller 1976[21]). Thus women are made to feel that they cannot challenge their subordinate position (Stiver 1983[25]).

As noted above, relationships based on mutuality are important for women. Therefore, isolation and lack of intimacy are more pathogenic for women than for men. Who creates the societal values that promote such isolation and are so traumatic? Society is dominated by men, and often women introject so-called male societal values. Yet women still bear the greatest responsibility in rearing their sons. Women who seem to delight in the narcissism of their 2- and 3-year-old boys, whom they allow and encourage to be "King of the World," may be angry at the narcissistic, empowered male adult into whom this child will grow. Mothers, as well as fathers, raise their sons to turn outward and be action-oriented, aggressive, and self-centered. Is this because of women's instinctive needs or rather because they have absorbed societal norms into their own self representation? The answer is not either/or, but varies from woman to woman depending on each woman's own childhood experiences. Developmental pathways arise out of the earliest mother/child relationship, and mothers often introject societal norms.

Adolescence is a time for reworking old conflicts and development of mastery. This process is quite a different experience for males than females. Adolescent boys form friendships in which competition is relegated to the playing field. For them, it is a time for honing abilities and skills, and for demonstrating prowess and mastery, both in general physical terms and in sexual terms. The transition for adolescent males is easier because their norms are dominant in society. For young women, it is a time when any unresolved issues of competition and control with the mother may resurface and consequently color interactions with friends. Old issues of sexual abuse may be exacerbated by budding sexuality. Relational needs may begin to conflict with those of a dominant male culture that stresses autonomy and achievement (Gilligan 1982[18]).

Adolescence is a time of self-doubt—about physical appearance, loyalty of friends, sexual desirability, and conflict about academic ability. For example, how smart can someone be in the classroom and still feel safe and be accepted? The boy who is the "class brain" is often admired. The girl who is the "class brain" is often teased, denigrated, and isolated. Girls enter the battle for the perfect body: they experiment between regression to childlike activities and a premature race toward sexual activity. The power struggle to separate from the mother is in ascendancy. During this period, bulimia and anorexia may develop. For those who are unable or not allowed to separate, and who do not control anything about their own lives, the only remaining control available is over what goes in and out of their body. Surrey (1985[16]) postulates another etiology for adolescent eating disorders: the conflict arising in the adolescent girl between her needs for intimacy and the cultural requirements for achievement and autonomy. Surrey feels that eating disorders occur when the adolescent must repress her own need and realities to conform to the cultural norms. We have discussed anorexia in terms of the relationship of the girl to her mother (see Chapter 2). Surrey may be pointing to yet another problem in terms of the adolescent girl's identification with the mother or her introjection of these values along with ones that she chooses to reject.

It is not enough for the adolescent girl to be just attractive, just smart, or just skilled. She must be all things to, for, and in place of her mother.[†] One resolution may be that the ego ideal is defensively overinflated to the detriment of the self representation. In this case, life progresses for the adolescent. Her accomplishments, however, will only "pump her up" temporarily and indeed may threaten either her real relationship with her mother or her internalized image of her mother. At a time when instinct and defense are precariously balanced (see Chapter 2), the maintenance of self-esteem and its regulation has already started to become the roller coaster that it will be for many women through the subsequent stages of development. Adolescents are given more leeway as far as fixed societal norms, but this changes as they become young adults.

Young adult women are more empowered today than ever before, yet many still have severe problems with self-esteem regulation. Women

---

[†]On "The Cosby Show," Dr. Huxtable refers to his son's infraction of the rules laughingly, "I remember when I once did something like that." In contrast, Ms. Huxtable says to her daughter, "I don't understand what has gotten into you," referring to a parallel infraction.

who accept the maternal role rather than strive for a career are often treated as second class and therefore feel guilty. Women who opt to channel their energies toward successful careers often feel that they have been cheated or have cheated themselves out of relationships and generativity. Women who opt for some compromise are often subject to severe role strain. In the resultant juggling act, balls are destined to fall, with subsequent episodes of doubting and loss of self-confidence and self-worth, and even episodes of self-denigration, clinical anxiety, and depression. As an example of this last scenario and its subsequent dilemma, we turn to the work of Edith Gilson (Gilson and Kane 1987[26]).

A portrait emerges from Gilson's survey (see Gilson and Kane 1987[26]). Women were found to like men and get along well with them. Women's greatest difficulties were in relationships with women, or arose because of avoidance of other women. It was the recognition of this aspect of her own life which led Gilson to design and conduct her study. She surveyed women with six-figure incomes in the so-called Fortune 500 companies. Twenty-five of these women participated in taped in-depth interviews. The vast majority of this group had educated mothers, many of whom had had careers. The mothers of the women in this group had been achievers and role models for their daughters. Despite the fact that these women felt successful in the world's eyes, most felt unhappy and had views of themselves that they knew were discordant with how they were perceived by others. The case might be made that those women who had chosen to be either unmarried or married but childless, or isolated from significant friendships, felt the loss, and some women acknowledged this in the survey. It also might be true that those women with families experienced role strain trying to bring perfectionism to two equally demanding and often mutually exclusive jobs. For example, no one can simultaneously attend a board meeting and be at open school. Most women interviewed complained of overwork at their jobs, a complaint in common with male colleagues. Most women also complained of overwork at home. The so-called double-shift phenomenon, in which women return from work to begin household tasks, is specific to women and not shared by most men. In addition, the majority of women felt guilty and/or sad about leaving their children. These feelings were not mitigated by obtaining excellent and reliable household help.

Men and women respond differently to the power hierarchy. Men feel enhanced and empowered by their position. Women, who structure their self-esteem differently, may feel fraudulent in "expert" and "power" positions (McIntosh 1985[27]). Faulty self-esteem regulation in women is more grave and goes further back historically than the availability of the "fast track." This dysregulation cannot totally be accounted for by realistic or factual explanations about the workplace or life-style.

Success approbation and validation do not work to reliably maintain self-esteem in women. Paradoxically, increasing success often worsens the problems of self-esteem. The daunting problem facing women can be accounted for by the "Alice in Wonderland phenomenon." As the Queen of Hearts questions Alice, the rules for answering the questions keep changing. The same is true of the behavioral and affective/affiliative norms for women. In bold terms, the lines between self-assertion, aggression, and unfeminine behavior are fuzzy and ever shifting from arena to arena and from task to task. The stakes grow higher with increasing success. The effects of a woman's behavior or emotional response often cannot be anticipated. Women are confronted moment by moment with a series of pass/fail tasks. Men pass if a task is accomplished accurately, independently or within a designated group, in a timely fashion. Women must maintain affiliative ties, be sensitively attuned and responsive, and avoid hurting or displeasing others while attaining or even surpassing all the other norms. This is (virtually) impossible on an ongoing basis. Failure or the threat of failure lurks at every turn. This threat of failure is overwhelmingly stressful and demoralizing, and destabilizes self-esteem.

To take a concrete example, men tend to have "regulation" work and play clothes. Women are expected to look feminine without being too frilly, seductive, or exhibitionistic. Short hair may be too masculine. Long hair may be too wild, messy, sexy, or unprofessional. An absence of jewelry and makeup may lead to accusations of being too plain or of being a "dyke." Jewelry and makeup may be taken as evidence of a lack of seriousness. Although expected to be sensitive, most women are accused of being too sensitive. The definition of too sensitive is often unclear or fluctuating. Thus, women find themselves in situations that they cannot control. Numerous authors (Dohrenwend 1973[28]; Gilligan 1979[29]; Miller 1976[21]) have pointed out that women are most stressed by situations that are beyond their control and by those in which they are held responsible for the well-being of others.

Obviously, education of women will not fully solve the problem of self-esteem regulation. In some cases the problem is unconscious and has genetically primitive roots. Robert Liebert (unpublished observations) has pointed out that therapy often does not help because male analysts tend to resist the maternal transference and are more comfortable with oedipal rather than preoedipal issues. In addition, many analytically oriented therapists still view penis envy as a biological given that necessarily accounts for poor self-esteem. Nor will the education of women or their treatment solve the problem of societal norms that, even if not introjected, are continuously stressful and often cause anxiety or depression. The attempts of women to get off the seesaw and feel reliably good have resulted in some maladaptive options. Many women use prescription or over-the-counter medications, or alcohol in an attempt to stabilize mood. Others become compulsive clothing shoppers, submit themselves to plastic surgery procedures, and/or spend large amounts of money on cosmetics in the search for youthfulness, beauty, and self-esteem. A more productive, less costly or damaging adaptation is the use of female support groups or the establishment of a female supportive network, and reliable friendships with women.

In presenting the case material below to show the vicissitudes of self-esteem regulation, we attempt to illustrate where on the psychiatric diagnostic spectrum the patients lie and which dynamics seem most pivotal.

Self-Esteem and Parental Regard

The patient, a 38-year-old successful partner in a prestigious law firm, was asked by her mother whether she could not get one of her male partners to help her father with his retirement contract and the investment and dispersal of his assets.

She told her mother that this was an area of her own expertise and that she would be glad to help. Her mother told her that she could never handle her father's board of directors. The patient angrily retorted, but to no avail, that she handles corporate directors whose net worth is twenty times her father's. So she obediently referred her father to the person requested, who then asked her advice.

While understanding the irrationality, the patient began to have doubts about her work and self-worth. She maintained the symbiotic relationship with her mother. For example, the patient was having most of her clothing made to order by a private designer, unconsciously shoring up her self-esteem to make her feel special. (No one else could have a similar dress.) At the same time there was a blurring of boundaries in terms of whose clothes these were. In the conversation about the impending clothing delivery, her mother said gratuitously, "I think you should stop ordering your clothes from G—— [the designer]"—she then used a peculiar phrase—"because the punishment does not fit the crime." This response made no sense except as a "burp" from the mother's unconscious. We gathered that the patient's "crime" was wanting to be special and separate; the punishment, paying for it. The patient's first association was, "I hate all my clothes; they don't make me feel pretty anymore, and I don't feel that I was functioning well at work this week." Her next concerns were about her son. Was she spending enough time with him? Within minutes her self-esteem had become like a tire with a slow persistent leak.

The Ego Ideal and Self-Esteem Regulation

A homemaker in her 40s who had once been a successful writer found that she could not write with predictable regularity or finish a project. Angry at herself for this, she berated her husband and family for failure to support her, love her, and be grateful for what she had sacrificed for them. Her failure to gain self-esteem through her vocation left her feeling depleted, needy, and angry. She was angry at her "objects" for not pumping up her self representation or assuring her that she meets her ego ideal.

[Jacobson (1964[9]) has used the failure of self-actualization and object relations in regard to writing as an illustration of the psychodynamics of self-esteem dysregulation. Jacobson, commenting on writing ability, noted that "writing will never proceed if the writer does not have sufficient self assurance" or "if the main incentive . . . is [gratification of] grandiose fantasies which surpass his [her] abilities" (p. 81). She contended that all ego activities aim at self-gratification and require that we withdraw our investment from objects and turn it into goal-directed activities. Overinvestment in objects or in the self brings about failure.]

Our patient is caught in a circular process. Failure to invest her ego activity turns her aggressively to her love objects. Her hostile demand discourages the expression of love and gratitude. She needs to feel self-assured enough to withdraw her investment from her objects and reinvest it in her chosen ego function. Unable to meet the requirements of her ego ideal, and unable to obtain enrichment of her self representation, she feels like a failure, like nothing, and she loses self-esteem, becoming despairing and depressed.

The two patients in the case examples above had damaging mothers and had serious self-esteem dysregulation but were able to become involved in psychodyamic therapy. There are a number of women who instead seek and receive treatment with prescription drugs or who self-medicate with over-the-counter medications or alcohol.

Abuse of Prescription and Over-the-Counter Drugs

The prescription drugs that are most commonly abused are the central nervous system (CNS) depressants, or "minor tranquilizers." These drugs, which act to dampen the excitable tissue of the CNS (Schuckit 1981[30]), fall into three categories: barbiturate-like drugs, benzodiazepines, and carbamates.

The barbiturate-like drugs ethchlorvynol (Placidyl), glutethimide (Doriden), methaqualone (Quaalude), as well as the benzodiazepines flurazepam (Dalmane) and temazepam (Restoril), are prescribed principally for insomnia. Diazepam (Valium) and meprobamate with aspirin (Equagesic) are prescribed for muscle spasm and lower back pain. Chlordiazepoxide and clindinium bromide (Librax) are commonly prescribed for "esophageal reflex" and "irritable bowel syndrome" when they occur in the absence of demonstrable tissue or infectious pathology.

The benzodiazepines are usually prescribed for the treatment of anxiety disorders. These drugs include alprazolam (Xanax), clorazepate (Tranxène), diazepam (Valium), lorazepam (Ativan), and triazolam (Halcion). In 1 year, over two billion tablets of diazepam were prescribed in the United States. Forty percent of the patients who had received or were receiving prescriptions for antianxiety or hypnotic drugs felt that they had been dependent on these drugs at some time during their lives. Outright abuse is estimated at about 5% to 10% ("Benzodiazepines" 1978[31]). The mechanism of action of these agents is partially understood. There are selective receptors in the brain for benzodiazepines (Greenblatt and Shader 1974[32]; Tallman et al. 1980[33]). These receptors interact closely with neurotransmitters in the gamma-aminobutyric acid (GABA) system (Masotti et al. 1981[34]).

Most clinicians believe that panic disorder and agoraphobia are more common in women than in men (Marks and Lader 1973[35]). In a recent review of epidemiological studies, Weissman (1983[36]) found that in three studies of patients with the diagnosis of anxiety disorder, discrete panic attacks were more common in women than in men. Other studies have found that all forms of anxiety disorder are more common in women than in men. The female-to-male ratio in panic disorder with agoraphobia has been estimated to be about 3.5:1 (Uhlenhuth et al. 1983[37]).

Despite an abundant literature that proves the superior efficacy of tricyclic antidepressants and monoamine oxidase (MAO) inhibitors in treating anxiety disorders and/or mixed anxiety and depression (Johnstone et al. 1980[38]; Kahn et al. 1986[39]; Kleber 1979[40]; Rickels et al. 1974[41]; Shammas 1977[42]), women tend to be treated with benzodiazepines. The dietary limitations and medical risks (such as malignant hypertension with the MAOIs) make it more "expedient" for the clinician to use the benzodiazepines.

Before we attempt to understand the etiology of the anxiety disorders in women, we must digress to briefly discuss the dangers of treating patients with the sedative-hypnotic drugs.

Tolerance is an important contributing factor to abuse of sedative-hypnotics and is due to increased metabolism of the drug and apparent adaptation of the CNS. When the drugs are used over months, the patient is apt to require higher and higher doses to produce the same degree of effect in combination with alcohol. Marks (1978[43]) studied 151 cases of patients who sometimes used excessive doses for the reasons already mentioned. He found that tolerance has another potentially harmful aspect. If a second CNS depressant is used, the two compete for metabolism and the toxic effects are additive. This, of course, applies to alcohol, which is also a CNS depressant. At the extreme we see accidental irreversible coma in patients who take their tranquilizers and then use a lot of alcohol, or in patients who first become intoxicated with alcohol and then take their tranquilizers. The other serious problems with the CNS depressants are the induction of sedation that impairs functioning (e.g., "falling asleep" at the wheel of a motor vehicle). Gorman et al. (1983,[44] 1984[45]), Hollander et al. (1987[46]), Pitts and McClune (1967[47]), and Skolnick and Paul (1982[48]) have ably reviewed the etiology of anxiety disorders. See Appendix D for biological theories related to anxiety disorders.

Psychodynamic theories of anxiety have had their vicissitudes. Freud (1896[49], 1898[50]) originally postulated a class of clinical entities that included anxiety neurosis and neurasthenia. Patients with anxiety neurosis sought treatment because of palpitations and other "physiological" complaints, and those with neurasthenia presented because of weakness, restlessness, fatigue, and general ennui. Freud (1893b[51]) grouped these patients together and described them as having actual neurosis anxiety resulting from dammed up libido. In 1926, Freud,[52] in changing his theory of anxiety, described anxiety as a signal to the ego of conflict. He postulated a series of intrapsychic events in which the conflict is repressed and additional defensive maneuvers in their aggregate could cause symptoms like phobias (Freud 1909a[53]). At that time Freud believed that castration anxiety was at the root of phobic symptoms.

Essentially Freud's view held sway until psychiatry became involved with biology, biochemistry, and physiology in the early 1960s. D. F. Klein (1964,[54] 1981[55]) postulated that agoraphobia with panic attacks represents aberrant function of the biological substrate that underlies human separation anxiety. Margaret Mahler (1963,[56] 1967[57]; Mahler and Furer 1963[58]; Mahler and La Perriere 1965[59]) studied early childhood development and described its many subphases. She observed separation anxiety and related it to the stages of separation-individuation. Since then, ego psychologists have linked separation anxiety, pathological dependence, and panic attacks.

We have described at length the evolving concept of the psychology of women as inexorably linked to the vicissitudes of their mother's bond to them. We have discussed the vicissitudes of self-esteem in the same regard. Before presenting case histories of patients with anxiety disorders and CNS depressant abuse, we address the abuse of prescription stimulants, over-the-counter drugs, alcohol, and food, and then discuss patients who were self-medicating because of anxiety, depression, or the inability to control eating behavior based on issues of narcissistic injury or failure of self-esteem regulation.

The stimulants encompass a wide variety of drugs that stimulate the CNS at many levels (Jaffe 1980[60]). Stimulants work by causing release of neurotransmitters such as norepinephrine in the CNS. Clinically, these drugs can cause euphoria, decreased fatigue and the diminished need for sleep, decreased appetite, and increased energy. As side effects these drugs can produce psychomotor restlessness, irritability, increased heart rate, and tremulousness. We are primarily concerned with the use of stimulants by women for appetite suppression, fatigue depression, and menstrual dysphoria.

The over-the-counter drugs with which we will concern ourselves next fall into several categories: antianxiety and sleep medications, antihistamines (used for CNS depression stimulants), and appetite suppressants (i.e., "diet pills"). It has been estimated that 18 million Americans have used over-the-counter hypnotics or sedatives. The use is higher in women. Two-thirds of the users are over age 35; 50% are over age 50 (Inciardi 1977[61]). These medications are used for their sedative side effects in the self-medication of anxiety or insomnia. Antihistamines are also often used for their sedative side effects.

Stimulants usually contain caffeine as their major ingredient. Individuals may respond with slightly increased thought flow, enhancement of motor activities, and decreased drowsiness and fatigue. Most of the users are male, but some women use these drugs to combat depression. Diet pills such as Dexatrim contain small amounts of Dexedrine and amphetamine (i.e., stimulants) that are addictive over time. Women use and abuse over-the-counter drugs to combat dysphoric states and to aid in their search for slimness, youth, and beauty. They anticipate that these attributes will bolster their self-esteem.

Panic Attack and Lorazepam Abuse

A 44-year-old mother of two college-age children was married to a physician. Eighteen years ago, after the birth of their second child, her husband, who did not want the child, went abroad to work for 2 months, leaving her with the two children. During that time she had her first panic attack, which included a variety of physical symptoms. Medical evaluation found no organic cause, and she was started on lorazepam. This was temporarily helpful, but she was phobic about driving and stayed close to home. She neglected her talents as a keyboardist and stopped doing volunteer work in her church.

Several years later, unbeknown to her, her husband went on a job interview in another city, accepted the job on the spot, and came home to announce that the family would be moving. Meanwhile, the patient had had the good fortune to be living in her dream house, which she was loathe to give up. Her widowed mother joined the family at the request of both the husband and the patient. After moving, her panic attacks accelerated in frequency and intensity. She was treated with increasing doses of lorazepam, which she could obtain at will without prescription because her husband was a physician. As her children grew older, money became an issue, and, in addition to playing the church organ, she took on a job managing an office for a group of physicians. When they took on a new partner without space or personnel expansion, her stress became unbearable. The turning point that led her to psychotherapy was attending a concert with her husband. She could not re-

member having seen the soloist before, which was notable because they had allegedly had on-stage seats to see that same soloist 5 years before. She felt that her mind had snapped or "was going."

She initially presented a Pollyanna version of her relationship with her husband. Her dreams, however, belied this depiction. Detoxification and psychodynamic treatment were begun. She "woke up enough" to realize that she must change jobs, which she did. For the first year she was unable to drive her own car to therapy. Although immaculately groomed, she was clinically depressed. Her denial broke down, and it became apparent that she was being treated badly by her husband, a fact with which her daughters and her mother concurred. With detoxification she became more lively and revealed herself to be a repository of talents heretofore unreported. She continued to have panic attacks, insomnia, and generalized anxiety while in the process of discontinuing lorazepam. Several tricyclic antidepressants brought no relief, but an MAO inhibitor did. Her husband was very derisive of her pill taking, but he never objected to the lorazepam. She felt progressively better, got another job, felt able to travel by train to see her daughters, and began to be more verbal in rejecting sarcasm and abuse. Her husband, however, became more difficult.

Feeling angry, lonely, and isolated, she wrote two novels and became involved in a very exciting music project. Every time she felt angry at her husband her response was panic rather than rage. When anger emerged she revealed literally murderous fantasies. This patient was expected to shut up, follow her husband's dictates, and reject her own needs and wishes. This she had accomplished only under a blanket of sedative-hypnotic medication.

The patient not only plans to be divorced but is thinking of remarrying. She is beginning to experience her sexual feelings and needs. Although initially reluctant to discuss these, she came to understand that her therapist was not her confessor and that in reality her own church was more permissive than the official party line of her religion. She continues to require small doses of an MAO inhibitor.

Sedative-Hypnotic Addiction

A single woman in her early 60s had a university appointment. She recalled adoring her father, whom she had lost as a teenager, and hating her mother, who, the daughter felt, was a very demeaning, critical, and self-involved woman. When her mother had a stroke, the patient's sister and brother-in-law, who was a physician, refused to take the patient's mother in or pay toward her placement in a nursing care facility. The patient, against her own wishes and with some help after her mother's discharge from the hospital, felt that the job of caring for her mother was thrust upon her. She resigned her university appointment and, more importantly, her position on the altar committee of her cathedral. She had to give up a room that she usually rented to a college student for whom she was a surrogate mother so that her mother could be accommodated. She began to deal with her anxiety and rage by dipping into medications designed to keep her mother sedated. Her mother lingered, incontinent and aphasic, for 5 years. After her mother's death the patient tried to detoxify herself but could not and so sought hospital admission.

After detoxification, she was more than willing to explore her history and seek psychodynamic relationships. She rejoined her altar group but was phobic about trying to regain her university position. She was welcomed back to that position, however, and invited to stay beyond the usual retirement age. In addition, she took on assignments with graduate students. She eventually rented out her spare room to a college student. She had never felt entitled to get married, and, in her view, her mother's illness put an end to any final chance. However, she had a steadfast male friend with whom she remained close up to and throughout his terminal illness.

Alcoholism

Alcoholism is defined as the occurrence of serious social or health problems related to alcohol consumption (Goodwin and Guze 1979[62]; National Council on Alcoholism 1972[63]; Schuckit 1973[64]). Alcoholism is categorized as primary or secondary. Primary alcoholism occurs in the absence of a major psychiatric disorder. Secondary alcoholism is alcoholism that results from a preexisting major psychiatric disorder. The highest rates of alcoholism are seen in men ages 39 to 50. Studies of alcoholic inpatients have revealed that 15% to 20% of female patients, compared with 5% of male patients, have had a prior affective disorder

(Haglund and Schuckit 1982[65]; Schuckit 1983[66]; Schuckit and Winbeur 1972[67]). Alcohol is known to be stress-inducing by initially lowering the threshold to a variety of stimuli (Haglund and Schuckit 1982[65]).

There are many theories about primary alcoholism, which we will briefly review. One set of theories about the onset of primary alcoholism is that alcohol removes discomfort and inhibition, enhances social interaction, and fulfills narcissistic needs to feel powerful or to abolish unpleasant memories (Haglund and Schuckit 1982[65]). A second set of theories revolves around sociocultural norms involving the acceptable use and the abuse of alcohol (Schuckit and Haglund 1982[68]). A third set of theories centers around biological factors that involve the ability of the liver to metabolize alcohol (Korsten et al. 1975[69]; Loebuck and Kessler 1971[70]; Schuckit and Rayser 1979[71]). A series of studies has confirmed a genetic hypothesis. Alcoholism occurs in families, with the best evidence coming from Scandinavian twin studies. Children of biological parents who were alcoholic adopted into nonalcoholic families have higher rates of alcoholism than those of nonalcoholic biological parents adopted into alcoholic families (Bohman et al. 1981[72]; Haglund and Schuckit 1982[65]). All of the theories have been reviewed by Haglund and Schuckit (1982[65]).

Conservative estimates indicate that between 6 and 11 million adult women (6% of the adult female population) have alcohol problems (Yandow 1989[73]). High-risk subgroups include younger women, never-married women, divorced or separated women, and unemployed women or those employed part-time (Wisnack et al. 1985[74]). Women's drinking is highly correlated with the drinking behaviors of significant others in their lives. There is a high association between alcoholism and eating disorders (Berny and Merry 1986[75]). As many as 75% of women in treatment for alcoholism have a history of childhood sexual abuse (Rohsenow et al. 1988[76]). In these cases women often resort to alcohol in order to engage in sexual activity. This is an example of secondary alcoholism in which incest or sexual abuse is the primary disorder. Our experience is that alcohol abuse is often secondary to stress, anxiety, or depression, or to a combination of any of these primary disorders. This is documented, as we have noted earlier, in women who have both an anxiety disorder and minor tranquilizer abuse. And we do not ignore the diagnosis of primary alcoholism in women for whom stress, anxiety, and/or depression is *secondary* to alcohol abuse.

Women "closet" drinkers often hide their alcohol in laundry baskets or briefcases. Often the alcoholism only becomes apparent when they are soporific or irritable, or when it is noted that they have become careless in personal appearance, in home care, or at work. These are patients who have not yet lost complete control of their alcoholism. They are in need of inpatient detoxification programs. If alcohol abuse is noted in a psychodynamic treatment of underlying anxiety and depression, the patient must be detoxified and drug free. Only then can pharmacological or psychodynamic therapy, or a combination of these two, be instituted.

Psychodynamic psychotherapy is aimed at the underlying anxiety, depression, or rage of the patient. Patients cannot be treated in psychotherapy while toxic from alcohol or during acute withdrawal because they have impaired cognition (comprehension and memory, particularly). Vaillant (1981[77]) makes a strong case against the dangers of psychotherapy without prior detoxification. He suggests that the reason for this is psychodynamic, postulating inadequate mothering as being causally related: "Psychoanalysis helps us love the parents we have, but does not provide the parents we never had" (p. 53). Vaillant points out that Alcoholics Anonymous (AA) can be that nurturing mother. Clearly, this is one aspect of the problem and its solution. More importantly, there are personality changes secondary to alcoholism. We cannot talk with patients who are intoxicated, withdrawing, or too deeply invested in getting their next drink.

Alcohol Abuse Due to Depression

A 40-year-old high school teacher began closet drinking when her husband had an affair and decided to leave her. It seemed to most people that the stress of the divorce accounted for her increased carelessness of appearance and the disorganization of her classroom. Her students complained that she had be-

come a sort of "loosey goosey," despite the fact that her reputation had been built on structure and a no-nonsense approach. Already in treatment for depression, she was helped to understand her passivity in the litigation and in other areas of her life. It emerged that she was aware of being a denigrated object for her husband and that he was spending nights elsewhere. She hypothesized that this was a result of her having had twins when her oldest daughter was 2 years old. As she described it, "Sure I was fat and sloppy. I had one baby in each arm and a toddler trailing behind. He came home expecting his dinner on the table, the children put to sleep, and his right to sit, read his newspaper, and go to sleep." Her own poor self-image as a result of her family's values, or rather devaluation, led her to see herself as unworthy. She used wine to handle sleep-onset insomnia and cessation of sexual relations.

Thereafter, she began to drink through the day to rid herself of her discontent and anxiety. It took a confrontation at work and a demand that she enter an AA program or else risk losing her job to pressure her to discuss her alcoholism in psychodynamic therapy. Intoxicated, she had been caught shoplifting. She saw herself as a dog.

In combination with the AA program, it was possible to work out the psychodynamics of her illness. Early narcissistic damage led to later willingness to accept domination and denigration that was socially sanctioned. Both thought that her husband, as a physician, had the right to be boss in his home, and the patient was expected to sacrifice her own needs, wishes, and talents to tend her household and single-handedly raise her children. Therefore she turned to alcohol.

Abuse of Food

We have discussed bulimia nervosa in the chapter on adolescence (see Chapter 2) because eating disorders are often manifested in childhood but become more apparent in their interference of adult functioning, and even survival, in adolescence.

There is a type of bulimia that does not involve the eating of vast quantities of unlikely combinations of foods to the point of nausea. Rather it involves nibbling, noshing, and snacking between meals, most frequently at night. Just as persons with secondary alcoholism drink until they are sedated, these bulimic persons eat until they feel soothed and/or soporific. The favored foods are ice cream and other sweets. Patients often spontaneously recognize it as mother's milk. Others talk about it as feeding the (angry) bear. When asked to pay careful attention to affects, many patients are able to report anger, tension, jitteriness, and "eating to calm down or to stay calm." Some bulimic patients are not obese. For obese bulimic patients, at some point a horrible cycle develops. The patients are obese enough to have to be on severely deprived diets (i.e., 800–1,200 calories maximum). This leads to further deprivation, jitteriness, and anger. Unlike patients who wish to lose 10 to 15 pounds and can do this by eating normal, nutritious meals and no high-caloric snacks or desserts, obese patients must literally starve to lose 40 to 50 pounds.

Bulimia, Anxiety, and Depression

A woman in her 50s was referred by her diabetologist and by the spa that she had attended for years. The counselor there was alarmed at her obvious depression and her newly manifested inability to finish sentences (because of her agitation). Although referred for medication, the patient refused "drugs." Her decompensation came when it was suggested that she might have to get divorced to lose weight. Very bright and psychologically minded, she began to give a clear history.

She was aware of the problem of denigration at the hands of her mother and husband and was able to look at her part in perpetuating this pattern. There was clearly a power struggle between the patient and her husband, to which she contributed. She kept their businesses enmeshed. During one trip out of town she asked her husband to go through her mail, even though he was known to be unreliable in this regard. (Her bookkeeper, on the other hand, could do this with great efficacy.) Her husband failed to notice something that needed her attention during her absence, and she came back furious at him. She also set things up so that she was responsible for getting to the cash machine for the two of them and seeing to it that his car had gasoline, and so forth. She would get angry when she let something slip through the cracks and he was sarcastic with her. She began to become aware that as soon as she felt hurt or "made to feel guilty," she would get something to eat. The same pattern emerged in her relationship with her mother: the more the patient did, the more she was expected to do, and the angrier she became, the more her anxiety increased. Unhappy and frustrated, she would eat. She was also aware of using food to get relaxed and sleepy.

Despite many achievements, she still did not feel entirely capable, and her husband's sarcastic and hostile comments still wounded her. She was also aware that whenever she dieted, he talked about how fat she was. In a slip she said, "He camouflages me," when she meant to say, "He sabotages me." She was being camouflaged in that her achievements were never credited. Steadfast in her resolve not to be verbally abused and denigrated, she began to diet. She stopped seeking food as solace but strengthened her resolve to stop taking undue responsibility for her husband and to get on with her own life.

The Abuse of Food as a Sedative-Hypnotic

A married professional woman, mother of three adult children, came to treatment because she had "never been as heavy as I am now." She sought to lose weight for an important family occasion. She denied any problem other than that she loved food. She overate and, unknown to others, participated in binge eating and purging. When her therapist used the word "vomit," the patient recoiled but began to recognize that this was a "major illness." She was given clonidine patches and fluoxetine (Prozac) for appetite suppression. She lost 12 pounds but rapidly regained them after the family party. She was rarely hungry but ate abnormally when she experienced "jittery feelings." She also became aware of depression.

She still gets nervous and overeats, but the binging and purging have stopped. She denies the obvious source of her anxiety. Her work is very stressful and leaves her exhausted. Her husband is retired. She works to keep her large home, where an adult son has "his own quarters." A would-be artist, he is not self-supporting. The patient's husband favors telling him he has to get out, but the patient could never allow this. She has barely begun to talk about guilt because this child was hyperactive, on medication, and in treatment as a youngster. Her self-esteem requires that she be a model's size. Clearly her ego ideal of thinness relates to her perception of her mother. In reality, her mother is petite, and the patient, like her father, is large-boned and tall. The determinants of her inability to get her adult son out on his own are unclear except for his childhood psychiatric history. Her husband correctly perceives that the problem is not her weight but her failure to accept herself as a slightly overweight but glamorous woman.

Cosmetic Repair: The Search for Youth and Beauty

Cosmetic surgery is defined by the American Medical Association as any operation designed to change a feature of the human body that would be considered in the range of normal for the person's age and ethnic background by an impartial observer (Beeson and McCollough 1986[78]). Several authors have recognized the psychological factors influencing the request for cosmetic repair (Hyman 1990[79]; Napolion and Lewis 1989,[80] 1990[81]; Wengle 1986[82]). Coleman (1990[83]) commented particularly on the disproportionately large number of patients with self-concept disorders. These authors point out that the number of patients receiving lipoplasty, 200,000 in 1986, had risen by 60% in 1987. The number of procedures performed by members of the Association of Plastic and Reproductive Surgeons in 1988 are shown in Figure 3–1. These figures do not include data about the number of similar procedures performed by licensed and trained dermatologists (Napolion and Lewis 1989[80]), non–specialty-boarded plastic surgeons, and general surgeons also doing these procedures.

Figure 3–1. *(At right)* Number of procedures performed by members of the Association of Plastic and Reproductive Surgeons in 1988. The authors wish to express their gratitude to Jane A. Petro, M.D., Director of the Burn Center at the Westchester County Medical Center, for making these data available to us.

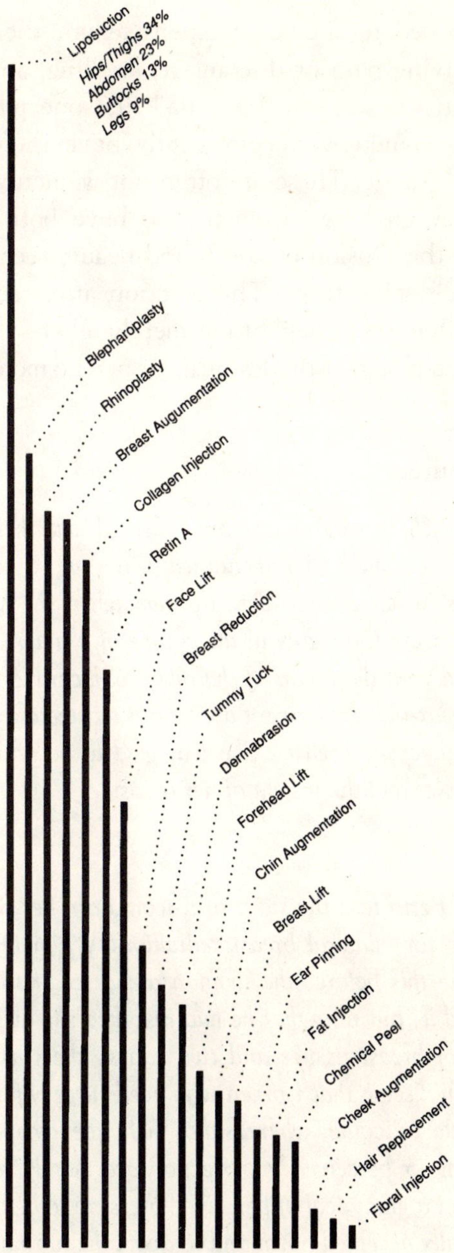

Physical Alteration Procedures

These procedures are not inexpensive, and there is a significant morbidity involving pain or discomfort, swelling, and ecchymosis. Yet we have known women who have had first one procedure and then another, and women who periodically have their blepharoplasties (or "face-lifts") redone. These are often not women whose lives are empty. In fact, they are often women who have both worked and raised a family. Yet the illusion of youth and beauty seems a necessary component of their self-esteem. The reaction after recovery from surgery is seldom excitement or delight but merely relief—the fat is gone from the thighs or buttocks, the wrinkles are gone, and no more "bags" under the eyes.

Cosmetic Surgery

Two women whom we treated were delighted with their outcomes. Each of the women had had medical indications. One, a 30-year-old, had ripped the pierced holes in her ears straight through when she had worn and slept with earrings that were too heavy in the course of a major depressive disorder. She was delighted with the repair of the bilateral lacerations. The other woman, a buxom 50-year-old, underwent a bilateral mastectomy for a midline cancer in pendulous polycystic breasts. She was glad to be rid of the pain of recurrent breast abscesses and the weight of her breasts.

* * *

Dr. Jane Petro tells the story of a woman in her 80s who came in on two canes asking for bilateral breast reduction. When Dr. Petro asked why she had not done this before, the woman answered that her husband would not have allowed it, but now that he had just died she was ready to proceed. Less 20 pounds of breast tissues and two canes, she was delighted with the outcome. It would seem that women who need surgery for medical indications are happy with the outcome, whereas those who feel compelled to rid themselves of signs of aging or perceived imperfection are merely relieved. This would appear to reflect a great deal of perceived pressure to be beautiful as measured by some culturally accepted norm and to avoid the normal aging process.

* * *

One divorced woman in her 50s was about to embark on a face-lift. Encouraged to examine self-esteem problems, she met and married a man with whom she fell very much in love and abandoned plans for plastic surgery.

* * *

Another patient, in her early 30s, had to sacrifice a promising, demanding career to care for her parents, each of whom died of cancer within a 3-year period. After the mourning process she intended to look for a job, but not before she underwent a lipectomy to remove fat from her buttocks and thighs. Objectively, she did not look a lot different, nor did her normally low weight decrease, but she had a sense of being relieved of a burden that she had felt since adolescence.

* * *

A woman in her 40s, who had been divorced several times, followed each of the divorces with a face-lift, as if convinced that her "aging face" had caused her marital difficulties.

* * *

One married woman in her 30s was overprotected by her parents and older sisters because of a birth defect. As an adult she tended to ignore this defect and her dyslexia. Instead, despite a statuesque model-like figure, she wished that she could have her legs cut off at the knees and be "petite and cute." It did not matter that her husband is tall and that the two make a stunning couple. The psychodynamics of this problem related to the woman's having been a tall, gawky child who had always been faulted for "not knowing better" because it was assumed that she was older. The patient is now just beginning to realize how much she still wishes to be an overprotected child. She has the fantasy that being small in stature would make her look younger and entitle her to special attention and to be taken care of by her husband and family. Her feelings are so strong that if there were a plastic surgical procedure to "shorten her," she would have the procedure done.

Less drastic but still symptomatic of underlying problems of self-esteem is the multibillion-dollar feminine cosmetic industry. Sanford and

Donovan (1984[84]) have studied women in therapy groups and have reported that nearly every woman in these groups suffered from negative body image. These authors assert that one reason so many women experience their appearance as a problem is that our culture sets up standards that are unhealthy and unattainable. Chernin (1981[85]) has elucidated the intrapsychic dynamics that influence the cultural norms of appearance. She speculates that out of the ecstasy and early experiences and frustration with the mother we develop an obsession with human flesh. Longing for security translates into longing for mother, which sustains the myth of female goodness and beauty. Anger at life translates into anger at mother and the myth of female physical deficiency. Thus, women become preoccupied with toning, softening, moisturizing, peeling, and covering up the skin with makeup. Many women need to color, wrap, tip, and manicure their nails. Hair must be conditioned, dyed, bleached, extended, curled, or straightened. As mentioned above, there is a hierarchy of psychodynamics that govern self-esteem regulation, and the psychodynamic that relates to faulty early mothering is one among many.

Freedman (1986[86]) has studied the beauty industry and women's never-ending quest for products that promise to beautify the woman and retard aging. Women spend $3 billion a year on makeup, $2 billion on hair products, $1 billion on nail products, and $800 million on feminine hygiene products. Stannard (1971[87]) pointed out that the beauty industry spends millions on telling women that they are in effect ugly—for example, their skin is too dry or oily, their complexion is too pale or ruddy, their lips are not bright enough, and they need lifting, shaping, dying, painting, curling, straightening, padding, and so forth.

Twice as many high school girls as boys want to change their looks (Musa and Roach 1973[88]). By college age, 75% of males report they feel good about their overall looks and facial features as compared with only 45% of females (Dacey 1979[89]). Adult males consistently place greater emphasis on good looks in the opposite sex than women do (Loombs 1982[90]). The actor Dustin Hoffman (1983[91]) described the realization that he could turn himself into a woman in the film *Tootsie* but not a beautiful woman, as shattering. In his role as a woman, men met and greeted him while looking over his shoulder to find an attractive woman.

He realized that men try to get a good looking girl next to them to get rid of bad feelings and reclaim beauty vicariously, the so-called rub-off effect.

Why do men, still largely raised by their mothers, regard attractive women as a prize? Has it to do with the early idealization of the mother by her son? Do mothers transmit a message that they expect their sons to marry women who will make up for their, the mothers', own perceived deficits? These are questions that our experience in treating the mothers of boys do not yet allow us to answer. Nevertheless, it seems clear that the pressure toward youth and beauty is not wholly intrinsic to the mother/daughter relationship but is fostered by the way in which mothers raise their sons. Virginia Woolf (1919,[92] pp. 35–36) provided one possible insight: "Women have served all these centuries as looking glasses possessing the magic and delicious power of reflecting the figure of man at twice its natural size. If she begins to tell the truth the figure in the looking glass shrinks." Is this the message women give their sons?

Compulsive clothes shopping is another way in which women seek relief from self-control deregulation. The popular motto aimed at women is, "When the going gets tough, the tough go shopping." Society recognizes this as an acceptable mechanism of repair except when the shopping becomes compulsive or turns to shoplifting.

Shopping

A patient in her 40s was facing a divorce that her husband wanted because of his involvement with a younger woman. The patient decided that she would go on a shopping spree to make herself over. She used credit cards to spend a fortune that she did not have and would not have under the terms of her divorce settlement. She had never, and did not plan to embark on, supporting herself. Her need to feel better about herself, to restore her self-esteem, outweighed any realistic considerations. She insisted on shopping in the most expensive boutiques and would not accept a friend's offer to take her places that sold designer clothes at discount prices.

* * *

Another patient, a married mother in her 30s, had always dressed well and rather flamboyantly. As her husband's career took off and he needed to spend increasing time out of town, she began to use her credit cards to buy thousands of dollars worth of clothing. She could not be persuaded to return anything or to promise to curtail her spending spree. Her husband decided to cancel her credit cards. Tired of being thought of as her husband's wife, she embarked on her own social whirl. This woman, who in times of economic struggle had been content to manage, clearly felt diminished by her husband's success.

There are other options for maintenance and repair of self-esteem. Self-esteem in women often rests as much on making and maintaining relationships and affiliations as on personal achievement. Women who manage self-esteem regulation fall along a spectrum of those who value achievement and vocational success almost exclusively, to those who add values of family relationships and/or friendships with other women, to those who find affirmation almost exclusively in nurturant relationships with family and friends. Surrey (1983[93]) has contrasted women, for whom she believes the self is organized and maintained in the context of relationships, and men, who place a high value on autonomy, self-reliance, independence, assertion, and self-actualization. We do not believe that such a clear dichotomy exists. We have already contrasted earlier in this chapter the differences in relationship of most mothers and their daughters with that of most mothers and their sons. On the one hand, the narcissistic relationship is closer and more prolonged and the female might find a positive prototype for relationships with family, friends, and other women. On the other hand, the relationship may be so invasive as to discourage its replication in other relationships. The potential for mutual undermining, competition, jealousy, and/or co-opting of power or achievement also exists. Clearly our data in relation to self-esteem show that women are less apt to benefit from a good relationship with their mothers than to suffer from a poor one.

The following vignettes illustrate the undermining of adult women by their mothers. Both of these women could benefit from expanding affiliative relationships that have already been established.

Undermining of Adult Women by Their Mothers

An unmarried social worker in her 30s reported the following episode. During a routine call to her mother, who lives in another city, the daughter reported an automobile accident in which her car had been "totaled." (She had miraculously escaped without major injury.) Her mother did not inquire about her physical status, inconvenience, or financial problems in getting a new car, but instead talked on and on about a minor fender bender she had had the week before. This patient's real difficulties had been reduced to the absurd. The patient stated correctly that she should not have bothered to mention it to her mother but should have discussed it with friends, who would have been more sympathetic and concerned.

* * *

A gifted attorney in her 30s would panic when shopping for clothing. She would hear her mother's criticisms in her mind. She hired a personal shopper to help her overcome her panic in department stores. This woman recommended three outfits that the patient disliked but nonetheless purchased, as if mesmerized. She noted quite accurately, "It is like shopping with my mother, or wearing anything new when I see her." The patient accurately perceived that she could not shop with an authority figure comfortably. She thought that she had to overcome the problem alone. The idea of shopping with a friend, of whom she has many, never occurred to her.

Networking

Women who are not dreadfully but only partially damaged by narcissistic mothers can be helped to see the value of friendship. We have seen a number of patients who need to dispose of friends who also need to merge or be independent, or who, on the other end of the spectrum, are envious, jealous, competitive, and undermining. There is a children's rhyme that says, "A friend is one who shares your woes and cuts them right in two; a friend is one who shares your joys and doubles them for you." Goldberg (1990[94]) discusses the history of the feminist movement in the context of "affirmative friendships." She starts with consciousness-raising groups that evolved in the 1960s and then addresses the evolving therapeutic effect of women's groups in the 1970s and 1980s. Goldberg notes the fact that many women lose something that is important for mental health: the closeness and bonding of women friends. She points to the value of women's psychotherapy groups in helping women find and regain the ability to relate to other women.

In those cases in which a psychotherapy group is not required, women have much to gain from women's networks. Bernstein and Warner (1984a[95]) have discussed the repetition of the old ambivalent struggles with the mother that are repeated in latency relationships between girls. Girls seem to reject the team spirit necessary for team sports in favor of latency intrigues involving female cliques and a changing hierarchical order of best friends. When the struggle remains unresolved through adolescence, there remains a legacy of ambivalence, competition, jealousy, and "cattiness" that results in recurrent reciprocal undermining of self-esteem.

Women are often able to organize effectively for altruistic and charitable pursuits. Yet very few papers or books are written by women as collaborators. When women organized feminist groups against men and male chauvinism, they found a target for their ambivalence and hostility. The backlash has unfortunately led to a loss in the initially promising advances for women.

If women need to create a supportive sisterhood, it is necessary to recognize the basic psychodynamic problems in relationship to self-esteem that paralyze their efforts. It is also necessary for women to categorize and learn to understand and cope with "problem" women who interfere in arenas where women are attempting to advance themselves and maintain their self-esteem. The authors have undertaken to present workshops for women in the medicinal professions in regard to this problem. The principles can be generalized to other careers, to schools, and to charitable and other voluntary organizations (see Appendix E).

Most women continue to have lines of development for self-esteem regulation, as well as affective and communicative styles, that are separate and distinct from those of most men. Women are still buffeted about by mixed messages concerning their femininity. We think that our data demonstrate the toll that is exacted in terms of a spectrum disorder of self-esteem regulation. We need to work with patients, colleagues, and friends—male and female—to encourage better, rather than more damaging, adaptations.

Notes

1. Freud S: Some psychical consequences of the anatomical distinction between the sexes (1925), in The Standard Edition of the Complete Psychological Works of Sigmund Freud, Vol 19. Translated and edited by Strachey J. London, Hogarth Press, 1961, pp 241–258
2. Horney K: Feminine Psychology. Edited by Kelman H. New York, WW Norton, 1967
3. Freud S: On narcissism: an introduction (1914a), in The Standard Edition of the Complete Psychological Works of Sigmund Freud, Vol 14. Translated and edited by Strachey J. London, Hogarth Press, 1957, pp 67–102
4. Winnicott DW: The theory of the parent-infant relationship. Int J Psychoanal 41:585–595, 1960
5. Reich A: Pathological forms of self-esteem regulation. Psychoanal Study Child 15:215, 1960
6. Spitz RA, Wolf KM: Anaclitic depression: an inquiry into the genesis of psychiatric conditions in early childhood. Psychoanal Study Child 2:313–342, 1946a
7. Erikson EH: Childhood and Society. New York, WW Norton, 1950
8. Freud S: Remembering, repeating and working-through (further recommendations on the technique of psycho-analysis III) (1914b), in The Standard Edition of the Complete Psychological Works of Sigmund Freud, Vol 12. Translated and edited by Strachey J. London, Hogarth Press, 1958, pp 145–156
9. Jacobson E: The Self and the Object World. New York, International Universities Press, 1964
10. Reich A: Narcissistic object choice in women. J Am Psychoanal Assoc 1:22–44, 1953
11. Bernstein AE, Warner GM: Women Treating Women. New York, International Universities Press, 1984b
12. Chodorow N: The Reproduction of Mothering: Psychoanalysis and the Sociology of Gender. Berkeley, CA, University of California Press, 1978

13. Friday N: My Mother, My Self. New York, Dell, 1978
14. Abelin EL: The role of the father in the separation-individuation process, in Separation-Individuation: Essays in Honor of Margaret S. Mahler. Edited by McDevitt JB, Settlage CF. New York, International Universities Press, 1971, pp 229–252
15. Klein M (with Joan Reviere): Love, Hate and Reparation. London, Hogarth Press, 1953
16. Surrey JL: Eating problems as a reflection of women's development. The Stone Center for Developmental Services and Studies, Working Papers, Wellesley, MA, 1985, No 83-06:l–7
17. Jordan JV: The meaning of mutuality. The Stone Center for Developmental Services and Studies, Work in Progress, Wellesley, MA, 1986, No 86-23
18. Gilligan C: In a Different Voice. Cambridge, MA, Harvard University Press, 1982
19. Rose R: Review of Tannen D: You Just Don't Understand: Women and Men in Conversation. *New York Times Book Review*, Aug 26, 1990, p 27
20. Stiver I: The meaning of "dependency" in female-male relationships. The Stone Center for Developmental Services and Studies, Working Papers, Wellesley, MA, 1984, No 83-07:1–12
21. Miller JB: Toward a New Psychology of Women. Boston, MA, Beacon Press, 1976
22. Miller JB: The construction of anger in women and men. The Stone Center for Developmental Services and Studies, Work in Progress, Wellesley, MA, 1983, No 83-01:l–7
23. Broverman IK, Broverman DM, Clarkson FE: Sex role stereotypes and clinical judgments of mental health. J Consult Clin Psychol 34:1–7, 1970
24. Nadelson CC, Notman MT, Bennett MB: Success or failure: psychotherapeutic considerations for women in conflict. Am J Psychiatry 135:1092–1096, 1978
25. Stiver I: Work inhibitions in women. The Stone Center for Developmental Services and Studies, Work in Progress, Wellesley, MA, 1983, No 82-03:1–11
26. Gilson E, Kane S: Unnecessary Choices: The Hidden Life of the Executive Woman. New York, William Morrow, 1987
27. McIntosh P: Feeling like a fraud. The Stone Center for Developmental Services and Studies, Work in Progress, Wellesley, MA, 1985, No 85-18:1–17
28. Dohrenwend BS: Social status and stressful life events. J Pers Soc Psychol 28:225–235, 1973
29. Gilligan C: Women's place in the man's life cycle. Harvard University Review 49:431–446, 1979

30. Schuckit MA: Current therapeutic options in the management of typical anxiety. J Clin Psychiatry 42(no 11, sec 2):15–26, 1981
31. Benzodiazepines: use, overuse, misuse, abuse (editorial). Lancet 1:1101–1102, 1978
32. Greenblatt DJ, Shader R: Benzodiazepines in Clinical Practice. New York, Raven, 1974
33. Tallman JF, Paul SM, Skolnick P, et al: Receptors for the age of anxiety: pharmacology of the benzodiazepines. Science 207:274–281, 1980
34. Masotti M, Guidotti A, Costa E: Characterization of benzodiazepine and gamma-aminobutyric acid recognition sites and their hydrogenous modulators. J Neurosci 1:409–418, 1981
35. Marks I, Lader M: Anxiety states (anxiety neurosis): a review. J Nerv Ment Dis 156:3–18, 1973
36. Weissman MM: The epidemiology of anxiety disorders: rates, risks, familial patterns. Paper presented at the National Institute of Mental Health Conference on Anxiety and Anxiety Disorders, Sterling Forest Conference Center, Tuxedo, NY, September 1983
37. Uhlenhuth EH, Balter MB, Mellinger GD, et al: Symptom checklist syndromes in the general population. Arch Gen Psychiatry 40:1167–1173, 1983
38. Johnstone EC, Cunningham Owens DG, Frith CD, et al: Neurotic illness and its response to anxiolytic and antidepressant treatment. Psychol Med 10:321–328, 1980
39. Kahn RJ, McNair DM, Lipman RS, et al: Imipramine and chlordiazepoxide in depression and anxiety disorders, II: efficacy in anxious outpatients. Arch Gen Psychiatry 43:79–85, 1986
40. Kleber RJ: A double-blind comparative study of desipramine hydrochloride and diazepam in the control of mixed anxiety/depression symptomatology. J Clin Psychiatry 40:165–170, 1979
41. Rickels K, Csanalosi I, Chung HR, et al: Amitriptyline in anxious-depressed outpatients: a controlled study. Am J Psychiatry 131:25–30, 1974
42. Shammas E: Controlled comparison of bromazepam, amitriptyline, and placebo in anxiety-depressive neurosis. Diseases of the Nervous System 38:201–207, 1977
43. Marks J: The Benzodiazepines: Use, Overuse, Misuse, and Abuse. Lancaster, UK, MT-P Press, 1978
44. Gorman JM, Levy GF, Liebowitz MR, et al: Effect of acute ß-adrenergic blockade on lactate-induced panic. Arch Gen Psychiatry 40:1079–1082, 1983

45. Gorman JM, Askanazi J, Liebowitz MR, et al: Response to hyperventilation in a group of patients with panic disorder. Am J Psychiatry 141:857–861, 1984
46. Hollander E, Liebowitz MR, Gorman JM: Anxiety disorders, in American Psychiatric Press Textbook of Psychiatry. Edited by Talbott JA, Hales RE, Yudofsky SC. Washington, DC, American Psychiatric Press, 1987, pp 443–491
47. Pitts FN, McClune JN: Lactate metabolism in anxiety neurosis. N Engl J Med 277:1329–1336, 1967
48. Skolnick P, Paul SM: Benzodiazepine receptors in the central nervous system. Int Rev Neurobiol 23:103–140, 1982
49. Freud S: Heredity and the aetiology of the neuroses (1896), in The Standard Edition of the Complete Psychological Works of Sigmund Freud, Vol 3. Translated and edited by Strachey J. London, Hogarth Press, 1962, pp 141–156
50. Freud S: Sexuality in the aetiology of the neuroses (1898), in The Standard Edition of the Complete Psychological Works of Sigmund Freud, Vol 3. Translated and edited by Strachey J. London, Hogarth Press, 1962, pp 259–285
51. Freud S: Extracts from the Fliess papers: Draft B, the aetiology of the neuroses (1893b), in The Standard Edition of the Complete Psychological Works of Sigmund Freud, Vol 1. Translated and edited by Strachey J. London, Hogarth Press, 1966, pp 179–184
52. Freud S: Inhibitions, symptoms and anxiety (1926a), in The Standard Edition of the Complete Psychological Works of Sigmund Freud, Vol 20. Translated and edited by Strachey J. London, Hogarth Press, 1959, pp 75–175
53. Freud S: Analysis of a phobia in a five-year-old boy (1909a), in The Standard Edition of the Complete Psychological Works of Sigmund Freud, Vol 10. Translated and edited by Strachey J. London, Hogarth Press, 1955, pp 1–149
54. Klein DF: Delineation of two drug-responsive anxiety syndromes. Psychopharmacologia 5:397–408, 1964
55. Klein DF: Anxiety reconceptualized, in Anxiety: New Research and Changing Concepts. Edited by Klein DF, Rabkin JG. New York, Raven, 1981, pp 235–265
56. Mahler MS: Thoughts about development and individuation. Psychoanal Study Child 18:307–324, 1963
57. Mahler MS: On human symbiosis and the vicissitudes of individualism. J Am Psychoanal Assoc 15:740–763, 1967
58. Mahler MS, Furer M: Certain aspects of the separation-individuation phase. Psychoanal Q 32:1–14, 1963

59. Mahler MS, La Perriere K: Mother-child interaction during separation-individuation. Psychoanal Q 34:483–498, 1965
60. Jaffe JH: Drug addiction and drug abuse, in The Pharmacological Basis of Therapeutics. Edited by Goodman LS, Gilman A. New York, Macmillan, 1980, pp 535–584
61. Inciardi JA: Over-the-counter drugs: epidemiology, adverse reactions, overdose deaths, and mass media promotion. Journal of Addictive Diseases 3:253–272, 1977
62. Goodwin DW, Guze SB: Psychiatric Diagnosis, 2nd Edition. New York, Oxford University Press, 1979
63. National Council on Alcoholism, Criteria, Criteria Committee: Criteria for the diagnosis of alcoholism. Am J Psychiatry 129:127–135, 1972
64. Schuckit MA: Alcoholism and sociopathy—diagnostic confusion. Quarterly Journal of Studies on Alcohol 34:157–164, 1973
65. Haglund RMJ, Schuckit MA: The epidemiology of alcoholism, in Alcoholism: Development, Consequences and Interventions. Edited by Estes N, Heinemann E. St Louis, MO, CV Mosby, 1982, pp 32–48
66. Schuckit MA: A study of alcoholism with secondary depression. Am J Psychiatry 140:711–714, 1983
67. Schuckit MA, Winbeur R: A short-term follow-up of women alcoholics. Diseases of the Nervous System 33:672–678, 1972
68. Schuckit MA, Haglund RMJ: Etiological theories on alcoholism, in Alcoholism: Development, Consequences and Interventions. Edited by Estes N, Heinemann E. St Louis, MO, CV Mosby, 1982, pp 16–31
69. Korsten MA, Matsuzaki S, Feinman L, et al: High blood acetaldehyde levels after ethanol administration: difference between alcoholic and non-alcoholic subjects. N Engl J Med 292:386–389, 1975
70. Loebuck JB, Kessler RG: The Etiology of Alcoholism. Springfield, IL, Charles C Thomas, 1971
71. Schuckit MA, Rayser V: Ethanol ingestion: differences in blood acetaldehyde concentrations in relatives of alcoholics and controls. Science 203:54–55, 1979
72. Bohman M, Sigvardsson S, Cloninger CR: Maternal inheritance of alcohol abuse: cross-fostering analysis of adopted women. Arch Gen Psychiatry 38:965–969, 1981
73. Yandow V: Alcoholism in women. Psychiatric Annals 19:243–247, 1989
74. Wisnack S, Wisnack R, Kassan A, et al: Drinking and drinking problems among women in a U.S. National Survey. Alcohol Health and Research World 9:3–13, 1985

75. Berny MD, Merry J: Alcoholism and eating disorders in women of fertile age. Br J Addict 81:685–687, 1986
76. Rohsenow D, Corbett R, Devine D: Molested as children: a hidden contribution to substance abuse? J Subst Abuse Treat 5:13–18, 1988
77. Vaillant G: Dangers of psychotherapy in the treatment of alcoholism, in Dynamic Approaches to Understanding and Treatment of Alcoholism. Edited by Bean HH, Zisberg NE. New York, Free Press, 1981, pp 36–55
78. Beeson W, McCollough E: Aesthetic Surgery of the Aging Face. St Louis, MO, CV Mosby, 1986, p 1
79. Hyman DA: Aesthetics and ethics: the implications of cosmetic surgery. Perspect Biol Med 33:190–202, 1990
80. Napolion A, Lewis CM: Psychological considerations in lipoplasty: the problematic or "special care" patient. Ann Plast Surg 23:430–432, 1989
81. Napolion A, Lewis CM: Psychological considerations in the elderly cosmetic surgery candidates. Ann Plast Surg 24:165–169, 1990
82. Wengle HP: The psychology of cosmetic surgery: a critical overview of the literature, 1960–62, Part 1. Ann Plast Surg 16:435–443, 1986
83. Coleman WP: Dermatologic cosmetic surgery. J Dermatol Surg Oncol 16:170–176, 1990
84. Sanford L, Donovan M: Women and Self-Esteem. Garden City, NY, Anchor Press/Doubleday, 1984
85. Chernin K: The Obsession. New York, Harper & Row, 1981
86. Freedman R: Beauty Bound. Lexington, MA, DC Heath, 1986
87. Stannard V: The mask of beauty, in Women in a Sexist Society. Edited by Gornick V, Moran B. New York, Basic Books, 1971, pp 118–130
88. Musa K, Roach M: Adolescent appearance and self concept. Adolescence 8:385–394, 1973
89. Dacey J: Adolescents Today. Santa Monica, CA, Goodyear, 1979
90. Loombs M: By Food Possessed. Women's Sports, February 1982, pp 12–18
91. Hoffman, Dustin. New York Times, December 21, 1983, pp 6–11
92. Woolf V: A Room of One's Own. New York, Harcourt, Brace, 1919, pp 35–36
93. Surrey JL: Self in relation: a theory of women's development. Presentation at The Stone Center for Developmental Services and Studies Colloquium Series, Wellesley, MA, November 1983
94. Goldberg MC: Women's friendships—women's groups. Psychiatric Annals 20:398–401, 1990
95. Bernstein AE, Warner GM: Female psychology and networking problems among female professionals. J Am Med Wom Assoc 39:156–158, 1984a

Chapter 4

Relationships, Careers, and Motherhood

Person (1989[1]) has commented that "many of us who are not in love long to be. We know only too well the glories we are missing. Friends and family are no protection against such loneliness . . . "(p. 39). She goes on to note the importance of being the most important person in someone else's life and says that this is one of the defining premises of passionate love.

Love is an extremely random and irrational experience. It can come at any time whether wished for or not. Falling in love, particularly "love at first sight," is a phenomenon of projection and projective identification. Faults are denied. Characteristics and attributes are idealized both before and even after the real qualities of the love object are known. The phenomenon of limerance involves obsessional idealized thinking, mood swings, and somatization (Person 1989[1]).

In Western culture, where we have been free to arrange our own liaisons, cohabitation, and marriage, we have not done well in terms of outcome. One estimate of the heterosexual divorce rate in the early 1980s was 49% (Glick 1984[2]). Research has shown that partners' stubborn commitment to maintaining their marriages and working out their problems is the primary factor in lasting marriages. At a 50th (golden) wedding celebration, someone asked one of the spouses whether divorce had ever been contemplated. The answer was, "Murder, maybe, but divorce, never." That thought had nothing to do with emotionally or physically battering relationships. It implied that divorce was not an option, and obviously neither was murder. Rage could be felt and managed without recourse to the thought of dissolution of the relationship.

Eastern cultures or subsets of western populations still rely on arranged marriages. In many cases bride and bridegroom never meet alone. These marriages are more stable. Happiness by Western standards is difficult to gauge. Authors writing about Moslem women have pointed out that happiness seems to depend more on reliability and the ability to provide the necessities of life than on any notion of romantic love (Bumiller 1990[3]; Friedl 1988[4]).

It is *not* true that women fall in love more frequently, blindly, or passionately than men. It *is* true that they seem more willing than their male counterparts to make sacrifices and accept difficulties for the sake of establishing or maintaining a committed relationship. Commitment appears to be more important to women, and it seems that many men actively try to avoid it.

Freud's contributions to the psychodynamic understanding of love have to do with the psychology of men (Freud 1910,[5] 1912a,[6] 1918[1917][7]) and with transference love (Freud 1915[1914][8]).

Kernberg (1974a,[9] 1974b[10]) reviewed the psychoanalytic literature in regard to both normal and pathological love and then formulated his own comprehensive theory. He categorizes the development of the mature capacity for falling and remaining in love into three developmental tasks that must be integrated. First, Kernberg states that infantile bodily erotism must be transformed into the tenderness of need-gratifying constant relationships. Citing the work of Jacobson (1964[11]), Bak (1973[12]), Bergmann (1971[13]), and Josselyn (1971[14]), Kernberg concludes that mature love requires both the ability to mourn the lost objects of childhood and the capacity for guilt and concern that results in a deepening awareness of the self and the other. In addition, one must have the capacity for empathy and for higher-level identifications. By these Kernberg means the capacity to empathize and identify with the love object in a way that, as Balint (1948,[15] p. 115) notes, the interests, wishes, feelings, sensitivity, and shortcomings of the partner attain, or are supposed to attain, about the same importance as one's own. A requisite for mature love is the integration of full genitality into the love relationship. For Kernberg it is this second factor that transforms *falling* in love into the state of *being* in love. To attain full genitality requires the complete integration of the primitive longing for contact with specific bodily surfaces into genitality. Arlow et al. (1968[16]) have written about the compulsive longing for specific body parts representing a regression to one or more split off infantile erogenous zones. This regression precludes a full range of sexual experience, which includes integration of pregenital erotism in the context of a total object relationship that is constant.

Kernberg (1974b[10]) described the sublimation of the oedipal phase of development into the love relationship and the acceptance of the value system and ideals expressed by the object. This latter task would seem to us to be particularly difficult in view of the real differences of values and goal orientation between men and women. May (1969[17]) has stressed the role of the capacity for tenderness and for full identification with the love object, without losing one's own identity. This is a point of difficulty for many women who otherwise do not have major psychopathology.

Another aspect of the emotional reaction that cements being and staying in love is the gratification derived not only from one's own orgasm but from the orgasm of the sexual partner. This requires the ability to identify with the partner. Kernberg (1974b,[10] p. 751) calls this the "capacity for transcendence." By this he means the ability to become one both physically and psychologically with another person. According to Kernberg, orgasm that binds two persons reflects the ability to achieve a level of fusion that is not so primitive as to obliterate one partner's individuality; rather orgasm in a mature love relationship represents a mature sexual identification with the partner while confirming one's own individuality and sexual identification. There is aggression involved in mature love relations. Partners, while making love, may occasionally enact pregenital needs using the other as an object for this enactment. If the other partner is able to collude and be empathic, then excitement and resolution are maximized for both partners. Of course, on another occasion the roles have to be reversed in terms of which partner is used as an object for the other partner's enactment of pregenital needs.

The most severely disturbed narcissistically disordered individuals are capable of transient infatuations and sexual excitement. Underlying unconscious elements of greed, exploitation, and the need to escape involvement preclude remaining in a mature love relationship. The Don Juan syndrome (i.e., compulsive sexual conquest of many women) has been described in the general and the psychiatric literature (Bernstein 1978[18]). This syndrome is not confined to men. Patients with borderline personality disorder cannot achieve mature love. They tend to develop intense love attachments, primitive idealization, splitting, and projection, all of which eventually destroy the love relationship. These patients are strongly motivated to seek help because their maladaptive defensive mechanisms cause problems in other areas as well (e.g., friendship, work).

Women patients with hysterical personality disorders accompanied by masochistic or self-sacrificial behavior have guilt over establishing mature love relationships with a man who unconsciously represents the forbidden oedipal object. Patients with other personality disorders need to conquer and devalue their love objects. This need to spoil what is good results in both loss of interest and loss of sexual excitement.

There are patients with severe personality pathology and problems in object relationships who experience a relative freedom in the expression of genital activity despite the absence of mature object relationships. This hypertrophy of genitality may represent a defense against frightening and frustrating oral needs. The infantile defensive splitting of overwhelming early oral needs may lead to a premature development of the Oedipus complex. This premature development interferes with the normal process of infantile polymorphously perverse sexuality. When integration of primitive sexuality occurs with integration of internalized object relationships before triangulation, a normal superego develops and prohibitions against primitive sexuality then develop. With this inhibition, romantic idealization develops. With the renunciation of the oedipal wishes at a normal time, total object relationships form in which guilt over aggression becomes tenderness and gratitude for love received. Residual guilt is repaired by giving love. Sometimes the deepening of a relationship may result in unconscious conflicts over oedipal issues that may prevent the individual from remaining in love.

Marriage

According to Erikson (1968a[19]), the marital relationship consists of two fully differentiated individuals, both with clear sex roles who work together to satisfy each other, themselves, and their responsibilities to society. Fairbairn (1954[20]) further elaborates this conception of mature dependence, stating that it "is a relationship involving evenly matched giving and taking between two differentiated individuals who are mutually dependent and between whom there is no disparity of dependence" (p. 145). This is a highly idealized concept of marriage. Many couples are not capable of sustained mutuality. In addition, radical changes in terms of society and individuals' concepts of sexual roles have generated a significant percentage of couples who view themselves as egalitarian within their gender roles in the marriage. Marriage is not always viewed as the opportunity to bear children and thus provide the next generation. Rather, it is frequently viewed as an opportunity for individual self-actualization within a partnership.

Ninety-five percent of contemporary Americans will marry at some time in their lives (Glick 1975[21]). A larger proportion of young adults reach the age of 30 without being married; however, the proportion of adults who reach 40 without marrying is lower than it has ever been before. It is unclear as yet whether this represents a new trend toward postponement of marriage until later in life or a new population of young people who will never marry (Nadelson and Notman 1981[22]). Goldberg (1982[23]) notes that we have remarkably high rates of marriage, divorce, remarriage, and divorce in remarriage. Marriage remains popular in the United States. In 1962 a study of unmarried college students revealed that only 2% of them had little or no interest in a future marriage (Bell 1971[24]). In 1972, however, 40% of senior college women stated that they were uncertain as to whether or not they would marry, and many viewed traditional marriages obsolete or inappropriate for them (Bird 1972[25]).

Numerous factors have contributed to this shift. The advent of safe and effective birth control has allowed both men and women to fulfill themselves sexually outside of marriage. Traditional sex roles are being questioned. Many adults are moving toward a more egalitarian pattern of relating with one another. Others have traditional values, and still others remain conflicted and caught between traditional and egalitarian roles. There has been a shift in contemporary values regarding women's roles at home and in the workplace. Since the 1970s more women have entered the workplace, and it is likely that they will remain in larger numbers for both economic and self-actualizing reasons. Institutions, corporations, and other employers have made no responsive change in their work policies to allow for marital and family life. Our institutions are therefore no longer supportive of the nuclear family. This process, combined with the uncertainty regarding what it is we should value, has led to what many have called the crisis of the family. Brazelton (1988[26]) has commented on this situation with regard to the lack of support married couples have in raising children. We will try to provide an overview of contemporary marriage, keeping in mind this broad range of possibilities.

Despite the wide variety of marital attitudes and structures we have outlined, there are some characteristics which, from a psychodynamic standpoint, are similar in all marriages. The intrapsychic factors involved in the choice of a mate are complicated. Freud (1915[1914][8]) contended that a person chooses a mate based on an anaclitic or narcissistic focus. An anaclitic choice is oriented toward nurturance and protection and the gratification of dependency needs, and a narcissistic choice involves a selection of a mate who represents the ideal self, a projected ego ideal, or a recaptured past self, a projected past self, or a person who was part of the self in the past. Nadelson (1978,[27] p. 105) has summarized the way in which couples are often drawn to one another via unconscious signals that enable them to recognize the possibility of resolving conflicts in each of them as individuals within marriage. Relief from past rivalries and repressed sexual feelings as well as identification with the loving aspects of parents can also be obtained via mate selection. Marriages can provide fulfillment from frustrated longings and offer new opportunities for self-realization and a successful reworking of unresolved issues with parents.

Marriage can also become a repository for unresolved conflicts, especially if mates project the hated aspects of themselves onto their partner and become locked into a sadomasochistic interaction. Marriages like these are psychologically stalemated because the partnership is based on a collusive process of mutual projective identifications (Main 1966[28]). In these marriages a joint ego boundary exists (Dicks 1963[29]), and instead of growth promotion with the strengthening of object relationships, the marriage is defensive in that it enables each partner to split off from unconscious objects that are perceived as potentially destructive. In contrast, mature partners can view each other as whole objects, and the aggressions can be tolerated without denial or projection and accepted by the other partner without loss of dignity or self-esteem. Marriage becomes the adult equivalent of a parent/child relationship. One can regress to a state of helplessness and lack of control without feeling threatened by annihilation, a situation that is crucial for adult sexuality as well as other adult interactions (Nadelson 1978,[27] p. 108).

In addition to the commonality of intrapsychic issues, each marriage has a life cycle related to the critical stages in the individual life cycle of each of the spouses (Berman and Lief 1975[30]; Blanck and Blanck 1968[31]). According to this concept of a marital life cycle, change or conflict can occur in a marital relationship at points of individual developmental change or crises. Tasks, expectations, demands, and experiences can vary through the course of the life cycle. Children are born, careers rise and fall, relationships with relatives and friends change, the physical environment varies, children leave home, and losses and illnesses occur. If the couple does not respond to these changes in a complementary fashion, conflict arises within the marriage (Nadelson 1978,[27] p. 104).

Several classifications of problematic marital relationships based on the interaction of mates have been reviewed by Nadelson (1978,[27] p. 112). The first classification, developed by Mittelmann (1948[32]), is described as follows:

1. One partner is emotionally detached, and the other craves affection.
2. Husband and wife engage in rivalry for aggressive dominance.

3. One partner is helpless, and the other appears overtly competent and strong but in reality is in a dependency role. (This situation is a quite common one given the characteristic way in which women have been socialized and because of their psychological development.)
4. One of the partners alternates between periods of assertiveness and dependency, and the other alternates between periods of helplessness and unsatisfied affectional needs.

Another set of conflictual marital patterns has been defined by P. A. Martin (1976[33]) and includes the following:

1. The relationship between a hysterical wife and an obsessional husband with limited intimacy
2. The relationship between a hysterical husband and an obsessional wife when dependency issues are prominent
3. The relationship between two people with similar rather than complementary dynamics in which each expects the other to be responsible for gratifying needs
4. The paranoid relationship, in which mistrust and jealousy are prominent

A third set of partner profiles—one that focuses on clarifying the interactional dimensions—includes equal, romantic, parental, childlike, rational, companionate, and parallel dimensions (Sager 1976[34]).

Most marriages in the United States begin with romantic love. Quadrio (1986[35]), drawing on the theories of Kohut (1971,[36] 1977[37]) and Mahler et al. (1975[38]), compares this stage of the marital relationship with that of the early mother/child relationship before self-differentiation has occurred. Couples who remain in this state have difficulty accepting children into the family because they disrupt the symbiotic dyad. These couples remain vulnerable to crises as either life circumstances or time eventually erodes this unrealistic symbiosis. Another typical way in which couples can become stuck in this phase of relating involves the wife's constant fulfilling of selfobject functions for her husband and later for her children. In true selfobject fashion she hears from people only when she has failed to meet their needs. Women combining this marital scenario with professional careers will most of the time experience burnout.

There is often a transitional period during which the couple are no longer passionately in love but are not yet settled into a pattern of sustaining love characteristic of successful long-term marriages (Fogarty 1985[39]). This period may be painful and unsettling, with each partner intermittently expressing anxiety and dissatisfaction with the marriage. Demands for closeness intersperse with demands for autonomy. Extramarital lovers are common during this period. The couple may progress to a more enduring form of love involving feelings of affection and loyalty with the capacity to internalize a constant, positively cathected internal image of each other and thus avoid the need to seek gratification outside the relationship. This level of interaction will allow periods of distancing and coming together. Mothers may be preoccupied with young children, fathers may focus intensely on work, dual-career couples may become involved or disillusioned with their work in cycles that do not exactly mesh, illness and aging occur, and the couple will still remain bonded. Quadrio (1986,[35] p. 2232) calls this "transmuting internalization."[†]

Marriage can play an important role in the self-actualization of women. A recent study by Inglis and Greenglass (1989[40]) found that, despite the belief that marriage involves much work, women are more motivated to marry. Women have always defined themselves in the context of relationships. Until recently society defined a woman's status according to her relationships, starting with her family of origin and then with her husband's status. The healthy, well-differentiated woman values herself for her capacity to make and maintain mutually satisfac-

[†]This mature, enduring love is characterized by Shakespeare's sonnet, "Love is not time's fool though rosy lips and cheeks within his bending cycles compass come. Love alters not with his brief hours and weeks, but bears it out even to the edge of doom."

tory relationships and for her capacity to be responsible and constructive to others. Therefore, many women give priority to the choice of a husband, marriage, and family rather than the choice of a career. Intimacy and generativity may actually precede or ultimately become intertwined with identity formation.

Some young women choose to postpone marriage until established in a career of occupation. Identity formation precedes intimacy and generativity. The value of relationships is still likely to be much higher for women than for their male counterparts. These women have a clearer definition of their own values, goals, satisfactions, and activities, and may be limited in their choices of a potential mate and constrained in childbearing by the "biological clock." Another group of women marry young but attempt to simultaneously establish career identities and identities as wives and mothers. Therapists can expect to see a continuum of women, ranging from those whose self-actualization is concentrated upon their marriages to that yet small group of women who meet Adams's (1971[41]) criteria for successful adaptation as singles—namely, they are economically independent and socially and psychologically autonomous, and have a preference to be single.

Contemporary families are more flexible regarding the expectations of marriage for their daughters. Some families actually stress career over marriage, and others struggle with their own ambivalent expectations for their developing daughters. Inheritance and succession, once highly valued by families, have also come to be less important, placing less pressure on females to marry because of familial expectations. A woman's sense of how to fulfill her gender role is also in a state of flux. Many women do not feel truly feminine unless they are providing for their husbands in all the traditional ways, caring for a home full time, and assuming primary responsibility for child rearing. Other women invested in traditional gender roles also have strong interests and drives toward career or work. Conflict may result, especially at times when the two value systems are mutually exclusive. Yet other women engage in partnerships with males who can adapt to their career goals. They may either remain childless or delegate child-rearing responsibilities to their mate or to a hired caregiver.

Women are handling their reproductive roles via a variety of pathways. Some women marry young and adopt the primary role of mother and housewife. Others return to school or work when their children are in school, and some return to work when their children leave home. These women at times discover and enjoy career aspirations for the first time in midlife. These women's goals may conflict with their husbands', who are focusing on retirement, relaxation, and enjoyment of their family. Another choice is to postpone childbearing until a career is well established (e.g., in the early 30s) and then attempt to combine career with parenthood. This may mean working on a "mommy track" until their children are somewhat older. Other women become pregnant for the first time in their late 30s or early 40s when contemporaries may be becoming grandmothers. Also, adoption is a choice at midlife and an option for single women who do not wish to marry.

The assumption of multiple roles is often a significant factor in marriage. Most women at some period are combining the roles of wife, mother, and career woman or worker. They achieve greater freedom of choice and greater economic strength and decision-making power within the marriage and a wider variety of potential satisfactions. These women are at risk because of increased stress from role overload and role conflicts. Working women perform a disproportionately high amount of household labor relative to their husbands (Krausz 1986[42]). Failure to reach an egalitarian balance may be either because men have been unwilling to accept responsibility for household labor or because women have been reluctant to relinquish this responsibility because of its connection to their role identity. Another conflict involves value and identity incongruity between work and home, where different behaviors, skills, and orientations are expected. A further area of conflict is socioeconomic. Some women define themselves and are defined by their husbands' or their own socioeconomic status. Others define themselves differently than society defines them.

Contemporary marriages may be traditional, transitional, or egalitarian. *Traditional marriages* are oriented toward child rearing and the solidity of the nuclear family, and sex roles are clear and complementary. Men are the breadwinners and primary authority figures, and women are the homemakers and mothers and fulfill the primary parental role. In *transitional families*, the husband and wife may both work but the wife's work is seen as secondary to the importance of the family life and adaptable to its needs. In addition, there may be some negotiating around sex roles and to what degree parenting and household tasks are shared. *Egalitarian marriages* are without strict gender roles. All tasks are shared and negotiated by the couple. There is equal commitment to job and child rearing.

Another way in which marital structures vary is with regard to the presence of children. Childless marriages may be viewed more positively and become more common than they were in the past. Childbearing occurs at variable stages of the life cycle, rather than just in early adulthood (Hunt and Hunt 1982[43]; Moore et al. 1984[44]; Ramu and Tavuchis 1986[45]; Veevers 1980[46]; Yogev and Vierra 1983[47]).

Marital structures can be defined in terms of the economic basis of the family in the following way:

1. Families in which only the husband works
2. Dual-earner families
3. Two-paycheck families (i.e., husbands work full time and provide the majority of the family income, and wife works part time or full time in order to maintain the family standard of living). If work shifts are alternated to provide for child care, the couple have little time together.
4. Dual-career families (i.e., work provides income and enhances career development and self-actualization for husband and wife). Conflicts arise when career goals cannot be synchronized with family needs or when career crises occur concomitant with family crises.
5. Commuter marriage, a form of dual-career marriage in which husband and wife reside part time in separate geographic locations to accommodate career goals, thus spending limited time together
6. Two-person careers in which one person, usually the male, is involved in a lucrative, time-intensive career and the spouse devotes full time to facilitate that career
7. House-husband families in which the mother works outside of the home

Some researchers have attempted to analyze longitudinal marital satisfaction. Schlesinger (1982[48]), reviewing the literature in North American families, found a positive correlation between the capacity to communicate, the capacity to share power, and the partners' mutual reports of respect and trust. Gottman and Krokoff (1989[49]), in a recent longitudinal study, found that the capacity to disagree and to express anger correlated positively with long-term marital satisfaction, while defensiveness, stubbornness, and withdrawal from interaction were found to be dysfunctional.

Marital conflict occurs because of differences in beliefs, interests, desires, values, or expectations, as well as from competition between the partners or differences in life stage or intrapsychic organization. Conflict does not necessarily mean that the partnership is threatened. If differences are communicated openly in the spirit of respect and trust, accommodations can generally be made, either immediately or over time.

Conflicts characterized by power struggles, coercion, deception, withdrawal, or repression of anger have a more negative outcome (Nadelson 1978[27]). Goldberg (1982[23]) has summarized common marital complaints as those involving 1) money, 2) sex, 3) child-rearing practices, 4) in-laws, 5) pregnancy and childbearing, and 6) alcohol and drug abuse. Green (1970[50]) conducted a survey that revealed the following conflicts: 1) lack of communication, 2) constant arguments, 3) unfulfilled emotional needs, 4) sexual dissatisfaction, 5) financial disagreement, 6) in-law trouble, 7) infidelity, 8) conflicts about children, 9) domineering spouse, 10) suspicious spouse, 11) alcoholism, and 12) physical attack or abuse.

Marital problems resulting from developmental life-cycle crises occur when one member of the couple is involved in a crisis and the other is not, or when both members of the couple are facing the same crisis but have different views regarding its resolution. Pivotal conflict points are 1) births of children, 2) children's departure to school, 3) children's leaving home, 4) problems with adult children, 5) adult children returning to live at home, 6) career spurts and successes that demand increased investment in career for either husband or wife, 7) career problems for either husband or wife, 8) retirement, 9) illness in the family, 10) deaths of parents, 11) geographic moves, 12) shifts in social relationships, and 13) losses and illnesses.

Difficulties around roles can occur whether or not the couple have different expectations of each of their fulfillment of gender roles or different expectations at different times. Although it has become popular to relate all marital distress toward role strain or multiple roles, the intrapsychic determinants of marital problems remain. H. Greenbaum (1983[51]) has discussed the way in which marital couples reenact the dysfunctional marital interactions of their parents or reenact patterns of significant childhood objects at specific times in their marriage in an "unfolding of identifications" (E. Greenbaum 1973[52]). Calogeras (1985[53]) and Finkelstein (1988[54]) have both discussed marital problems in terms of object-relations theory and the negative interaction of individual character styles. Individuals with more primitive defenses have fluid ego boundaries, and there is much projection and projective identification between the partners, resulting in a collusive, defensive style that prohibits further differentiation and improvement for either member of the couple. These mechanisms exist in higher-functioning individuals as well and determine how well a couple can manage conflicts.

In approaching treatment for women with marital problems from a psychodynamic viewpoint, the therapist needs to be aware of several factors, as summarized by Nadelson (1978,[27] pp. 114–115). An individual approach can be taken if the woman has intrapsychic issues contributing to her marital problems that can be changed and if her partner changes in response. This approach allows individuals to assume responsibility for their own personal growth and change and permits independent work if a divorce is being contemplated. It also protects the confidentiality of the woman. Couples work is indicated if the individual therapy has failed, stalemated, or cannot be utilized; if the woman has a sudden onset of symptoms related to marital conflicts; if the couple together request treatment; or if it appears that an improvement in the woman's individual psychopathology will create such a disequilibrium in the marriage that the couple will not be able to manage it without assistance.

A variety of techniques for psychodynamically oriented marital therapy have evolved and been elaborated by Nadelson (1978,[27] pp. 114–116). Either a supportive, directive approach stressing current life issues and crises and sociocultural factors or a more long-term approach focusing upon the unconscious conflictual elements of the couple's relationship may be appropriate. Resolving crises and ordering the environment optimally, resolving individual psychopathology, and understanding and improving reciprocal interactions are important aspects of the therapeutic approach. The couple may be seen separately or together. Co-therapists or groups may be utilized.

Borderline Narcissistic Psychopathology

A 28-year-old mental health professional sought treatment, wishing a divorce because her husband refused to have children. The two had had unsuccessful sex therapy for his impotence. She was involved in a serious love affair with a married man that had been going on for 2 years. She divorced her husband and continued her love affair, hoping that her lover would divorce his wife. When this seemed a possibility, she became panicky and broke off the relationship. She went on to a series of lovers who functioned as part objects for the patient. Some were good in bed, while others took care of her but were immature and/or unsuccessful in their own lives. She was unstable in her work relationships. She was estranged from a chaotic family with a profoundly disturbed and abusive older sibling with whom her mother sided, although her father favored her. She had long-standing mutually supportive friendships with women. During her father's protracted illness prior to his death, a reunion was achieved. In dreams the patient understood her father's cruelty, which she had denied in favor of a formulation about his passive compliance.

She became involved with a man who exhibited lack of constancy and even cruelty to his divorced family. Exciting sex, frightening and demeaning because it was polymorphously perverse, accompanied the expectation of financial security and physical shelter. A depressive episode and a period of almost indiscriminate promiscuity followed the breakup of this relationship. Her guilt and rage about her mother, who had reversed the mother/child caretaking relationship, were analyzed. The patient handled her next heterosexual relationship in a calmer, more reflective way. She began to feel attractive instead of seeing herself as merely being "able to give off sexual vibes." She valued her work, her intelligence, and her specific ability to empathize and understand the psychology of others. She had been a person with borderline functioning and narcissistic depletion whose demands played out most disastrously in love relationships. By mourning the mother she never had, the patient allowed herself to develop a mature love relationship.

Dependent Personality Disorder

A 24-year-old single patient came to treatment after an affair with a married man ended when his wife became pregnant. The patient was the "baby" in a family of brothers. She had relied on her parents and siblings for emotional support despite her own attractiveness and intellectual and artistic talents. She left therapy to accept a geographically distant opportunity in her field. She met a man younger than herself and became so preoccupied with him and with an intercurrent physical illness that she rationalized not working toward her goal of actualizing her artistic potential. As the "girl" whom her parents expected simply to marry, as her mother had done, the woman experienced a conflict between realizing her artistic and intellectual goals and having a committed relationship. Eager for a full object relationship and a gratifying sexual relationship, she sacrificed these goals for her dependency needs. Shy and timid in her relationships, she was unable or unwilling to assert herself as an equal for fear of object loss. The ability to form a mature love relationship awaits her ability to mature, individuate, and develop a stable self representation and concomitant self-esteem.

Control Issues

A patient in her 50s came to treatment when her second husband moved out. She was unsatisfied with his income, especially because so much of it went to support three adult children with major problems who were not making it on their own. The patient needed to prove in therapy that her philosophy of cutting them loose was correct, and she had a difficult time envisioning the fact that each time she attacked these children, her husband redoubled his defensiveness. She was controlling both in the transference in therapy and at work. After interpretation she agreed to meet with her husband and listen to what he would say about their problems. As she began to look at her own angry and disappointed feelings in her father and his failure to provide for her mother, whom she had to support, she came to understand her husband's problems better. When she "got off his back," her husband discussed his anger and disappointment with his children in an atmosphere in which she could refrain from "rubbing it in." He acted to improve his business and get his children to be independent. She began to look back at her first marriage and say that she had tried to be the boss and that her first husband had openly resented her attempt to control. She wondered if she was responsible for her own children's unorthodox adaptations. When her grandchildren visited, she negotiated visiting times with her ex-husband without the rancor that had usually accompanied those occasions in the past. She remained relaxed and rational. This patient worked in a limited area of her pathology and was able to give up a critical and controlling attitude so that she could maintain a loving and gratifying relationship.

Failure or Oedipal Resolution

A woman in her mid-40s, a married mother of four grown children, was a recent professional school graduate and sought help because of work-related difficulties. These difficulties were a result not of her psychopathology but rather her status as an upper-class, highly sophisticated, educated member of what was generally considered a lower socioeconomic group. A second problem was the failure of her sexual relationship with her husband, for which she compensated by a series of extramarital affairs. She admired her husband's professional achievements and his functioning as a father. Her father had died before her birth. Although she had chosen her imagined oedipal object for marriage, she selected to go elsewhere for sexual gratification.

In joint therapy there was an attempt to work out some of the couple's interpersonal problems about her inheritance that she refused to share. The couple resumed sexual relationships, which she experienced as satisfying, but she nevertheless plunged headlong into another affair. Shortly thereafter her husband was killed. A year later she began another relationship, this time with a more appropriate man from the point of view of age and availability for a long-term relationship. Asked if she would marry him, the patient said, "Oh, but I was married." She unconsciously understands that marriage would interfere with her sexuality.

A Woman Pressured by Her Husband to Retire With Him

A 52-year-old married employed mother of grown children was arrested for driving while intoxicated. Initially she rationalized her behavior. She later revealed that she was a very regular social drinker and that in recent months she had begun drinking a shot of hard liquor upon arrival home from work so that she could "handle her husband." This patient had returned to work some 10 years before when she had finished raising her children. Her husband, some 10 years her senior, had opted for early retirement in the past year. He had steadfastly refused to return to any kind of work, either paid or voluntary. She continued to work and to travel for work-related matters. Her husband became increasingly resentful and pressured her to move with him out of state to a retirement community. For her this meant losing her job, her friends, and physical proximity to her children. She stopped drinking. The couple were seen jointly, and friends supported her wish to remain active. Her work did allow for travel time with her husband, and a plan was made that was acceptable to both.

A Woman Whose Midlife Career Resulted in Divorce

A patient in her mid-40s had had a difficult first marriage and had been abandoned by her husband. Left with two small daughters, she put a patchwork of jobs together for income. She met an older wealthy man, himself divorced, who agreed to marry her and to adopt her daughters. When her children went away to school, she wearied of her job as hostess, decorator, and manager of a staff of household help. She obtained a voluntary job, which led, in a year, to an offer of employ-

ment. Her husband was very unhappy and unsupportive of her. She began a love affair, and when this seemed to offer the promise of marriage if she were to divorce her husband, she sought psychiatric help. She seemed caught between her guilt about the man who had become her children's father and her resentment of him for obstructing her career. The patient and her husband decided to divorce. She was able to begin her own business. During the course of a succession of unhappy affairs, she realized that she was choosing flamboyant, unreliable men who were like her father. After work on oedipal issues, she met a widower whose wife had been a traditional homemaker. He enjoyed her growing business successes, was supportive of her, and was not troubled by her rather hectic hours. The two have had a successful and loving marriage as well as separately successful business lives.

A Woman Whose Marriage Forced Her to Return to Work

A 50-year-old married mother of two grown children had left the business world when she needed surgery and chemotherapy. Upon recovery she could not seem to get her life together and appeared to be depressed. Initially she stated that she wished to return to work so as to support herself and leave her husband. She did not then know that he was on the verge of bankruptcy. She did not recognize that his "sloppiness in paying bills" and his failure to communicate were due to near-panic levels of anxiety. She was able over time to feel less resentful toward him and about her need to seek new employment.

Commuter Marriage

A medical student, mother of two school-age children, applied for her postgraduate hospital training. Her husband's corporation moved its headquarters, and although he was given a year's grace to relocate because of his wife's status, he was expected to move to another city. She interviewed in both cities and considered giving up her household help, leaving her home, and taking her children out of school. She interviewed at hospitals near her husband's new assignment but found these programs in her chosen specialty inferior. The arrangement was made that her husband would relocate and commute home on weekends. She agonized over her choice, realizing that the strain of weekend commuting would be difficult for him and would leave him little time for her and the children. She also worried about the "single parenting" by a mother who would have to work on a rotating schedule involving nights and weekends. The couple, however, made their arrangement work.

Career

The issues confronting women in the establishment of a career are complicated and different from those confronting men. Therapists attempting to help women with career issues must understand a number of complex and interrelated issues:

1. Intrapsychic and psychodynamic issues that include not only intrapsychic structures and conflicts typical of women but also relevant developmental stage issues and familial issues
2. The negative input of sex role stereotypes
3. The realities of discrimination and lack of opportunity
4. The impact of situational and contextual factors that affect women
5. The structure and division of parenting

Early theories developed to explain women's conflicts around work were groundbreaking and important in the attention that they drew to this subject, although somewhat unidimensional. Horner's (1972[55]) classic "fear of success" model and Hennig and Jardim's (1977[56]) writings regarding women's lack of knowledge of the ground rules of the work world have been amplified by more sophisticated models of both the intrapsychic and the external factors at work in inhibiting women's career development. Women often attempt to externalize intrapsychic conflicts by attributing their difficulties to discrimination and sex role stereotyping. In contrast, they may also internalize blame and responsibility for discrimination and other external factors and become immobilized and depressed if their therapists are unable to help them make these differentiations. (Sexual harassment, one of the most common forms of illegal gender discrimination against women, is discussed in detail in Chapter 6.)

The ways in which women's minority numerical status in many professions and work organizations contribute to group dynamics and processes that impede their career development have been outlined by Moss-Kanter (1977a,[57] 1977b[58]). Drawing on the work of Simmel (1950[59]), who analyzed the significance of numbers in social life, Moss-Kanter (1984,[60] pp. 53–54) elaborated four types of organizational groups:

1. *Uniform groups*, which have only one kind of person or social type.
2. *Skewed groups*, which have a large preponderance of one "dominant" type that controls the group and its culture. In this type of group, "tokens" (as the nondominant members are called) are seen as symbolic stereotypes, that is, as representatives of their class rather than individuals. Even if there is more than one token, these individuals can seldom form an alliance that is powerful enough to affect the group.
3. *Tilted groups*, which are those that have less extreme distributions and effects between tokens and "dominants" and in which the tokens constitute a significant minority (approximately 35%) and form a coalition that affects the group. Tokens can also be seen as individuals, not just as symbols in tilted groups.
4. *Balanced groups*, which have a 60%/40% or a 50%/50% typographical ratio and are characterized by subgroups. Individuals are differentiated by clear roles and abilities in this type of group.

In skewed groups, dominants harbor assumptions regarding the culture status and behavior of tokens. If these ancillary assumptions run counter to the requirements of the work task, they will impede the tokens' acceptance, despite any realistic innate ability and accomplishments. In skewed groups, two factors may heighten the dynamics that we have previously described: 1) if the token's social category is physical or obvious as in the case of sex, and 2) if the token's social type is new to the work setting or position level. Laws (1975[61]) has described how token women can be accepted into the group via the sponsorship of a dominant male.

In a field study of women employees of a Fortune 500 company, Moss-Kanter (1977a,[57] p. 58) documented the pressures that male dominants imposed on token women as well as the women's characteristic responses to these pressures. Moss-Kanter noted that the token women were more visible and that the dominants tended to both polarize the token women's differences in relation to the majority group and assimilate them into stereotypes that distorted the token women's real individual characteristics. Moss-Kanter also noted that the three characteristics of visibility, polarization, and stereotyping of token women were each associated with specific interactional dynamics that resulted in typical responses from the token women.

Moss-Kanter's (1984,[60] pp. 59–72) findings may be summarized as follows.

First, women's high visibility resulted in performance pressures that included the following:

1. *Public performance*: Token women's work was closely scrutinized, and there was a high visibility of mistakes and a lack of privacy.
2. *Extension of consequences*: Women's work was received not as an individual performance but rather as an indication of the performance of their entire sex.
3. *Attention to discrepant characteristics*: Token women were noticed for their ancillary characteristics (e.g., physical appearance and dress) rather than their work performance.
4. *Fears of retaliation*: Token women feared retaliation if their performances and achievements were outstanding and perceived as humiliating to the dominants.

Token women tended to respond to these pressures via overachievement, which often set them up for retaliatory maneuvers, usually described as "cutting them down to size." Token women's second characteristic response was to assume an invisible and avoidant stance by dressing mannishly; by avoiding public forums, meetings, and leadership positions; or by minimizing their competence or allowing it to be attributed elsewhere. This often helped these women avoid retaliatory maneuvers but also limited their recognition within the organization and therefore interfered with promotion and advancement of other kinds.

Second, polarization or exaggeration of the token women's characteristics in relation to the dominants' led to the following performance pressures:

1. *Exaggerations of the dominant culture*: Males asserted group identity via exaggerating their maleness through typical male behaviors in the token women's presence. Examples of such behaviors were talk of drinking, sports, and sex and displays of aggression and potency, which perhaps accounts for Klein's (1984[62]) observations showing that the highest rate of sexual harassment occurs in skewed groups (see Chapter 6).
2. *Interruptions*: Males made token women the focus of interruptions in the group flow by asking them questions such as, "Can we still swear? tell jokes? go drinking?" These types of questions put women in the uncomfortable position of either asking the majority of people to change (and thus be seen as imposing an inconvenience and at the same time be reminded of their difference from the dominants) or asserting their cultural roles.
3. *Overt inhibition and informal isolation*: Token women were informally quarantined by keeping them away from the informal activities during which many business dealings and rules of the game were discussed; keeping them away from certain meetings; keeping corporate secrets; and failing to provide them with important initiation information. (This dynamic is related to Hennig and Jardim's [1977[56]] early writings about women being unaware of the rules of the game.) In some instances dominants even avoided giving women information regarding their performance and the women were not warned of their risk of being fired.
4. *Loyalty tests*: In this instance dominants sought reassurance that tokens would not turn against them by asking a token to join or identify with the dominants against competing groups, often the

token group itself. In other words, women were pitted against women. This was done in several ways. They could either silently accept or participate in derogatory statements, or they could accept the dominant view fully and actually vocalize it, thus taking over the gate-keeping role for the dominants. Another variation of this phenomenon is requesting that women allow themselves to bear the brunt of derogatory humor against them. The reward for passing these loyalty tests is permission to move closer into the dominant group; punishment involves further isolation. Responses to these polarization pressures are very limited. Tokens can either accept the isolation-risking exclusion and lack of opportunities for promotion or try to become insiders by defining themselves as exceptions or turning against their own group.

Third, and finally, tokens tended to be assimilated—that is their individual characteristics were distorted to fit stereotypes of their sex, forcing them to play rigid and caricatured roles. Performance pressures in this category included *status leveling*, in which the token women were perceived not in their professional role but rather in the position that would be expected given their sex (e.g., doctors being perceived as nurses, saleswomen being perceived as mistresses or secretaries). A second performance pressure involved stereotype role induction in which dominants forced women into four classic role traps that men could respond to in highly ritualized ways that severely limited the women's activity:

a. *Mother*: The woman is not vulnerable to sexual pursuit but is not rewarded for her job performance but rather for her service in taking care of people. The mother was not permitted to be critical or objective. The mother is seen as a specialist in feeling but largely devalued for this.
b. *Seductress*: The woman is seen as highly desirable and is very visible but is also the focus of considerable tension. She may bear the brunt of unwanted sexual pursuits, or she may be protected by a high-level dominant male who then is resented by the other males in the group.

c. *Token pet*: The woman is expected to bear the brunt of much humor and is devalued in terms of her competence in the sense that any achievement is considered a surprise, which prevents her from realizing or demonstrating her own competence.
d. *Iron maiden*: This stereotype is characteristic of women who avoid and resist overtures of the other three stereotypes and insist on full rights in the group. Such women are stereotyped as being tougher than they are and are thus trapped into more polarized militant stances than they actually feel. Several other stereotypes somewhat similarly have been described as the "maiden aunt" and the "kid sister."

Characteristic responses to role entrapment lead women to minimize their stranger contact in the work world and to take very low risk positions. They find it easier to accept the stereotypical roles because it offers them some acceptance in the group. However, the price that is paid is in personal distortion. Moss-Kanter notes that women who accept token positions often take on the exaggerated characteristics attributed to them and suggests that this may have skewed studies of women's work behaviors when token women were studied rather than women who were in more tilted or balanced groups.

A second and somewhat related model relevant to external discriminatory factors is the model of microinequities developed by Rowe (1990[63]). She defines *microinequities* as interactions that occur in the workplace at the level of individual decision-makers and that are not always illegal but negatively impact morale, job performance, and opportunities for promotion and training. Rowe notes that the impact of these microinequities is cumulative, like drops of water collecting in a bucket. Utilizing the motivation of the perpetrator, Rowe divides microinequities into four categories:

1. *Unconscious slights and invisibility problems*: Women's work is not seen in the same way as that of their male colleagues. Women are left out of both formal and informal work networks. They often do not perceive any conscious malice intended on the part of the per-

petrator, which makes them somewhat confused regarding whether they should be angry and how to handle the situation.

2. *Conscious slights and harassment*: In this type of microinequity the perpetrator clearly directs hostility toward the woman, either sending messages that she cannot handle the job and should not be in the job, or assaulting her with unwanted and devaluing attention based on her gender.
3. *Poor service*: This phenomenon refers to the way in which women either are not noticed and are not put forward for promotional, training, and educational opportunities, or are overtly discouraged from these opportunities because they are women.
4. *Outright exploitation*: The woman is paid less, not given credit for work done, and/or placed in a position where she cannot deliver work that would lead to her own promotion but where her training and abilities are utilized in the intentional service of promoting someone else.

Etiologies for the negative impact of these phenomena include

1. The power of negative reinforcement is present such that women will begin to perform at the level expected of them and perceive themselves in a negative way, particularly if the negative feedback comes from persons in authority.
2. Microinequities make it impossible for female employees to perform quality work at the level of their ability by overloading them with routine or personal work that does not allow room for their creativity to be expressed.
3. Microinequities have negative input via the mechanism of intermittent reinforcement—that is, they are irrational and intermittent and do not occur in the context of merit or striving for excellence. Laboratory studies have shown that such intermittent, unpredictable negative reinforcement creates high levels of anxiety and a sense of helplessness.
4. Microinequities are difficult to address. If a woman ignores them, she permits a situation to continue that may damage her career. But if she responds at every instance, she will be pegged as a trouble-

maker. It is not always clear to the woman that she has been discriminated against or that any negative impact was intended, making it more difficult for her to speak up and address the issues.

5. Microinequities take up time and energy.
6. Microinequities exaggerate the polarity between men and women, making it harder for them to work together.
7. Women have few role models to help them deal with methods for redress. Women supervisors often react with a sense of denial, helplessness, or identification with the aggressor.
8. Power politics are at play in microinequities in the sense that often the perpetrators are in authority positions and the women victims are in junior positions.
9. Microinequities have an especially detrimental effect if a woman is just in the process of developing her career identity or if she is trying to consolidate her identity as a mother at the same time.
10. Because microinequities directed against women often take a sexist form, they do more damage to women's morale. This is because the microinequities are not focused on job performance or more randomly applied.
11. Women have been socialized to be sensitive to any anger or disapproval directed at them and are inhibited in their abilities to assert themselves in many cases. Therefore, the impact of the microinequity may be greater on a female than on her male colleague.
12. Microinequities are particularly hard to stop in skewed groups for reasons that we have previously elaborated.

Rowe feels it is more difficult for minorities and women to find adequate support in dealing with racism and sexism than it is for white males to find help in dealing with general inhumanities and generalized work harassment. Continued experiencing of these types of destructive situations can lead to unhappy cycles of avoidant behavior, declining self-esteem, withdrawal, resignation, poor work, and fantasies of violence. These difficulties cannot be legislated out of existence. Workshops, support groups, mentoring programs, and education of management are helpful.

In *role stereotyping*, a third model explaining external work inhibition, women are seen as women rather than as professionals. They are seen either as feminine and therefore good or as not staying in their place and therefore bad. They are viewed as being in a woman's role rather than as an individual. These difficulties stem from an unconscious feeling of what is correct or proper. Examples include a female student being complimented on her looks rather than her work. Another example would be the rewards sent to women who act in traditional ways and the labels of "abrasive" or "bitchy" presented to women who do not act in such ways. A third example would be a woman physician who is introduced as the wife of another physician. There are common gender stereotypes for women, including "incompetent," "emotional," and "fragile." Some stereotypes are more positive (e.g., "warm," "maternal," and "flexible"). If a woman is not in a skewed group, it may be possible to address these stereotypes via rational discourse. However, women are sometimes ambivalent and uncertain of how they feel about these stereotypes themselves, which adds to the problem.

Klein (1984[62]) noted that negative behaviors do not diminish until women constitute almost 75% of the work group. Because this is unlikely to be accomplished soon, and perhaps never in some professional settings, it is likely that any patient approaching a therapist will be encountering some of these difficulties and will require help not only in identifying the internal conflicts that she may be experiencing over career issues but also in not internalizing guilt or blame for these difficulties. Therapists should evaluate their female patients as individuals and be cognizant of the complex interplay between intrapsychic, developmental, familial, social, cultural, parental, and environmental issues.

Applegarth (1976[64]) has noted that severe external obstacles could mask the presence of internal problems and that gratifying alternative routes of marriage and motherhood, with strong familial and societal support, may distract a woman from her career goals. Both of these obstacles can be used defensively in the service of denying internal disturbances. Pathological narcissism can lead women to avoid situations because of fear of failure combined with unrealistically high expectations for which they constantly reproach themselves. Narcissistic women often value illusions of glamour or admiration rather than the discipline and perseverance to acquire certain new skills. They feel entitled to success and often respond with rage at any obstacle. Pathological narcissism results when a child is admired in a grandiose fashion and perceived to be perfect, or when a child's mother feels narcissistically injured and communicates this sense of self to her young daughter.

Applegarth applies the hypothesis of penis envy to women who are envious and have doubts regarding their capacities as well as specific convictions that some necessary ingredient for success is missing. They often experience a strong sense of being deprived or injured. They admire men and are frequently contemptuous of women. These women may attempt either to form an alliance with a powerful man or to have a child. Women may enact oedipal conflict via attempts to get closer to their father with their intellectual work or to surpass their mother. Occasionally, women cannot assert themselves at work. Sadism or aggression of pregenital origin, often threatens to intrude into consciousness at the moment of self-assertion. Passivity keeps unresolved sadism and aggression of pregenital origin unconscious for these women. Some women struggle with competition and aggression and often experience themselves as bad for expressing these traits. Superego traits such as curiosity and exploration are more discouraged in women and influence women's difficulty in pursing work-related tasks alone.

Applegarth also feels that women have difficulties giving up their role of being cared for. Although her work focused on the internal problems to career development, she did not minimize the realities and the legitimate competition between the demands of motherhood and career.

Person (1982,[65] p. 68) has reexplored some of the above issues and elaborated on new ones. She points out that professional ambition in women is often mislabeled as masculine and a derivative of penis envy. She also comments on the female "fear of success" notion popularized by Horner (1972[55]), lamenting its use as a catchword to describe all work inhibitions and its obscuring of some more important dynamics. Person suggests a classification of work problems and inhibitions for women that includes the following: 1) role conflicts, 2) ambition with no clear-cut goals, 3) fear of failure, 4) fear of deviance, 5) fear of success, and 6) some special problems among successful women. Person recommends that all views of women's work problems be analyzed via a frame of reference that includes the contemporary shift in values, gender role socialization, female developmental psychology, and the specificity of an individual's life history. She notes the importance of role conflicts and observes that many women are caught between the traditional role of nurturant helpmate and the autonomous world of work, with no guarantees for protection, with no clear role models in either area, and without some of the psychological skills necessary for achievement.

Ambition without clear-cut goals is another factor that Person believes is necessary for understanding work-related problems in women. We have discussed women who have narcissistic fantasies of becoming famous or well known. The problem of ambition combined with passivity is exacerbated by a series of highly visible role models who indeed achieve success and obtain recognition through beauty or status but not because of acquired skills.

Fear of failure is noted by Person to be associated with a history of low self-esteem and shame. Person does not attribute this to penis envy but instead defines such self-esteem issues as most likely being related to an identification with a mother figure who is devalued and to the socialization patterns of women in which competition and mastery are not encouraged. Success is often attributed to key relationships, luck, or chance.

Beginning with a discussion of Horner's (1972[55]) landmark study on success inhibitions in women, Person elaborates the fourth factor: fears of deviance in women that affect self-valuation and an accompanying fear of losing highly valued relationships and dependent gratification. This approach shifts the notion of success away from internal developmental issues to inhibition based on realistic assessment of negative consequences. Persons notes that the threat of rejection, particularly by men, is especially noxious for women who are socialized to define their worth by their acceptability to males and their ability to make and maintain relationships. As these values are internalized into their own ego ideals, the boundaries between what is an internal problem and what is an external problem become more complicated.

Person identifies fear of success as a fifth factor in work-related problems. Inhibition of assertion and competition stems from childhood experiences in which the woman perceived rivalries as potentially murderous. This may come from the child's fantasy life or be the result of intimidation from primary adults. The focus of the inhibition is the individual's fear of retaliation or sense of guilt at the potentially damaging aspects of any assertive act. Other theoreticians have felt this difficulty to be a reflection of a woman's guilt at surpassing her mother.

Person also notes several special problems encountered by successful career women:

a. *The fear of public speaking and public exposure*: This fear seems to stem from fears regarding either sexual exhibitionism or assertiveness. In Persons' opinion, the inhibition of libidinal impulses rather than of the aggressive ones is primary in this context.
b. *The personalization of work*: Women tend to place high value on affiliative ties and may therefore not distinguish situations that are personal from situations that have nothing to do with personal feelings but are simply workplace related. A woman may have trouble leaving mentors, or she might merge her goals with those of her supervisors or company.
c. *The misunderstanding of power*: Some women confuse relationships to powerful people with power that they themselves hold, or they may confuse status with power. This confusion again results from the focus on affiliative ties that obscures the value of power relationships.
d. A *sense of fraudulence and fear of exposure*. McIntosh (1985[66]) explains this fear by noting that women sometimes feel fraudulent because they are not accustomed to the traditionally male hierarchical standards that define competence in terms of status.

Person concludes with the statement that women's work inhibitions are closely linked to the importance of affiliative ties in the development of girls and women.

Stiver (1983[67]) presents a slightly different version of some of these core issues with some additional points. She focuses less on a deficit model of female development than on a different value system that places affiliative ties at the forefront and often leads women to make choices that are not conducive to their promotion at work. The solution is not solely dependent on taking more power or being more task oriented and impersonal. Women's valuing of relationships is often misinterpreted as dependency. Hennig and Jardim (1977[56]) have noted that one difference between men and women is women's not knowing the ground rules and their failing to recognize challenges and opportunities. Stiver's view is that women simply make choices according to their own value system and that there would be great losses for women in not maintaining their integrity. Women, for example, may choose to compromise because of very legitimate family ties and the demands of household tasks that are still unevenly distributed. These women may be labeled as unprofessional because of their affective styles despite the reality that cognitive effectiveness and affect can be harmoniously integrated. Stiver believes that competitive skills are overrated and the value of facilitative skills underrated in current literature regarding working women. She notes that women may be forced to accept the masculine norms, thus breaking, rather than reworking, important and legitimate affiliative bonds, especially with nonworking or nonsuccess-oriented mothers. Stiver points out that fears of success in women are probably related to the fear of not being able to stay related to other persons. Women need to feel entitled to pursue work interests without feeling held back by beliefs that the needs of others are always more important, without feeling selfish and destructive, and without giving up valuable relationships but rather working to change the relationships to accommodate the more competent aspects of themselves. Stiver cautions against psychotherapists' pushing women to accept and integrate values that may run counter to their intrinsic sense of worth; instead she emphasizes integrating these values into the existing work structure.

Lerner (1980,[68] 1983,[69] 1987[70]) also connects work inhibitions in females to complexities in their valuing of relationships and in their difficulties with expression of anger. She emphasizes important aspects of familial bonding and familial experiences with work. Lerner describes the way in which a mother who has been blocked from her own self-development and growth may ignore or devalue her daughter's attempts to establish a career, or, conversely, may encourage her daughter to be special and vicariously enjoy her successes. Such women can be caught in the conflicting messages of mothers who say, "Be independent but also be like me." Lerner considers such difficulties as distortions of the mother-daughter bond stemming from family and cultural patterns that may be dysfunctional for women's development. Young women attempting to establish careers for themselves when previous generations of women in the family have not may experience profound anxiety and guilt that needs to be explored within the context of these very important female-to-female relationships. Lerner calls this *multigenerational guilt* and notes its extreme prevalence in families who have emigrated, often requiring the loss and disruption of valuable emotional relationships. Like Stiver, Lerner feels these difficulties should be worked out in the context of relationships.

Lerner (1980[68]), paralleling Bernardez-Bonesatti (1978,[71] 1988[73]) and Miller (1983[72]), points to the way in which women tend to be overly inhibited in the expression of anger and aggression, traits that are often necessary in the workplace. Lerner believes that the locus of this inhibition is with fears of omnipotent destructiveness or in separation-individuation difficulties in the mother-daughter relationship. She notes that there is a progression from anger to hurt, from "I" to the relational "We," in that hurt draws the object closer and emphasizes the object's importance to the self. Expression of legitimate anger places women at risk for standing alone and being perceived as unloving and unlovable, both of which run counter to their core sense of identity and values. Women must be helped to separate and differentiate so that they can become free to express their anger in response to legitimate concerns.

Lerner (1983[69]) explores the context of female dependency and states that there is often a distinction between a woman's passive dependent behavior and her actual level of differentiation. Many times her behavior serves as a protective function in the maintenance of primary relationships (with mothers and then husbands), underfunctioning to allow another person to overfunction. Lerner notes the ironic generalization that although women are often accused of being overly dependent, they are not dependent enough in the sense that they are far better at identifying and attending to the needs of others than in identifying and claiming their own needs. This can be especially problematic for a woman who is attempting to establish her career at a time when she is also parenting and being a wife. Lerner joins Surrey (1985[74]) in establishing the problem that occurs when the relationship does not support the continued growth and independence of the woman and the woman is forced to make a choice between the relationship and her own growth.

Additional writers have noted some single, salient feature in women's work inhibitions. Symonds (1986[75]) has described a depression occurring in highly functioning career women that results from sexism in their families of origin, in which mothers rejected and devalued their daughters and idealized their sons. Girls respond to this rejection of their own needs with a sense of blame. The double burden of rejection—because of gender and suppression of self in order to care for others—results in an unentitlement and a sense of isolation.

Lebe (1986[76]) calls attention to some female ego ideal conflicts in adulthood. She notes four developmental factors that lead to later internal conflicts:

1. The special bond between mothers and daughters, consisting of mutual interaction and relatedness and resulting in an ego ideal that includes caring for and relating to others
2. Body image development in which girls are not able to touch or visualize their own sexual organs, which leads to later experiences of their bodies as inner, unknown, and diffuse
3. Differences in experiences of bodily injury that seem more prevalent in women and that may later result in trouble with aggression and assertion
4. The importance of the father's encouragement of the daughter's differentiation

Lebe believes that these four early developmental issues can lead to adult internal conflicts as follows:

1. *Breaking the early mother/daughter emotional bond.* Stepping out of the mother/daughter relationship in part to create a new self-image is experienced by many women as an aggressive act toward their mother, or it may leave them feeling alone and unsupported, or unactualized in their capacity to relate.
2. *The superwoman syndrome.* Women's healthy needs for dynamic relationships can provide a motivating force toward establishing both career and family. Strong commitment to these often conflictual needs may either discourage women from their careers or lead to increased conflict among their choices. Such commitment often places them in the position that in order to meet their own ego ideals as a feminine woman, they must perform an inordinate amount of the household and child-care tasks.
3. *Difficulties in expressing anger.* Suppression of anger takes energy and can lead to depression and physical symptomatology. Lebe notes that women also are more upset when others perceive them as insensitive, even if this perception is based on the authority role these women have been given. Women therefore feel more personally injured by common criticisms of bosses.
4. *High expectations.* Lebe notes that women often have high expectations that involve providing infinite care to others in their careers and in their personal lives. There are no accompanying ideals that involve expressing the same care toward their own well-being.

In addition to these dynamic models illuminating career issues for women, several authors have also pointed to some similarities in career issues between men and women. Kaplan (1989[77]) notes that the unconscious factors influencing adult career decisions for both sexes can include positive and negative identifications with important childhood objects and fears, and/or needs for competitive struggle, narcissistic needs, the expression of otherwise unacceptable instinctual drive derivatives, parental and internalized superego values and demands, unconscious guilt and/or shame, and reversals from passive to active. Sublimation and reaction formation via career routes have also been noted in both sexes. Both men and women frequently change careers multiple times during early adulthood, and these changes can represent either a positive working of issues toward a stable identity or the repetitive and fruitless expression of ego diffusion.

Citing the work of Michels (1980[78]), Viederman (1986[79]) notes that both men and women can experience personality changes through life experiences, often leading to vocational change or the development of a career. Viederman contends that the mechanism for this is the same for men and women. Individuals who have been haunted by perceptions of defectiveness or badness may choose to test out these self representations via making a life decision that involves taking risks. The patient's taking of these risks, which could lead to either positive outcome or repetition of narcissistic injury, requires that another person with a special status assist in the consolidation of the positive view of the patient and serve as an object of identification. This consolidates the modified self representation. This particular model is of special interest in terms of midlife women who often, in the context of identifying with their younger career-oriented daughters, begin spontaneously to take college courses or to decide to work. This would be a positive outcome of the mother-daughter bond, one in which both parties would grow in the service of the relationship.

Perosa and Perosa (1984–1985[80]) discuss midlife career crises, observing that both male and female adults incorporate new information concerning the self throughout life. Individuals thus rework their identity based on new information or fully differentiate from points of lesser differentiation. Read et al. (1988[81]) have noted an interesting phenomenon in reentry women who return to the work world, particularly those women who are divorced or separated with children and have never established careers prior to this time in their lives. Financial concerns are often paramount to this group of women who define their occupational careers in terms of the financial rewards that can be brought into the family. Rosenwald and Wiersma (1983[82]) point out that many women in midlife present establishment of careers as rebirths or ruptures rather than viewing it in the context of their lives. The authors present these distorted self-accounts as a coping device, a kind of alibi or press release to help a woman escape the cultural retribution and potentially negative responses from significant others that would come if she laid out more clearly her frustrations and the assertive autonomous wishes that led her to the establishment or change of her career.

Gooden and Toye (1984[83]) have noted that both men and women become depressed when they are pressured to give up a valued occupational dream in young adulthood because of difficulties with an authoritative mother, or if their options are limited by this same authoritative figure. Archer (1989[84]) has proposed that men and women may respond similarly if, in men, the formation of a career goal or occupational dream appears to be in strong conflict with their primary nurturant object.

Nadelson et al. (1978[85]), in discussing the actual treatment of women for career-related disturbances, note that therapists often have the same conflicts and must work hard in differentiating what is objectively healthy. Therapists need to take biological timetables into consideration in their psychotherapy. Nadelson et al. relate a series of problems for which patients often present at various times in their life cycle—namely, career choice, career development, and midlife issues.

Career choice issues often present for treatment as difficulty in exceeding or competing with the mother's achievements and other concerns regarding the rupture of the mother-daughter bond. Career development issues often present as patients' unrealistic notions of what the demands of developing their career will be; unconscious sabotaging of others' efforts to help them; inability to make long-range plans; or concerns that these women's career advancement will interfere with their relationships with men. These women may react with depression, anxiety, marital discord, or difficulties in asserting themselves or in completing work that would lead to advancement. Difficulties in handling the anger associated with recognizing discontent with an unreasonable situation are often present. Anger may conflict with a sense of self as a nonaggressive feminine person. Externalization of internal conflicts onto family, bosses, and peers, or on work demands and discrimination, may also occur. Women may punish themselves by actions in their career pathways as retribution for their inability to form a relationship. Others handle the relational conflict by foregoing relationships and attempting to become "one of the boys." A husband may respond to a wife's career success with impotence or withdrawal. Children may respond with a sense of loss and abandonment. Reentry women may present with difficulties in obtaining proper credentials, in competing with younger colleagues, and/or in mobilizing a sufficient degree of self-assertion to establish the role, resulting in depression and anxiety, or again in depression and anxiety if their assertive aspects are mobilized and they experience this as damaging aggression.

Midlife career issues involve difficulties facing the closure of the choices made to have careers or the compromises made careerwise in order to have a family. Divorces, deaths, and children's leaving the household may complicate these difficulties. Highly committed career women may actually do better during midlife. Nadelson et al. (1978,[85] p. 1095) make some therapeutic suggestions regarding referrals, reality-based factors, and countertransference issues. Women therapists are often requested as a basis for a positive alliance. Crisis-oriented, supportive, or long-term psychoanalytic approaches should be based on the realities of the patient's situation.

Countertransference issues can arise when the therapist's rather than the woman's personal priorities guide the therapy (e.g., therapist pressures woman to have children or forge ahead for a doctoral degree, or discourages the wish to have children or to give up successful careers later). Therapists may also misinterpret regressive behavior as primitive character pathology rather than low self-esteem. They may overidealize competent professional women and fail to see their areas of deficit. Therapists also may overinterpret patients' legitimate concerns and questions regarding therapists' orientation about, for example, penis envy or the misuse of psychoanalytic theory in interpreting work aspirations in women as pathological.

A Later-Life Career With Spousal Support

A pregnant patient in her early 30s had come from a lower socioeconomic class background and had been professionally trained in a situation where there was a financial incentive to spontaneously obtain a college degree. She then accompanied her husband to two separate cities where his corporation had assigned him. Upon return to a large metropolitan center, she worked and obtained an advanced degree in a field recommended by her husband that did not interest her.

The patient had in the past been treated for a borderline personality disorder with affective dyscontrol. Now pregnant and entering treatment, she entertained the notion of pursuing a career in medicine. Although she met great resistance from family and friends, her husband was very supportive. The patient took her therapist's silence as support for her goal and began a pre-med program. She was enormously successful, and her youngster adjusted well with household help. She applied to and was accepted at a medical school. Her husband was willing to incur debt in order to pay for her schooling and household help.

She explored many psychodynamic issues related to both parents and a younger, but favored, sibling. She was happy in pursuit of her new career but wondered if she would devalue it, much as she was devalued in childhood, as soon as she was successful. As therapist and patient worked on issues of gender ambiguity, the patient began to look more feminine. She agonized about whether she ought to become a psychiatrist in identification with her new mother-therapist. In an atmosphere of neutrality she selected another specialty and did not devalue her new career.

A Patient Whose Husband Was Verbally Abused Because of Her Job-Related Stress

A married professional and mother of two college students sought treatment because she was verbally abusive to her husband on several weekend occasions when she had had a second glass of wine. She felt very anxious because of pressures at work. She was both drinking a lot of coffee and taking Valium to get through her mornings. There were two factors that combined to make her job suddenly almost impossible: she earned a high salary and she had been contributing to her children's education. Her husband suggested an easier job that would, however, involve accepting a decrease in salary and a loss of a valuable benefits package that would accrue in 2 years. There was a history of alcoholism and suicide in her family of origin. She was fearful for herself because of this, but did not want to give up wine, because she and her husband were collectors and their social life revolved around this shared hobby. A contract was made to limit her total wine intake on weekends and to limit intake of decaffeinated coffee, and not to take Valium.

For a while she used the sedative side effect of a tricyclic antidepressant to sleep on Sunday night, prior to the work week. She talked about the chaotic relationships in her family, her pride in her success, and her appreciation that her husband was low keyed and supportive. What she was failing to recognize at work was that staff stress produced splitting and projection against her. A parallel process was taking place, helped by alcohol, in her marriage. She feared firing anyone until the fear of replicating violent anger and abandonment in her own childhood was derepressed. She then took the helm of her ship. Her anxiety diminished and she was relieved at the improvement in her behavior at home. Her husband responded by providing a supportive atmosphere in which she could talk through work-related issues.

Homosexual Love Relationships

Historically, views of homosexuality have evolved in the literature since the terms *homosexual* and *heterosexual* were first used in 1869, when Carl Maria Kertbeny, also know as Benkert, published them in a newspaper article advocating sexual law reform in Prussia (Money 1990[86]).

Freud (1905b,[87] 1909a[88]) based his model of female sexual development upon the theories he had constructed for men. He stated clearly that the negative Oedipus complex, and thus homoerotic wishes and fantasies, are an integral part of the Oedipus complex in both men and women. For Freud, homosexual object choice represented either a failure of development or a regression to a safer stage of development.

In a clinical study of female homosexuality, Freud (1920b[89]) discussed a young woman, 18 years old, who adored an older woman. The young woman's adoration occurred at the time of her mother's pregnancy and the birth of a male sibling when she was 16. Freud conceptualized her homosexual attraction in oedipal terms. She wished to bear her father's child and was embittered and turned away from men and from the love of a man. It is difficult to accept this formulation for two reasons. The first reason is that in women in whom homosexuality has been presumed to have a psychogenic cause, the more likely formulation is in terms of loss of and search for the mother. This is supported by Freud's patient's choice of an older woman. The second reason is that homosexual fantasies and behavior usually originate earlier in childhood. When affectively invested heterosexual fantasies have predominated and change suddenly, this represents a regression.

Socarides (1962,[90] 1963[91]) has reviewed both the clinical aspects of female homosexuality and its developmental concepts from a psychoanalytic point of view. These concepts represent the view of classical psychoanalysis, namely, that constitutional factors do not allow us to automatically dismiss psychological factors. That view, however, is open to some question in the light of more recent data. Socarides cites a great deal of work that verifies the longer attachment of the daughter to her mother in contrast to that of the mother/son relationship. He points out, quoting the work of another author, the role of oedipal rejection by the father in causing "libidinal" regression to the mother. He also notes the role of the daughter's identification with the father. Socarides reviews Freud's postulates about the need to renounce the clitoris as the primary sexual organ in favor of the vagina, and the unwillingness to do this, as causal in a homoerotic object choice. Current psychological research already cited (see Chapter 1) does not support this theory. Socarides also reviews ideas about female castration anxiety and female masochism as being genetic to female homosexuality. We have, however, refuted the idea that women are intrinsically masochistic in Chapter 3. Socarides discusses the work of other analysts about the role of projection in female homosexuality. As we stated earlier in this chapter, we feel that projection initially contributes to infatuation and idealization in heterosexual relationships.

In presenting the work of the 1962 symposium, Socarides exhaustively reviews and references "classical" psychoanalytic theory about female sexual development as well as the structuralization of the female psyche and female psychology in general. While this history is interesting, later knowledge and contributions make the theories anachronistic. In the 1963 review, Socarides (1963[91]) discusses the contributions of Jones (1927[92]), which include formulations about intense oral erotism and sadism. If the infant girl who later becomes homosexual has these characteristics, we would have to wonder if they were innate or rather a response to maternal deprivation. Jones also raised the issue of identification with the father, and we would have to ask if this is a result of, on the one hand, the need to break away from the mother or of, on the other, the mother's rejection. Because these phenomena are postulated to occur early in development, we must wonder if they are constitutional.

Deutsch (1932,[93] 1933a,[94] 1933b[95]), who wrote extensively about female sexuality, emphasized preoedipal issues, citing female homosexuality as almost a reenactment of the active-passive roles of the mother/child relationship. This occurs before the triadic relationship of mother, father, and child. The active-passive mother/child paradigm exists for men as well, and one would be hard put to explain male homosexuality as similarly related to this paradigm.

Socarides (1963[91]), in his extensive review of the contributions of ego psychology to female homosexuality, proposes a number of explanations of female homosexuality as a defense against a variety of problems attributed to women (e.g., penis envy, masochism, and oral sadism, to name a few). This view of female psychology as well as the prerogatived labeling of homosexuality as a perversion is no longer acceptable to us in view of current research.

One of the present authors (Bernstein and Warner 1984b[96]) has written about female homosexuality in terms of the search for a good mother. The author has described the treatment of two young women who sought treatment for depression. Neither woman wished to have her sexual preference changed, and no attempt was made to do so. A psychoanalytic process was used in the hope of resolving symptoms, improving family and love relationships, and helping the women to make career choices. In each patient an erotic maternal transference developed and was resolved. In the resolution heterosexual love objects were sought.

Several authors have described the firm development of gender identity prior to the age of 18 months (Money and Erhardt 1972[97]; Stoller 1964,[98] 1968[99]). They believe that gender identity is a learned or taught phenomenon. It is not clear what percentage of homosexual women are gender dysphoric.

Homosexual men have been studied more carefully in the psychiatric and psychological literature (Friedman 1988[100]; Isay 1989[101]) than have homosexual women. Women have been, and are, in general, more emotional and more physically expressive. It has never been unacceptable for women to walk arm in arm or hand in hand and to kiss each other in greeting. Great controversy exists, however, regarding claims that lesbianism is better than heterosexual relationships, or that women can only overcome male political domination by renouncing men. Emmore (1980[102]) notes that female homosexuality is considered a threat to the formal societal and religious investment in family life and that female homosexuality allows and fosters financial autonomy of women.

Homosexual women often become patients for reasons both external and internal. In their discussion of the psychiatric treatment of homosexual women, Cohen and Stein (1986[103]) note the problems that homosexual women face in creating a positive identity. The creation of a positive identity, or self representation, and self-esteem regulation are complicated by the lack of social affirmation and the presence of social stigmatization. The second problem is that "coming out" seldom takes place in a linear fashion but occurs in bits and pieces at various stages of psychosocial development. The influence of the fragmentation of coming out molds each phase in ways that are often complicated. The struggle for identity in any phase will create both positive and negative feelings. The positive aspects are the diminution of anxiety, the relief of depression, and the finding of an accepting peer group.

Kleinberg (1986[104]) points out that the process of disclosure involves disclosure to the self, cognitive transformation recreating the past (i.e., understanding and reinterpreting old feelings, thoughts, and behaviors), and self-labeling and disclosure to the parents. Each of these processes may be painful and conflicted. She notes that many homosexual women choose not to come out to their parents and will not necessarily suffer in terms of solidifying their identity. What is necessary for identity solidification is coming out to those important people in the individual's life who will be supportive, nurturing, and helpful to her in evolving her sense of herself. A homosexual woman must recognize that the choice of not coming out to her parents will have an impact on her ability to relate to them because of the barriers caused by this secrecy. Both Kleinberg (1986[104]) and Gartrell (1984[105]) point out that the main issues that homosexual women face are issues of femininity, the way women relate, and the special needs that they have (concerning their biology and in relation to a male-dominated culture), which do not differ from those of their heterosexual sisters except by virtue of their sexual object choice.

Another problem is homophobia, which is often a regressive response to the increasing consciousness of homosexuality and the wish to ward it off. Homophobia may also be a defensive response to conflicts around intimacy, dependency, and regression. Gartrell (1984[105]) focuses on coming out and homophobia as the major issues in psychotherapy with homosexual women.

The area of sexuality and sexual behavior may be a difficult one for both patient and therapist to explore partially due to the erotization of the transference. Both patient and therapist may unconsciously conspire to avoid this.

Homosexual couples have problems that are distinct to their relationship. Burch (1986[106]) has discussed the problem of merger between members of the couple. This process may be pressured by social isolation outside the relationship. The pressure for merger is also a problem in the transference. Blumstein and Schwartz (1983[107]) have discussed another problem in female homosexual couples: the decrease in sexuality in the relationship. These authors believe that this decrease has several determinants, one related to the problems all women have with sexuality and body image, and another that merger, when it occurs outside the sexual relationship, also discourages sexuality.

The frequency of problems related to merger brings us full circle to the psychoanalytic observation that female homosexuality is related to the early maternal relationship.

Motherhood

Motherhood, which has traditionally been viewed as crucial to a woman's sense of identity and self-esteem, is both idealized to the point of worship and at the same time devalued in American culture. Images of female fertility goddesses exist, yet caretaking functions receive no pay, little notice, and little prestige, as exemplified by the lower status of the housewife. The importance of motherhood as a central theme in women's development of identity and self-actualization is changing somewhat. Many young women are ambivalent regarding motherhood. Some choose to remain childless; others are combining work with motherhood; and still others continue to place their mothering role as primary.

Demographic work, recently summarized by Gerson et al. (1984,[108] pp. 436–437), documents these shifts in attitude and identity. These authors point out seven characteristic changes in women's childbearing patterns:

1. There has been a marked decline in the number of children that women are planning. In 1980, 11% of all 18- to 24-year-old women expected to have no children. When college-educated women were isolated as a subgroup, the percentage rose to 17%. In 1955, 37% of young women expected to have four or more children. Only 8% of young women anticipated this in 1974.
2. There has been a sharp decline in unplanned or unwanted births.
3. The time frame in which mothers are bearing children and actively parenting is shrinking as women are having fewer children. As women live longer, a significant percentage of their lives will be spent without children at home.
4. Women are having children later in life. In 1960, 76% of women ages 20 to 24 already had children. By 1977 the rate had dropped to 57%. A correlation between delayed childbearing and higher education and labor force participation has also been established. A 1983 study showed a 67% rate of childlessness among young professional women.

5. There has been a rise in the incidence of families that are headed by a single parent. In 1970 the percentage of single mother–headed households was 8.7%. By 1983 it was 11.3%. By 1981, 18.8% of all families with minor children were headed by a single mother. For blacks the rate was even higher (47.5%) (Mednick 1987[109]).
6. Female employment of mothers outside the home has been on the rise, particularly among mothers with preschool children. Work participation rate for mothers with children under 6 years of age was 18.2% in 1955, 25.3% in 1965, 38.9% in 1975, 49.9% in 1982, and 77% in 1992.
7. During the last 15 years there has been an increase in alternate structures for mothering. These include single-parent households headed by women, cohabitation among heterosexual couples and among lesbian and gay couples, communal living arrangements, and forms of the postdivorce nuclear family such as stepfamilies and joint custody, as well as an increase in the rate of adolescent mothers (see Chapter 2).

All of these changes impact on the meaning and experience of motherhood for women today. In this context we provide a historical overview of the psychodynamic literature of motherhood. We discuss current motivations for motherhood, transition to motherhood, and the developmental phases of motherhood, as well as some special issues relevant to contemporary mothers.

Notman and Nadelson (1982a,[110] pp. 32–37) have reviewed the psychodynamic literature of motherhood, which we will summarize.

Freud's (1925,[111] 1950[112]) concept of motherhood consisted of two sources that accounted for the wish for a baby. One, which he termed "the anal baby," was associated with a passive feminine attitude, and one was derived from the phallic phase and was termed "the penis baby." This latter concept, though now refuted, remained the uncontested formulation of motherhood for many decades—that is, that a woman's original wish for a penis was replaced by a wish for a child. Deutsch (1945[113]) essentially accepted Freud's formulation of motherhood but added to the literature in terms of her elaboration of the concepts of feminine passivity and receptiveness. A further evolution of this theory was elaborated in the writings of Kestenberg and Benedek, who focused on the instinctual origins of feelings associated with pregnancy and motherhood. For these authors the wish for children and associated maternal feelings were not the result of penis envy or the pressures of males for heirs, but rather a biological requirement of the species and a primary organizer of women's sexual drive and personality. Kestenberg (1956b[114]) viewed the source of maternal affect as arising from sensations in the libido that were derived from the vagina and experienced by very young females. Benedek (1970c[115]), drawing on Deutsch's dual characteristics of passivity and introversion, connected the feelings associated with pregnancy and motherhood with the postovulative phase of the menstrual cycle. Benedek's position was in essence that there was a biological need for motherhood accompanied by psychodynamic correlates of receptiveness and introversion. Later work by Stoller (1976[116]) based on direct observational studies of the process of gender identity formation in young female children resulted in the concept of *primary femininity*, a term that was used to describe a nonconflictual first stage of female development wherein a young girl establishes a sense of being female based on a combination of factors that include bodily sensations, biological factors, sex assignment, and parental attitudes and conditioning.

Current work on the biological determinants of motherhood has stressed the relationship between hormonal status and behavior and has demonstrated the importance of biological correlates via empirical and cross-cultural data (Chodorow 1978[117]; Maccoby and Jacklin 1974[118]). Additional research based on observations of early mother/infant bonding (Klaus and Kennell 1976[119]; Spitz and Wolf 1946b[120]; Stern 1974[121]) indicates the importance of the mother's capacity to become involved in an active, affective mutual relationship rather than to act on a preset series of maternal behaviors. Although focusing on the biological and instinctual origins of motherhood, Benedek also served as the bridge between the biological and the more recent psychodynamic formulations for motherhood. She conceptualized the importance of the developmental identification with one's mother in the maternal experience (Benedek 1970a[122]). Benedek also elaborated on the potential for a woman's growth through parenthood (Benedek 1952[123]). She spoke of parenthood as a developmental phase and emphasized that the parent also matures in response to the child's growth (Benedek 1959a[124]). Bibring (1959[125]) also conceptualized motherhood in terms of a potential for growth. She defined pregnancy as a developmental crisis resulting in a loosening of defenses and the potential for reworking old identifications and conflicts and establishing a new sense of self-confidence through the experience of successful mothering.

Current psychodynamic theoreticians join Horney (1926[126]) and Thompson (1950[127]) in refuting Freud's early theory of the wish for a child as a substitution for an anatomical deficit. Current theory has been derived from work on the following:

1. Maternal-infant bonding, which emphasizes the intense dynamic affective relationship that occurs between an infant and his or her primary caregiver (Brazelton and Keefer 1982[128]; Stern 1974[121])
2. Maternal-infant separation, in which significant developmental deficits occur when infants are separated from primary caregivers (Klaus and Kennell 1976[119]; Spitz and Wolf 1946a[129])
3. The existence of a separate but parallel line of female psychological development that differs from male development primarily in its emphasis on the establishment of dynamic and mutually empathic relationships between mother and child (particularly mother and daughter) that change and accommodate to the growth of the child in ways that are empowering to both mother and child (Surrey 1985[74])

In young girls this relationship with mother continues throughout all stages of development, changing to accommodate the girls' differing developmental needs but always stressing closeness and mutual empathy and thus preparing them for motherhood. For young boys the relationship is somewhat different in that they are encouraged to break this affective tie and become more involved in competitive and assertive task- and skill-oriented behaviors. Although pregnancy obviously prepares females by its very nature toward close and intimate ties with their infants, there are some data (Coltrane 1989[130]) which suggest that fathers who are actively engaged in the care of young infants are also capable of bonding intensely with them and demonstrating many of the behaviors commonly associated with "mothering."

Several authors have recently reviewed the intrapsychic and sociocultural motivations for motherhood, as summarized below. Domash (1988[131]) has designated the expression of primary creativity as one of the most healthy motivations for wanting a child. By this she means the acceptance of the child's unique personality and the creativity of the mother to sense the child's native inclinations and enhance them yet leave them the exclusive property of the child. Building on Chodorow's (1978[117]) notions of a mother's wish to reestablish her bond with her own mother, and Winnicott's (1980[132]) conception of transitional relatedness of the good-enough mother who actively and creatively adapts to her child's needs and provides a nonpathological selfobject tie, Domash describes the term of "transitional relatedness," which includes the ability on the part of the mother to be with the child, to understand, to empathize, to nurture, and to provide this support without the need for personal confirmation from the child. The pathological equivalent of this healthy motivation would be a woman who wishes to mother as a means of creating her own selfobject within her baby, someone who will always love and be what she wants it to be in order to help her repair her own early narcissistic injuries.

Focusing on more sociocultural motivations for motherhood, Robinson and Stewart (1989[133]) note that women choose to become mothers to

- Confirm their status as women
- Solidify their self-esteem
- Escape from difficult situations or avoid career crises
- Keep a boyfriend
- Please their husband
- Attempt to solidify unhappy marriages
- Fulfill valued sociocultural norms

- Culminate a joyous, successful, and happy union with their husband
- Establish a means of separating themselves from their family of origin
- Replace a lost object.

Bergmann (1985[134]) provides an interesting study demonstrating that women who were forced prematurely to care for their own mothers or for younger siblings often opt to remain childless. However, there is also evidence that voluntarily childless women are not unhappy (Bernard 1972[135]; Campbell 1975[136]; Campbell et al. 1976[137]). Veevers (1979[138]), in her extensive review, notes the striking career success of childless women. Some women may choose childlessness because they have a firmly established identity forged through a career or they have managed to express their affiliative nurturing traits via other appropriate means (e.g., by mentoring young people or through nurturing relationships with other people's children).

The transition to motherhood is a complex intrapsychic task that is complicated by a variety of sociocultural factors prevalent today. Pines (1972,[139] 1982[140]), drawing on Bibring's concept of pregnancy as a developmental crisis, has elaborated the way in which the task of separation-individuation is reviewed and completed during pregnancy.

Lester and Notman (1986,[141] 1988[142]) and Raphael-Leff (1982[143]) have elaborated the way in which pregnancy provides an intrapsychic transition to motherhood and the ways in which difficulties with the pregnancy may mirror latter difficulties in the early infant/mother relationship. These authors divide pregnancy into a fusion phase, a differentiation phase, and a separation phase that provide the woman with an opportunity to rework her separation-individuation from her own mother as well as to prepare to mother her own baby. The *fusion phase* starts with awareness of pregnancy and lasts to approximately the fourth month. During this period the mother experiences a distortion in her own body image and a fusion with her fetus. This awareness of the fetus growing inside her reactivates old primitive fantasies of both violating her own mother's body and being incorporated by an overpowering mother. Any unresolved conflicts regarding these issues are available for reworking at this time. The *differentiation* phase of pregnancy begins 3 to 4 months into the pregnancy and is triggered by the quickening of the fetus. With these first-felt movements of the fetus comes the pregnant woman's capacity to differentiate between herself and the baby, and at the same time the wish to nurture and promote the baby's growth is triggered. This stage also enhances the creation of firmer boundaries between the pregnant woman and her own mother and her identification with her mother's maternal behavior. The *separation* phase occurs during the last 4 to 6 weeks of the pregnancy and consists of the reactions to the physical condition, the anticipation of labor, and essentially the separation between baby and mother. The woman visualizes the baby as viable outside herself and has fantasies regarding what that experience will be like. Overly ambivalent or overidealized versions of her own mother have been sufficiently differentiated and placed into perspective to enable her to identify positively and realistically with the mothering role. Primitive fantasies regarding the damaging aspects of childbirth may be reexperienced at this time, focusing on anxieties regarding the labor and delivery.

Raphael-Leff (1982,[143] pp. 8–13) describes four risk factors that may occur in pregnancy and, if identified in treatment, assist the woman in her transition to motherhood:

1. *Overvalued pregnancies*: Pregnancies following abortions, habitual miscarriages, previous stillbirths, perinatal death of a baby, and pregnancies in women with prolonged infertility problems and previous deliveries of abnormal babies may create a syndrome in which the woman oscillates between hope and distrust, elation and detachment, idealization and investment, and dread and conviction of failure. Untreated, this syndrome can result in overly anxious mothers.
2. *Ambivalent pregnancies*: Unwanted pregnancies, pressured late-life pregnancies, women in feminine revolt, unsupported women, and adolescent vacillations regarding pregnancy can entail ambivalence that interferes with the normal progression of intrapsychic work necessary for successful transition to motherhood.

3. *Pregnancies interrupted by traumatic life events*: Accidents, serious illnesses in the family, bereavement, divorce, eviction, and emigration are common etiologies. The confusion, anxiety, and distress created by these events interrupt the psychological work and present intrusive and conflicting demands.
4. *Historical sensitization*: This risk factor is defined by the history of some unusual occurrence during either the woman's previous pregnancy, her mother's pregnancy, a sibling's pregnancy, or the pregnancy of another close relative or relation that results in the woman being highly aroused during her own pregnancy and fearful via identification of a recurrence. Examples are a mother's death in childbirth, a father's death prior to the patient's birth, a stillbirth or abnormality of a sibling, the patient's own adoption, and eating disturbances such as anorexia and compulsive eating that result in preoccupation with body image and size. These women are also hindered in the normal progression of intrapsychic work during the pregnancy.

In addition to the reworkings of the woman's early relationship with her own mother and her establishment of positive identification with the mothering role already elaborated, we are, via our own clinical work, aware of some other complexities arising regarding the establishment of positive maternal identifications. The inability to rework a deficient early relationship with the woman's own mother can be one cause of difficulties in transition to motherhood. The complexity of today's sociocultural setting, however, has resulted in some additional problems regarding the identification with mothers. Working women who have had a very good early relationship with their own mothers and are positively identified regarding maternal behaviors may still have difficulty in becoming mothers if their own mothers have not worked. In this instance these women's very positive and solid identifications with their mothers can be experienced as conflicting with their current status. Their ego ideal regarding maternal behavior may also demand the all-inclusive preoccupation with child rearing demonstrated by their own mothers. Working women with nonworking mothers who were devalued, although adequate mothers, can be the source of another type of identification problem whereby the woman experiences a sense of loss or devaluation as she steps back from her work role to become more actively involved in her mothering. Working women who have identified strongly with their fathers who have been supportive of them up to this point may experience difficulties if their fathers become ambivalent about their working during their child-rearing years or if their fathers become overly invested in their daughters' maintaining a strong commitment to their working identity.

A second important aspect of the transition to motherhood involves mother/infant bonding and attachment. Maccoby and Jacklin (1974[118]) and Chodorow (1978[117]) were among the first to highlight the relationship between maternal behavior and concentrated exposure to infants. Brazelton and Keefer (1982[128]) have documented that the infant is complex and competent in ways that are particularly suited to eliciting caregiving behavior and to learning about and making adaptations to maternal behaviors. Within the first 4 months after delivery, a reciprocal interactional pattern has been established that allows the baby to be affectively and cognitively fueled by the reaction with the mother, and that allows the mother to have a strong sense of the identity of her baby and to be positively fueled regarding her competency as a mother. The absence of extended family and clear cultural values, poor support systems, and premature and excessive work demands make this bonding more difficult to accomplish and sometimes encourage mothers to defend against attaching to their babies (Brazelton 1986,[144] 1988[26]). Women who are securely attached will be able to remain actively involved with their children despite separations induced by work or other causes.

Motherhood has been defined by Benedek (1970b[145]) as a lifetime occupation, a psychobiological process that ends only with the death of the parent. Benedek was among the first to elaborate the ways in which mothers develop and mature concomitant with their child's sequential developmental phases. These phases are classically defined as the first year of life, the toddler years, the oedipal years, latency, adolescence, and the adult child.

These phases also fall into the larger categories of the early, middle, and late phases of parenthood. The early phase of parenthood extends from birth to adolescence. The years from birth to school age are considered the time of total parenthood, a time when a mother has the most complete possessing of her child and almost exclusive influence over him or her. Then, as school coincides with the end of the oedipal phase, a socially required and regulated partial separation takes place. Latency is a period of part-time parenthood. It tests a mother's capacity to share her influence and help her child to adapt to the world. The middle phase of parenthood begins with adolescence and the sexual maturity of the child and extends through the marriage of the child. Its major characteristic is the mother's involvement in and preoccupation with her child's sexual life, during which time she reassesses her own sexuality. The late phase of parenthood is characterized by the old age of the parent and is often accompanied by a role reversal. The need to adapt to a reasonable dependence on the child with concomitant issues of jealousy and competition is the major issue.

The early phase of parenthood includes the stages of infancy and toddlerhood, and the oedipal period of children. During *infancy*, communication is dominated by a response to the child's biological needs. This can be a time of anxiety as the mother learns to adjust to the child's cues and if the baby does not always respond positively to the mother's nurturing. It is also a time of pure pleasure when the child's early speech and verbalizations are broadly enjoyed by the mother. It is a relatively nonconflictual time for many mothers, as it most closely resembles their own symbiotic period with their mothers. During the *toddler* years the mother needs to learn to adapt to the child's need for individuation and separatism. This involves her reactions to the child's developing early personality. Her task is to deal with the loss of the symbiotic object and accept a new object relationship with an individuating child. She must deal with a sense of progressive and developmentally related loss of symbiosis and physical closeness, and accept and find pleasure in the child's achievements. During the *oedipal period* there is further diminishing of physical intimacy and the need for the mother to help her child incorporate societal rules and prohibitions. It is a period of growing maturity and settling down. The mother must deal with the child's seductiveness to the father or her, and a reactivation of her own oedipal wishes that are often projected onto her child. It is a period in which she must tolerate some rejection from her female children.

Latency is a time of great change in the sense that the mother has to give up the child that she knew. Separation anxiety may be experienced by the mother as well as feelings of resentment toward her child's school. The mother may experience a wish to slow down the growth of her child. She may feel threatened by the scrutiny of the school system and fearful that criticisms of her child are a reflection on her parenting. It is a period of regret and pride in her child's growing advancement. Releasing her children to teachers' influence can lead to the feeling of childlessness even as the mother must help her child feel self-esteem as an achiever and self-identity as a student. Parents often reorganize their own learning patterns during this period. For example, hobbies are revived along with other childhood interests. Career-oriented mothers of latency-age children may feel released to pursue more work goals. The prepubertal period coming at the end of latency is characterized by the mother's need to deal with the child's burgeoning sexuality and wishes to ignore this in order to cling to the peace of latency.

During *adolescence*, a mother needs to avoid responding to her child stereotypically as either an object of envy and a victimizer of the adult, or as a sexual object. She must also avoid treating her adolescent as a replacement for her own lost objects. There is a need for empathy derived from the mother's own adolescence, a relative freedom from her own transference projections, and a relative happiness with her own life.

The *adult child* phase is dominated by the child's marriage, which presents a new developmental task for the mother. She must include the child's mate into the family's own psychic system. Reactions of overinvolvement and intrusion are possible negative consequences. There is a need for the mother to adapt to the alienation of her children, which involves more distancing and a sense of not being needed in the same way. With the birth of her children's child and the entry into grandparenthood, the mother again may have a chance to rework developmental issues. (These later-life tasks are summarized in Chapter 7.)

There are some special issues concerning motherhood in contemporary society. This first issue is the conflict of autonomy versus nurturance. These two traits are perceived as somewhat polarizing for women today, and to some degree they are. Work often represents the need for autonomous strivings and motherhood represents the need for affiliative ties and nurturance. The issue is in fact more complicated. One of the present authors has had extensive experience in working with mothers' groups, some of which have met for as long as 3 years on a regular basis. One of the repetitive themes appearing in these groups has to do with the establishment of a satisfactory identity as a mother in a sociocultural climate that is unstable and changing and that no longer provides the traditional supports for motherhood.

Over half the mothers of young children under the age of 6 are currently in the work force (Gilbert and Rachlin 1987[146]), and yet the structure and norms of the workplace remain rigidly adherent to models that were established for male workers who had no active or conflicting parenting or maternity responsibilities. Women invested in career development must follow pathways that demand large investments of time and energy in their career at the same time that most women are parenting young children. Part-time or flexible-time opportunities are still a rarity and come with negative consequences. Women who wish to pursue their career but take maternity leave are perceived as less serious, lose valuable career development opportunities, and find reentry into full-time work complicated and problematic. Women working primarily for salaries usually are paid disproportionately low for flexible- and part-time work. Mothers staying at home receive negative messages questioning their choice to remain as full-time mothers. Questions such as, "What else are you doing with your time?" imply that this is not a wise investment or that they must somehow justify their decision.

Economic pressures forcing women into the workplace create problems in these women's ability to mother as they would like and sometimes create tensions between the mothers and spouses who do not ultimately approve of their working but must adjust to this for economic reasons. Reliable, affordable, high-quality child care is not well established in the United States. Extended families are often unavailable. Cultural values are unclear regarding the valuation of family life and parenting. Support systems for new mothers are limited and poorly defined, and role models are hard to find because women's mothers often parented in a totally different era via a very different pathway, and because each woman is forging her own route. Peer support is not as available as it should be, especially for working women who are often separated in the workplace and do not have the energy and time to establish relationships with other working mothers.

Speaking about family issues in the workplace is not yet acceptable work behavior. It would seem, given the complexity of this situation, that the woman who would be most effective in achieving a maternal identity would have to be a highly autonomous individual who feels free to construct her own role for herself. Guttman (1983)[147] has elaborated on this concept and its relationship to motherhood. A recent study by Robinson et al. (1982[148]) indicates that only a small percentage of working mothers exhibit the high degree of autonomy necessary to forge their own pathway amid this variety of options and conflicting expectations. Therapists working with mothers should therefore keep in mind that what ultimately needs to be fostered is the autonomous ability of the woman to determine her parenting needs, her personal needs, and her work needs, and to forge her own pathway toward adequately addressing these needs.

A second issue relevant to contemporary motherhood is the significant presence of single mothers. Mednick (1987[109]) has recently reviewed the literature on single mothers, noting the changing beliefs and values regarding this group. Studies have moved from assumptions about deviant family forms and psychopathology to the consideration of the possibility for good adjustment, well-being, and satisfaction for single mothers. The determinants of good outcome for these mothers have not been well established but are being explored. More sophisticated research has led to new interpretations of depression and stress in this group as being related to poverty and its concomitants rather than simply being due to single parent status. Support systems, coping styles, and life conditions have also been shown to be related to good adjustment to this status. In single mothers, enjoyment of their work and receiving of adequate pay to support their life-style have been correlated with positive mental health consequences. However, many researchers continue to be biased by traditional gender roles and do not ask sufficient questions about women's work status and satisfaction. In some studies, working single mothers reported more satisfaction and less depression than nonworking single mothers, especially if the former were able to assert their needs as mothers in the workplace. For example, refusing to work overtime because a child had to be picked up from day care signaled that role overload was preferable to a sense of helplessness and inability to care for oneself and one's family. Help with child care and household responsibilities generally correlated with a positive impact on single mothers, although, interestingly, time pressure stress was found to be less for single mothers because of absence of demands from a spouse. Autonomy, authority, and power were well correlated with positive feelings for single mothers, and perceived competence at self-support was a strong predictor of life satisfaction—even more so than perceived competence in the parenting role. The effect of sex role stereotypes that relegate women to supportive roles and create negative expectations regarding their competence in traditionally male functions (e.g., serving as the head of a household) has not been well studied. There is, however, reason to believe that single mothers are probably particularly undermined by gender role expectations.

Mednick (1987[109]) has also discussed the debilitating effect on single mothers of boys who do not affiliate, do not obey, and do not attend to their mother. There are several hypotheses, none of which are well established, to explain this. When single parenthood represents a positive choice for the mother, this would presumably have a positive impact, although this scenario has not been studied. Mednick notes that there are data to support the idea that single mothers enjoy being parents and are generally satisfied. Biases toward single mothers are declining but still exist, especially within the school system. Mednick concludes that much more research and clinical reporting on the interactions of single mothers and their children will be necessary in order to establish relevant clinical themes.

The next critical issue involving contemporary mothers is the relationship of the mother with the parenting father and with other substitute caregivers. Several authors (Casler 1961[149]; Murray 1975[150]; Rutter 1974[151]) have reported on the infant's ability to make multiple attachments and have emphasized consistency in caregiving, as opposed to a single primary caregiver, as being of paramount importance. Notman and Nadelson (1982b[152]) have emphasized that maternal separation is not equivalent to maternal deprivation. If, however, more and more young and developing children are coming in contact with multiple caregivers in the form of actively parenting fathers, day care workers, au pairs, housekeepers, family day care workers, and live-out baby-sitters, some attention should obviously be paid to the relationship between the mother and these ancillary caregivers.

Our experience with this issue is that mothers establish very complicated relationships with the persons who provide substitute care for their children and that these relationships can be either very positive or very negative for the mother in enhancing her experience of herself as a mother. Baby-sitters can be supportive of the mother in the sense that they can provide good substitute care with which the mother is comfortable and therefore is able to leave her children without undue anxiety. Supportive sitters also communicate well enough with the mother to convey important developmental information regarding her children. Additionally, these sitters may be supportive to the mother in her work role as well, helping her with household tasks and in other ways making her job easier, and at some points actually caring for her when she is ill or stressed. Other sitters are able to care well for the children but become antagonistic toward the mother when their pathways cross. Some mothers and sitters establish competitive relationships that are uncomfortable for both. Some mothers abdicate to their sitters, especially if the sitters are older than the young mother and perceived to be more capable mothers, if the young mother is defensively disengaging from her baby, or if she is under undue pressure to fully engage in the workplace with little flexibility to attend to her children. The relationship between mothers and young au pairs, a common form of substitute care, is often like that of a mother to an adolescent daughter, and the employer-mother often inherits all of the unresolved problems between the au pair and her own mother. Babysitting arrangements with extended family have proved very positive for many parents in terms of reliability and a sense that their child is being cared for by an invested person. Intergenerational competitions and conflicts may, however, interfere with what would otherwise be a positive arrangement. Sensitive mothers often change their form of child care even when it is not unsatisfactory because of awareness of the changes in the developmental needs of their children. Day care situations or family day care situations may work well for a toddler but do not always work well for older children or provide sufficient opportunities for development. Day care programs may vary in their quality with regard to the age groups that they serve, and so forth.

It is the present authors' impression based on following numerous mothers over time that invested mothers spend a great deal of time and energy establishing a positive and mutually supportive relationship with their substitute care providers. There are ample periods during the day when these mothers discuss and exchange information with the babysitter as well as work on improving the relationship between the two.

A growing number of fathers, by choice and by necessity, have become actively involved in the parenting of very young children. As noted previously (Coltrane 1989[130]), fathers who are exposed in a continuous way to young infants develop the capacity for what would traditionally be called sophisticated maternal behavior. For some mothers, this is intensely gratifying, but for others there is real difficulty in relinquishing and sharing their child and their primary role with the father, and to some degree with any babysitter. Some other mothers are frustrated and overstressed by their husband's reluctance to engage in active parenting of infants and children.

A final issue of importance is the mother's relationship with the school and, if she is employed, with her workplace. Working mothers especially appreciate sensitivity to their need for advance notification of school events and opportunities for involvement with the school system that do not conflict with their work role. Workplaces that allow little discussion of women's maternal activities and adhere to rigid structures that are incompatible with parenting needs are very stressful, especially for new mothers. In contrast, work situations with some flexibility and respect for the mother's role as well as respect for her value as a worker, and workplaces that allow for some collaboration and opportunity for the working mother to share with other working mothers, can be extremely enhancing.

Improving Help With Child Care as a Result of Increased Self-Esteem

A 35-year-old attorney who had already opted out of the large law firm rat race in favor of teaching law became a full professor during her first pregnancy. She found daily baby-sitting help for her daughter. Her selection was an older woman with infant care experience who initially planned to stay several months but agreed to remain on. The patient's husband, a busy professional with long hours, always made time to play with his daughter, although child care was left to the patient on weekends. After some debate and in line with her husband's expressed wishes, the patient again became pregnant. She managed a prestigious visiting professorship and assignment to important faculty committees. After the birth of her son she found herself chronically exhausted, awakening with him at night for the first few months. Although her sitter had some flexibility, the patient was caught, upon return from work, with driving her sitter to the train, preparing dinner for herself and her daughter, feeding her son, and keeping a late dinner ready for her husband. She was also asked to take on extra classes as a substitute for a colleague on sabbatical leave. Her husband accepted some writing obligations and had difficulty making time for his baby son. After a lot of work on self-esteem and poor feelings about entitlement, the patient was able to engage a weekend baby-sitter and contemplate hiring live-in help over her husband's initial objections.

The patient had spent a lot of time left on her own as a young child while her mother completed advanced studies. It also seems that in spare time her mother retreated to her own room behind a locked door. The patient was sent to boarding school. She fortunately had a very warm and loving relationship with her father despite his long hours attempting to save a failing business. She determined not to lock herself away from her children except on brief occasions during which her work required concentration. Always afraid to anger her husband or to argue with him because her parents had always fought, she was able to confront him and demand that he spend some time with their son.

Pregnancy Repairing a Damaged Sibling Relationship

A 36-year-old attorney left law practice in the city to move into her parents' home in a suburb after they had died. Her husband renovated the house and worked at his business while the patient took a position with a small suburban law firm, where she had a hectic, time-consuming job as a litigator. She hoped to make herself invaluable so as to secure an adequate maternity leave followed by a period of return to part-time work. This patient was bereft of family except for her mother's older sister in a distant city and a sister 2 years her junior. She had been estranged from this sister, who had been busy with an extramarital love affair during their father's terminal illness. The sister had divorced her husband and married her lover. She never visited. The patient recalled bitterly that she had taken her sister into her apartment after the sister graduated college and during the time her sister was unemployed. The two had had a bitter time over the settlement of their parents' estate. Her sister did not attend the patient's wedding.

The patient had a difficult pregnancy, including "9 months of morning sickness," and a difficult labor terminated by cesarean section and subsequent sepsis. With the baby's birth, the patient's sister came to help her out. The patient reported not only that her sister was enamored with and caring of the baby, but that she was caring of the patient as well. It seems as though the baby will be the catalyst for the reworking and resolution of these sisters' unresolved problems.

Change of Type of Caregiving to Suit the Working Mother's Needs

A 50-year-old physician mother of four children had made two successive excellent child care choices. The women chosen were older grandmotherly women whose primary task was child care. In addition, the patient had additional part-time help for baby-sitting on weekends or to do heavy cleaning. The patient cooked for her family. She did not have to take care of these women or be responsible for their social lives or affective states. She was willing to defer to both of these caregivers in terms of decisions about a variety of household matters. Both caregivers eventually retired because of age and failing health. With two children at home—one employed and ready to move out, the other about to attend high school—the patient elected a different choice. She hired a widowed woman her own age who was able to assume complete care of the house and do laundry and cooking as required. Being waited on for dinner was a pleasant and acceptable change for the patient, not regarded as a putdown by either woman. The employer-mother now makes household decisions. The housekeeper is flexible about time and is eager to help the mother and the children, even the older ones who visit.

Marriage, Career, and Motherhood Combinations

One of the most profound sociological changes of the last 20 years has been the increase in the number of women who have chosen to combine work, marital, and mothering roles for both economic and psychological reasons. Larger numbers of women today consider work in combination with motherhood as the most viable route for their self-actualization. In the early 1950s, 60% of American families contained a male breadwinner, a female homemaker, and several children; today, only 17% of all families fit that stereotype (Akabas 1984[153]). In 1980, 42% of all mothers with children under 3 years of age were employed. By 1986 this figure had risen to 51%, and it is expected to rise to above 60% in the 1990s. In fact, 52% of married women with infants under 1 year of age are currently employed (Schachere 1990[154]).

Research on this phenomenon of concurrent work and motherhood began in the late 1960s. In order to understand this phenomenon of *multiple roles*, some terminology has been developed that is helpful for therapists in dealing with women in these situations. Women involved in these types of work/family arrangements perform the roles of worker, parent, and spouse, usually simultaneously, thus the term multiple roles. *Role accumulation* is defined as the total number of roles an individual is embarking upon, and *role strain* is the perceived difficulty in performing the obligations of a role. Roles involve activities, identities, obligations, rewards, and relationships (Voydanoff 1987,[155] p. 78).

An early presumption regarding role strain was that the accumulation of multiple roles would automatically result in greater stress. However, this has not been proven to be the case. Some studies (Barnett and Baruch 1983[156]; Pugliesi 1988[157]; Wolfman 1984[158]) have shown that women with multiple roles have better psychological health when they are allowed to be autonomous in regard to how they perform the roles and when the roles are satisfying to them and assigned according to their own preference. In these studies the role of mother, not the role of worker, was noted to be most stressful. In general, however, the greater the role accumulation, the greater the possibility for potential role strain (Burr et al. 1979[159]).

Another etiology of role strain proposes that such strain occurs only when the demands of the roles outweigh the rewards and privileges; it is further noted that with some role accumulation the privileges that are accrued actually assist in the management of multiple roles (Sieber 1974[160]). Examples of this phenomenon are status enhancement, status security (in which success in one role compensates for failure in another), personal enrichment, and ego gratification.

A third approach to role strain (Marks 1977[161]) notes that for some persons, multiple roles create, rather than deplete, energy and vice versa. According to this theory, when all roles have equal positive or negative value, role strain will not occur. However, when there is a variation in the level of positive commitment, this encroaches on the time and energy available for the undercommitted interests (e.g., middle-class men overcommitted to work and undercommitted to family).

Some authors propose that women's increased entrance into the work force while men remain culturally sanctioned to being undercommitted to family life has created a special burden for women, who must now pick up and perform well in both roles. A different perspective is presented by Thoits (1983[162]), who proposes that multiple roles result in multiple identities that help to organize behavior and enhance well-being. Role conflict occurs 1) when an overload exists in which the total demands of time and energy for the various roles are too great to perform comfortably or adequately, or 2) via interference when conflicting demands make it impossible to fulfill the requirements of multiple roles. There are two types of interference: 1) interference that occurs when role expectations are contradictory or vague, and 2) role incompatibility in which the person is unable to perform the prescribed roles because of conflicts in scheduling or demands (Voydanoff 1987,[155] p. 83).

Difficulties with multiple roles affect women more than men because women have traditionally, and continue to be, expected to perform more of the household and child-rearing roles, and also because their gender roles and early socialization are more in conflict with the norms of the workplace than the gender roles and early socialization of men. Women may deal with these role stresses via two techniques (Voydanoff 1987,[155] p. 83). The first technique involves the manipulation of the role structure and relationships via compartmentalization and delegation of role obligations, elimination of role relationships, extension of role relationships to provide scarcity excuses for not performing in other roles or to facilitate role performance, and the creation of barriers against intrusion from role partners. The second technique for dealing with role conflict is negotiation of the terms of the relationships with others involved in a role. In this instance, the woman may bargain with her role partner, usually her spouse, to negotiate the standards of quality for their role performances. For example, how will we parent? What degree of household disarray will we tolerate in order to decrease the stress of additional housework?

Another set of coping strategies, which was developed by Douglas Hall (as cited in Voydanoff 1987,[155] p. 84), consists of the following:

1. *Structural role redefinition*, which is exemplified by obtaining role supports from inside and outside and changing society's definitions of the roles

2. *Personal role redefinition*, which includes eliminating roles, establishing priorities, compartmentalizing demands, and altering one's personal attitudes toward the role
3. *Reactive role behavior*, which includes working harder; planning, scheduling, organizing, and using time management techniques; and attempting to meet all external role demands [Many women engage in this latter behavior and become exhausted and overly stressed in an attempt to keep everyone happy with them.]

Another technique for role conflict involves *role cycling*, which is a common technique for two-career families in which one of the partners will pull back on a work or home commitment to allow for a pickup in another role commitment. Putting oneself on the "mommy track" is an example of role cycling.

In addition to these problem-focused strategies, Elman and Gilbert (1984[163]) define an emotion-based strategy involving modifying the woman's emotional response to the conflict via relaxation techniques, etc. Although understanding the concept of role behaviors and demands is important to mental health professionals treating working women, it cannot be seen as a substitute explanation for the full exploration of intrapsychic determinants of difficulty.

A woman's ability to structure her roles or arrange a pattern most compatible for her is greatly enhanced by her capacity for autonomous thinking. Lynn (1980[164]), in discussing women's intellectual development, notes that first-born females or females who are only children, or eldest daughters in families lacking sons, were likely to be socialized best for high achievement. Lynn suggests that fathers who relate to daughters as persons rather than as embodiments of feminine roles enhance intellectual development as well as encourage independence. A number of fathers who have been very helpful to their daughters in this respect early on in their daughters' professional development become ambivalent at the time their daughters become mothers and sometimes withdraw support. In addition, if a daughter is positively identified with her own mother, which is a desirable reaction as she becomes a mother herself, but her own mother has had traditional feminine values, this may cause undue conflict for the daughter if she is also working at the time she becomes a mother. Mothers who were devalued can create problems for daughters who work and become pregnant in that the daughter may perceive that by assuming a positive identification with her mother and paralleling her own mothering, she will lose the status that she has accomplished via working.

Lynn (1980,[164] pp. 62–65) further notes that creativity in women is correlated with a number of factors, as follows. Higher cultural level in the women's homes, professional status in their father's role, and a disparity in education between fathers and mothers in these families are positively associated with creativity. Creative women also seem to flourish in those families in which the socioeconomic position of the family was insecure relative to the actual professional status of the father. Mothers parenting daughters who are creative have higher levels of formal education, are more likely to work outside the home, and are more egalitarian in their child rearing. In the case of creative genius in women, mothers are unduly devoted to their daughters, force precocious development, and generate an unusual drive for creativity. Intense focus on the development of the daughter by one parent or the other is also typical in the childhood of creative women.

Lynn (1980[164]) also discusses a study (Hennig and Jardim 1977[56]) of high-achieving managerial women in which were reported the daughters' having a special relationship with their fathers, the daughters' engagement in vigorous physical activity, the fathers' sharing of their workplace with their daughters, and the family's explicit or tacit permission for a less-than-rigid adherence to the feminine model. Adolescence for these high-achieving women was felt to be difficult because of the impingement of peer models upon the adolescent female, making it harder for these women to utilize the support of their parents in establishing nontraditional roles for themselves.

Sefton (1987[165]) has described some of the characteristics of the dual-career family life cycle. Marriages tend to be postponed until later in life for dual-career couples. These couples often opt for a role-sharing mode. They also are often separated from their extended families either because of the geographic necessity of their work roles or because their families do not approve of the dual-career status and the couples, in order to cope with this disapproval, feel it is necessary to maintain a separation. Sexual equality and an egalitarian role-sharing mode for household work are characteristic. However, there continues to be a discrepancy even among couples who espouse to this method in that the majority of women, even in dual-career marriages, do more housework than their spouses. Some separation from families of origin is helpful in this respect in that it enables the new couple to attempt to negotiate a more balanced role sharing within their own marriage and frees them up, to some degree, from the dictates of learned dysfunctional patterns in their families of origin. The entry of a child into the dual-career family usually causes increased stress for the woman in that her definition of motherhood and femininity may require her to assume primary responsibility for child rearing, or her husband may be unwilling to assume these responsibilities. The present authors are aware of multiple studies documenting this phenomenon for women physicians (Association of American Medical Colleges 1988[166]; Bennett and Nickerson 1990[167]; Greganti and Fletcher 1985[168]; Sayres et al. 1986[169]).

It is still quite difficult to obtain appropriate child care in the United States. The supply of high-quality child care is very limited. It falls usually to the woman to negotiate difficulties and roles with child care substitutes. Strain on the family tends to decrease to some extent as the children become older and more autonomous; however, there is a danger that the parents may withdraw too much from the children and not provide adequate support at these later stages of development. Johnson and Johnson (1980[170]) described a particular form of parenting, common in dual-career couples, that stresses too much internalization of the parental norms and does not allow enough opportunity for the child to differentiate himself or herself from parental norms and expectations. Dual-career couples tend to do better at midlife in particular, with women having a less intense response to menopause and to the departure of children from the home. Difficulties with career balance can occur at this point, however, if one of the spouses is looking toward retirement or his or her career is peaking and the other's is beginning to take off.

Skinner (1980[171]) has elaborated a number of stresses common to dual-career families. She defines internal stresses as including overload issues, identity issues, role cycling issues, and family characteristics. Overload issues are particularly prevalent among dual-career couples who insist on maintaining high standards of domestic living and placing a high priority on both work and family. Identity issues stem from a discontinuity between current wishes and practices on the one hand and early identifications and gender role socialization on the other. Women have the burden of proving themselves and debunking myths regarding female workers by overachieving in their work roles, finding increased demands on their time and energy and still facing discrimination and lack of positive feedback for their high output. Another type of internal demand is a role-cycling problem involved in pivotal transitional points in the family life cycle when the woman structures her role to accommodate others. Further internal strain results from the lack of family support and relationships. Dual-career couples are in many cases isolated from their families and extended families, and they often do not have the time or opportunity to form supportive relationships. In addition, the rigid separation of work and family does not make it professionally permissible to talk about home issues in the workplace and therefore to readily establish networks with colleagues. Help can be found in network groups for working mothers (see below). Skinner also discusses normative issues that involve the bucking of the traditional norms for both family life and traditional roles of the workplace.

Dual-career couples have difficulty finding time and energy to create a social life. Poloma (1972[172]) outlined four techniques used by dual-career women to relieve tension: 1) redefinition of their situation in a more favorable light via cognitive restructuring, 2) reestablishment of priorities within each role, 3) compromise, and 4) compartmentalization of work and family roles. O'Neill et al. (1987[173]) define a group of dilemmas for dual-career couples, including career dilemmas involving conflicts in coordinating two vocations, gender role dilemmas (as previously described), and marriage family norm deviation. Gilbert (1984[174]) describes sources of stress around the question of whether and when to become a parent, child care arrangements, the combination of occupational and family roles, and occupational mobility and job placement requirements. Gilbert weighs these against the sources of satisfaction and fulfillment that come from intense spouse support and shared values and the flexibility for self-actualization within the structure.

Dual-paycheck families differ from dual-career families regarding their special issues (Stromberg and Harkess 1978[175]; Voydanoff 1987[155]). Dual-paycheck families tend to be traditional, and conflicts do not occur for the woman around career development and satisfaction. Instead, the lack of economic resources, along with limited child care options and increased pressures to work for family income, is prevalent. The rigidity of the workplace, with little opportunity for flex time and part-time work, or lack of satisfaction within the job because of its mundane nature or its perceived low status, can also be a source of stress for these women. Hochschild (1989[176]), in describing some of the outcomes of this difficulty, points out that couples either attempt to deny that they are not living according to their value system, or tend to develop problems around the inability to follow through on a value system that they both prefer. Two-paycheck families tend to fall into blue collar and the middle-class socioeconomically. They also tend to utilize and enjoy a better relationship with extended family and are more supported by the extended family in general than are dual-career couples. The disproportionately large amount of housework performed by women in dual-paycheck families is in line with traditional family values. Women have trouble asking for help, and men have trouble providing it. Lewis and Cooper (1988[177]) reported greater stress in the women in dual-paycheck families in transitioning to parenthood, presumably because of the increased demands. The dual-paycheck families reported greater distress over child care, which is often limited by these families' financial resources.

One of the present authors has had extensive experience in working with groups of career mothers over the past 6 years. Several of these groups met for more than 3 years, several as few as 3 months. However, some general themes evolved in all of these groups:

1. *The notion of a critical balance point*. Most of these women establish some form of equilibrium in balancing rather creatively a number of complicated demands and appear to be functioning at full capacity most of the time. An unexpected increased demand in work or an unanticipated illness at a time when no backup is available would often have the impact to the observer of upsetting some kind of critical balance, at which point the couple seemed unable to adapt creatively. This is similar to the tension lines described by Rapoport and Rapoport (1971[178]), which involved the points at which the couple felt if they overstepped their limitations there would be damage to themselves or to their marital state. The issue seems to speak to the degree to which working parents are operating at full capacity most of the time.
2. *The search for role models and the difficulty in accepting the need for autonomous definition of individual pathways*. Women consistently looked to the group facilitator to provide answers as though there were some right way to do things. There is a resistance to autonomous solutions in terms of each unique situation.
3. *The tendency to overfunction in an attempt to gratify and meet the needs of children, husbands, and workplaces at the expense of the women themselves*. This theme was coupled with a tendency for the women to devalue their own creativity and competence. The majority of women in these groups were operating at very high levels and quite creatively and adaptively, but they most often seemed preoccupied with concerns about ideals that they were not meeting. They had difficulty setting limits on colleagues and family members on their own behalf and tended to treat the group leader as a selfobject, as they were treated in their home and in their workplace. Interpretation of these issues over time usually resulted in a remarkable spurt of professional and personal growth of participants.
4. *Problems involved with the introversion of anger*. Discriminatory practices at work or in academic settings, as well as critical and unreasonable demands were commonly reported. Often anger at being placed in this situation was not experienced directly but projected

in the group. Interpretation of this difficulty was repeatedly necessary in order to assist these women in directing their anger more productively rather than devaluing themselves and the group leader.

5. *Competitive issues*. Competitive issues were complicated and delicate matters within each group. The initial group response was of great relief and a sense of pleasure at finding a supportive network of peers, so most of the competition was denied or directed toward the group leader. Overt competition between group members only appeared in well-established groups in which a certain level of comfort had been attained; the competitive behavior usually led to enriching discussions of the dilemma of competing with those you also wish to support.
6. *The occurrence of crisis points*. In general, in each group at least one developmental crisis occurred because of too many stresses appearing concurrently. High-achieving, competent group members seemed to have difficulty acknowledging that at times there would be periods of feeling overwhelmed. Overreacting and considering themselves complete failures was a common response.
7. *Issues around work discrimination*. Most of the groups began on a fairly optimistic note regarding the possibility for women to work hard and advance via their own merit. At some point, however, in the long-term groups, the issues of job discrimination and career arose, and there was usually a period of intense depression around the recognition of the existence of these difficulties and the amount of time it would take for change to occur.
8. *Acceptance of exaggerated responsibility for the well-being of children*. Most of the women in these groups, though performing very well at both work and at home, were quick to accept almost sole responsibility for the well-being of their children and constantly needed reassurance and reinterpretation of the multiple etiologies for any disturbances their children might be encountering.
9. *Relationships with child care providers*. Types of child care, changes in child care, child care crises, and relationships with substitute caregivers were constant focuses of attention.
10. *The establishment of critical time with the children*. Each mother needed a certain amount of unencumbered time with her children

in order to feel securely bonded. The amount of time this required differed and was to some degree related to their identifications with their mothers. That is, women who had full-time working mothers seemed to require less time at home with their children to feel connected than those women whose mothers had been home with them full time. What was important was not a specific amount of time but the autonomy and entitlement of the mother in creating the time that she needed to feel in touch with her child.

Change of Career and Child Care in a Patient Who Had Been Denying the Realities of Societal Prejudice

A patient came to treatment for depression secondary to Epstein-Barr virus, for which she had had a hospital admission. She had been working for a voluntary organization and was raising her young children. The patient supplemented the family income by caring for a racially and ethnically mixed group of children in her home. She developed a relationship that crossed ethnic lines and was appalled by having been requested to resign from the voluntary organization in which she had worked. Needing money very badly, she was unable to pick up the pieces of her life until her complex family-of-birth relationships had been worked out. She was a product of a mixed marriage. One of her parents had children of a previous single-race marriage. These single-race step-siblings left her out of family plans. As a favorite child she denied that her mother had never opposed the prejudice of her other children. Her job and service to a mixed community was a failed attempt to rework her family's life. She finished her dissertation, then planned on a part-time job, which required putting her children into full-day private school programs and abandoning the "little United Nations" she had created at home. This part-time position will lead, the patient expects, to full-time employment.

Support of Husband Allows for the Combination of High-Power Career and Motherhood

One patient was married to a commercial artist and pursuing her law career on the fast track. She was hoping to become pregnant and perhaps switch to a less demanding job. Her husband hated his work and expressed the desire to acquire a studio and paint full time. He did not want to have children, and this threatened their marriage. She told her therapist that she would stay married but would end up never forgiving her husband. Her mother had been the controlling figure in three marriages, all of which had ended in divorce. Through her treatment the patient was able to be less demanding and controlling of her husband. He quit his job to pursue his artistic career. The patient's husband was able to devote himself full time to art and, with her help, to explore his abusive childhood. Gratification in his own work and exploration of his early life as an abused child and of his fear of becoming an abusive parent allowed him to consider having children. The patient arranged to re-position herself at work to be more efficient and improve her hours. She had a baby, obtained household help, and returned to work full time. Her husband has some good prospects for his work and is very productive and helpful at home. The patient is willing to continue as the major family breadwinner.

Unwillingness to Return to Work After Delivery of a Baby and Resultant Marital Dissolution

A 28-year-old successful attorney married a man, a college graduate and a heavy marijuana user, who was in and out of satisfactory employment. She was able to prevail upon him to get treatment. During his treatment he gave up the drug abuse and began a professional graduate program. She became insistent on having a child. Her husband wanted to wait until he was employed, but she was very insistent and threatened divorce, and he gave in. The patient worked throughout her pregnancy and was able to arrange a 6-week maternity leave with pay. When her son was 6 weeks old, she had not arranged for household help and asked for another 6 weeks of leave without pay. Her husband became panicky because of the loss of income. He found it difficult to bond to the baby and had doubts about the viability of his marriage. When his wife decided at the end of 3 months that she could not leave her son and return to work, he obtained a divorce. His family of origin helped him with tuition funds and minimum maintenance. Out of necessity the patient must now return to work and obtain household help. She has hoped for a marital reconciliation. Her husband, however, feels strongly that she sabotaged his plans and still feels unready to accept the responsibility of raising a child. He is, however, committed to his son's financial support after finding employment.

Role Cycling

One physician, who had married in college, had career support from her husband, who was already employed in industry. He was especially helpful with child care and in bringing their three children for meals with her when she could not leave her hospital because she was on call. Her husband's engineering career led to a position with a company making biomedical equipment. He engineered a product with special usefulness in patients with a specific chronic disease. He did major research studies that demonstrated the value of patient education in regard to managing their own care. Learning that his credentials would not be adequate to "sell" his plan to physicians, he wondered what to do. His wife suggested that he, in his mid-40s, obtain a medical degree. He began premedical courses and applied to medical school. During the course of his education, she increased her income, assumed the major role in child care, and helped him to prepare for his examinations. After his postgraduate years he opted to practice close to home. Because his practice was slow to start and he was geographically closer to the children, he once again assumed a major child caregiving role. The couple are both authors of books in their specialties and have alternated their writing years.

When Love Fails: Uncoupling, Separation, and Divorce

Person (1989[179]), in writing about falling out of love, discusses the kinds of outcome in terms of apathy, boredom, and restlessness, as well as the development of rage and resentment. She points out that falling out of love can occur gradually or quite suddenly and that it can happen to one or both members of the dyad. Problems of exploitation, loss of autonomy, failure of mutuality, betrayal, and rejection are very painful. Overt arguments, violence, sexual involvement outside the marriage, and clinical depression are not uncommon consequences.†

The rate of divorce of heterosexual couples was 5.3 per 1,000 in 1981 (National Center for Health Statistics 1981[180]). Glick and Norton (1973[181]) projected that eventually 25% to 29% of young women in their late 20s and early 30s were likely to end their first marriage in divorce.

Qualitatively there has been a change in the kinds of people who become separated and divorced with a shift toward the more educated and affluent. All but one quarter of the women eventually remarry (Carter and Glick 1976[182]). For those women who remarry, the median duration between marriages is 4.7 years (U.S. Bureau of the Census 1977[183]). The median duration for women ages 14 to 29, ages 30 to 39, and ages 40 to 75 was 3.4, 5.8, and 6.5 years, respectively. Divorce rates are still highest in the black and Hispanic populations. The association between education and the divorce rate is a complicated one. The divorce rate is highest for high school dropouts but decreases for high school graduates. It rises again for college dropouts and falls again for college graduates. For women the divorce rate rises among those who have one or more years of postgraduate education (Carter and Glick 1976[182]).

The attractiveness of a pair partnership is directly proportional to the perceived rewards and inversely proportional to the perceived cost (Thiebault and Kelly 1959[184]). This perception may shift over time. When a relationship is more costly than rewarding, it has moved closer to dissolution. Involved in the reward-cost balance are factors such as income, status, similarities of interests, companionship and mutual esteem, sexual enjoyment, and commitment to children.

Variables Impacting on the Divorce Rate

Among the variables that impact on the divorce rate are 1) income, 2) social class and status, 3) similarities of interest, companionship, and

†The reason for focusing on heterosexual marital dissolution is simply that this is the source of the most data and the situation most studied.

mutual esteem, 4) independence and self-actualization, 5) desire for increased or decreased intimacy, 6) sexual enjoyment, 7) commitment to children, 8) legal and religious considerations, 9) availability of preferred alternatives in terms of sexual partner or life-style, and 10) intergenerational models for divorce.

The higher a woman's income, the more likely it is that she will have been divorced. Women earning their own income are three times more likely to obtain a divorce than are women without income (Carter and Glick 1976[182]).

Income

The role of the welfare systems in terms of encouraging divorce is unclear. Hornig (1973[185]) found that welfare payments were not statistically significant for white persons. Cutright and Scanzoni (1973[186]) showed no effect of benefit levels between 1950 and 1970 on the percentage of women living with a spouse present. Ross and Sawhill (1975[187]) found that predictors of female-headed families included several welfare benefit variables, women's earnings, and husband/wife family income. The value of welfare benefits plus food stamps as compared with male earnings was associated with a larger proportion of non-white women heading families.[†]

Social Class and Status

Social class is closely related to divorce. Divorce was once only fashionable and acceptable for the rich and glamorous and thus first became respectable in the highest social classes (Bernard 1970[188]). Some time after the 1920s the association between social class and divorce became

[†]In all of these studies, widowed and unmarried women were counted, so none of the data can be solely attributed to marital dissolution. It is beyond the scope of this chapter to consider the many limitations like the one just cited, which influence studies that are based on census.

inverted. Marital unhappiness has always existed in the lower social classes partly because of the greater economic stress of daily living.

Social status is a separate issue, however, if by this term we mean an investment in the status of being married. It is our experience that women may ignore their husbands' sexual affairs, their own needs for intimacy, and even their self-esteem in order to remain married. There is an entire population of women who are willing to remain financially dependent, accepting male decisions about money and its expenditure. This population may even include women who earn as much or more than their husbands. We see no shortage of women who are unwilling to risk "tipping the marital boat." For these women, marriage at any cost is preferable to being single. In addition, we have seen women who elected to divorce and are sorry that they did so, despite the fact that their marriages were at best untenable and at worst outrightly abusive.

Similarity of Interests, Companionship, and Mutual Esteem

Kerchoff (1974[189]) has noted that people marry others similar to themselves both because they encounter them more frequently and because they prefer social similarity and seek it out. Many studies show a similarity in the race, age, educational levels, religion, and socioeconomic backgrounds of marital partners, as well as similarities in physical health and interests. Blood and Wolfe (1960[190]) and Kirkpatrick (1937[191]) found that satisfaction with marital companionship was linked with satisfaction in marriage.

Mutual esteem as manifested by positive reporting about a spouse was linked with marital stability by Locke (1951[192]) and Kelly (1941[193]). Conversely, spousal criticism and complaints were linked to poor marital outcome by Good (1956[194]), Harmsworth and Minnis (1955[195]), and Locke (1951[192]).

It is apparent that studies about the above factors are old and were done while divorce was unusual rather than usual. Although we agree that divorce is related to many interpersonal factors, it seems that more of our women patients focus on issues of self-esteem, companionship, intimacy, communication, independence, and self-actualization.

Intimacy and Sexual Enjoyment

The need for independence and self-actualization along with the desire for intimacy has already been discussed (see Chapter 3). In recent years, women have tended to expect and demand sexual enjoyment. It is well accepted that there are several sources of disordered sexuality in both men and women that prevent such enjoyment (Kaplan 1979[196]). Sex therapy/counseling has become a specialty of social workers, psychologists, and physicians (see Chapter 5 for discussion of disorders of sexual functioning).

Problems in intimacy, companionship, communication, and self-actualization often masquerade as sexual problems. When women are hurt because of problems in the relationship, it is not uncommon for them to become unavailable or passive receptacles for sexual intercourse. It is common knowledge that most women are aroused by romance, fantasy, intimacy, and caring much more than by the sight of the male genital or pornographic representations of sexuality. Women are not major consumers of pornography but are instead drawn to materials such as the "Gothic Romance" novel, in which often the only physicality mentioned is the embrace in the final pages of the book.

Commitment to Children

Commitment to children is also a complicated question that has elicited contrary findings in studies. Hunt and Hunt (1977[197]) reported that 60% of all divorcing individuals had children still at home. Thus, a common belief that children hold a marriage together is shown to be false. Meade (see Bohannon 1970[198]) hypothesizes that the increase in divorce rate is related to a decline in the extended family, which once was a support system in terms of marital stability, specifically in regard to helping in the provision of child care.

There is information that links severe illness in a child with the tendency for parents to divorce (Beigleiter et al. 1976[199]; Lansky 1974[200]; Tew et al. 1974,[201] 1977[202]). Another contributing factor to the high rate of divorce is premarital conception (Davis 1972[203]).

The issue of divorce as regards children is an increasingly complicated one. There are an increasing number of custody battles, with each parent wanting to keep the child. In addition, parents are often willing to endure an ongoing bitter relationship with former spouses as complicated arrangements are made for joint or alternate custody. Some parents split up the week, and others alternate weeks, months, or even years in these custody arrangements. We have noted that blended families are becoming more common than fractured families. "His" and "Her" children often reside with the second marital pair simultaneously. The time, effort, and energy spent on making arrangements and helping these half-siblings to establish good relationships often disrupt the current marital partnership.

Legal and Religious Considerations

The upsurge in divorce has come at least in part because of the growing acceptance of divorce as an alternative to an unhappy marriage. The legal and economic constraints of obtaining a divorce had already begun to slacken in the mid-1960s (Levinger 1965[204]). Most states now have "no fault" divorce laws. In addition, the time of required residence in a particular state, as well as the required time of separation, has also decreased. Some states have community property laws that mandate the splitting of assets.

Religious interdictions against divorce are becoming less of an influence. Hunt and Hunt (1977[197]) found that there was no longer a significant difference in divorce rates between major American religious groups. The unwavering stance of the Catholic church may influence remarriage, especially in the newly emigrated Catholic population. Although the concepts of happiness and personal fulfillment remain loosely defined, they have become an expectation in a marriage that often supersedes religious convictions or edicts. In increasing numbers, young people are composing their own marriage vows that pledge mutual help, esteem, respect, and equity. Even those that take the traditional vow (i.e., "for better or for worse") seldom consider what worse would be and determine nevertheless to keep their marriage intact.

Availability of Preferred Alternatives

There is an ever increasing availability of alternatives to an unhappy marriage. As more women work full-time, economic considerations seem less of an obstacle, certainly to the middle and upper socioeconomic classes. Single parenting no longer dooms a woman either to a life of celibacy or to hopelessness about remarriage.[†] The alternative of a homosexual partner, while still socially unacceptable in "Bible Belt" communities, causes less difficulty in large population centers. Women get together to raise children. The experience of an all-female family, including mother, grandmother, aunts, cousins, or any combination of the above, is commonplace in both the black and the Hispanic populations. Some women elect to live alone without obligation to a partner.

Intergenerational Models for Divorce

Pope and Mueller (1977[205]) have carefully considered the intergenerational transmission of marital instability. The authors feel that broken parental marriages make these parents' children's marriages more susceptible to instability. The reasons for this are, first, the absence of role models for marital stability and, second, the disruptive effect on the lives of children when parents separate and divorce. Yet

---

[†]Those women who wish to continue a heterosexual life are at increasing risk because of the AIDS epidemic. Data from the Centers for Disease Control show a shift in the pattern of infection away from the male homosexual community toward intravenous drug–abusing persons and their partners and children. Women are exposed because of personal drug abuse or drug abuse by partners who are HIV-seropositive. The community of drug-abusing prostitutes is at highest risk. Some of our divorced patients have told us that the slogan frequently heard in the singles scene is, "Remember, if you sleep with that guy, you are also sleeping with everyone he has slept with in the past 10 years." Women have been purchasing and carrying condoms. Our more highly educated patients comment that they know intellectually that their heterosexual choices ought to be celibacy or monogamy. They also tell us that this is more easily said than done.

studies reporting data relevant to the transmission theory are not consistent. Duncan and Duncan (1969[206]) found no transmission. Bumpass and Sweet (1972[207]) found increased transmission in white women. Heiss (1972[208]) found little transmission in black metropolitan families.

The Context of Divorce

The usual perception about divorce is that it represents a failure that results in loss, grief, anger, and mourning sometimes made worse by the legal processes involved in separation, division of assets, custody issues, and eventual divorce. Conversely, anger and feelings of betrayal and loss often complicate the necessary formal processes. We will discuss these in some detail and then briefly present work that has been done around the concept that divorce is a developmental process that can contribute to individual growth and maturity.

It was Freud's view (Freud 1895,[209] 1918[1917][7]) that other people (i.e., objects) were important for the gratification of instinctual needs and that the pain of loss was secondary to the interruption of gratification of those needs. In considering mourning and abnormal mourning reactions, Freud theorized that the problem was one of ambivalent attachment to the object of gratification. When experiencing loss, the individual internalizes the negative part of the ambivalence onto the mental representation of the self (i.e., self representation). The positive part of the ambivalence is directed to the object representation that is then preserved in an idealized state. (See Chapter 7 for a detailed discussion of the psychodynamics of mourning.)

Bowlby's formulation (Bowlby 1973[210]) of the dissolution or loss of a relationship was that such loss involved attachment. For Bowlby, attachment needs are instinctual, beginning with the primary attachment of mother and infant, which he conceptualized as being fundamental to all future attachments. For Bowlby, mourning is for the loss of attachment.

Bergler (1970[211]) makes the case for the psychoanalytic position that divorce is the result of neurotic problems and that the divorcée, if not treated intensively, will repeat the problems in a subsequent marriage(s).

The sociological view of divorce is based on several concepts. The first is Dunkheim's concept (Gove 1973[212]) of a coefficient of protection afforded by marriage. This does not explain why divorced individuals should feel more unprotected than widowed persons. The concept that role transition is more easily accomplished by the widowed person than by the divorced individual (Jacobson 1983[213]) occurs because of the widow's right to grieve about death, the perceived guiltlessness of the widow, and her right to be supported and comforted. In our experience the perceived rights of the widow to emotional and financial support and the assumption of her guiltlessness mobilize a support network to which she feels entitled. Kitson and Zyzanski (1987[214]) have found that widows have significantly higher scores on measures of grief and that divorcées have higher levels of anger. Widows are more likely to seek help because of distress secondary to psychiatric symptoms rather than for symptoms related to grief. Divorcées, on the other hand, are more likely to seek help because of anger.

The process of divorce is a complicated one. The easiest divorce is the uncontested one in which both parties reach an agreement on all relevant issues. These may include custody of minor children, visitation, child support, spousal support, and division of marital property. The courts tend to rubber-stamp these agreements in a process that takes between 3.5 to 5 minutes (Kressel 1985[215]). Often the term *uncontested* is used from the perspective of the court and hides many hours of often acrimonious dispute involving psychiatrists, psychologists, or social workers who have served as marital counselors as well as the family and their legal representatives.

Contested divorce cases are in the minority (i.e., about 10%). About two-thirds of these concern custody disputes, and the remaining one-third are related to issues of finances, property, and support (Caron and Doyle 1979[216]). Kressel (1985[215]) points out the appalling lack of literature on the nature and extent of destructive conflicts during and after divorce settlement negotiations. Equally sparse are any large studies in the state of relations during the period of separation and negotiation. Because there are more than one million negotiations per year, Kressel finds the absence of data startling. As we have already noted, researchers tend to avoid painful subjects, especially those related to loss.

Kressel's estimate of 20% to 30% of high conflict in couples with children, based on studies of small numbers of subjects, seems low to us based on our work with patients who do not come with problems around divorce but who in the course of treatment for other problems review their divorce experiences. It may be that divorced mothers are more frequently aggrieved than divorced fathers.

Data from studies of divorced parents whose initial settlement was unsatisfactory, embittered, and difficult reveal a 50% chance of return to court for further contest in the postdivorce period (Ahrons 1981[217]).

The problem of noncompliance vis-à-vis child support is a very serious one in the case of noncustodial fathers: 50% pay little or nothing of the child support to which they are legally obligated. Even jailing in the most punitive county studied still resulted in only 40% compliance (Chambers 1979[218]). Other problems in postdivorce families have to do with unkept promises, angry scenes at visiting times with children, missed visits, and a deep reservoir of recriminations.

Kressel (1985,[215] pp. 26–27) believes that a constructive divorce settlement can ameliorate many of these problems. He outlines the key elements of a constructive settlement:

1. Resolution of *all* relevant issues
2. Tolerable financial and emotional costs
3. Technically correct agreements
4. Agreements that are fair and equitable (in line with the prevailing norms of the community)
5. Agreements that protect the rights, interests, and welfare of affected third parties [Kressel mentions children; we would include grandparents.]
6. Creative agreements (flexible, innovative, and suited to the needs of the spouses and their families)
7. Satisfaction with overall results
8. Experience of a sense of control over the agreement (rather than a sense that it has been imposed)
9. Parties complying with the agreement
10. Spouses who are better able, rather than less able, to cooperate

Certainly these are important aspects of an ideal resolution and should be the goal of both health care professionals and attorneys. However, given the predispositions that will end in separation and divorce, as well as the disappointment, anger, and mourning that interfere with negotiations, it is difficult to envision a process that can be "easy" psychologically for the majority of individuals who must negotiate from a yet raw and painful emotional stage.

Spanier and Casto (1979[219]) have addressed the issues of divorce outcome. In addition to the problems we have already mentioned, these authors call our attention to adjustments related to dealing with one's family and with social and work-related networks. In the family social network and in work-related networks, the individual becomes a single person rather than a member of a couple. The individual again becomes a sexual object, a person in need of "pairing up," an object of pity, and sometimes a competitor to a same-sex married friend or associate. Another set of adjustments relate to finding a new residence, living on less money, getting a job, and single parenting. The divorcée often needs to find new friends or to give up friends held in common with the spouse. This is not a problem for the widow. Both the widow and the divorcée must often find new affectionate and sexual partnerships. Spanier and Casto's study suggests that the transition to separation and the establishment of a new life-style are more problematic than the dissolution of the marriage.

The Distress of Divorce

Gove (1973[212]) found that married people are better off than the unmarried population in terms of their psychological functioning. Among the currently unmarried, the never married, and the married, the married function best psychologically, followed by the widowed, the divorced, and the separated. Gove especially studied suicide, motor vehicle accidents, cirrhosis of the liver, and lung cancer because of the linkage of those occurrences with alcoholism and smoking. This contrasts with the finding of no correlation between marital status and leukemia. Gove found the suicide rate for single women to be 1.5 times as great as for married women. Widowed women were more than twice as likely to commit suicide than married women. Separated and divorced women were found to have 3.5 times the rate of suicide than that for married women. Mellinger et al. (1978[220]) also studied psychological distress in women and found the best psychological health in those never married. This is in contrast to men, for whom marriage decreases the prevalence of psychic distress.

Avoiding Divorce as an Outcome

Glick (1980[221]) explains that psychoanalytic theory does not deal with a patient's disturbed feelings or behavior that is a response to someone else's disturbing actions. It can, however, help us to understand, in terms of the psychogenetic history of the individual, why certain kinds of behavior on the part of others adversely affect patient A more than patient B. For Glick, marital therapy is interpersonal and requires a systems approach. We agree that this modality of treatment may be helpful in that it focuses on the characteristic repetitive behaviors between marital partners and family members that are repeatedly frustrating and lead to distress. For example, the designation of one person as "sick," "crazy," or "impossible" leaves others in the position of not examining their own behavior. If the needs of the individuals in the dyad or family can be expressed, ways can be found for gratification that leave significant others feeling good or better.

Jacobson and Bussod (1983[222]) point out that distressed couples tend to exhibit low rates of pleasing behavior and/or high rates of displeasing behavior. They note the role of poor communications and the problems of intent versus impact. Jacobson and Bussod also feel that the existence of conflict per se is not what differentiates distressed from nondistressed relationships. Rather, it is the couple's response to conflict that is pivotal.

Bornstein and Bornstein (1986[223]) have pointed out that ongoing relationships cannot function well unless there is a mutually agreed upon division of responsibility, obligations, and rules. It is often when one member of the dyad unilaterally changes the system that couples begin to become distressed. Bornstein and Bornstein provide a concise outline of what they call the "principles of relationship change." They discuss the tactical skills of therapists that aim toward building a working relationship between partners and helping many to develop the tools to maintain this working relationship. Couples are helped to understand behavior and to speak the language of behavioral change rather than the language of criticism, complaint, and anger. According to these authors, then, the therapist's work involves cultivating reciprocity and compromise.

We have not seen large studies that document the success of marital therapy. Our experience is that persons who seek help early on and stick with it can accomplish the task. On the other hand, we do not feel optimistic when couples seek help as a last-ditch effort to save a marriage from dissolution. By this time there is a long history of hurt and rage. Often the bitterness is so great that the couple cannot cooperate even in the presence of the therapist. These marriages will dissolve, and the dissolution will be painful for the same reason.

"Divorce as a Developmental Process"

The phrase "divorce as a developmental process" has been borrowed from the title of a book edited by Gold (1988[224]). The authors in this book show that although divorce is often stressful and traumatic, it can eventually result in growth for the individual.

As Dickstein (1988a[225]) notes, divorced women are more likely to seek psychiatric help than are divorced men. They are able to integrate their new assertiveness and their rejection of the role of traditional wife, feel relief from role strain, and be open to the pursuit of career, more satisfying sexual relationships, and egalitarian marriages. Very often personal illnesses, addiction disorders, overeating, phobias, anxieties, affective disorders, and personality disorders can be treated once a marriage has been dissolved. Dickstein makes the point that women have often married because of the need for security, dependency, or escape; because of social or parental pressure; or because of pregnancy or the desire for a child. These motivations have little to do with love, self-actualization, self-esteem, or the need to share oneself with another. Kirkpatrick (1988[226]) calls attention to the opportunity for middle-aged divorced women to proceed with the delayed process of separation-individuation and to find new adaptive capacities, despite the economic strain and the frequent loss of a social support system.

In terms of sexual development, women may regain self-esteem because of the discovery that other men find them desirable. They may experiment in creative ways. These women may for the first time insist on and obtain satisfaction of their own needs. They may look to other women for fulfillment of their sexual needs. They may develop a network of women where this subject is no longer taboo. Some divorced women report masturbating for the first time (that they can remember) without guilt and in ways in which they can learn what feels good and satisfying to them.

Many divorced women expand their horizons in terms of avocational interests. Women who have neglected their physical health, appearance, and body begin to exercise, learn to use makeup, experiment with hairstyles, and dress differently. Thus they feel better, resolve depression, and undergo other positive personality changes. Economic pressures often force them to take jobs and careers more seriously. They may change jobs and careers or get promoted.

When these benefits accrue from divorce, these women become better role models for their daughters and free up both sons and daughters who have felt responsible for staying close and helping to ensure a precarious emotional balance or to relieve a previously dysphoric state.

Unfortunately there are women who remain permanently embittered, angry, and isolated. We think that there is a great deal that therapists can do to reverse this tragic outcome.

Divorce as a Developmental Process

Drug Abuse

A mother of a 3-year-old son was married to the childhood love of her life. The two came from very wealthy families who were in effect supporting them. During her pregnancy and after her son's birth, she had stopped the use of recreational drugs, which had at one time or another included marijuana, cigarettes, alcohol, and LSD. Her husband continued to be a nonworking drug user and abuser. In the course of resolving family issues, the woman realized that her relationship and her pregnancy were efforts to escape what was a nightmarish, though privileged, childhood. She obtained an entry-level production position. Although she had not been educated past private high school, she learned the trade and was rapidly promoted. She was an excellent parent.

After establishing an independent financial base and seeing no change in her husband, to whom she was still attracted, the patient decided on separation and divorce. Despite mourning connected with her decision, she continued to move forward with her life. She felt terribly guilty as her former spouse got more and more heavily into "hard drugs," but she learned that she could not rescue him any more than she had been able to rescue her birth family. She devoted herself to her work and raising her son. She refused to date until her son was 8 years old and she felt mature enough to make a rational decision about choosing a husband and a father for him.

The Search for Oedipal Victory

A married mother of four children first sought treatment after an affair that her husband knew about. He then became suspicious of all her comings and goings. Although he was a successful professional with a very masculine hobby, she regarded him as passive, lazy, and unambitious.

The patient was the only daughter of a father and mother who struggled for minimum financial security. Her father was unsuccessful, and therefore her mother had to work. Their marriage had been difficult. The father was alleged to have had several affairs, and the patient was intimately involved in "discovery operations."

The patient felt pressured to abandon her marriage, go to work, and find a more suitable partner. Her husband, although reasonably generous about child support, clearly was able to establish a more affluent life-style. He remarried very quickly to a traditional woman. The second wife came to accept the children that one by one elected to live with their father, which resulted in the patient's perceiving the second wife to be more maternal than she. In addition, another child was born into the second marriage.

The patient persevered in pushing a new career forward and becoming financially successful. However, her subsequent love affairs were unfulfilling. At first she had a dangerous but exciting liaison with a married man who helped her financially. In a series of relationships, she rejected men whom she felt were too passive, and she was involved more than once with men who were attractive and exciting but abusive in some way.

The patient came in and out of treatment as a reflection of the problems in her relationships. Her career progressed, she made friends, and developed good relationships with her grown child and a more pleasant negotiable relationship with her former spouse. Ultimately, the working out of the oedipal nature of her choices and her unresolved dependency needs led to her ability to break off a troubled relationship and be able, for the first time, to live alone.

Devaluation

A 32-year-old architect entered therapy for depression perpetuated by her recent divorce from a prominent novelist who, despite his charming and accomplished exterior, was cold and devaluing within the marriage. Although she had initiated the divorce proceedings for clear and legitimate concerns, she was filled with a sense of helplessness and failure. She had turned down a prominent fellowship to marry what her mentor had termed "the catch of the century." In the 5 years that ensued, her career became stalemated while she provided the emotional support and social entertaining necessary to promote her husband's career. Her affair with a work mentor, who took her talents seriously, clearly precipitated the divorce. Although she did not miss her husband, she was anxious regarding her decision and guilty for having disappointed her mother, who was openly critical of her decision.

The patient alternated between regressive flights home and assertive but brief forays into searching for a better job. Her anxiety symptoms escalated when she was offered a position with a prestigious firm and was unable to enjoy the substantial increase in salary that came with her new position. Dream images of herself as ugly and defective emerged in the context of her mother's critical and unempathic stance toward her. This was in striking contrast to her mother's subservient stance toward her aloof and imperious husband.

While working through these issues the patient was able to expand her creativity at work, compete for and win a promotion, and buy herself an attractive condominium. She engaged in several brief devaluing affairs but remained phobic toward marriage. During the third year of treatment she was able to move beyond affairs and establish an intimate and loving relationship with a young widower that eventually led to marriage.

Abandonment

A 36-year-old college graduate and mother of three entered therapy after her divorce from her 42-year-old husband of 16 years, a very prominent surgeon and civic leader in the small community in which they lived. Married at 20 and devoting her life to homemaking and social entertaining for her spouse, she was completely devastated when she discovered that her husband, who was Chief of Staff at the local hospital, was having an affair with his 23-year-old office nurse who, he maintained, brought him youth and excitement and whom he wished to marry. Although agreeable to a divorce, the patient was unprepared for the losses ahead. She cited social ostracization from friends, devaluing behavior from the judge when she attempted to address her ex-husband's failure to make child support payments, and abrupt decline in socioeconomic status. Her degree in liberal arts was not marketable, and when she finally gained employment, it was at an entry-level position with few benefits and no vacation time. Her children were deeply disturbed at their father's rapid remarriage and perceived displacement by his young wife who was now pregnant. The patient struggled to meet the emotional and economic challenges of single motherhood. Her mother, a wealthy widow, initially refused financial support, chastising her for failing at her marriage. She later provided some funds for housing and educational expenses but dispersed this help in a controlling, withholding manner.

At the time she was referred for treatment, the patient was intermittently suicidal but certain she would never act on her thoughts because she would never abandon her children. In treatment she was gradually able to respect her capacity in surviving her experience and was able to resume a relationship with a younger sister from whom she had been estranged. Her sister had recently been divorced and had remarried. With a loan from her sister, the patient was able to return to graduate school in a neighboring state. With her therapist's help, she located a therapist in her new location and moved herself and her children to a university apartment, where she initiated a peer support group for divorcées, established a baby-sitting cooperative, and obtained her master's degree. Two years later her former therapist received an announcement of her marriage to a faculty member at the university where she worked.

Settling Versus Falling in Love

There are many women who have postponed marriage until their 30s and who are then unable to find available men with whom they can fall in love. In addition, there is a pool of divorced women in their 20s, 30s, and 40s who do not look forward to spending years alone. After a period of the "singles scene" in which they feel too old because like-aged men are looking for women in their 20s, these women decide that it is unlikely that they will fall in love and they are willing to settle for men who seem kind and companionable but with whom they have not fallen in love. Sometimes settling is done under the pretense of being in love, and sometimes it happens as a rational decision made by the individuals involved. The AIDS epidemic has made the sampling prospect more unpalatable to more mature adults of both sexes than it seems to persons still in their 20s. This is a topic that the psychiatric and psychological literature has ignored.

Settling Because of Grief

The patient, a victim of early traumatic widowhood, remarried in a relationship where both she and her partner consciously settled, rather than falling in love. The couple thought that they could manage a blended family together. The patient resolved constant sadness and returned to postgraduate work and a successful career. When the children were grown, the couple divorced. The marriage had accomplished its purpose. In addition, settling represented a wish not to reinvest again in a profound love relationship and be at risk for loss.

Settling for Security

A 40-year-old divorced, childless florist had about given up on marriage. Through her work she found a man who was the father of three high school–age daughters. His wife had "discovered her homosexuality" and had moved out, leaving the children behind. The man was a very successful businessperson with no financial postdivorce obligations. The florist and her newly found acquaintance enjoyed each other's company. She sought help when she realized that he wanted to marry her. On a cognitive level she found him attractive and interesting but realized that she was not in love with him, although she felt she might begin to love him. She contrasted her present feelings with the tempestuous feelings she had had in her first, chaotic, and short-lived marriage.

The patient felt secure and even proud at the thought of accepting a marriage proposal. She welcomed the opportunity of acquiring children. His children were eager to have a mother in their home. She felt guilty about marrying someone whom she perceived to be in love with her when she did not reciprocate those feelings. She was afraid to discuss her doubts with this man because she might lose him. In fact, she had lost her father prior to her first marriage, of which he had not approved. Psychodynamic issues focused around guilt and loss. Finally, she discussed her feelings with her partner and he responded by saying that she would feel more loving toward him as time went on. Falling in love was not a major issue for him because an "in love" relationship had failed him. Indeed, the two were married and raised the daughters who always remained attached to both of them. In addition to their work, the couple developed a joint hobby.

Settling Because of the Need to Support Two Young Children

A homemaker in her late 40s sought treatment because she wished to leave her husband. She had two daughters in college. The patient had a new work opportunity to which her husband objected. In her early 20s her first husband had committed suicide after discharge from a psychiatric hospital. She was left with his children, two toddlers, and very little money, in a city far from her own parents. Her first husband's parents abandoned her after his death and never saw their grandchildren again. The patient had married a second time, to an older man who had been divorced and was well-to-do. Her second husband adopted and supported her children. He was a kind person but very obsessional and still a workaholic. She felt that she was dying in her fancy apartment and worried about what he would do should she now divorce him. She felt that she had never been free in her life since her childhood, so she decided to work and try to make a life for herself.

After their divorce, her second husband found a new partner and was soon remarried. The patient spent some years working her way up to an excellent position and dating some unpromising men. She then met a recent widower who was successful, helpful in her career, and had a variety of interests and many friends. With her children now adults, she decided that this would be a suitable marriage that would not only offer security but allow her freedom to work and a chance for fun in the form of entertainment, travel, and a social network. For the first time, the patient began to laugh and enjoy herself. Her children, although they loved their adoptive father, found her new husband, their "stepfather," easier and nicer to be around.

Settling for the Picture-Perfect Life

Another patient married a man whom she called her childhood sweetheart. She was a bright, obsessional student from a fractured family. Her father had had many love affairs and several marriages. He was intellectual and entertaining. Her mother was described as not too bright, a stay-at-home housewife who eventually married a laborer. As a child this patient had picked out a stable, comfortable, intelligent family and man whom she felt had great potential. His family had helped finance her education.

She came to treatment because she "could no longer do without sex." Her husband felt severely wounded by the need to pursue her and because of her lack of sexual responsiveness. She did love him but had a profound disorder of desire. She had never had conscious sexual fantasies and had never masturbated. (Moreover, she was unwilling to masturbate.) Despite a long analysis and an understanding of her need to avoid her father's open sexuality, the patient really was never able to become sexually stimulated. Her husband did very well financially and they bought a beautiful house. He felt unwilling to "screw just to have kids," nor did he wish to be merely accommodated. Her wish to have children, her fantasies about a loving relationship with them, her reparative fantasies about the perfect family, and the acquisition of family pets allowed her to become interested in and focused on the loving aspects of lovemaking. Her husband felt better, and she felt relieved of the demand to become a sexual person. She had succeeded in settling for a life without sexuality, although not without sex.

She has one child and hopes to conceive again. She is active in her community and has the "normal, comfortable life" for which she had chosen her husband.

The "Sandwich Generation"

The generation of women who have assumed primary responsibility for the care of dependent children and for the elderly has been dubbed the "Sandwich Generation."† Some of these women are also managing work or careers. The elderly not only may be these women's own parent or parents, but may be grandparents, aunts, and uncles of their own as well as parents, grandparents, aunts, and uncles in their husband's family. Women are more frequently burdened with this responsibility than men, regardless of equal work status, because it is demanded of them and because they value relationships and find it more difficult than men to walk away.

In the first chapter of our book, we discussed the narcissistic attachment of mothers to their daughters. Deutsch (1925,[228] 1930,[229] 1944,[230] 1945[113]) noted that women seem more inner directed, intuitive, and empathic than men. Greenacre (1952b[231], 1953a[232], 1953b[233]) pointed out that the fear of loss of love seems more important in female develop-

†We are unsure where the descriptive phrase "Sandwich Generation" originated. It appeared in quotation marks in a paper by Notman (1990,[227] p. 151). We first heard this phrase at a meeting of the Dependent Care Task Force of the American Medical Women's Association.

ment than other sources of anxiety. Bernstein and Warner (1984b[96]) have noted that the fantasies, identifications, and selfobject representations arising from the preoedipal mother/daughter relationship are responsible for otherwise unintelligible problems of the life cycle, including the stress of the "Sandwich Generation." The preoedipal narcissistic relationship of mother and daughter may be displaced or replayed in relation to the care of elderly parents or parent surrogates. Gilligan (1982[234]) focuses on the tendency of women to take a broad view in terms of the consequences for many individuals with whom they have relationships. She proposes that women consider loyalties, the well-being of a group, and the value of a concept or project in an altruistic way.

In publications by The Stone Center for Developmental Services and Studies, a theory of female development based on the primary importance of relationships has been elucidated. Surrey (1985[74]) discusses the mutuality of growth of mother and daughter by which a collaborative, flexible life-style evolves. Jordan et al. (1983[235]) points out that in the context of this kind of relationship, empathy evolves. Women who have not had the advantage of such a relationship get depressed because they hold themselves responsible for the failure of a relationship. A relationship may seem "failed" if the parent or parent surrogate is not well, is depressed, or is disappointed in his or her care and maintenance.

Lerner (1985[236]) has elucidated the tendency of women to express their anger against introjected selfobjects. By this she means that self and object representations remain merged and that anger mobilized against the object is therefore directed against the self representation. Therefore, the resentment of the elderly person who is failing and requires care may cast its shadow over the self representation, causing self-hatred, loss of self esteem, and depression.

Particularly pertinent to the problem of the "Sandwich Generation" is the fact that women are supposed to be sensitive, pleasing, and attuned to and responsible for the emotional needs of others, even when these needs are overwhelming and regressive. Women are expected to avoid displeasing others while attaining or even surpassing other norms.

It has been noted (Dohrenwend 1973[237]; Gilligan 1982[234]; Miller 1976[238]) that women are especially stressed by situations that are beyond their control and by those in which they perceive themselves to be responsible for the well-being of others. In situations such as these, failure causes a marked lowering of self-esteem.

Many women become depressed not because of psychogenic or genetic/biochemical abnormalities but because of the burden of this severe role strain. Working inside or outside of the home and caring for dependent children are tasks that require a high degree of flexibility, stamina, and good physical health. Adding the burden of elder care can often overwhelm mental and physical resources. In addition, when elderly persons are ill and often deteriorating in overall physical status, they themselves frequently become depressed. The sadness and helplessness of many elderly persons and their depression are often contagious and pass on to the caregiver. Problems of elder care are predominantly dealt with in articles about nursing homes and nonfamily home-rendered care. Even in these cases little note is taken of the fact that a family member must still supervise the care and must often contribute to the finances of the elderly person.

Some authors have dealt specifically with the nature of the role strain and the specific psychodynamics of intergenerational relationships. Brody (1979,[239] 1981[240]) has noted that middle-age women, with their changing life-styles and responsibilities, may be at high risk for stress-related health problems. Shanas (1980[241]) points out that neither older adults nor their adult children have been socialized adequately to cope with increased longevity and fewer caregivers. Although the consequences of aging are a fact, our culture provides little guidance to help make decisions associated with planning for complex health-related social and economic issues of elderly persons. Some authors (Arling 1976a[242]; Getzel 1981[243]; Seelback 1978[244]) reported that neither the elderly person nor the adult child caregiver was prepared to accept the shift in roles. Adult children achieve their independence, establish their own way of life, and develop careers. In short, their lives are full. They, as well as their elderly parents, have memories of how their relationship had once been and how this has colored their ability to see the nature of each other's life-style, needs, and health in the present (Johnson 1983[245]).

Cohler and Greenbaum (1981[246]) suggest that adult women and their mothers continue to be dependent on each other. In contrast, Bromberg (1983[247]) describes the mother/daughter relationship as potentially becoming characterized by mutuality and interdependence, whereas the father/daughter relationship seems more often to remain a relationship of unequals, with the father in the authoritarian role.

Geographical distance also enters the caregiving equation. Daughters at more distant geographical locations report emotionally negative effects, such as feeling helpless, drained, and overwhelmed, and having difficulty in setting priorities, particularly related to their mother's need for help (Schoonover et al. 1988[248]).

Streib and Beck (1980[249]), in their decade review of elder care, point out that there is a paucity of published work related to ethnicity.

Reinhardt and Fisher (1989[250]) have found that in studying social adaptation in elderly women, the primary factor was not marital status but the relationship with a daughter. The effect of daughters working outside the home versus daughters working in the home relative to providing care to widowed mothers was studied by Brody and Schoonover (1986[251]). These authors found that patterns of help provided to disabled elderly widows were no different in the group of daughters working outside the home and in those daughters who were homemakers.

It is apparent that all of the research that we have cited (and that which we could cite) has focused on the role of daughters in elder care, especially in care of mothers. Daughters' care of mothers is of greater importance because women outlive men. It is the daughter who most frequently provides care for her aging parent and other relatives, both biological and in her husband's family, as we will show in our case histories. It is also true that daughters care more about all of these aging relatives than do sons.†

†Note the old adage, "A son is a son 'til he gets him a wife; a daughter is a daughter for the rest of her life."

Care of Extended Family

One patient in her 50s who worked out of her home as a freelance artist already was burdened by the need to render some physical care for an adult disabled child. In addition, she had partial responsibility for the financial support of her elderly mother. The mother's bachelor brothers (i.e., the patient's uncles) helped with this obligation. They were schizoid individuals who never welcomed anyone to their home. When one had to be hospitalized and the patient went to see how she could help, she found an apartment that looked as if it had not been painted or cleaned in 40 years. The uncle remaining at home clearly required physical assistance, which the now-hospitalized uncle had once given him. The hospitalized uncle required funding for his care. The patient thus became responsible for these two elderly men. She found and engaged a housekeeper as well as an around-the-clock caregiver. After the hospitalized brother died, the one remaining uncle became clinically depressed and required hospitalization and antidepressant medication. This uncle was then able to return to home. The patient now finds herself balancing, along with her uncle's care, her career, extended visits from cross country, visits with grandchildren, and visits to her mother who lives out of state.

* * *

A patient in her mid-30s, after acquiring her M.B.A., had a responsible position that did not require her to travel. When her husband's brother committed suicide, she found herself responsible for helping her widowed mother-in-law, who lived in another state, cope with the loss. The patient did this despite the fact that she was finally pregnant with her first baby, after operative and biochemical procedures and hormonal treatment.

* * *

A patient in her 50s had been divorced for 3 years, during which time her ex-husband had remarried. He ultimately divorced his second wife after she lost a child and became depressed, and remarried the patient, his first wife. The second wife became alcoholic. During one of her husband's business trips, the ex–second wife developed liver disease as well as bleeding from esophageal varices. The patient suddenly found herself responsible for arranging hospitalization for the woman she referred to as her "step-wife."

Care of Mother and Siblings

One patient in her 20s suddenly lost her father in her junior year in college. Her father, in a spiteful rage over reimbursement for minor surgery, had canceled his life insurance that he had held with the same company. The family was thus left virtually penniless. The patient took on the responsibility of helping to support her two younger brothers even though she was not earning a great deal. She was devoted to her widowed mother. Her fiancé, who had worked his own way through college and graduate school, was very upset that she did not wash her hands of the situation. He felt that the patient's brothers were very spoiled. She felt very sad for the youngest brother, who had lost his father when he was 12, and she knew that her help meant a great deal symbolically.

Care of Dying Parents

A young attorney who had a very promising career with a major law firm forfeited her career in the following context. Her father developed prostatic cancer and her mother felt unable to cope. Surgery brought a remission, but his very bitter moods worsened because of his impotency. Her mother neglected a problem in swallowing, thinking that it was "just nerves." Upon evaluating the patient's mother, it was found that she had inoperative gastric cancer. The patient devoted her life, during the year her mother lived, to her mother's chemotherapy and to helping her mother keep up appearances so that she could continue to work. Her mother was the family breadwinner. After a period of grieving and just when the patient was attempting to put her life and career back together, a routine checkup revealed that her father had bone metastases. Although very angry at this man, who had not been kind to her and had withdrawn from her mother's care, the patient nevertheless dedicated herself to his terminal care. The young woman has since returned to her career, married, and is expecting a baby.

Care of a Dependent Widowed Parent

One of the authors has worked with two women who verbalized that they had lost the wrong parent. Each nevertheless went on to assume responsibility for the remaining parent not out of guilt but because they felt that they were doing what the favorite parent would have expected of them. Each of these patients initially presented with panic attacks and forms of somatization—symptoms that lasted until they could identify their resentment due to the task they had undertaken. They also had to understand their identification with the deceased but preferred parent.

Parent Care in a Dysfunctional Family

A divorced woman in her 30s, who was a mental health professional, severed her relationship with both parents and a psychotic older sister. She felt that her mother had always teamed up with her older sister to protect the sister at the patient's expense. The patient had been physically abused by the elder sister. Only careful review of the family history revealed that the older sister had once been treated in a residential setting for schizophrenic children, a fact that both parents denied. The patient had very much been her father's daughter even though, when it came down to siding with her, her father bowed to his wife's pressure. She tended to her father during his terminal illness but refused to have anything to do with her manipulative mother.

The mother announced her intention to keep smoking despite repeated hospitalizations for emphysema. The patient's attitude was "Let her smoke herself to death." Her mother eventually succumbed to emphysema, but the patient did not attend her funeral. In marked contrast was her attachment to and care of her mother's brother, an irrascible old man with a long history of psychiatric treatment. Clearly he loved her and understood her adaptation to her family of origin. She spoke with him daily, visited him, and saw that he had household help to tend to his daily needs.

Care of Both a Disabled Parent and a Sibling

A 33-year-old unmarried attorney who was up for partnership in her firm presented because of a serious depression. A number of years earlier her father had had a stroke that necessitated care in a nursing facility. Her older brother, who lived with her mother, suffered from a painful degenerative disease. She, her younger brother, and his wife visited the father and took him out of the nursing home every weekend. The attorney had not taken a vacation in years and had all but given up her social life. She felt that she would lose her chance to achieve her desired professional aim if she did not put more of her energy toward this goal and less into her family. She felt guilt ridden and duty bound to her father's demands and to relieving her mother's burden. In fact, the patient was afraid that her father would deteriorate and die if she were not at his beck and call. Obviously behind the fear lay the wish: Her father had been a very narcissistic and demanding man who had never cared to understand the wishes, needs, and plans of his children. Her mother was very locked into her husband's perceptions and therefore really emotionally unavailable to the patient. The patient had been badly assaulted in the context of a job she had held between college and graduate school. She had never shared this experience or its sequelae with her parents, feeling that they would blame her, even though she had been the sleeping victim.

In her treatment she was helped to understand her anger, and her wish for a life of her own was supported. She took a first vacation, a share in a summer house, and went out of town to visit with college friends on occasional weekends. Her father survived her absences. At a time when her mother had to be out of town because elderly grandparents were ill, and her younger brother could not be available, she decided to go on with her own life. Her chronically ill older brother managed his own care. He managed to visit the father in the nursing home. When her mother had a fall and broke some bones, the daughter was helpful but did not move in to take over. She worked hard toward advancing her own career and pursuing a social life. She became more lively and assertive, and established her credibility as a litigator who could not be coerced or manipulated.

A not altogether unpredictable outcome was that the patient's father became less regressed, learned to manage his own bodily functions, and could be moved to a more ambulatory functioning unit that was less depressing. The patient's mother was planning to retire and move with the patient's father and older brother, feeling that the change of climate would benefit her son. In this location there would be availability of living units where a patient could more easily be transferred from a family living unit to a skilled care floor as needed.

It is often difficult to discriminate between the perceived (i.e, guilt driven) demand of the "sandwich woman" and the reality. The case of the woman who had to care for her mother with gastric cancer because her father would not have done so emphasizes the reality aspect. The woman who attended her father's nursing care facility on his demand is on the other end of the spectrum.

One of the authors has treated a woman, a married mother and teacher, who was very attached to her husband's parents. When they elected to give up their home and move to a multilayered facility where they could live together or could have more intensive care as needed, she had trouble accepting their decision because of severe hostility to her own parents and attachment to these "good surrogate parents" to whom she felt indebted. Nevertheless, her husband's parents' decision was made, and she was forced to accept it. Had they been ambivalent or guilt-producing parents, they would have found a willing caregiver in their daughter-in-law, anyway.

Care of a Spouse's Family

A woman professional in her 50s was in psychoanalytic treatment because of difficulties in actualizing her career potential. She had problems in self-assertion both at work and at home. She had agreed to a financial investment by her husband even though she did not approve of it. After this she took more control of family finances.

Her husband had never had a real attachment to his family of origin, and over the years she had often taken over social obligations, helped her mother-in-law on occasion, and visited regularly. When it was clear that her mother-in-law needed outside help to clean, prepare meals, and help with shopping and laundry, the patient found such an employee, whom her husband paid out of his earnings.

Her husband began to have some financial difficulties. The couple had already committed themselves to furnishing a baby's room for the grandchild they expected. Her husband was unable to pay for his mother's helper, and the patient felt called upon to meet this obligation out of her paycheck, although this money was already allotted to household expenses. She felt depressed in a way she had not been for over a year. She made the decision to review family finances with her husband and to insist that his brother begin to assume some responsibility for their mother. She also decided to reassess the extent of their promised gift for their grandchild.

Women feel the need to be physically and affectively present, even if this presence is not required in reality. Men feel the obligation to see that everything is properly managed, ordered, and arranged. This represents a good partnership of effort, each sex doing what they conceptualize as their role. If this can be done with mutual support and respect, it can work well.[†] One could argue that the "feminine style" is more stressful because of the requirement for physical proximity regardless of obligation to work or family. It is difficult to judge whether the overt affective involvement is more stressful than its displacement or perhaps its sublimation into the cognitive system. If the elderly persons needing care are panicky or depressed, certainly physical proximity to the affective storm makes the panic or depression more likely to be contagious. It might be, however, that hearing it by telephone or secondhand might be more stressful than being directly involved in the care.

Notes

1. Person ES: Dreams of Love and Fateful Encounters: The Power of Romantic Passion. New York, WW Norton, 1989
2. Glick PC: How American families are changing. American Demography 6:20–27, 1984

[†]As this book was being written, the authors both had instances of an elderly parent-in-law becoming suddenly seriously ill. The authors' husbands, both of whom are very caring persons, handled the events logically, making good arrangements during the crises. Both sisters-in-law, having careers and families of their own, physically went to be with the ailing parent. One of the daughters-in-law did the same. These, we felt, were good indicators of nonpathological but quite different styles of caring illustrated by men and women in two families, each of which have good relationships with parents and parents-in-law.

3. Bumiller E: May You Be the Mother of a Hundred Sons. New York, Random House, 1990
4. Friedl E: Women of Deh Koh: Lives in an Iranian Village. Washington, DC, Smithsonian Institute Press, 1988
5. Freud S: A special type of choice of object made by men (contributions to the psychology of love I) (1910), in The Standard Edition of the Complete Psychological Works of Sigmund Freud, Vol 11. Translated and edited by Strachey J. London, Hogarth Press, 1957, pp 163–175
6. Freud S: On the universal tendency to debasement in the sphere of love (contributions to the psychology of love II) (1912a), in The Standard Edition of the Complete Psychological Works of Sigmund Freud, Vol 11. Translated and edited by Strachey J. London, Hogarth Press, 1957, pp 177–191
7. Freud S: The taboo of virginity (contributions to the psychology of love III) (1918[1917]), in The Standard Edition of the Complete Psychological Works of Sigmund Freud, Vol 11. Translated and edited by Strachey J. London, Hogarth Press, 1957, pp 191–208
8. Freud S: Observations on transference-love (further recommendations on the technique of psycho-analysis III) (1915[1914], in The Standard Edition of the Complete Psychological Works of Sigmund Freud, Vol 12. Translated and edited by Strachey J. London, Hogarth Press, 1958, pp 157–173
9. Kernberg O: Barriers to falling and remaining in love. J Am Psychoanal Assoc 22:486–511, 1974a
10. Kernberg O: Mature love: prerequisites and characteristics. J Am Psychoanal Assoc 22:743–768, 1974b
11. Jacobson E: The Self and the Object World. New York, International Universities Press, 1964
12. Bak RK: Being in love and object loss. Int J Psychoanal 54:1–8, 1973
13. Bergmann MS: Psychoanalytic observations on the capacity to love, in Separation-Individuation. Edited by McDevitt JV, Settlage CF. New York, International Universities Press, 1971, pp 15–40
14. Josselyn IM: The capacity to love: a possible reformulation. Journal of the American Academy of Child Psychiatry 10:6–22, 1971
15. Balint M: On genital love, in Primary Love and Psychoanalytic Technique. New York, Tavistock, 1948, pp 109–120
16. Arlow J, Freud A, Lampl–de Groot J, et al: Panel discussion. Int J Psychoanal 49:506–512, 1968
17. May R: Love and Will. New York, WW Norton, 1969
18. Bernstein AE: A psychoanalytic contribution to the etiology of "back pain" and "spinal disc syndromes." J Am Acad Psychoanal 6:547–556, 1978
19. Erikson EA: Identity, Youth, and Crisis. New York, WW Norton, 1968a

20. Fairbairn WRD: An Object-Relations Theory of the Personality. New York, Basic Books, 1954
21. Glick P: A demographer looks at American families. Journal of Marriage and the Family 37:15–26, 1975
22. Nadelson CC, Notman MT: To marry or not to marry: a choice. Am J Psychiatry 138:1352–1356, 1981
23. Goldberg M: The dynamics of marital interaction and marital conflict. Psychiatr Clin North Am 5:449–467, 1982
24. Bell R: Marriage and Family Interaction. Homewood, IL, Dorsey Press, 1971
25. Bird C: The case against marriage, in The Future of the Family. Edited by Howe LK. New York, Simon & Schuster, 1972
26. Brazelton TB: Stress for families today. Infant Mental Health Journal 9:65–71, 1988
27. Nadelson CC: Marital therapy from a psychoanalytic perspective, in Marriage and Marital Therapy: Psychoanalytic, Behavioral, and Systems Theory Perspectives. Edited by Paolino TJ Jr, McCrady BS. New York, Brunner/Mazel, 1978, pp 89–164
28. Main TF: Mutual projection in a marriage. Compr Psychiatry 7:432–449, 1966
29. Dicks HV: Object-relations theory and marital studies. Br J Med Psychol 36:125–129, 1963
30. Berman EM, Lief HI: Marital therapy from a psychiatric perspective: an overview. Am J Psychiatry 132:583–592, 1975
31. Blanck R, Blanck G: Marriage and Personal Development. New York, Columbia University Press, 1968
32. Mittelmann B: The concurrent analysis of married couples. Psychoanal Q 17:182–197, 1948
33. Martin PA: A Marital Therapy Manual. New York, Brunner/Mazel, 1976
34. Sager CJ: Marriage Contracts and Couple Therapy: Hidden Forces in Intimate Relationships. New York, Brunner/Mazel, 1976
35. Quadrio C: Analysis and system: a marriage. Aust N Z J Psychiatry 20:219–224, 1986
36. Kohut H: The Analysis of the Self: A Systemic Approach to the Psychoanalytic Treatment of Narcissistic Personality Disorders. New York, International Universities Press, 1971
37. Kohut H: The Restoration of the Self. New York, International Universities Press, 1977
38. Mahler MS, Pine F, Bergman A: The Psychological Birth of the Human Infant: Symbiosis and Individuation. London, Hutchinson and Company, 1975

39. Fogarty TF: The role of romantic love in marriage, in Contemporary Marriage: Special Issues in Couples Therapy. Edited by Goldberg DC. Homewood, IL, Dorsey Press, 1985, pp 19–34
40. Inglis A, Greenglass ER: Motivation for marriage among women and men. Psychol Rep 65:1035–1042, 1989
41. Adams M: The single woman in today's society: a reappraisal. Am J Orthopsychiatry 41:776–786, 1971
42. Krausz SL: Sex roles within marriage. Social Work 31:457–464, 1986
43. Hunt JG, Hunt LL: The dualities of careers and families: new integrations or new polarizations? Social Problems 29:499–510, 1982
44. Moore K, Spain D, Bianchi S: Working wives and mothers. Marriage and Family Review 7:77–98, 1984
45. Ramu GN, Tavuchis N: The valuation of children and parenthood among the voluntary childless and parental couples in Canada. Journal of Comparative Family Studies 17:99–116, 1986
46. Veevers JE: Childless by Choice. Toronto, Butterworths, 1980
47. Yogev S, Vierra A: The state of motherhood among professional women. Sex Roles 9:391–396, 1983
48. Schlesinger B: Lasting marriages in the 1980s. Conciliation Courts Review 20:43–49, 1982
49. Gottman JM, Krokoff LJ: Marital interaction and satisfaction: a longitudinal view. J Consult Clin Psychol 57:47–52, 1989
50. Green BL: A Clinical Approach to Marital Problems: Evaluation and Management. Springfield, IL, Charles C Thomas, 1970
51. Greenbaum H: On the nature of marriage and marriage therapy. J Am Acad Psychoanal 11:284–297, 1983
52. Greenbaum E: Unfolding of identifications: repetition and change in identity formation. J Am Acad Psychoanal 1:125–143, 1973
53. Calogeras RC: Early object-relations conflicts in marital interaction. Psychoanal Rev 72:31–53, 1985
54. Finkelstein L: Psychoanalysis, marital therapy, and object-relations theory. J Am Psychoanal Assoc 36:905–931, 1988
55. Horner MS: Toward an understanding of achievement-related conflicts in women. Journal of Social Issues 28:157–175, 1972
56. Hennig M, Jardim A: The Managerial Woman. New York, Anchor Press/Doubleday, 1977
57. Moss-Kanter RM: Men and Women of the Corporation. New York, Basic Books, 1977a
58. Moss-Kanter RM: Some effects of proportions on group life: skewed sex ratios and responses to token women. American Journal of Sociology

82:965-990, 1977b [Reprinted in Rieker PP, Carmen EH (eds): The Gender Gap in Psychotherapy: Social Realities and Psychological Processes. New York, Plenum, 1984, pp 53–78]

59. Simmel G: The Sociology of Georg Simmel. Translated by Wolff KH. Glencoe, IL, Free Press, 1950
60. Moss-Kanter RM: Some effects of proportions on group life: skewed sex ratios and responses to token women, in The Gender Gap in Psychotherapy: Social Realities and Psychological Processes. Edited by Rieker PP, Carmen EH. New York, Plenum, 1984, pp 53–78
61. Laws JL: The psychology of tokenism: an analysis. Sex Roles 1:51–67, 1975
62. Klein F: Sexual harassment in federal employment: factors affecting its incidence, severity, duration and relationship to productivity. Doctoral dissertation, Brandeis University, Waltham, MA, 1984
63. Rowe M: Barriers to equality: the power of subtle discrimination to maintain unequal opportunity. Employee Responsibilities and Rights Journal 3:153–163, 1990
64. Applegarth A: Some observations on work inhibitions in women. J Am Psychoanal Assoc 24(suppl):251–268, 1976
65. Person ES: Women working: fears of failure, deviance and success. J Am Acad Psychoanal 10:67–84, 1982
66. McIntosh P: Feeling like a fraud. The Stone Center for Developmental Services and Studies, Work in Progress, Wellesley, MA, 1985, No 85-18:1–17
67. Stiver IP: Work inhibitions in women. The Stone Center for Developmental Services and Studies, Work in Progress, Wellesley, MA, 1983, No 82-03:1–11
68. Lerner HE: Internal prohibitions against female anger. Am J Psychoanal 40:137–148, 1980
69. Lerner HE: Female dependency in context: some theoretical and technical considerations. Am J Orthopsychiatry 53:697–705, 1983
70. Lerner HE: Work and success inhibitions in women: family systems level interventions in psychodynamic treatment. Bull Menninger Clin 51:338–360, 1987
71. Bernardez-Bonesatti T: Women and anger: conflicts with aggression in contemporary women. J Am Med Wom Assoc 33:215–219, 1978
72. Miller JB: The construction of anger in women and men. The Stone Center for Developmental Services and Studies, Work in Progress, Wellesley, MA, 1983, No 83-01:1–7
73. Bernardez-Bonesatti T: Women and anger: cultural prohibitions and the feminine ideal. The Stone Center for Developmental Services and Studies, Work in Progress, Wellesley, MA, 1988, No 88-31

74. Surrey JL: Self in relation: a theory of women's development. The Stone Center for Developmental Services and Studies, Work in Progress, Wellesley, MA, 1985, No 85-13
75. Symonds A: The dynamics of depression in functioning women—sexism in the family. J Am Acad Psychoanal 14:395–406, 1986
76 Lebe DM: Female ego ideal conflicts in adulthood. Am J Psychoanal 46:22–32, 1986
77. Kaplan EH: Career change in early adulthood: developmental considerations. Adolesc Psychiatry 16:259–277, 1989
78. Michels R: Adulthood, in The Course of Life: Psychoanalytic Contributions Toward Understanding Personality Development, Vol 3: Adulthood and the Aging Process (DHHS Publ No [ADM]-81-1000). Edited by Greenspan SI, Pollock GH. Washington, DC, National Institute of Mental Health, 1980, pp 25–34
79. Viederman M: Personality change through life experience (I): a model. Psychiatry 49:204–217, 1986
80. Perosa SL, Perosa LM: The mid-career crisis in relation to Super's career and Erikson's adult developmental theory. International Journal of Aging and Human Development 20:53–68, 1984–1985
81. Read NO, Elliot MR, Escobar MD, et al: The effects of marital status and motherhood on the career concerns of reentry women. Career Development Quarterly 37:47–55, 1988
82. Rosenwald GC, Wiersma J: Women, career changes and the new self: an analysis of rhetoric. Psychiatry 46:213–229, 1983
83. Gooden W, Toye R: Occupational dream, relation to parents and depression in the early adult transition. J Clin Psychol 40:945–954, 1984
84. Archer SL: Gender differences in identity development: issues of process domain and timing. J Adolesc 12:117–138, 1989
85. Nadelson CC, Notman MT, Bennett MB: Success or failure: psychotherapeutic considerations for women in conflict. Am J Psychiatry 135:1092–1096, 1978
86. Money J: Androgyne becomes bisexual in sexological theory: Plato to Freud and neuroscience. J Am Acad Psychoanal 18:392–413, 1990
87. Freud S: Three essays on the theory of sexuality (1905b), in The Standard Edition of the Complete Psychological Works of Sigmund Freud, Vol 7. Translated and edited by Strachey J. London, Hogarth Press, 1953, pp 123–245
88. Freud S: The analysis of a phobia in a five-year-old boy (1909a), in The Standard Edition of the Complete Psychological Works of Sigmund Freud, Vol 10. Translated and edited by Strachey J. London, Hogarth Press, 1955, pp 3–149

89. Freud S: The psychogenesis of a case of homosexuality in a woman (1920b), in The Standard Edition of the Complete Psychological Works of Sigmund Freud, Vol 18. Translated and edited by Strachey J. London, Hogarth Press, 1955, pp 145–172
90. Socarides CW: Theoretical and clinical aspects of female homosexuality. J Am Psychoanal Assoc 10:579–592, 1962
91. Socarides CW: The historical development of theoretical and clinical concepts of overt female homosexuality. J Am Psychoanal Assoc 11:386–414, 1963
92. Jones E: Early development of female homosexuality. Int J Psychoanal 8:459–572, 1927
93. Deutsch H: On female homosexuality. Psychoanal Q 1:484–510, 1932
94. Deutsch H: Homosexuality in women. Int J Psychoanal 14:34–56, 1933a
95. Deutsch H: Motherhood and sexuality. Psychoanal Q 2:476–488, 1933b
96. Bernstein AE, Warner GM: Women Treating Women. New York, International Universities Press, 1984b
97. Money J, Erhardt A: Man and Woman, Boy and Girl. Baltimore, MD, Johns Hopkins University Press, 1972
98. Stoller RJ: A contribution to the study of gender identity. Int J Psychoanal 45:220–226, 1964
99. Stoller RJ: The sense of femaleness. Psychoanal Q 37:42–55, 1968
100. Friedman RC: Male Homosexuality: Contemporary Psychoanalytic Perspectives. New Haven, CT, Yale University Press, 1988
101. Isay RA: Being Homosexual: Gay Men and Their Development. New York, Farrar, Straus & Giroux, 1989
102. Emmore E: Lesbian Women and Society. London, Routledge & Kegan Paul, 1980
103. Cohen CJ, Stein T: Reconceptualizing individual psychotherapy with gay men and lesbians, in Contemporary Perspectives on Psychotherapy With Lesbians and Gay Men. Edited by Stein TS, Cohen CJ. New York, Plenum, 1986, pp 27–54
104. Kleinberg L: Coming home to self, going home to parents: lesbian identity disclosure. The Stone Center for Developmental Services and Studies, Work in Progress, Wellesley, MA, 1986, No 86-24:1–16
105. Gartrell N: Issues in psychotherapy with lesbian women. The Stone Center for Developmental Services and Studies, Work in Progress, Wellesley, MA, 1984, No 83-04:1–12
106. Burch B: Psychotherapy and the dynamics of merger in lesbian couples, in Contemporary Perspectives on Psychotherapy With Lesbians and Gay Men. Edited by Stein TS, Cohen CJ. New York, Plenum, 1986, pp 57–71

107. Blumstein P, Schwartz P: American Couples. New York, William Morrow, 1983
108. Gerson MJ, Alpert JL, Richardson MS: Mothering: the view from psychological research. Signs 9:434–453, 1984
109. Mednick MT: Single mothers: a review and critique of current research. Applied Sociological and Psychological Annals 7:184–201, 1987
110. Notman MT, Nadelson CC: Changing views of the relationship between femininity and reproduction, in The Woman Patient, Vol 2: Concepts of Femininity and the Life Cycle. Edited by Nadelson CC, Notman MT. New York, Plenum, 1982a, pp 31–42
111. Freud S: Some psychical consequences of the anatomical distinction between the sexes (1925), in The Standard Edition of the Complete Psychological Works of Sigmund Freud, Vol 19. Translated and edited by Strachey J. London, Hogarth Press, 1961, pp 241–258
112. Freud S: Female sexuality, in Collected Papers. London, Hogarth Press, 1950, pp 225–243
113. Deutsch H: The Psychology of Women, a Psychoanalytic Interpretation, Vol 2: Motherhood. New York, Grune & Stratton, 1945
114. Kestenberg JS: Vicissitudes of female sexuality. J Am Psychoanal Assoc 4:453–476, 1956b
115. Benedek T: The psychobiology of pregnancy, in Parenthood: Its Psychology and Psychopathology. Edited by Antony EJ, Benedek T. Boston, Little, Brown, 1970c, pp 137–152
116. Stoller R: Primary femininity. J Am Psychoanal Assoc 24(suppl):59–78, 1976
117. Chodorow N: The Reproduction of Mothering: Psychoanalysis and the Sociology of Gender. Berkeley, CA, University of California Press, 1978
118. Maccoby E, Jacklin C: The Psychology of Sex Differences. Stanford, CA, Stanford University Press, 1974
119. Klaus MH, Kennell JH: Maternal-Infant Bonding: The Impact of Early Separation or Loss on Family Development. St Louis, MO, CV Mosby, 1976
120. Spitz RA, Wolf KM: The smiling response: a contribution to the ontogenesis of social relations. Genetic Psychology Monographs 34:57–125, 1946b
121. Stern P: Mother and infant at play: the dyadic interaction involving facial, vocal, and gaze behavior, in The Effect of the Infant on Its Caregiver. Edited by Lewis M, Rosenblum M. New York, Wiley, 1974, pp 187–215
122. Benedek T: Motherhood and nurturing, in Parenthood: Its Psychology and Psychopathology. Edited by Anthony EJ, Benedek T. Boston, MA, Little, Brown, 1970a, pp 153–166

123. Benedek T: Infertility as a psychosomatic defense. Fertil Steril 3:527–541, 1952
124. Benedek T: Parenthood as a developmental phase: a contribution to the libido theory. J Am Psychoanal Assoc 7:389–417, 1959a
125. Bibring GL: Some considerations of the psychological processes in pregnancy. Psychoanal Study Child 14:113–121, 1959
126. Horney K: The flight from womanhood: the masculinity-complex in women as viewed by men and women. Int J Psychoanal 7:324–339, 1926 [Reprinted in Miller JB: Psychoanalysis and Women: Contributions to New Theory and Therapy. New York, Brunner/Mazel, 1973, pp 3–16]
127. Thompson C: Some effects of the derogatory attitude towards female sexuality. Psychiatry 13:349-354, 1950 [Reprinted in Miller JB: Psychoanalysis and Women: Contributions to New Theory and Therapy. New York, Brunner/Mazel, 1973, pp 65–74]
128. Brazelton TB, Keefer CH: The early mother-child relationship: a developmental view of woman as mother, in The Woman Patient, Vol 2: Concepts of Femininity and the Life Cycle. Edited by Nadelson CC, Notman MT. New York, Plenum, 1982, pp 95–109
129. Spitz RA, Wolf KM: Anaclitic depression: an inquiry into the genesis of psychiatric conditions in early childhood. Psychoanal Study Child 2:313–342, 1946a
130. Coltrane S: Household labor and the routine production of gender. Social Problems 36:473–490, 1989
131. Domash L: Motivations for motherhood and the nature of the self-object tie, in Critical Psychophysical Passages in the Life of a Woman: A Psychodynamic Perspective. Edited by Offerman-Zuckerman J. New York, Plenum, 1988, pp 93–102
132. Winnicott DW: Transitional Objects and Transitional Phenomena in Playing and Reality. New York, Penguin, 1980
133. Robinson GE, Stewart DE: Motivation for motherhood and the experience of pregnancy. Can J Psychiatry 34:861–865, 1989
134. Bergmann MV: The effect of role reversal on delayed marriage and maternity. Psychoanal Study Child 40:197–219, 1985
135. Bernard J: The Future of Marriage. New York, World, 1972
136. Campbell A: The American way of mating: marriages, children only maybe. Psychology Today, May 1975, pp 37–43
137. Campbell A, Converse P, Rodgers W: The Quality of American Life: Perceptions, Evaluations and Satisfactions. New York, Russell Sage, 1976
138. Veevers J: Voluntary childlessness: a review of issues and evidence. Marriage and Family Review 2:261, 1979

139. Pines D: Pregnancy and motherhood: interaction between fantasy and reality. Br J Med Psychol 45:333–343, 1972
140. Pines D: The relevance of early psychic development to pregnancy and abortion. Int J Psychoanal 63:311–319, 1982
141. Lester EP, Notman MT: Pregnancy, developmental crisis and object relations: psychoanalytic considerations. Int J Psychoanal 67:357–366, 1986
142. Lester EP, Notman MT: Pregnancy and object relations: clinical considerations. Psychoanalytic Inquiry 8:196–221, 1988
143. Raphael-Leff J: Psychotherapeutic needs of mothers-to-be. Journal of Child Psychotherapy 8:3–13, 1982
144. Brazelton TB: Issues for working parents. Am J Orthopsychiatry 56:14–25, 1986
145. Benedek T: Parenthood during the life cycle, in Parenthood: Its Psychology and Psychopathology. Edited by Anthony EJ, Benedek T. Boston, MA, Little, Brown, 1970b, pp 185–206
146. Gilbert LA, Rachlin V: Mental health and psychological functioning of dual-career families. The Counseling Psychologist 15:7–49, 1987
147. Guttman HA: Autonomy and motherhood. Psychiatry 46:230–235, 1983
148. Robinson GE, Perrotta M, Burne S: Autonomy in mothers with careers. Can J Psychiatry 27:270–274, 1982
149. Casler L: Maternal deprivation: a critical review of the literature. Monogr Soc Res Child Dev, Vol 26, No 2, 1961
150. Murray AD: Maternal employment reconsidered: effects on infants. Am J Orthopsychiatry 45:773–790, 1975
151. Rutter M: The Qualities of Mothering: Maternal Deprivation Reassessed. New York, Jason Aronson, 1974
152. Notman MT, Nadelson CC: Maternal work and children, in The Woman Patient, Vol 2: Concepts of Femininity and the Life Cycle. Edited by Nadelson CC, Notman MT. New York, Plenum, 1982b, pp 121–134
153. Akabas SH: Workers are parents too. Child Welfare 63:387–399, 1984
154. Schachere K: Attachment between working mothers and their infants: the influence of family processes. Am J Orthopsychiatry 60:19–34, 1990
155. Voydanoff P: Work and Family Life. Newbury Park, CA, Sage, 1987
156. Barnett RC, Baruch GK: Women's involvement in multiple roles, role strain and psychological distress. The Stone Center for Developmental Services and Studies, Work in Progress, Wellesley, MA, 1983, No 83-107
157. Pugliesi K: Employment characteristics, social support and the well-being of women. Women Health 14:35–58, 1988

158. Wolfman BR: Women and their many roles. The Stone Center for Developmental Services and Studies, Work in Progress, Wellesley, MA, 1984, No 83-03
159. Burr WR, Leigh GK, Day P, et al: Symbolic interaction and the family, in Contemporary Theories About the Family, Vol 2: General Theories and Theoretical Orientation. Edited by Burr WR, Hill R, et al. New York, Free Press, 1979, pp 42–111
160. Sieber SD: Towards a theory of role accumulation. American Sociological Review 39:567–578, 1974
161. Marks SR: Multiple roles and role strain. American Sociological Review 42:921–936, 1977
162. Thoits PA: Multiple identities and psychological well-being. American Sociological Review 48:174–187, 1983
163. Elman MR, Gilbert LA: Coping strategies for role conflict in married professional women with children. Family Relations 33:317–327, 1984
164. Lynn DB: Intellectual development of women, in Dual-Career Couples. Edited by Pepitone-Rockwell F. Beverly Hills, CA, Sage, 1980, pp 55–71
165. Sefton MS: Dual-career families and the family life cycle. Australian Journal of Sex, Marriage and Family 8:118–123, 1987
166. Association of American Medical Colleges: Women and Minorities on U.S. Medical School Faculties. Washington, DC, Association of American Medical Colleges, 1988
167. Bennett NM, Nickerson KG: Women families and academic medicine. N Y State J Med 90:284–285, 1990
168. Greganti MA, Fletcher SW: House staff pregnancy in internal medicine residencies. Ann Intern Med 102:123–125, 1985
169. Sayres M, Wyshak G, Denterlein G, et al: Pregnancy during residency. N Engl J Med 314:418–423, 1986
170. Johnson CL, Johnson FA: Parenthood, marriage and careers: situational constraints and role strain, in Dual-Career Couples. Edited by Pepitone-Rockwell F. Beverly Hills, CA, Sage, 1980, pp 143–161
171. Skinner DA: Dual-career family stress and coping. Family Relations 29:473–481, 1980
172. Poloma MM: Role conflict and the married professional woman, in Toward a Sociology of Women. Edited by Safilios-Rothschild C. Lexington, MA, Xerox College Publications, 1972
173. O'Neill JM, Fishman DM, Kinsella-Shaw M: Dual career couples' career transitions and normative dilemmas: a preliminary assessment model. Counseling Psychologist 15:50–96, 1987

174. Gilbert LA: Understanding dual-career families. Family Therapy Collections 10:56–71, 1984
175. Stromberg AH, Harkess S: Women Working: Theories and Facts in Perspective. Palo Alto, CA, Mayfield, 1978
176. Hochschild A (with Machung A): The Second Shift. New York, Avon Books, 1989
177. Lewis SN, Cooper CL: The transition to parenthood in dual-earner couples. Psychol Med 18:477–486, 1988
178. Rapoport R, Rapoport RN: Dual-Career Families. London, Penguin, 1971
179. Person ES: Dreams of Love and Fateful Encounters: The Power of Romantic Passion, New York, WW Norton, 1989, p 39
180. National Center for Health Statistics: Monthly Vital Statistics Report, Vol 29. U.S. Department of Health and Human Services, Public Health Service, Office of Health Research Statistics and Technology, 1981, p 13
181. Glick PC, Norton AJ: Perspectives on the recent upturn in divorce and remarriage. Demography 10:301–314, 1973
182. Carter H, Glick PC: Marriage and Divorce: A Social and Economic Study. Cambridge, MA, Harvard University Press, 1976
183. U.S. Bureau of the Census: Current Population Reports, Series P-20:31C: Marriage, Divorce, Widowhood and Remarriage by Family Characteristics, June 1975. Washington, DC, U.S. Government Printing Office, 1977
184. Thiebault J, Kelly H: The Social Psychology of Groups. New York, Wiley, 1959
185. Hornig M: The impact of welfare payment levels on family stability, in The Family Poverty and Welfare Programs: Factors Influencing Family Instability (Studies in Public Welfare 12). Edited by Joint Economic Committee. Washington, DC, U.S. Government Printing Office, 1973
186. Cutright P, Scanzoni J: Income supplements and the American family, in The Family Poverty and Welfare Programs: Factors Influencing Family Instability (Studies in Public Welfare 12). Edited by Joint Economic Committee. Washington DC, U.S. Government Printing Office, 1973
187. Ross HL, Sawhill IV: Time of Transition: The Growth of Families Headed by Women. Washington, DC, The Urban Institute, 1975
188. Bernard J: No news but new ideas, in Divorce and After. Edited by Bohannon P. New York, Doubleday, 1970, pp 1–29
189. Kerchoff AC: The social context of interpersonal attraction, in Foundation of Interpersonal Attractions. Edited by Huston TL. New York, Academic, 1974, pp 61–78

190. Blood RO, Wolfe DM: Husbands and Wives: The Dynamics of Married Living. New York, Free Press, 1960
191. Kirkpatrick C: Community of interest and the measurement of adjustment in marriage. The Family 18:133–137, 1937
192. Locke HJ: Predicting Adjustment in Marriage: A Comparison of a Divorced and Happily Married Group. New York, Henry Holt, 1951
193. Kelly EE: Marital compatibility as related to personality traits of husbands and wives as rated by self and spouse. J Soc Psychol 13:193–198, 1941
194. Good WJ: After Divorce. New York, Free Press, 1956
195. Harmsworth HC, Minnis M: Non-statutory causes of divorce: the lawyers' point of view. Marriage and Family Living 17:316–321, 1955
196. Kaplan HS: Disorders of Sexual Desire. New York, Brunner/Mazel, 1979
197. Hunt M, Hunt B: The Divorce Experience, New York, McGraw-Hill, 1977
198. Bohannon P (ed): Divorce and After. New York, Doubleday, 1970
199. Beigleiter ML, Burry VF, Harris DJ: Prevalence of divorce among parents of children with cystic fibrosis and other chronic diseases. Soc Biol 23:261–264, 1976
200. Lansky SB: Childhood leukemia: the child psychiatrist as a member of the oncology team. Journal of the American Academy of Child Psychiatry 14:499–508, 1974
201. Tew BJ, Payne H, Lawrence KM: Must a family with a handicapped child be a handicapped family? Medical and Childhood Neurology 16 (suppl 32):95–98, 1974
202. Tew BJ, Lawrence KM, Payne H, et al: Marital stability following the birth of a child with spina bifida. Br J Psychiatry 131:79–82, 1977
203. Davis K: The American family in relation to demographic change: report of the U.S. Commission on Population Growth and the American future, in Demographic and Social Aspects of Population Growth, Vol 1. Edited by Westoff CCT, Raske R Jr. Washington, DC, U.S. Government Printing Office, 1972, pp 235–266
204. Levinger G: Marital cohesiveness and dissolution: an integrative review. Journal of Marriage and the Family 27:19–28, 1965
205. Pope H, Mueller C: The intergeneration transmission of marital instability: comparisons by race and sex, in Divorce and Separation: Context, Causes and Consequences. Edited by Levinger G, Mole O. New York, Basic Books, 1977, pp 89–113
206. Duncan B, Duncan OD: Family stability and occupational success. Social Problems 16:271–306, 1969
207. Bumpass L, Sweet L: Differentials in Marital Instability. American Sociological Review 37:754–766, 1972

208. Heiss J: On the transmission of marital instability in black families. American Sociological Review 37:82–92, 1972
209. Freud S: Melancholia (1895), in The Standard Edition of the Complete Psychological Works of Sigmund Freud, Vol 1. Translated and edited by Strachey J. London, Hogarth Press, 1966, pp 200–206
210. Bowlby J: Attachment and Loss, Vol 2: Separation. New York, Basic Books, 1973
211. Bergler E: Divorce Won't Help. New York, Harper, 1970
212. Gove WR: Sex, marital status and mortality. American Journal of Sociology 79:45–67, 1973
213. Jacobson GF: The Multiple Crises of Marital Separation and Divorce. New York, Grune & Stratton, 1983
214. Kitson G, Zyzanski S: Grief in widowhood and divorce. Psychiatr Clin North Am 10:369–386, 1987
215. Kressel K: The Process of Divorce. New York, Basic Books, 1985
216. Caron W, Doyle P: Contested custody intervention: an empirical assessment, in Child Custody: Literature Review and Alternative Approaches. Edited by Olsen D. Minneapolis, MN, University of Minnesota, Child Custody Research Project, 1979
217. Ahrons CR: The continuing co-parental relationship between divorced spouses. Am J Orthopsychiatry 52:415–428, 1981
218. Chambers DL: Making Fathers Pay: The Enforcement of Child Support. Chicago, IL, University of Chicago Press, 1979
219. Spanier FR, Casto RF: Adjustment in separation and divorce, in Divorce and Separation: Context, Causes and Consequences. Edited by Levinger G, Moles O. New York, Basic Books, 1979, pp 211–227
220. Mellinger GD, Barter MB, Manheimer DI, et al: Psychic distress, life crises and the use of psychotropic medication. Arch Gen Psychiatry 35:1048–1052, 1978
221. Glick ID: Marital and Family Therapy. New York, Grune & Stratton, 1980
222. Jacobson MS, Bussod N: Marital and family therapy, in The Clinical Psychology Handbook. Edited by Hussen M, Kazdin AE, Bellard AS. Elmsford, NY, Pergamon, 1983, pp 611–630
223. Bornstein H, Bornstein M: Marital Therapy: A Behavioral Communications Approach. New York, Pergamon, 1986
224. Gold JM: Divorce as a Developmental Process. Washington, DC, American Psychiatric Press, 1988
225. Dickstein L: The psychosocial effects of divorce on young adults, in Divorce as a Developmental Process. Edited by Gold JH. Washington, DC, American Psychiatric Press, 1988a, pp 3–26

226. Kirkpatrick M: Some clinical perception of middle-aged divorcing women, in Divorce as a Developmental Process. Edited by Gold JM. Washington, DC, American Psychiatric Press, 1988, pp 81–97
227. Notman M: Menopause and adult development. Ann N Y Acad Sci 592:92–151, 1990
228. Deutsch H: The psychology of women in relation to the functions of reproduction. Int J Psychoanal 6:405–418, 1925
229. Deutsch H: The significance of masochism in the mental life of women. Int J Psychoanal 11:40–60, 1930
230. Deutsch H: The Psychology of Women, a Psychoanalytic Interpretation, Vol 1. New York, Grune & Stratton, 1944
231. Greenacre P: Some factors producing different types of genital and pregenital irrational development, in Trauma, Growth and Personality. New York, International Universities Press, 1952b, pp 293–302
232. Greenacre P: Certain relationships between fetishism and faulty development of body image (1953a), in Emotional Growth. Edited by Lowenstein M. New York, International Universities Press, 1971, pp 9–30
233. Greenacre P: Penis awe and its relation to penis envy (1953b), in Emotional Growth. Edited by Lowenstein M. New York, International Universities Press, 1971, pp 31–49
234. Gilligan C: In a Different Voice. Cambridge, MA, Harvard Universities Press, 1982
235. Jordan J, Surrey J, Kaplan A: Women and empathy: implications for psychological development and psychotherapy. The Stone Center for Developmental Services and Studies, Work in Progress, Wellesley, MA, 1983, No 82-02
236. Lerner HE: The Dance of Anger. New York, Harper & Row, 1985
237. Dohrenwend BS: Social status and stressful life events. J Pers Soc Psychol 28:225–235, 1973
238. Miller JB: Toward a New Psychology of Women. Boston, MA, Beacon Press, 1976
239. Brody EM: Social, economic and environmental issues related to aging with some thoughts about "women in the middle." Aging: Research and Perspectives 3:37–45, 1979
240. Brody EM: Women in the middle and family help to older people. Gerontologist 21:471–480, 1981
241. Shanas E: Older people and their families: the new pioneers. Journal of Marriage and the Family 42:9–15, 1980
242. Arling G: The elder widow, her family, neighbors and friends. Journal of Marriage and the Family 38:757–768, 1976a

243. Getzel GS: Social work with family caregivers to the aged. Social Casework 62:201–210, 1981
244. Seelback WC: Correlates of aged person's filial responsibility, expectation and realizations. Family Coordinator 27:341–350, 1978
245. Johnson CL: Dyadic family relationships and social support. Gerontologist 23:377–383, 1983
246. Cohler BJ, Greenbaum H: Mother, Grandmothers and Daughters. New York, Wiley, 1981
247. Bromberg EM: Mother/daughter relationships and later life: the effect of quality of relationship on mutual aid. Journal of Gerontological Social Work 6:75–92, 1983
248. Schoonover CB, Brody EM, Hoffman C, et al: Parent care and geographically distant children. Research on Aging 10:472–492, 1988
249. Streib GF, Beck RW: Older families: a decade review. Journal of Marriage and the Family 42:937–956, 1980
250. Reinhardt JP, Fisher CB: Kinship versus friendship: social adaptation in married and widowed elderly women. Doctoral dissertation, Fordham University, Bronx, NY (New York, Haworth Press), 1989
251. Brody EM, Schoonover CB: Patterns of parentcare when adult daughters work and when they do not. Gerontologist 26:372–381, 1986

Chapter 5

Disorders Linked to Reproductive Functioning

Numerous psychiatric syndromes have been identified that relate to women's reproductive functioning, including 1) problems associated with menarche (see Chapter 2); 2) dysmenorrhea, premenstrual syndrome (PMS), or late luteal phase dysphoric disorder; 3) disorders of sexual functioning; 4) sexually transmitted disease; 5) infertility and the search for a baby; 6) problems associated with pregnancy; 7) abortion; 8) postpartum depression and infanticide; 9) the loss of a child; 10) post–genital surgery and depression; and 11) menopause or involutional depression (see Chapter 7).

Dysmenorrhea

Women have always been aware of disorders of menstruation and have considered them part of an expected physiological pattern. Difficult or painful menstruation or difficulty before the onset of menstrual flow in the absence of demonstrable anatomical or infectious disorder was often considered to be psychosomatic or functional. Recent research has attempted to account for symptoms in terms of excessive endometrial prostaglandin production resulting in uterine hypercontractility (Budoff 1982[1]). *Dysmenorrhea* is a spectrum disorder that can vary from the presence of mild to severe cramping, all the way to "dysmenorrhea syndrome." Dysmenorrhea syndrome may include headache, vomiting, diarrhea, and syncope. This syndrome is the single greatest course of missed school and work days. In 20% to 30% of patients, prostaglandin antagonists or nonsteroidal anti-inflammatory medication will bring relief. *Sec-*

ondary dysmenorrhea is a separate syndrome that can be shown to have a variety of medical causes. Relief of secondary dysmenorrhea requires treatment of the primary medical or surgical cause (Ylikor Kala and Dawood 1978[2]).

Gitlin and Pasnau (1989[3]), in reviewing four syndromes related to reproductive functioning, pointed out that in recent years PMS has received the greatest amount of attention and yet is the least understood. These authors have underlined the methodological difficulties, which include poor definition, few controlled treatment trials, and conflicting treatment results. For the purpose of their review, Gitlin and Pasnau have defined PMS as "a constellation of mood, behavior, and/or physical symptoms that have a regular cyclical relationship to the luteal phase of the menstrual cycle; and are present in most (if not all) cycles" (p. 1416).

Premenstrual syndrome is marked by a cluster of physical, affective, and behavioral changes occurring in a cyclical fashion that affects most women. The common complaints are breast tenderness, bloating, fluid retention, craving for sweet or salty food, acne, sleep disturbance, changes in bladder and bowel function, and, usually, frequent urination and constipation (Green and Dalton 1953[4]; Reid and Yen 1981[5]). Psychological changes include emotional lability, anxiety, depression, lethargy, or irritability and aggressiveness. Symptoms may begin to occur as early as 14 days prior to menstruation. Although PMS was once believed to end with the onset of menstrual flow, we have seen patients who continue to feel disrupted for 2 or 3 days into menstruation.

Abraham (1981[6]) has studied the frequency of the occurrence of dysfunctional symptoms. The frequency of the report of anxiety, irritability, tension, and emotional lability is 70% to 90%. The frequency of food craving, fatigue, dizziness, palpitations, and increased appetite is 30% to 40%. From 1% to 20% of women report depression with crying, withdrawal, forgetfulness, confusion, and insomnia; 60% report breast tenderness, fluid retention, bloating, and weight gain (see Appendix F).

It is the recommendation of the DSM-IV Committee that the diagnosis of premenstrual dysphoric disorder be moved from Appendix A of DSM-III-R (American Psychiatric Association 1987[7]), where it appeared as late luteal phase dysphoric disorder, to the body of DSM-IV and that it be defined as a psychiatric disorder. There is a subset of women with premenstrual syndrome who experience a disturbance of emotions severe enough to qualify as an affective disorder. (See Appendix F for metabolic mechanisms believed to underlie PMS, late luteal phase dysfunction, and premenstrual dysphoric disorder.)

We can only conclude that PMS has a complicated physiological and neuroendocrinological basis and that it has no single etiology. These biological factors create an added burden for women who have psychological disorders. It has been our experience that any disorder of physiology or any single (or group of) physiologically determined symptom(s) is burdensome for patients who already have affective or psychotic disorders.

Some attention has been paid in single studies to psychosocial factors such as type of personality, education and profession, and severity of personality disturbance. Stress is generally agreed to aggravate symptoms, but that can be said of any medical disorder. There have been attempts to correlate PMS with underlying affective disorder (Yankauskas 1990[8]). Again, it seems obvious to us that depression makes illness worse and that illness provokes depression.

Increased psychiatric hospitalization and criminal activity have been documented during the premenstrual period. Keye et al. (1986[9]) reported increased rates of major psychological, medical, and marital problems as well as child and spouse abuse, and suicide. The British criminal justice system recognizes the insanity defense for murder that occurs in the premenstruum.

For some women, changes in diet and exercise, including the elimination of alcohol and caffeine, decreased intake of simple sugar and salt, and vitamin supplementation, are helpful. Vitamin B_6 seems to ameliorate headache and breast tenderness (Abraham 1981[6]). Other investigators recommend vitamin E supplementation to decrease anxiety headache, sugar craving, and depression (London et al. 1987[10]). Because premenstrual symptoms often seem worse with stress, a variety of methods such as relaxation exercises, meditation, biofeedback, and physical exercises are sometimes helpful (Prior 1987[11]).

One of the present authors learned while in residence training that cathartics and diuretics had been used informally and pragmatically to relieve premenstrual constipation and edema since the 1940s (S. L. Feder, Unit Chief, Mount Sinai Hospital, personal communication, 1964). For patients who become severely ill, a variety of psychotropic and other medications have been tried. Yankauskas (1990[8]) has tabulated these medications, their dosages, and the target symptom(s). The most recent psychotropic medications to be tried are the serotonin agonist D-fentulamine (Wurthman 1990[12]) and the antidepressant fluoxetine (Stone 1990[13]). Until the pathophysiology of PMS is understood, pharmacological treatment is by trial and error.

We now present case examples of the treatment of women with late luteal phase dysfunction.

The Role of Stress

One patient, a 42-year-old health care administrator, was undaunted by union negotiations and managed to calmly help her daughter through emergency surgery. In the 2 to 3 days when the administrator-patient was premenstrual, however, she always struggled to stay in control of her emotional lability (e.g., being close to tears or angrily irritable). When seen during one episode, she had pitting pretibial edema but denied other physical complaints. Caffeine contributed to headache and breast tenderness and was eliminated from her diet. The patient also discovered the salutary effects of exercise. She was unable during the premenstruum to control some nibbling at nonchocolate sweets. The patient described her inability to control tears, and indeed she cried. Her hands were tremulous. Some minor and routine work problems seemed insoluble, and she questioned continuing at her present work site or even continuing to work at all. The third day after her menstrual flow was established, she could recognize her temporary depression and said, "I feel I am two people, the usual me and the me who becomes unglued for 3 to 5 days once a month." This patient responded to treatment in the premenstruum with a tricyclic antidepressant just before sleep and a diuretic.

* * *

Another patient, who had graduated from a professional program and was preparing for her licensing examination, appeared in hysterical tears. She had not been a somatizing patient. (In fact, she jogged in all weather regardless of whether she had a cold.) She had a staggering headache with photosensitivity continuously for 3 days. Her condition defied usual medication and it also interrupted her sleep. She refused a sedative-hypnotic that was prescribed by her internist. The symptoms did not occur with every menstrual cycle and seemed to be worse when she used the birth control pill. No psychologically disturbing events could be discerned.

* * *

A 40-year-old divorced patient with an important stressful administrative job and a busy social life remarked wryly that she got PMS only when she took some time off. Her symptoms were impatience, irritability, breast soreness, and obvious bloating, as well as sleep disturbance. She said that perhaps when she worked 12-hour days she did not have time to notice her physical complaints.

* * *

Obviously, psychodynamic treatment was not the treatment of choice for these patients. Their symptoms were obviously amenable to medical intervention.

* * *

The patient, a married mother of two who had returned to graduate school, was being treated psychodynamically for generalized anxiety and a somatization disorder. The latter included a fluctuatingly positive review of all systems—respiratory, gastrointestinal, genitourinary, and musculoskeletal. She also experienced irritability and weepiness in the premenstrual period. Analysis of the anger underlying the generalized anxiety brought these latter symptoms into remission. Her somatic complaints decreased in frequency and intensity, as did her PMS. None of these symptoms has been debilitating for well over 2 years, but they are not yet gone.

Identification With a Somatizing Mother

An analytic patient diagnosed with borderline personality disorder was treated five times a week in a classical analysis. Her presenting symptom was depression with headache, nausea, and vomiting, but she also complained of PMS and severe dysmenorrhea. It was revealed that the patient's mother had PMS and severe dysmenorrhea and had in fact been forced to take to her bed for one week monthly ever since the patient could remember. With analysis of her identification with her sick and generally dysfunctional mother, the patient recovered, went on to complete graduate school, and had a baby. Postpartum, she no longer experienced either PMS or dysmenorrhea.

Failure to Become Pregnant

A patient complained of bloating and feeling ugly in the premenstruum. Much work had to be done around her symbiotic and rageful attachment to her mother before she could divorce from an arranged marriage, become a successful professional, remarry, and have a first child. This first child, a son, was identified with her privileged brother. Subsequent attempts to become pregnant with a fantasized daughter proved futile. She was being treated with infertility drugs, which cause discomfort and bloating. She felt fearful, desperate, and irritable as her body changed, signaling the onset of menstruation. Her difficult premenstruum was accounted for by the use of hormones as well as her feelings of failure at not becoming pregnant. After starting adoption proceedings, her premenstrual symptoms abated.

Paternal Identification

An analysand was fully conscious of her resentment at being a woman. Unfeminine in dress and behavior, she was the daughter of a successful father and a chronically depressed and sick mother, and the youngest of her siblings, the two brothers both doctors. Interested in medicine herself, she was guided toward nursing but decided on social work. During premenstruum and menstruation she always felt enraged, and her depression and irritability were often out of control. During her analysis, she identified with the analyst as a successful woman who was making great strides in her own career. The patient became more feminine in appearance and began dating. She masturbated for the first time. [The need to deny her female genitalia had always stopped her.] She acknowledged the need for direct clitoral stimulation during intercourse and lost her premenstrual and intramenstrual symptoms.

Disorders of Sexual Functioning

Female sexual functioning is a complex phenomenon requiring interplay of the neurological, hormonal, vascular, and psychological systems.

The four stages of sexual response in women are the appetitive phase (i.e., the phase of desire), arousal, the orgasmic phase, and resolution. Frank et al. (1978[14]), in a survey of 100 normal couples from the middle and upper socioeconomic classes, found that 63% of the women reported either arousal or orgasmic dysfunction. Kaplan (1979[15]) recognized, treated, and reported on sexual dysfunction, including dysfunctions of desire, arousal, and orgasm. Imboden and Urbaitis (1978[16]) listed the most common forms of sexual dysfunction in women as 1) anorgasmia, 2) dyspareunia, and 3) vaginismus.

Medical Factors

Before proceeding to a psychodynamic formulation of disabilities in sexual functioning, we must first rule out medical and surgical causes and the effects of drugs, both prescribed and illegal. The most simple psychological causes are inadequate stimulation, poor communication with the partner, and a history of prior sexual harassment, rape, or sexual abuse.

Dyspareunia, or painful sensations in the vagina that make intercourse or the enjoyment of it impossible, usually has a medical explanation. Anxiety or other psychosomatic etiologies seldom play a major role in the genesis of this disorder. Causes are vaginal inflammation or infection involving the vagina or vulva, and endometriosis. This condition can often be treated hormonally. In later-age multiparous parents, anatomical dislocation or even prolapse of the uterus or bladder may cause dyspareunia. Surgery is often the cure. One of the authors saw a young woman with dyspareunia secondary to severe and chronic constipation that caused the frequent presence of a hard bolus of feces in the rectum—a condition that could be corrected medically.

Vaginismus is defined as involuntary contraction of the vaginal outlet, which prevents entry of the penis. The use of graduated dilators by the patient and then by the patient and her partner usually results in a cure of this disability.

Anorgasmia is the inability to experience orgasm in a relationship with a partner. Anorgasmia may be primary or secondary (i.e., once capable of orgasm, the patient has lost this ability). Secondary anorgasmia can usually be traced to difficulties in the relationship with the partner. Some women climax with self-stimulation but not with intercourse; others have never had an orgasm in their lives (contradicting Freud [1931,[17] 1933[18]]). Masters and Johnston (1970[19]) dispelled the myth that the friction of penile thrusting alone should be sufficient to bring about orgasm. The clitoris is the main organ of stimulation for the woman. Sherffy (1966,[20] 1973)[21]) reaffirmed that physiological evidence does not distinguish "clitoral orgasm" from "vaginal orgasm." She established that clitoral stimulation, direct or indirect, is the prerequisite for orgasm in the female.

There are women who can masturbate to orgasm but hesitate to admit to, or ask their partners for, direct clitoral stimulation. Many women imagine that "men must know" or that a male partner would do it if he wanted to. Underlying these two assumptions are pathological fantasies—for example, the wish to be gratified without taking the responsibility for asking, or the assumption that the partner should be like the mind-reading mother of infancy. In addition, some women are concerned with vaginal odor. The odor of the vagina should not be noxious. A chronic malodorous discharge is a medical problem often related to sexually transmitted disease. Unfortunately, practitioners who dismiss complaints of vaginal odor without obtaining adequate smears and cultures and treating the disease process are not practicing good medicine.

Still another determinant of failure of sufficient sexual arousal for orgasm occurs in the many women who have difficulties in self-assertion. In many arenas, not only sexual, these women have trouble in asking for what they want, need, or deserve, or for anything that has not been spontaneously volunteered. This condition is suitable for psychodynamic treatment.

Psychodynamic Factors

The problem of primary anorgasmia is rooted in development. Either masturbation never occurred or else it disappeared entirely in latency for serious psychodynamic reasons. The rapprochement subphase of separation-individuation coincides with the oedipal conflict (Bernstein and Warner 1984b[22]). Galenson and Roiphe (1976[23]) observed that boys are affected by this temperal coincidence and handle maternal loss by turning to their penis as a transitional object. Girls turn inward. This turning inward reflects a period of fantasy. The fantasy of an illusory penis with resultant castration anxiety is a reparative fantasy of this period. Masturbation might allow reality (i.e., of not having a penis) to interfere with the fantasy, which might provoke intense castration anxiety. Thus, masturbation is relinquished forever. Danger is inherent in the choice of a fantasized oedipal object, and this may end in the renunciation of masturbation. The psychodynamic treatment of women who have not masturbated or do not masturbate involves the resolution of the oedipal conflict and the result of masturbation. Masturbation is often the prerequisite to orgasm with a partner.

Sexual arousal involves nipple erection, flushing, the buildup of muscle tension, vaginal lubrication, and the retraction of the cervix higher into the vaginal vault.

Disorders of sexual arousal are generally the by-product of anxiety, depression, or anger. When these arise only in the context of the sexual relationship with a partner, they are often resolved with various kinds of sexual therapy using sensate focus exercises. Patients may report intrusive, diverting thoughts. These thoughts may be rather simply solved, or they may involve serious psychodynamic issues.

Maternal Identification

A married 30-year-old mother of three reentered therapy after terminating a long-term therapy a year before. Her reentry was prompted by depression, which continued to plague her despite the achievement of all the long-term goals she had set for herself: to obtain a fine home, to find a fine husband, and to accomplish three pregnancies resulting in "beautiful children." Her history was of rebellious promiscuity. Five months into the treatment, she began having nightmares, panic attacks, and a remarkable inhibition in her libido that both she and her husband found extremely disturbing, having enjoyed an active sexual life prior to this time. During this period the patient noticed that she was constantly turning herself off to her husband's advances by focusing on his shortcomings or on financial problems or other sources of anxiety during any attempts at lovemaking. In this context, she began to re-explore her childhood, uncovering first memories of her mother's coldness, abusiveness, and neglect, and later memories of sexual abuse by her father in the context of a marital separation.

Some patients cannot respond to behavioral intervention until the psychodynamic meaning of their interfering fantasies has been explored. Others can respond to directed thinking (i.e., the substitution of unwanted thoughts by fantasies that contribute to arousal). Sado-masochistic, incestuous, and pedophilic fantasies are most anxiogenic. Disorders of desire are often rooted in incest or other abuse either in childhood or later in life (Becker 1986[24]). Sexuality can become threatening because it may open the box of these memories of conflicted or unpleasant experiences. Sherkow (1990b[25]) reported the psychoanalytic treatment of an adult woman who had been abused as a child and who therefore had an impulse to flee that was pervasive in her life and manifest in her sexuality by the momentary resistance to foreplay when approached by her husband.

The failure of the stage of resolution in which sexual feelings temporarily recede and in which there may be sleepiness or afterplay has several determinants. For example, women who can be repeatedly orgasmic with little or no resolution time often require this to avoid experiencing anxiety, agitation, sleeplessness, or depression. Other women have an insatiability that is displaced to the sexual sphere of functioning.

The literature—popular, medical, and psychiatric—is replete with treatment strategies that are not psychodynamic but seem to have a high success rate (except for disorders in the appetitive phase). These involve conditioning positive responses and deconditioning negative ones, relaxation techniques, and the extinction of nonsexual fantasies during loving.

Schreiner-Engel (1990[26]) states that 24% to 64% of all women presenting at marital dysfunction clinics report hypoactive sexual desire, which the author defines as loss of interest in or motivation for sexual experiences or cognitive awareness of stimulation and of sexual thoughts and fantasies. This may be the first symptom of marital problems.

Contributing conditions to sexual dysfunction may be neurological, hormonal, or metabolic, or may be related to drugs and medication or to genital surgery. Among the psychological disorders that are causal or contributory are anxiety, depression, borderline personality disorder, psychosis, and sexual abuse. These conditions may require pharmacological intervention or a combination of pharmacological and psychodynamic intervention, or psychodynamic treatment alone.

The clinical material below is confined to issues that are clearly psychodynamically determined and that respond to dynamically oriented therapy.

Anxiety About Genital Integrity

A patient felt empty, damaged, and consciously aware of her negative feelings about her vagina. She never desired her husband but could be aroused and reach orgasm. During the course of a pregnancy, her appetitive behavior blossomed, much to her husband's delight. Close to delivery she had dreams of being ripped apart and left with a gaping hole. Delighted with the birth of a son and aroused while breast feeding, she again lost desire for her husband. Her unconscious rage at her husband and at her son for having penises, in addition to her open competition with and belittling of her husband as a narcissistic reparative maneuver, had to be analyzed before she could again become desirous of sex. The psychodynamics pertinent to her rage at men involved the recollection of her father's love affair and her mother's depression through the transference, in which she felt like a frustrated, neglected child.

The Loss of the Father

A woman college student who lost her father ignored the loss. She had a major retarded depression upon her return to her parental home and during her attempts to establish a career. She met a man senior in age to her whose character reminded her of her father's positive characteristics. Her father was idealized, and she refused to discuss her failure or mourn his death. She felt very aroused by her boyfriend but put down by comments about her sexual inexperience and youthful demeanor. Impending marriage confronted her with the loss of her father. She began to avoid sex. Reviewing her experiences that she had had with her father, she acknowledged several negative characteristics that she had repressed. In addition, she became painfully aware that her boyfriend seemed like the repository of all those negative characteristics. She now is beginning to see that perhaps she has provoked criticism in her current relationship to recreate her life as "Daddy's girl." She concedes that if she continues to perceive her boyfriend as her father and to provoke his criticism, she will never feel sexually attracted to him.

Depression

A woman in her 40s with grown children and a career sought help for her depression and low self-esteem. She and her husband had a very gratifying sexual relationship despite being unhappy in many other areas. Her husband took the side of her children against her. Even while overtly agreeing to joint decisions about wedding plans and financial support, he went behind her back to pacify the children. He became clinically depressed at one point in his own treatment. He also made gross financial blunders. Still their sexual relationship remained fulfilling but rare. She began to understand that her unconscious identification was with a depressed mother who was subservient to a narcissistic father. The patient saw how that impinged on her own ability to work successfully and maintain a position of equality with friends and colleagues and to enjoy sex. Disidentification with the mother returned the patient to a more frequent sexual life, involving her initiation and activity.

* * *

A young divorced woman who was very depressed after the breakup of her marriage fell "in love at first sight" with a man whom she met on a blind date. The man clearly reciprocated her feelings. Her marriage had been long and sexless. This new relationship had begun after a lengthy period of promiscuity during which she had a chance to explore and become comfortable with her sexuality. As her new boyfriend began to get closer and more committed, she felt less aroused and less in love with him, fearing a repetition of her marital experience. Her fears of rejection and of making yet another mistake were repeatedly interpreted to her until she was able to become more comfortable in experiencing her sexual feelings.

Devaluation of Self

Another analytic patient was desirous of her husband and was orgasmic, but kept saying to her analyst, "So what? It feels like nothing." This odd phenomenon seemed difficult to understand until it became apparent that she extended her devaluation of herself to the devaluation of all her life experiences. [LaFarge (1989[27]) has conceptualized such emptiness as a defense against severe regressive states.] A borderline patient with a psychotic father and a depressed mother, she feared regression to either the paranoid or depressive positions she felt in identification with her parents.

Primal Scene Exposure

A patient sought treatment for anxiety and depression because of the temptation of a work-related love affair. She and her husband never had had a satisfactory sexual life, although he was clearly trying. The patient complained of a very striking fear that her children would find her in some state of undress. Her dreams indicated repeated exposure to the primal scene. Finally, she could remember being in her crib, soiled and frantic for help and solace, while her parents were involved in their own sexual relationship. Her clandestine "love affair" (it was never consummated) had many of the characteristics of her parents' sexual relationship. In treatment her sexual life dramatically improved and her depression lifted, and she became more assertive and outspoken (i.e., exposed) at work, which led to her promotion. She felt less shy with her husband but never lost a morbid fear that her children might see her undressed.

Maternal Abandonment and Substitute Attachment to a Male Sibling

Another patient who presented because of a somatoform disorder had a good enough sexual relationship with her husband, although it was never as exciting as a love affair that had preceded her marriage. As her anxiety abated, she went to work and fell in love with a colleague. It turned out that both he and her first lover reminded her of her older brother. She and her brother had been left alone to manage most of their lives while their parents worked. They had shared the same bedroom until her brother went to college. With the analysis of her unconscious sexual fantasies about her brother, her extramarital amorous feelings cooled, and she again became desirous of her husband.

Sexually Transmitted Disease

Medical Factors

Sexually transmitted diseases are often contagious or systemic and, especially if they result in permanent damage to health, cause many psychological repercussions for afflicted women. Sexually transmitted disease in women can be divided into several categories: lower genitourinary infections; genital ulceration, with or without systemic manifestations; pelvic inflammatory disease; and systemic infections (Isselbacher et al. 1980[28]). Disorders related to lower genitourinary infection are characterized by itching and irritation, vaginal discharge, dyspareunia, and frequency and burning on urination. A full discussion of the diagnosis and treatment of these infections, as well as other lesions of the reproductive system, is given in Appendix G.

We are currently in the midst of an epidemic of acquired immune deficiency syndrome (AIDS). This disease is communicated through the exchange of bodily fluids, usually sexually, or by the practice of sharing needles for the injection of "recreational" drugs. A specific blood test for the presence of the causative virus is available and is administered in most localities on a voluntary basis. The virus eventually compromises the ability of the immune system to deal with intercurrent infections. There are two drugs, zidovudine (AZT) and pentamidine, that are often palliative, but there is no cure. Ten percent of AIDS patients are women, infants, and children (Guinan and Hardy 1987[29]). Whether human immunodeficiency virus (HIV) occurs in pregnant women or newborns, it disproportionately affects disadvantaged women of color. Seventy percent of female AIDS patients are either African-American or Hispanic ("Coolfront Report" 1986[30]). The Working Group on HIV Testing of Pregnant Women and the Newborn (1990[31]) clearly relates poverty and social isolation to drug dependency in women.

In Chapter 3 we discussed the "toss over" phenomenon (i.e., the exchange of sex for drugs) among prostitutes. In addition, women are becoming infected through unprotected sex with either intravenous drug-abusing men or bisexual men. The best protection against AIDS is the condom. The most resistance to condom use occurs in the populations at greatest risk. Women in the high-risk groups hesitate to insist that men use condoms or are reluctant to provide condoms for them. Studies are currently being conducted under the auspices of the National Institutes of Health on a female condom (Fourcroy 1990[32]).

Human immunodeficiency virus infection can cause a myriad of neurological symptoms. Of especial concern to readers of the present volume are three issues: 1) the phenomenon of "fr AIDS" (i.e., fear that AIDS has been contracted), 2) the depression that often follows the knowledge of being seropositive for the HIV virus, and 3) the complications, such as cognitive deficits and dementia, that are caused by the effects of the virus in the central nervous system.

Patients with "fr AIDS" present with anxiety, depression, and guilt. Patients who become phobic when there is little or no reality to their belief that they may have AIDS are treated with all the modalities—cognitive, behavioral, and/or psychodynamic—applicable to any phobic patient.

Patients at risk for HIV infection have to be treated psychodynamically and supportively. There is conflict about advising these patients to have HIV testing. One the one hand, those who are HIV-seropositive can be medically followed and treated prophylactically when prodromal signs of immunodeficiency appear. On the other hand, HIV-seronegative patients can convert at any time. Also, the knowledge of HIV seropositivity often causes anxiety and depression. The issues of confidentiality, fear of discovery, loss of family ties, and loss of jobs and benefits are very real. In addition, it is estimated that 30% to 70% of HIV-seropositive patients have some cognitive or neuropsychological deficits at some point during the course of the disease (Kertzner 1989[33]). These deficits are due to what Tucker (1986[34]) describes under the general rubric of frontal release signs. These are marked by either pathetic passive unconcern or alternatively low frustration tolerance, hostility, aggressive behavior, temper tantrums, paranoia, delusion, psychotic thought, anxiety, and affective lability. Diagnostic studies include the electroencephalogram, which may show diffuse slowing, and the computed tomography scan, which may reveal cerebral atrophy and ventricular enlargement.

The treatment for psychotic symptomatology involves the use of low-dose medications like haloperidol or thiothixene that have low anticholinergic activity The low doses avoid sedation, orthostatic hypotension, and lowering of the seizure threshhold. Medications with low anticholinergic activity also help to avoid the occurrence of disorientation, memory deficits, and toxic psychosis. In addition, potent anticholinergic agents often cause dry mouth and drying of nasal passages. Normal secretions are the first-line defense against opportunistic infections that need to be avoided in immunocompromised individuals. The same logic applies to the prescription of antidepressant or antianxiety medications. Trazodone and alprazolam are the preferred medications. Benzodiazepines are to be avoided because they tend to increase confusion and depress higher cortical functions.

In addition to the need to treat the psychiatric effects of HIV infection, we must treat the psychosexual complications. HIV-seropositive females should avoid procreation. Shame and blame are often the lot of both herpes- and HIV-infected individuals.

For AIDS patients, the final dimension is what Cohen (1988[35]) calls the "biology of hopelessness" (p. 102). By this he means that hopelessness and depression cause changes in the CNS and its connections to the immune system. The model that Cohen uses is of "voodoo"—when individuals who believe themselves cursed and doomed to die sometimes die of no biologically discernable cause. Cohen cites the work of Cousins (1979,[36], 1983[37]) in terms of the curative effects of hope (e.g., in cancer patients). Although we feel that Cousins' formulations are scientifically questionable in terms of both the prolongation of life and the production of cure, it is clear that hope changes the quality of life, and thus it is something for which we must aim in any event.

In addition to hope, the availability of a support network for white homosexual men has beneficial impact on the length and quality of their lives. These groups, such as Gay Men's Health Crises and ACT UP, are beginning to reach out to nonwhite homosexuals; more gradually (because of socioeconomic class differences) to persons who abuse drugs; and not at all to women and children, especially those of color who are most affected (Fullilove and Fullilove 1989[38]; Fullilove et al. 1990,[39] 1991[40]).

The psychiatric assessments and treatment recommendations that apply to AIDS come from the study and treatment of men and can only be extrapolated to women. This bias is especially damaging because of the concurrence of pregnancy and the AIDS epidemic in the newborn. We have yet to appreciate the problem of poverty-stricken, drug-addicted women who give birth to children with HIV infection. More and more frequently the children are abandoned and are unadoptable, even though only 30% of these children eventually develop AIDS.

Psychodynamic Factors

We now discuss the psychodynamic issues that involve sexually transmitted diseases and provide illustrations from patient treatment whenever possible.

The discovery of infection with a sexually transmitted disease is always distressing, leading to feelings of guilt, mistrust, anger, depression, and despair, all related to the severity of the disease. Sexually transmitted diseases often destroy committed relationships, and even marriages, because of the feeling of betrayal. Pelvic inflammatory disease threatens fertility; herpes limits sexual relationships. AIDS affects every aspect of life, with the individual being confronted with the specter of severe prolonged illness and death.

Incest and Systemic Infection

A 22-year-old single conservatory student entered therapy because of unremitting depression consisting of tearfulness, sleep disturbance, poor concentration, intermittent suicidal ideation, and obsessive ruminations of worthlessness and self-disgust. Also significant was a sexual history revealing severe dating anxiety, sexual inhibition, and a significant dissociative episode.

Early in her second year of treatment outside of the hospital she shamefully and anxiously (but in graphic detail) reported to her therapist vaginal discharge, pruritus, and labial tenderness. She minimized the significance of these symptoms, and only upon the persistent recommendations of her therapist did she visit a gynecologist. Her symptoms persisted and she made several gynecology clinic visits, with repeated diagnosis and treatment of monilial and bacterial vaginitis. The patient consistently denied the possibility of a connection between her gynecological condition and her psychological issues but became increasingly anxious during her sessions.

Ten months after the onset of her vaginal symptoms, she arrived for therapy in a state of panic. During the session she dissociated and stated, "There are little men in my vagina." Further exploration of her dissociative episode revealed that the patient had been putting objects in her vagina and retaining them for periods of up to 1 week. Eventually the patient derepressed a history of persistent and sadistic incest dating back to age 3 years when her father persuaded her to play a game involving the insertion of two miniature toys into her vagina that progressed to the painful and sadistic insertion of brush handles.

Psychosis

A 32-year-old single unemployed writer and researcher entered therapy because of persistent control struggles with her male therapist and persistent psychotic episodes that required emergency hospitalization and disrupted her life. A college graduate who held a M.A. degree in library science, the patient came from an upper-middle-class family with hidden and denied major psychotic illness. The patient's mother was alcoholic, her father had multiple episodes of depression, and her brother suffered from paranoid schizophrenia and was abusive toward her during his psychotic episodes.

The patient had a history of eczema and of sexual promiscuity resulting in pelvic inflammatory disease. She received a full course of antibiotic treatment but was told that her fertility status was uncertain due to severe scarring. She was diagnosed as having major affective disorder. Over the course of 18 months of treatment she was helped to stabilize her life. Despite her preoccupation with children, she remained too anxious and ambivalent to permit an evaluation of her fertility. She became preoccupied with obtaining a high-status job. Utilizing her academic credentials, attractive appearance, and superficial social poise, she obtained a series of positions but either left or was fired when she was unable to sustain her performance. With each impending job disaster she would return home or join her family in an exotic escape vacation. At home, she would begin barhopping and invariably engage in an intense and impulsive sexual relationship with an abusive man of lower socioeconomic status.

The patient was graphic and provocative about both her pleasure and pride in being "so good at sex" and her fears that her promiscuity would result in further genital infection. Obsessed with contracting AIDS, she alternated binges of unprotected sex with frantic visits to her gynecologist for HIV testing. During these 2 years she was diagnosed with gonorrhea but never contracted AIDS. In therapy the patient was able to acknowledge a profound sense of defectiveness and rage stemming from her family's emphasis on superficial appearance and profound neglect and denial of her mother's alcoholism, her brother's psychosis and abuse of her, and her father's depression. As her self-esteem improved, she was able to take better care of her own psychotic illness and to stop using her sexuality to express her anger and to compensate for feelings of inadequacy. She has stabilized in all areas of her life but remains ambivalent in regard to having children and has never confirmed her fertility status.

Failure of Self-Actualization

A single young artist had a series of affairs with inappropriate, unavailable men. During one affair she developed abdominal pain. The diagnosis of pelvic inflammatory disease with Staphylococcus aureus, an unusual pathogen, was not made until laparoscopy. With the discovery of this disease, the patient became enraged with her lover, whom she had assumed had lied to her about prior promiscuity and had given her gonorrhea. The relationship deteriorated and then was broke off, resulting in the patient's depression and job loss. Major psychodynamic issues centered around the patient's anger at her lover, displaced from feelings of failure at work. She was the only one of her siblings to choose a nonstandard profession, which has caused problems in her earning a living and taking care of herself, and which made her failure so much more glaring.

Denial

A health care professional entered analytic treatment because of her inability to form a relationship with a man. She was one of three children, the only daughter of a physician and a homemaker. Her father wanted all three children to study medicine, which her brothers went on to do, but the patient enjoyed an active social life in college and did not obtain the grades for a medical education.

She had never had intercourse or masturbated in her adult life. She stated that she had "nothing to masturbate with." She felt like a failed woman (i.e., castrated male) rather than a successful woman. She had the unconscious fantasy of having a hidden penis. Her mother, who had wanted a daughter, held her too close and demanded that she fulfill her mother's definition of the female role (e.g., being asexual and passive). Separation, sexuality, and even socialization were discouraged. The patient's adaptation was a compromise both intrapsychically and in reality.

During her analysis she began to masturbate to orgasm and to become heterosexually active. She contracted gonorrhea (prior to the AIDS epidemic) and was given penicillin for this infection. She had not been tested for syphilis, having dismissed the test as unnecessary. The analyst told her that there would be no further analysis unless she was tested for syphilis. The patient became enraged and stormed out, but indeed had a blood test, which was positive. Treated with massive doses of intramuscular penicillin, she was enraged at the analyst (i.e., mother) for controlling her, for being right, and for causing the painful treatment. She was grateful to the analyst, however, for risking "losing the case," being concerned, and sparing the patient's health. In the context of departure from classic psychoanalysis, the maternal transference in all its ramifications became analyzable.

Guilt About Sexuality

A professional divorced mother of two sons was depressed. She was under considerable stress because of a complicated joint custody arrangement, because her mother had cancer, and because her career was demanding. Circumspect in her sexual relationships, with serial relationships lasting months to a year, she contracted herpes, which was adequately treated with oral medication. She believed that she had a recurrence every time she had now-protected intercourse. Despite a subjective feeling of pain, no lesions were documented. She felt compelled to tell all possible lovers about her herpes, which was a form of masochistic self-punishment. The compulsion only eased when she worked out complex issues relating to the loss of her father when she was a teenager.

fr AIDS

A divorced woman in her 40s became counterphobic about AIDS and somewhat carelessly promiscuous, as part of a life pattern of borderline and exaggerated behavior. Subject to allergic reactions of several kinds, she worried about some skin lesions. She was encouraged to seek HIV testing. For the first time, her fear became real. She had often histrionically threatened suicide.

Her fantasies were violent ones. She stated that if she developed AIDS, she would commit suicide. She confided her fears to a female physician friend who promised to help her not to suffer. Fortunately, she was HIV-seronegative. At that point her careless sexual behavior stopped, as did her threats of violent suicide. Work had been done around genetic issues that made her behave as if she was as "crazy" as her psychotic sister and psychotic mother. She had already become more stable in work-related behavior and in her choice of men for long-term relationships.

Infertility and the Quest for a Baby

Infertility

One out of every six couples of childbearing age is unable to achieve pregnancy (Lalos et al. 1985[41]). Medical, social, and psychological dimensions contribute to infertility, and often the interaction of these factors is very complex. Some simple social and medical factors are as follows:

1. More women who are from upper or middle socioeconomic classes tend to marry at an older age and defer first pregnancies until their mid-30s.
2. Women wish to avoid the "mommy track" (i.e., a lower rate of occupational progression due to maternity and child care leave). Many women want to get established on the fast track before starting a family.
3. Rising costs of living and increasing costs of housing, education, and child care, as well as the scarcity of acceptable, affordable day care, household help, and prenursery/nursery school care, prompt many couples to save first and begin a family later.
4. Many women who have deferred marriage have had a number of sexual partners and severe venereal disease that often compromises fertility.
5. Intrauterine devices often lead to infertility.

Initially, there was an attempt to divide sterility into organic sterility and psychogenic sterility. *Organic sterility* meant that a physical or physiological mechanism could be identified. *Psychogenic*, or "functional," sterility was defined as sterility for which no such mechanism could be found (Bydlowski and Dagan-Lintzer 1988[42]).

Many authors agree that there are psychic components of sterility (Karahanasoglu et al. 1972[43]; Kraft et al. 1980[44]; Pennington and Atlay 1972[45]; Wasser and Isembert 1986[46]). A number of authors have discussed these components from the standpoint of relatively negative attributions toward the would-be mother. Menninger (1943[47]) referred to infertility as if it were due to psychic conflicts sailing under a gynecological flag. Kraft et al. (1980[44]) spoke of infertility in terms of a basic flaw in self concept that provides unjustifiable hurt. Sandler (1961[48]) speculated on infertility as a symptom arising from conflict between career ambition and motherhood. Benedek (1952[49]) thought infertility was a psychosomatic defense against a feared pregnancy and motherhood. Rubenstein (1951[50]) studied infertility as a psychosomatic defense, arising from the unconscious, against feared postpartum psychosis. Hall (1985[51]) reported on cases in which the women were found to not want a child.

Sarrel and DeCherney (1985[52]) studied 20 couples who had already conceived one child together but were subsequently infertile. In 10 of the couples the authors found marked psychological conflict. "Mother-fusion" was defined as the inability of the would-be mother to break ties with her own mother. Other conflicts were the fear of pregnancy based on a prior difficult experience, interpersonal marital problems, and sexual dysfunction. In this investigation, psychotherapy was studied in terms of achieving pregnancy. Bresnick and Taymor (1979[53]) wrote about successful counseling for sexual disorders in infertile patients. Downey et al. (1989[54]), in a study of infertile women and control subjects, found no significant differences between groups on psychological tests, as contrasted with a high self-perception of depression and dysphoric difficulty with intimacy, sexual activity, and self-esteem.

Other authors have noted the role of stress in infertility (Mahlstedt 1985[55]; Seibel and Taymor 1982[56]). For example, there is stress associated with the awareness of "the ticking of the biological clock."

We report below on patients in whom clinical anxiety and depressive syndromes follow quickly upon the suspicion of infertility and worsen through the period of diagnostic evaluation and treatment. Infertility is a spectrum disorder. That is, its causes run the spectrum from purely organic to purely psychological with mixed proportions of etiology in between. Eighty percent of infertile couples will be found to have an organic lesion (Lalos et al. 1985[41]). Even rudimentary knowledge of the interaction of the neurotransmitters and neuroendocrine systems would tell us that these abnormalities of neurotransmitters and the neuroendocrine system in the latter are associated with anxiety, depression, and stress (Seibel and Taymor 1982[56]). Platt et al. (1973[57]) have written extensively on the very complex neuroendocrine hormonal aspects of the process from cyclic ovulation to fertilization to implantation of the fertilized egg in the female.

The expressed wish to have a child has many meanings.[†] It begins with the wish to perpetuate oneself and not be physically obliterated, about which the patient is often conflicted. The wish for and the fear of having a child are deeply rooted in the unconscious. One fantasy revolves around the wish to have one's father's child and the fear of displacing mother. Another fantasy involves reestablishing the tie to the preoedipal mother.

Many women develop psychological problems secondary to their infertility (Denber 1978[58]; Kipper et al. 1977[59]; Mai et al. 1972[60]; Menning 1977[61]). Daniluk (1988[62]) points out that depressive symptoms arise commonly in infertility patients during the course of evaluation and treatment. These symptoms are noted to be more frequent in the female

---

[†]The desire to have a child is different than the wish to be pregnant. The latter often involves fantasies about being special, full, or repairing a prior narcissistic injury or poor self-image and about permission to be dependent and to enjoy the special privileges perceived as accompanying pregnancy. One patient who had mastered adolescent obesity was frightened and disgusted by the idea of once again having a big belly. She reported that she often failed to notice that other women were pregnant. Her first impression was to think, "Look at that fat slob."

partner. Eck Menning (1980[63]) has noted the presence of grief, periodic depression, irritability, guilt, and inferiority. Jessner et al. (1986[64]) have commented on the feelings of self-worth and femininity that are affected by infertility.

McGuire (1975[65]) noted that women who are undergoing treatment for infertility often have to put their lives on hold, postponing crucial decisions about career, life plans, adoption, and confrontation with childlessness. Berger (1977[66]) has pointed out the role of the psychiatrist in the infertility clinic, and Walker (1978[67]) has highlighted the role of the psychiatrist in treating secondary sexual dysfunction. Behavioral treatment of sexual dysfunction, supportive treatment for persons undergoing medical and surgical procedures, and counseling of patients about life decisions and adoption are all important. (See Appendix H for details of the medical workup and treatment.)

The Unconscious Wish to Avoid Pregnancy

One patient, who had been married for 6 years and had a successful career in journalism, presented with depression, agitation, and insomnia, as well as anorexia. These symptoms started 1 year after the couple had amassed enough savings to purchase a home in a distant suburb, which required that she move away from her assigned "beat" and commute. The unspoken agreement between her husband and herself was that she would try to become pregnant, which she was unable to do, and take a leave of absence from her work. She felt unsure of the quality of her work, but she planned to move, continue her career, and become pregnant.

In therapy she began to feel better about her work; she felt more comfortable in the newsroom and was able to make friends. She sought consultation with an infertility expert but was sluggish in following the recommended course of treatment. Confronted with her ambivalence, she had no insight into the reasons behind her sluggishness but did begin to follow instructions. She went for several diagnostic procedures as scheduled but rationalized about asking her husband to furnish a sperm sample for analysis. Her husband furnished a sperm sample, which was normal. She had no obstructive pathology and was ovulating. But because she was allergic with eczema and intermittent asthma, artificial insemination with her husband's sperm was recommended. She found every excuse to avoid this procedure. When analysis of this resistance was attempted, she decided to leave therapy. She agreed to call back as needed. One year later she sent a long letter detailing the progression of her and her husband's careers and her psychiatric recovery. She had not yet talked with her husband about artificial insemination and thought that she might one day do so. She was 36 years old at the time of the letter.

Organic Determinant of Infertility

One patient with a degree in business administration came to therapy at the recommendation of her husband's therapist. This couple were high school sweethearts and had attended college and business school together. She held a job close to their suburban apartment and took charge of managing their activities and finances. She was referred because she was anorgasmic and disinterested in sex. She was perceived by her husband as very uptight and cold. He had expected this to change after the stress of school was over. However, she needed to work through conflicts related to her fractured family—her father's love affairs and her mother's remarriage and second pregnancy when the daughter was in college. The couple agreed that in a few months, despite her problems with sexual disinterest and anorgasmia, she would have her intrauterine contraceptive coil removed and would attempt a pregnancy. With the coil in place she accidently became pregnant. Her husband was adamant about discontinuing the pregnancy because it was not part of the deal they had made about the timing of her pregnancy. The coil had to be removed because of the danger that it might rupture the uterine wall during pregnancy. Removal of the coil would inevitably result in abortion. The patient lost the pregnancy.

The patient subsequently lost her job but found a new position. She clearly wanted a pregnancy, and she anticipated working part time. She found an infertility specialist, began to put her cyclic data on her personal computer, and faithfully pursued her workup and her husband's. Initially she was found to be ovulating and unobstructed. She was later found to have a bicornuate uterus that required surgical repair. She then was cycled on drugs to produce multiple ova. This very private person, after analyzing this charateristic in light of her father's public affair, agreed to be the subject of an article on infertility. She was determined to become pregnant and to have the first male child to carry her husband's family name, which she accomplished.

Struggle to Obtain Medical Help: Six Patients

A patient who had completed psychoanalytic treatment reached her career apogee and was married, and gave birth to her son, who was now 2 years old. After trying for almost a year to become pregnant again, the woman returned to treatment for depression. She researched her problem and found an infertility expert. She found herself pushing him every step of the way, reminding him of parts of the evaluation he had forgotten and pressuring him for appointments and sonography, and yet being put off by his approach. She talked with other infertile women who also had an uphill struggle to get help and information.

* * *

A successful businesswoman was referred by her infertility physician because of depression and fearfulness. She had been attempting to conceive for 3 years. Although a basic workup was done and everything was "fine," she had not been offered artificial insemination with her husband's sperm or in vitro fertilization. Although angry, helpless, and infantilized, she had not confronted her physician. Her personality disorder kept her passive.

* * *

Another patient came to treatment because she felt obligated to stop smoking before attempting a pregnancy. The patient was indeed able to stop smoking. She became pregnant but had an early miscarriage followed by difficulty in conceiving. Her physician had a laissez-faire attitude. The patient began to get depressed. As the head of a large social welfare agency she was no stranger to arm twisting. When she realized what would be needed, she did not feel conflicted and actively pursued her goal.

* * *

The wife of one patient had had surgery as an adolescent because of peritonitis. She failed to conceive within a reasonable time. As a physician's wife she was evaluated in a timely fashion. When her workup ground to a halt, she became insomniac and tearful and had difficulty functioning at her job. Her husband, at his therapist's suggestion, did the research, saw her X rays, and decided she probably needed reconstructive surgery on her fallopian tubes. At her husband's suggestion, she had artificial insemination with his sperm and became pregnant.

* * *

A patient who was having difficulty conceiving had also had abdominal surgery, allegedly for "pylonephritis." Her gynecologist concluded that this could not have led to an obstruction in her reproductive system. Months went by and she became depressed. When her therapist pointed out that surgery is not done for pylonephritis unless it is done accidently, she agreed to try to get her hospital records. The record, which she was able to obtain, showed ruptured appendicitis and peritonitis. Pelvic insufflation led to pregnancy.

* * *

A sophisticated woman, active in the art and business worlds, had tried unsuccessfully for 7 years to conceive but had not pressed her gynecologist for a workup beyond ascertaining that she was ovulating. She had never been studied for obstruction; her husband had never been asked to provide a sperm sample. The woman was becoming disinterested in sex and depressed.

It is clear that infertility per se causes depression. Most of the patients we have studied had some depression and a passive adaptation to their physicians[†] despite dramatic business and career success. The patients often became passive and vulnerable in the context of failure to master infertility, in sharp contrast to the mastery they demonstrated in other areas of their lives.

[†]An incidental finding is that of long trials of labor in older primiparas who had transverse shoulder or breech presentations.

Adoption

For those patients who elect or feel resigned to seeking adoption, the road is filled with many obstacles and hardships. There is an appalling paucity of recent data about adoption. Lazare (1984[68]) found that it took 3 to 6 years from the time of deciding on adoption for a Caucasian family to get a healthy Caucasian child. Therefore, a woman in her middle to late 30s may be 40 before she can adopt a child, and her husband may be significantly older. In our experience privately arranged adoptions can cost anywhere from $10,000 to $15,000 in the South and Midwest, to $50,000 on the East and West coasts. Paying exorbitant costs beyond the health costs for the mother is considered the "purchase" of a child. Although illegal, this practice continues nonetheless. Legitimately, it might cost up to $20,000 to fly to South America or Asia to bring back an infant. It is easier to adopt a child of 3 to 10 years old. These children have often been acculturated differently or have had multiple prior foster care placements, hospitalization, or institutionalization. Infants known to be ill are readily available for adoption. These illnesses, such as AIDS, may be fatal. Fetal alcohol syndrome or intrauterine drug addiction often result in stunted physical and mental development.

There is a broader literature on the adoption of special children. The adoptive parents frequently have children of their own.

Ironically, while infertile couples pine for a child, there is a glut of "boarder" babies living in hospitals who are not legally free to be adopted. The psychiatric literature fails to deal with the plight of these youngsters or the anguish of their caregivers. Nor does it attend to the stress and conflict individuals experience in dealing with the adopting process, whether it is legal or clandestine. Patients report about the stress of interviewing with adoption agencies and the home visits in which they feel that their entire life-style is being graded pass/fail. No matter how gently and professionally adoption agencies deal with their clients, the stakes are high and the probabilities of a client adopting a given child are low.

The importance of "passing the examination" has been noted by Andrews (1970[69]) in an attempt to understand why parents frequently conceive after adopting:

1. An authoritative agency has given permission to a couple to achieve parenthood.
2. Agency approval is an ego-supportive process helping couples to relax and to attend to the libidinal aspects of their lives.
3. Agency workers often help prospective parents ventilate and sort out dammed up feelings about earlier life experiences.
4. Feelings about sterility and the accompanying failed treatment procedures are also ventilated.
5. Sterility is no longer a secret or a private disgrace.

Another scenario follows: The couple hires an individual (usually an attorney) who guides them to advertise in impoverished rural areas. A second phone is installed at home for the purpose of anonymity while negotiating with a birth mother. These private adoptions often have to be made without an adequate birth history or an attempt to match the expected child with any of the physical characteristics of the adoptive family. The difficulty that this may cause is illustrated by a case currently in litigation in New York City. A man with cancer deposited semen in a sperm bank, hoping that if he became sterile his wife could be impregnated with that semen. Accidentally, his wife was impregnated with the semen of a man of a different race. She has been accused of sexual relations outside her marriage while her husband was ill and dying. Her child is being taunted by schoolmates because of her race. These types of reactions can happen in the case of any obvious physical mismatch. Couples who make the conscious decision to adopt a child of another race also have problems but have generally prepared themselves to face them.

Even adoptive parents who are struggling to love their new baby endure a delay in the final signing of the adoption papers. Therefore, they are put in the position of fearing to love too much and lose the child.

Adoption

A much sought after baby failed to feed properly or thrive. Without a medical history the infant had to be hospitalized and studied for genetic or congenital disease. The adoptive mother had no idea how to help this infant. She devoted herself night and day to its care but could not seem to comfort the baby. The mother had a serious psychotic depression. She was seen by a therapist first with her infant for support and instruction, and later on in therapy for herself. In a few months, the baby became well. No medical diagnosis had been made. The mother has continued in psychotherapy to resolve issues of self-confidence and loss of self-esteem.

* * *

A mother of one child moved to adopt. Her biological child was as gifted as his parents. The mother was somewhat fearful that an "average" child may be overwhelmed and thrust aside by his or her older brother.

* * *

A menopausal health care professional who had lost an 8-year-old son to a fulminating viral disease moved within months to adopt. She anticipated waiting at least 5 years. She was just coming to terms with this when she received a call that her "birth mother" was in the delivery room. She and her husband had 24 hours to set up a nursery and purchase clothing, formula bottles, and assorted baby paraphernalia. She had made no arrangements at work for maternity leave. The joy and surprise of the parents helped them through what might otherwise have been a difficult situation.

Adoptive Experimentation: Withheld Information

Psychiatrists at one agency, realizing that adoption carries a risk of psychiatric morbidity and that twinship carries the same risk, decided to separate one set of twins and place them in homes in each of which a prior adoptee was doing well. However, they withheld this information from the adopting parents. The psychiatrists did periodically evaluate these separated twins, their adopted siblings, and the families. Later, one of the twins, Lynn, in treatment, recalled a sister named Kim, whom her parents took to be an imaginary companion. A neighbor who had moved called to say that she had met Lynn's double. After the two met, Lynn became depressed and Kim manic. The agency revealed the experiment and data on the birth mother. With the help of both adoptive families the girls found the birth mother. She met with them for one visit. Both girls recovered from their psychiatric illness. Although both adoptive families were angry at the withholding of data, neither was interested in anything but the well-being of their daughters.

The Search for the Birth Mother

A gifted college student, the older of two adopted sisters, came to treatment because of a crisis in identity and in future goals. The patient had decided to find her birth mother. Knowing what effect this decision would have on her adoptive mother, who opposed such a search, the patient opted to use trust money from her grandmother's estate. The biological mother, who had married the birth father and had two other children, was eager to meet the daughter whom she had given up at birth. The patient found nothing in common with her biological mother's family, who were of a different socioeconomic class and had very different interests. Despite the uncovering of physical abuse by the adoptive mother and the fact that the adoptive father knew that he was infertile and had lied to his wife, the adoptive daughter preferred her adoptive parents.

Surrogate Mothering

Surrogate mothering has received a lot of attention in the media and some vague editorializing by physician-ethicists. Yet there are no reports in the medical or psychiatric literature on the subject.

The fields of infertility, adoption, and surrogate parenting involve money and sexuality, the very subjects most persons are hesitant to discuss. There is no paucity of literature on the development and problems of both adopted and foster children. Yet we continue to ignore the problems, emotional distress, and overt psychiatric illness that are often the legacy of the quest for a baby.

Pregnancy

Pregnancy may be burdened because of the following: 1) it may have been difficult to achieve; 2) it may have happened outside of a committed relationship; 3) it may have happened within a stormy relationship; 4) it may have been unplanned; 5) it may present problems vis-à-vis employment; and 6) it may be a great financial burden. In addition, pregnancy may, even in good circumstances, cause psychological problems secondary to medical ones. It is a stage in development in which unresolved but heretofore quiescent conflicts may be rekindled. When a patient becomes pregnant, it is possible to study her fantasies, progressions, and regressions.

Pregnancy involves many physiological changes. The way in which these changes are processed often pertains to both the present life of the mother-to-be and her prior adaptation. In the first trimester, physiological changes include nausea and vomiting (i.e., morning sickness), frequency of urination, vaginal discharge, painfully swollen breasts, edema of the legs, and lethargy. In the midtrimester, some patients report gastric reflux. In the last trimester, there may be difficulties in locomotion, sleeping, urinary frequency, and constipation. Throughout pregnancy women must undergo repeated gynecological examination, change in body image, and fluctuations in both sexual desire and the mechanics of sexual behavior.

Expectant mothers develop a set of fantasies about unborn babies. These fantasies begin between the awareness of conception and the feeling of fetal movement (Bernstein and Warner 1984b[22]). The fantasies involve the sex of the child and the anticipation of the repetition of the relationship that the future mother had with her own family. A female child is wished for when the woman seeks unconsciously to replicate or repair her tie to her mother. Wishing to reenact an oedipal relationship with her father, a woman may wish for a son. When a male sibling had been a favored child, a woman also may wish for a son. For example, one patient who had unresolved unconscious issues around the loss of bodily products and parts wished for a daughter whom she anticipated keeping close to her. Self-esteem issues affect fantasied object choice (see Chapter 3).

The mother-to-be has a set of fantasies, conscious and unconscious, that will allow greater or lesser flexibility in facing the inevitable loss of her baby as part of her own body. Fantasies involve the dependent state that an obvious pregnancy traditionally allows in our society. Women who take care of themselves will often accept proffered courtesy and help, both from men and from other nonpregnant women. Some patients experience inner fullness and euphoria that may be related to reunion with the mother of early childhood and to filling the inner genital space. Other women may react with rage and depression because their pregnancy threatens their unconscious fantasy of being male. Changes in breasts and in bodily shape and weight have not only real but fantasized meaning.

The following case examples are of patients whose pregnancies were observed during treatment. In these examples we focus on the effect of unconscious fantasies on medical realities. Patients whose primary issues during pregnancy were psychodynamically determined are also discussed.

Physiological Illness

A 30-year-old attorney longed to be pregnant. Initially she sought treatment for marital difficulties and problems of passivity in her job. She became pregnant at first trial. The couple were so ecstatic that they cast aside an initial decision to wait for the first trimester to pass before informing their out-of-town relatives. Postpartum arrangements were secure. She had solved her work problems and had become more assertive and comfortable.

The mother-to-be suffered not only "morning sickness" (not a major problem in her family or among her friends), but also nausea and vomiting all day long. She continued to work despite this and took a planned vacation in Europe with her husband. Visibly weak and depleted yet overjoyed with her pregnancy, she determined to carry on her activities. Her illness did not abate until her sixth month of pregnancy. Determination to have a family and a career clearly carried her through an illness that would have taken a greater toll on someone who was ambivalent.

Ambivalence

Another patient, who had marked ambivalence about her gender identity (the result of incest), reported an obsessive preoccupation with a "swollen belly."

She compulsively watched her diet so that she could be "as small as possible." She was unhappy through both of two pregnancies despite the fact that she "looked good."

Symptoms Reactivating Past Conflicts: Three Patients

One patient, a saleswoman who was delighted with her pregnancy, became clinically depressed in the last trimester when her legs "swelled like balloons" and she had to stay home with legs elevated. She was reminded of a time when she had broken a leg and had been forced to be immobilized and had felt helpless. Uncovering this connection helped psychologically. A second patient was plagued during pregnancy by issues of adolescent obesity. A third patient who had felt burdened during childhood and adolescence by a mother who thought her daughter was too fat literally starved herself during her pregnancy and required treatment for anemia.

Sexual Difficulties Secondary to Readjustments During Pregnancy

A patient who highly valued her sexual relationship with her husband became depressed when intercourse in the male superior position became impossible. Trying other positions raised issues relating to the aggression she perceived in assuming the female superior position. She also risked increased exposure of her "shameful" sexual needs and responses. The only acceptable physical position was side to side.

Two Patients Whose Euphoria Carried Them Through Difficult Pregnancies

Two employed nonobese patients with tall husbands carried large babies in the transverse position. Each woman was well except for seventh-month problems in lying down. One husband described his wife as a "beached whale." Once supine, neither could get up unassisted. One of the women, during her husband's absence for a week, had to sleep sitting. Both women were euphoric with their pregnancies and did not lose self-esteem. Both had the fantasy of being pregnant with a son, in families where a first-born son was a priority.

Regressive Projection of Rage in Three Patients

A patient, a very deprived and lonely child, devoted all her energy toward academic and career success. Her aggressive fantasies toward her mother were sublimated to intellectual achievement. Her dreams were of a destructive cancer that would eat her up from the inside. This dream was interpreted as a projection of her rage at her mother onto an imagined female fetus.

* * *

Another patient fantasized pregnancy with a son who would be born either dead or with a deformity. She felt guilty about a favored brother (whom as a child she had wished dead or deformed) who had died. Her male fetus also represented her father's penis. She felt panicky about delivery because of the fantasy that she would be ripped apart and mutilated because of her baby/penis equation and fear of castration. Intense separation anxiety emerged after analysis of these fantasies. Nursing, she experienced a sense of satiety and orgasmic pleasure. The intersecting paths of separation and castration anxiety, oedipal guilt, and issues around separation-individuation were worked through, resulting in weaning with pleasure in her son's separateness and masculinity and her own competence as a mother.

* * *

Yet another patient, a psychiatrist, was reported on by one of the authors (Bernstein and Warner 1984b,[22] pp. 146–147). This woman sought supervision because she had had two miscarriages, secondary to a genetic abnormality transmitted by her mother. The patient had difficulty in coping with verbal attacks that were made upon her and her unborn fetus by several very sick patients. Because these attacks threatened derepression of her rage at her mother, the patient handled them by countertransference withdrawal. The psychiatrist-patient again became pregnant. She continued to work and ar-

ranged a maternity leave. Patients reacted with rage and dangerous behavior. She successfully confronted and enabled them to manage the impending separation. The psychiatrist-patient was conflicted about the defect in her and in her mother. Learning via amniocentesis that she was pregnant with a daughter, she managed the rest of her pregnancy and therapeutic work with ease.[†]

Self-Hatred Because of Femininity During Pregnancy

A patient presented with a severe depressive disorder precipitated by the loss of an important friendship with someone who had helped her to negotiate her children's adolescence and a new career. A routine gynecological examination led to treatment for a yeast infection and referral for mammography. She felt enraged and spoke of how much she hated being a woman. In the past she had postponed and tried to avoid pregnancy because of the "financial burden." Through education, she had struggled out of poverty. She had perceived that having too many children had kept relatives impoverished and depressed. She spoke retrospectively with startling vehemence about her hatred of her pregnant state and her rage at bodily changes and at her husband who inflicted them.

Pregnancy is a pivotal time in a woman's psychological life. It often exacerbates old conflicts, but it also provides an opportunity for reworking conflict either spontaneously or while in therapy. In many cases, but not all, the woman may emerge with increased psychic growth.

Abortion: Spontaneous and Induced

It has been estimated that approximately one out of five women in the United States has had a legal abortion (Forrest et al. 1979[70]). The vast majority of these women report that their pregnancy was accidental (Henshaw and O'Reilly 1983[71]). In a study commissioned by the Ameri-

---

[†]The analysis of three pregnant patients was reported in detail by Bernstein and Warner (1984b[22]).

can Psychological Association, it was found that voluntary first-trimester abortions rarely resulted in severe psychological trauma (Adler et al. 1990[72]). Some studies have indicated that 5% to 10% of women who have abortions will experience long-term negative effects (Adler et al. 1990[72]; Ashton 1980[73]).

Major et al. (1985[74]) reviewed studies on postabortion adjustment. In most of these studies, minimal psychiatric stress was reported (Adler 1975[75]; Belsey et al. 1977[76]; Bracken et al. 1978[77]; Shusterman 1979[78]). These authors have noted certain risk factors, as follows:

1. Young age (Adler 1975[75])
2. Weak social support systems (Bracken et al. 1978[77]; Shusterman 1979[78])
3. Conflicted decision making around the abortion (Adler 1975[75]; Bracken et al. 1978[77])
4. Lack of psychological stability before the abortion (Belsey et al. 1977[76])

Other authors have correlated the following factors with negative postabortion outcomes:

1. Premorbid psychiatric illness (Whittington 1970[79]; Ford et al. 1971[80])
2. Medical indications dictating abortion (Niswander and Patterson 1967[81]; Simon et al. 1967[82])
3. Lack of family support (Moseley et al. 1981[83])
4. Ambivalence (Patt et al. 1969[84]; Payne et al. 1976[85])
5. Coercion (Friedman et al. 1974[86])
6. Conflicting social values (Freeman et al. 1980[87])

Multiple abortions seem to increase the amount of dysphoria (Niemela et al. 1981[88]). Franco et al. (1989[89]) have profiled dysphoria in postabortion women as it relates to premorbid psychiatric illness, lack of support, ambivalence, and coercion.

Mueller and Major (1989[90]) found that better outcome related to better self-efficacy, low "self-blame," and ratings in "other blame" quotients. They also felt that expectation was related to outcome. Mueller and Major attempted to briefly precounsel women, anticipating a better outcome. The immediate outcome was better but lasted only temporarily.

Fisch and Tadmor (1989[91]) have reported on posttraumatic stress disorder after abortion. Even in patients who do not experience posttraumatic stress disorder after abortion, we see the sequelae reexperienced as the abortion is discussed in therapy. In addition, guilt, mourning, anxiety, and depression may arise when a desired pregnancy is being planned, when infertility is discovered or an infertility workup is in progress, and when a patient expects a grandchild.

Childhood Sexual Abuse

A 31-year-old divorced business executive sought treatment for anxiety attacks and trichotillomania. She engaged in a series of promiscuous sexual relationships with men who either mistreated or abandoned her. The patient eventually became pregnant and obtained an elective abortion. She handled it in "businesslike" fashion. Later, memories of repeated childhood sexual abuse experiences with her uncle were derepresessed. During the analysis of a dream, she reexplored additional earlier elective abortions.

Substance Abuse Secondary to Coerced Abortion

A 32-year-old single college graduate was admitted for long-term inpatient treatment for severe polydrug and alcohol abuse, social isolation, vocational failure, multiple passive suicide attempts, and intermittent bulimia with chronic feelings of numbness and emptiness. Prior to her hospitalization, the patient had lived in a series of chaotic communal, drug-dominated settings. She had several heterosexual relationships with men who were drug addicted and/or physically abused her. She contracted hepatitis and her parents intervened, moving her back to her hometown and financially supporting her. She was hospitalized after a 2-week bout of continuous cocaine abuse followed by a severe bulimic episode. She suffered severe panic symptoms and a sense of complete loss of control.

Long-term hospitalization focused on detoxification, structured living, and psychotherapy. She actively explored childhood experiences in which she had been a narcissistic extension of her mother. She had a nightmare in which she was being haunted by the corpse of a dead baby who resembled her. She derepressed memories of a therapeutic abortion at age 15 that her mother had coercively arranged. The father was someone the patient truly loved, and her decision to have intercourse had represented the rare assertion of feelings independent of her mother. She had undergone the abortion alone and had been distraught. Her mother had later said, angrily, "How could you do this to me?" In reviewing the incident, the patient remarked, "It was as though she had killed me along with the baby."

Negative Reaction to Voluntary Abortion

A 25-year-old single woman on the "fast track" became involved with a married father of two children. The man began the process of divorce. In the meantime she became accidently pregnant. She felt unwilling to begin a family and opted for an abortion. The father reluctantly agreed. The woman became easily tearful and insomniac for several weeks thereafter. Her career success continued. Her ardor for her former lover cooled, and she attributed this to the abortion.

She became involved with another man for several years. She had anniversary (i.e., of the abortion) depression. She cried at her friends' baby showers. She began another affair with a married man, much her senior, in a very intimate and loving relationship. She explored the oedipal etiology of her inability to find and marry a suitable available man. Her beloved father died. Her mourning reaction was not as painful as her continued mourning about her aborted fetus.

Identification With Daughters Who Aborted

A married professional mother of two grown children presented with anxiety and depression secondary to failure in career advancement. The recall of her own mother's premature death, the subsequent loss of her father, and the very premature loss of a beloved nephew did not evoke the same affective response as the recollection of two elective abortions, about which she cried bitterly. She had a major depressive reaction to the news that one of her children had had a spontaneous first trimester abortion. Her daughter's second pregnancy was rapidly achieved. The patient was very tearful at the thought that this infant either might or might not be of the same sex as she imagined her fetuses had been. She thought of this upcoming grandchild as the one she lost. Her fantasies included taking over the mothering of this child.

* * *

A married professional mother of several children, the youngest still in latency, became enraged and then depressed when her oldest married daughter elected to have an abortion. Associations were to her feelings about being the only obligatory child of her family of origin, and she explained why she herself had chosen to have many children. Later, after the birth of a grandchild, she mourned the loss of the first conceptus.

Acting Out of the Transference

An unmarried patient became pregnant while denying her analyst's pregnancy. The patient aborted and felt depressed and weepy but asserted that this had to do with sudden hormonal changes. She had weepy spells on the abortion anniversary. Involved in a serious relationship, she had guilty ruminations about infertility. Confronted with her guilt, the patient said, "Why should I be guilty; I didn't kill a baby." She had, however, considered the fetus a baby. Her rage that the analyst had delivered a baby emerged, and it was revealed that the patient, in unconscious identification with the analyst, had felt pregnant before she had actually become pregnant. The patient also wanted to be the analyst's baby. She wished that the analyst's baby would be killed as she had killed her own baby. A period of mourning followed.

Unconscious Resistance to Pregnancy

A childhood-onset diabetic mother of a 3-year-old child sought treatment for depression after a spontaneous early abortion that she believed was due to her neglect of her diabetes. Her first pregnancy had been very difficult. Scrupulous in following her medical regimen, she had become unconscious because of low blood sugar on many occasions. She and her family feared another pregnancy, but she felt determined to try. She had not mourned her miscarriage. Everyone around her was relieved that it had happened. When the mourning process began, her menstrual flow returned. She no longer felt so distraught even though her infertility continued.

The Desire to Adopt a Child of the Same Sex as an Aborted Fetus

A married mother in her early 30s came for treatment after a depression secondary to a medical illness. She had marital and career problems. She had chosen to work as a volunteer from her home while baby sitting and managing care of a foster child. It was only possible to understand the choice she made after unlocking a history of two abortions, one before her marriage and the second after her two children were born. She declined employment outside of her home. She disclosed her fantasy of adopting an older child of the same sex as the aborted fetuses.

Abortion for Genetic Reasons Without Apparent Psychiatric Side Effects

A young married woman had her first child in her early 20s. Her one older sister had been chronically hospitalized since adolescence. This sister was finally diagnosed as having manic-depressive psychosis. A family genealogy revealed a large number of family members who had manic depression. The patient accidently became pregnant. She and her husband, both well educated, decided that this pregnancy should be terminated. She anticipated that either she and/or her son might require psychiatric care. In order to amass funds, she took a job. She never felt depressed or guilty about the abortion. She was enraged that her sister, now stable, was considering pregnancy rather than adoption.

Abortion of an Unplanned Pregnancy

A patient in her 20s who had a prolonged hospitalization for self-mutilation and suicidal ideation established a good relationship with a man who had been her private-school classmate for years. In the course of their engagement they had protected sex. Nevertheless, she became pregnant and suicidal, and sought an abortion, which immediately relieved her. She married the man she had chosen and started a family. Five years later she had no regrets about the abortion.

Postpartum Depression

Infants die suddenly from a variety of diseases, including sudden infant death syndrome (SIDS), the etiology of which remains uncertain. Mothers who have lost an infant to SIDS remain aggrieved regardless of the number of healthy children born before or after an infant death.

Postpartum depression is a spectrum disorder. In its most severe manifestation (i.e., postpartum psychosis), it may lead to infanticide. In its mildest form (i.e., postpartum depression or "the blues"), it is a transient period of mild depression characterized by mood lability and anxiety. It begins from 2 to 4 days after delivery and is estimated to affect 50% to 80% of all mothers (Alfonso and Domino 1984[92]; Cox et al. 1982[93]; Hopkins et al. 1984[94]; Pitt 1973[95]; Yalom et al. 1968[96]). Postpartum depression is a depressive episode that is characterized by depressed mood, lethargy, and the vegetative signs that are described in DSM-III-R (American Psychiatric Association 1987[7]) as characteristic of a major depressive episode. Rates for postpartum disorder vary from 3% to 27%, with most authors citing a 10% figure (Alfonso and Domino 1984[92]; Cox et al. 1982[93]; Harding 1989[97]; Jamison et al. 1978[98]; Kumar and Robson 1984[99]; Pitt 1968[100]). Some studies suggest that stressful life events and less spousal support may be factors (O'Hara 1986[101]; Paykel et al. 1980[102]). A previous depressive history is significantly related to the incidence of postpartum depression (Garvey and Tollefson 1984[103]; Hopkins et al. 1984[94]; Kendell 1985[104]). Postpartum depression is predictive of future postpartum depressive disorders and of depressive disorders such as postmenopausal depression and depression after the birth of grandchildren (see Chapter 7).

Psychosis occurs more frequently during postpartum depressive episodes than during other depressive disorders (Dean and Kendell 1981[105]; Meltzer and Kumar 1985[106]; Oates 1986[107]). Psychotic episodes include delusions, hallucinations, agitation, and loosening of associations. Incidence of postpartum psychosis is 2 in 1,000. This entity is not a cultural artifact (Cox 1988[108]).

Asch (1968,[109] p. 215) gave a clear explication of postpartum "blues," conceptualizing this condition as a universal reaction to an emotionally significant loss and relating it to the depression not uncommonly seen in all postoperative patients. The postpartum loss is the loss of the pregnant state along with the feeling and fantasies surrounding the mental image of the fetus. Asch pointed to fantasy of acquisition of a phallus and or reunion with the mother.

Infanticide

Cherland and Matthews (1989[110]) have addressed themselves to issues of teenage pregnancy, lack of family support systems for handling problems (often the pregnancy itself is hidden), and panic at the child's birth. Resnick (1970[111]) observed other characteristics, including the young, unmarried status of the mother; the mother's not wanting a child because of its paternity; and the mother's perception of the child as an obstacle to her ambitions. D'Orbán (1979[112]) reviewed 76 cases and found that the perpetrators tended to come from large families with a family history of mental illness, alcoholism, and early criminality. D'Orbán recognized the role of the mother's having been separated from her own family prior to the age of 15, as well as the roles of social stress (financial and housing related) and marital discord.

Scott (1973[113]) discussed the sources of the impulse to kill one's own child and grouped them in four categories: 1) parents who eliminate an unwanted child; 2) parents who kill the child out of mercy; 3) parents whose uncontrolled aggression is related to gross psychopathology; and 4) parents who displace their anger onto the victim. Scott also recognized the role of battering of the mother during her childhood.

Asch (1968[109]) pointed out that the parturient state inevitably stimulates memories and fantasies of old mother-child relationships. The expectant mother often fantasies herself as both the child she was in the past and the mother she is about to become. Delivery interrupts this mother-child unity and revives experiences associated with the earlier experiences of painful separation from the mother in childhood.

The ability to make a good adjustment to motherhood is an outcome of the stable identification with one's own mother and her positively perceived nurturant functions. Postpartum depression occurs in mothers who cannot deal with separation.

Suicide is a danger in postpartum depression. This act symbolically represents an undoing of the birth and separation or, alternately, the expression of the wish to be rid of the bad, hateful parts of the self. Suicide also represents in this context a symbolic reunion with the wished-for good mother of early childhood.

In patients in whom splitting takes place, the splitting results in the projecting of the bad parts of the self onto the baby. At this point the infant may become the target of the mother's hostile impulses. In the epilogue to the extremely frightening book by Joyce Egginton, *From Cradle to Grave; The Short Lives and Strange Deaths of Marybeth Tinning's Nine Children* (Egginton 1989[114]), Dr. Asch, in his discussion of the case, tells us that he had to abandon the study of the causes of infanticide begun in the 1960s because the opposition was overwhelming.

Infanticide is a psychiatric entity that has been underreported and underaddressed by the legal and medical professions in the United States. The rising incidence of battered and abused children has forced us to attend more seriously to infanticide. The British have recognized this entity for years and have established a period of a year and a day after childbirth in which a woman may not be judged criminally liable for killing her child (Levan 1982[115]). A letter to the editor of the *New York Times Magazine* on July 11, 1988, written by an individual who was familiar with the British position on infanticide, stated that "it is wrong for American courts to imprison mothers who kill their babies. They suffer from a mental illness."

One of the authors had the opportunity to treat a woman who had had previous hospitalizations for paranoid schizophrenia. During one psychotic episode the patient threw her baby with her garbage down an incinerator. Several weeks after psychiatric hospitalization and treatment with phenothiazines, her hallucinations and delusions ceased and she wondered when her baby was due. She had no recollection of labor and delivery or of taking her infant home. When confronted with what had happened, she was at first incredulous and then suicidally depressed. She could not recall the episode.

The diagnosis of the perpetrators of infanticide may run the gamut of psychiatric diagnostic categories, from the psychoses through multiple personality and schizoid, paranoid, borderline, or sociopathic personality disorders.

Some women without psychopathology may have the fantasy or wish for infanticide in special circumstances.

The Resentment of the Million Dollar Baby

A premature infant resuscitated artificially emerged with many major medical problems. His mother became seriously depressed and felt unable to visit the child, bond to him, or assume any hands-on responsibility for his care as the hospital prepared to send him home. In therapy she could reveal her rage over the resuscitation and at the unexpected burden that almost destroyed her career, upon which the family depended for its sustenance. She felt like a terrible person because she considered her son as a "million dollar monster." Ventilation of these feelings and their acceptance allowed her to buy some items for his crib and become able to administer his medication in the hospital.

There are two instances of infanticide extensively reported in the literature. Neither mother was psychotic but both shared several characteristics in terms of public presentation and affect.

In 1987 a woman in New York State was convicted of infanticide (Egginton 1989[114]). She was convicted on one count, although she had confessed to three, because there was medical evidence in only one case. She most probably murdered nine children, three of whom were not infants and one of whom was adopted. The mother was known to make herself seem important and to lie about past events. (The fabrication of a different self for different occasions is reminiscent of patients with Munchausen syndrome.) This mother was also guilty of petty thievery and was known to buy and hoard things she did not need and to chronically overspend the family budget. She appeared affectless.

Siegel (1990[116]), a journalist for the *Los Angeles Times*, reviewed the circumstances of the conviction of an adoptive mother 22 years after the death of her 3-year-old son. Many disturbing questions are raised about the circumstances that allowed this woman to adopt and abuse four more children who were eventually taken from her. She had been treated, evaluated, and even hospitalized on many occasions for anxiety, depression, and absolute insomnia, and one physician posited that she might "turn paranoid schizophrenic." None recognized either her severe character disorder or her sadism. Her history of having been an abused child was only known by her own birth family.

British physicians have observed mothers with infants at risk via video camera. Before the act of smothering, these mothers are observed to be careful lest anyone observe them (Wilkins 1985[117]). After the episode, they successfully block it out so that it is not available to their memory. In psychiatric terms this implies denial rather than lying. It is not yet understood whether this behavior takes place during a dissociative state or the dissociated state supervenes.

Regardless of the stance of the American criminal justice system, we have several obligations in regard to nonpsychotic perpetration of infanticide. The first is not to overlook the diagnosis of infanticide. The second is to keep our minds open to the possibility of infanticidal behavior in all our pregnant women patients and to assess their fantasies, their own childhood relationships, and their prior psychiatric history as regards psychosis or major affective disorder. Third, we must be able to make the proper psychiatric diagnosis of a suspected perpetrator and then offer appropriate treatment. This may include hospitalization or separation from the baby.

Certain cultures—for example, the Nesilik Eskimo, the Tickopia of Polynesia, and the very civilized Japanese culture in the 18th and 19th centuries—have used infanticide as a way of paring population down or protecting limited food supplies (Post 1988[118]). Western tradition differs from other societies that may elect to commit infanticide for purposes of sex selection, population control, and even ridding society of the burden imposed by handicapped individuals. Therefore, for us, infanticide is a major deviation from our cultural norms. Infanticide, like incest, violent abuse, battering, and rape, must no longer be considered impossible or unknowable. Children must be protected and perpetrators treated for their disorder.

The Loss of a Child

The loss of a child is unlike any other loss or bereavement and often results in severe grief (Clayton 1982[119]; Clayton et al. 1968[120]; Sanders 1979–1980[121]; Schwab et al. 1975[122]; Shanfield and Swain 1984[123]; Shanfield et al. 1984[124]; Singh and Raphael 1981[125]). This grief is often complicated and long lasting (Osterweiss et al. 1988[126]), with a major fluctuation in symptomatology over time (Fish and Whitney 1983[127]; Levan 1982[115]; Rando 1983[128]).

The loss of a child impacts the individual parents, the marital dyad, the family system, and society. No matter what the age of the deceased child, he or she has already been imbued with hopes, expectations, wishes, and fantasies. Parents experience the loss as a loss of part of themselves, of part of each other, and of part of the family. With the loss of a child comes the threat of the loss of the fantasy of immortality (Schwartz 1977[129]).

The loss of a child presents special issues of grieving for his or her mother that depend on the age of the child, the manner of his or her death, when the death occurs in the mother's life cycle, and the mother's social role conditioning. The mother's prior unresolved problems shape her grief. The sense of helplessness and tendency toward regression may cause issues that were once well defended or resolved to resurface. For example, one mother of a son involved in the Desert Shield operation in the Persian Gulf War began to discuss the time 20 years before that an older son had been hospitalized and near death with an overwhelming infection. The other children had never heard this story before. Clearly, the agony of that earlier wait that she had mastered and probably repressed resurfaced in the face of a current life-or-death uncertainty involving a different child.

We have already discussed the reaction to abortion, planned or accidental. When ultrasound confirms the diagnosis of a dead baby, there is the medical question of whether to induce labor or to wait for natural labor to ensue. One patient who was advised to let natural labor ensue in another 6 weeks felt forced to carry a dead baby and was embittered by this burden. She felt a great desire for riddance and also resented the loss of time in attempting a new pregnancy. Fetuses who must await natural labor become macerated, and often they are not shown to the mother, who is deprived of mourning for a "real baby."

The death of a baby in the peri- or intrapartum period often leaves the parents no time for preparation. Shock supervenes and the mother misses the opportunity for anticipatory grief. One physician, mother of three sons, felt convinced that she was pregnant with a daughter. At term, she had some spotting and asked for a cesarean section but her request was denied. The baby was lost intrapartum. Although she went on to have a daughter, she never recovered from the loss of her "baby girl." Whenever people referred to her as the mother of four children, she corrected them to state that she had had five children but one little girl had died.

The problem of stillbirth is even more difficult for the woman with an infertility problem or for the older woman who wishes to have a child or children. A replacement baby may not be a good substitute for an unresolved loss. With proper help the task of grieving may be accomplished in a shorter time span (Worden 1982[130]). The grief of a mother who is unable to have another infant is clearly more difficult to manage. This grief is compounded for a woman who loses her uterus at the time she loses her baby.

Loss of a Baby After Having Had Several Children

A 40-year-old Italian Catholic pregnant mother of seven children of mixed sexes experienced a ruptured uterus with the onset of labor. She was brought to the hospital unconscious with an unobtainable blood pressure. The mother miraculously recovered without complications. She appreciated that her life had been saved and was relieved that the baby was dead before any intervention had been made. Yet she became depressed. She felt guilty that her life had been saved at her baby's expense, although this was not true, and sad at the loss of her child, which she imagined would have been her last. For many years she had difficulty when seeing babies.

When a baby dies, there are a variety of mourning reactions ranging from normal grief to feelings of unreality, somatization, and clinical (and even psychotic) depression. Mothers seem to be more severely affected. They must be helped to grieve and to avoid the negation and denial of individuals who, in other situations, would be supportive. Parents of the couple and other family members need to be encouraged to persist despite rebuff by the grieving mother. Irrational guilt must be explored.

Sudden infant death syndrome describes the sudden death of any infant that was unexpected by history and in which thorough autopsy fails to demonstrate a cause of death. SIDS accounts for more than one-half of all infant deaths between the ages of 3 and 4 months (Beckwirth 1975[131]). The grief reaction is compounded by the sudden and unexpectedness of the loss. Severe guilt may supervene because of insinuations about the adequacy of care. The loss occurs just as bonding has been established. SIDS robs the mother of her infant just at the time when breast-feeding may have been established, when the mother and child have learned each other's rhythms, when the infant's gaze is fixed on the mother's face, and when the baby may have begun to smile or to quiet at the sound of the mother's voice or footsteps.

Yet another issue is that of family bereavement. The baby is lost just as he or she may have become a real person to family members. Taylor et al. (1986,[132] p. 167), who have had extensive experience in treating survivors of SIDS, provide an outline of treatment issues to be addressed, which we have consolidated as follows:

1. Communication of feelings
2. Life-style resumption
3. Use and perception of family and community support and family solidarity
4. Information on SIDS
5. Preventability
6. Subsequent children
7. Religion
8. Family morbidity and emotional health
9. Infant centrality and functional role of the deceased infant in the family

---

Death of an Especially Beloved Child

A woman in her early 30s, the eldest of three daughters in her birth family, identified with her mother in the maternal role. She had three sons. She had longed for a daughter, and her fourth pregnancy produced an "utterly beautiful little girl." When the daughter was 4 months old, she was left in the care of both the housekeeper who had taken care of her brothers and the child's grandparents. With the caretakers in the house, the baby was found by the housekeeper to be unarousable from an afternoon nap. The overt expression of grief and guilt by all concerned parties was apparent and communicated. Despite receiving psychological help and having enthusiastic interest in her sons and their activities, the mother did not lose the sadness in her eyes for a full 10 years.

The accidental death of a child, no matter what the age, presents all the problems of what Parkes and Weiss (1983[133]) have called the "unexpected loss syndrome." They describe the following characteristics of this syndrome, to which we add from our own experience:

1. Difficulty in believing that the death occurred, with delay in processing the loss

2. Social withdrawal
3. Close attachment to the deceased long after this is intelligible to others
4. Re-exacerbation of acute grief around holidays, the child's birthday, the date of expected school graduation, etc.
5. Marital discord, separation, and even divorce (Schiff 1977[134])

Death of an Infant With Heart Defects

One of the authors worked with the family of a 2-year-old child who was born with multiple heart defects and who, despite surgical and medical intervention, developed increasing heart failure. The mother was so distraught over her daughter's condition that she swore never to have another child, although her daughter's disease was not hereditary. This decision threatened her marriage. Prior to the child's certain death, the mother was helped to begin the mourning process. Unconscious, the child clung to life for many months, her mother by her side and unrelenting in her resolve not to try to have another child. Her interest in other children who were more responsive was encouraged and she began to help children who were recovering and whose parents were less available. Her husband joined her after his work and became involved with her in the care of other children. The mother became pregnant. Her daughter died with both parents present. A healthy daughter was born 7 months later.

Death of an Infant From Leukemia

A 40-year-old mother of an 8-year-old daughter, a 5-year-old son, and a 1-year-old son noticed that her baby did not seem to be recovering from bronchitis despite antibiotic therapy. The child was found to have acute leukemia. With chemotherapy he was brought into remission, only to relapse rapidly. He spent his last 9 months hospitalized and was well cared for. The mother began to grieve in preparation for his death. After the baby died, she spent a lot of time with his siblings. She became pregnant after the mourning period. She did not allow her oldest daughter to go away to camp with her friends, insisting that she needed this child at home to help her. It was only after the birth of another son that she admitted to her fears and her need to keep her surviving children close by. Birth anniversaries and holidays are still hard for her.†

The Death of an Adolescent

One patient, a 55-year-old woman and the mother of four children, was seen because of depression and bulimia. She stated, "My trouble began 5 years ago, when my beautiful little daughter was killed. It was for no reason. It was no one's fault, and none of that matters. She is gone. What use is there for me to live anymore?" The mother had looked forward to this dead child's potential for achievement and her vicarious enjoyment of the easy, better life she had imagined for her daughter. Despite treatment and symptom remission, the mother remained inconsolable.

The death of a child from a serious illness that is predicted to be fatal poses other problems. Parents struggle to find a cure. When a cure is not found, some feel satisfied that they did their best. Others become angry at the medical staff and other caregivers. Often parents are caught between the perceived obligations to the dying child and the needs of their well children. Still others accept the inevitable and prepare for it by pulling back from their child. When children are older, often parents and children are able to discuss and prepare for death. The most common adaptation, however, is the vacillation between denial and despair. The opportunity to intervene with the family of a dying child is very valuable. It gives the therapist the opportunity to strengthen and support the relationships within the family and between spouses. It is helpful for the therapist to help prevent the withdrawal from the dying child and thus the guilt that may follow.

†One of the most poignant descriptions of what it is like to endure the dying and death of a young, but not infant, child is furnished by Gunther (1949[135]).

Perhaps the worst grief is that experienced when a child dies by suicide. This death often has the characteristics of being sudden and unexpected, with no time for anticipatory preparation. In addition, there are issues of guilt of a unique kind. When a child commits suicide, we recognize it as an act not only against the self but possibly against the parents. That this may have nothing to do with the realities of parental care or caring but rather with the misconceptions of the child about the parents, is often lost to friends, family, and the community. Sue Chance, M.D. (1991[136]), has written eloquently on this subject—the reaction of shock and disbelief, the painful feelings and fears, the physical symptoms and negative signs, the anorexia and insomnia, usually associated with depression. She understands how suicide often disrupts marriage because of the misunderstandings about the different rates and styles of mourning in spouses. Suicide may also precipitate the dissolution of an already tenuous marriage.

Often, after the initial grief, guilt, and lowering of self-esteem, anger emerges at self, at God, and finally at the child. The survivor may also feel anger at other parents who complain too much of the burdens of child rearing or who criticize or punish their child, because the survivor thinks that they fail to appreciate how lucky they are that their child is alive.

With the recent frightening increase in murder of children and adolescents in inner cities, we are just beginning to learn about mourning in these cases. It would seem that parental activism against drugs, weapons, and racism is often palliative.

The loss of an adult child in war is a special problem, with which we, in the United States, are only beginning to come to grips. Operation Desert Storm in the Persian Gulf War has resulted in a vast supportive network for families, many of whom have reached out to the parents of victims of the Vietnam War who suffered from lack of support.

The grieving process for adult children who die contradicts the expectation that parents will die first (Gorer 1965[137]). Fish (1986[138]) found that this is the one instance in which there is less incongruence between the grief experienced by mothers and fathers. Rosenblatt (1983[139]) differentiated the grieving over lost hopes from the grieving over memories. The older the adult child, the more intense the grief over memories. There are other concerns for elderly parents. They have often cared for their children and anticipate some dependence, or may already have some dependence on them, in time of illness or in contemplation of their own death.

One mother of a divorced woman with two children had a difficult time around the suicide of her estranged former son-in-law who had joint custody of his sons. Ill herself, this woman got more ill and regressed. Her demands on her daughter, who now had to manage her children alone and had less time to devote to her mother, were increased.

There are a couple of unique kinds of loss, the cases of which involve ambiguity. We are particularly referring to the cases of missing children, hostages, and soldiers missing in action. Although many of the issues of mourning are similar, the inability to find closure and certainty postpones definitive mourning.

The loss of the child who is the favorite child, even if not overtly favored, has its special problems, as does the loss of the least favorite child. However, mothers who have lost an only child do feel as if they have lost everything, both past memories and future expectations. The loss of an only child may constitute an increased jeopardy in a marriage. This loss has been described by Gurdus (1978[140]), who, along with her husband, attempted to resolve this loss in a not unusual way—by caring for other children.

The single mother's loss of a child, even if the child is one of several, will necessarily have the added dimension of the mother not having a partner in the grieving process. Conversely, we have mentioned previously that the child or children of unwed mothers are at higher risk for abuse, neglect, and infanticide or murder. This abuse is often at the hands of the mother's current boyfriend. This may be because the child is his competition for the girlfriend-mother's attention.

Genital Surgery

Genital surgery causes more severe psychiatric repercussions in women, even when the indication is not cancer. The female genital organs, particularly the uterus, are identified with mother. The persistent desire to have a baby so as to maintain the tie with the mother of early childhood has long been recognized as a pervasive fantasy in women (Deutsch 1944,[141] 1945[142]; Kestenberg 1978[143]). Bernstein and Warner (1984b[22]) have extensively reviewed the literature on female genital surgery.

Mastectomy

A married, nulliparous woman in her 20s underwent a radical mastectomy for a cancer in situ. The woman, who was in psychoanalytic treatment at the time, was angry about what she regarded as an unnecessary surgical procedure; she denied that she really had cancer. Her marital relationship did not deteriorate as it often does when a mastectomy patient is in denial about cancer and is angry about the surgery. Shortly after her surgery, her mother died. Her first reaction was, "First I lost my breast, now I lost my mother." Against medical advice, she proceeded to become pregnant. She would hold and feed her baby thinking of being held and fed by her own mother. After the birth of her second child, she began to mourn the loss of her breast and to become frightened that she had had cancer and that, like her mother, she could die.

* * *

A 40-year-old woman analysand discovered a lump in her breast shortly after the death of her twin sister. She had a modified mastectomy and chemotherapy. She initially reacted with bravery, which was quickly followed by a panicky depression. Analysis of this depression revealed that she, "the brave twin," had spent a long symbiotic period with her mother, who was phobic. The mother had been unable to care for her daughters when they were ill, and her father had had to reassure the mother that her children would not die. When the patient perceived death as a real threat to her, she identified with her mother's panicky and phobic reaction.

Mastectomy patients are seeking breast reconstruction more and more frequently. Often the obsession with what appears to be a matter of vanity may mask a denial of the fear of a life-threatening illness.

Breast Reconstruction

A 50-year-old married mother of three children had lost a sister as a result of metastatic breast cancer. Three neighbors had undergone mastectomy in the past several years. The patient had carefully avoided any inquiry and denied any concern about them. When a mass was discovered in this patient's breast, she was hospitalized for biopsy. She signed a consent form for a simple mastectomy only because she desired immediate reconstructive surgery. This was done several months later, a period during which she mercilessly hounded her surgeon, who was not prepared to operate until he felt that adequate healing had taken place. After the reconstructive surgery the patient was entirely preoccupied with a 3 cm difference in the size of her breasts. She underwent another operative procedure to correct this, despite the opposition of her family. This patient denied her fear of dying and displaced her anger and frustration onto what she regarded as unsatisfactory reconstructive surgery. She later developed infiltration of the mediastinum, which required radiation and chemotherapy. She lost all her hair but nevertheless attended her daughter's wedding wearing a wig. She was without concern about her wig, but still upset with the appearance of her breasts.

[Interviews with family members after this woman's death revealed that in the closing days of her life, she had been very panicky and required the constant presence of family members at her bedside. She could not be left alone. Had anyone understood her psychology, she could have been treated, and she and her family might have been spared a great deal of additional and unnecessary pain.]

This patient's daughter, a professional married mother of two young daughters, discovered a minute lesion in one of her breasts. At mammography she was told that the lesion "looked benign." Heeding the advice of a college friend who became an obstetrician and gynecologist, she demanded an excision biopsy. The biopsy revealed carcinoma. The lesion was excised with wide margins. Refusing to let it go at that, the daughter demanded bilateral simple mastectomy along with the bilateral excision of axillary nodes. The nodes were free of disease, as were her bones, lungs, liver, and brain. Nevertheless, she insisted on and received an extended course of chemotherapy. She suffered the attendant side effects, including complete hair loss. With psychotherapy and the support of her physician-husband she maintained her good spirits and optimism. She celebrated the end of her chemotherapy with a champagne party for family and friends. She then read an article ("Breast Cancer" 1989[144]) that resulted from a large outcome study at a major medical center. In the article researchers stated that 8 to 10 women without evidence of metastases at the time of surgery will die within 10 years from the onset of the disease. In reality, then, breast cancer has become a lethal disease with a relatively long-term survival. The patient is dealing with what she accepts as reality in a better way than we would dare to have expected.

* * *

Another patient, the married mother of mature children, was carefully followed with mammography because her mother had survived breast cancer and later lung metastases. A "suspicious looking" mammogram led to frozen section biopsy and immediate mastectomy, including node excision. There was no evidence of spread. She received a full course of chemotherapy. One year later she developed headaches. She went immediately for a computed axial tomography brain scan, which was positive, and the growth was located in such a way that it was inoperable. She hoped to survive as her mother had, but succumbed to her disease. She received intravenous Demerol and Valium, which made her stuporous in her last weeks. She was not given any morphine.[†]

* * *

One young patient, who already has a son, has not been able to become pregnant again. She has had two bouts with osteosarcoma that required surgery, leaving her with an inflexible leg. She also has had lung surgery and chemotherapy for metastases. She understands that her long-term prognosis is guarded, and she does complain of her physical disability. However, she seems to have no problem with body image, self-esteem, or the threat of recurrent

[†]This is in contrast to a male patient with prostate cancer and painful liver metastasis who was given morphine and traveled abroad on a business trip.

cancer. This is not because she makes use of the psychological defense of denial. Rather, it seems that mutilation and the threat of death (as in the case of Sigmund Freud) do not have the overwhelming valence that genital surgery has for women. That is, cancer that affects the female genital organs and requires mutilation is more traumatic than cancer and surgery of other organs in either men or women.

Oophorectomy

A businesswoman, the mother of four children, had already had a fibroidectomy and a tubal ligation (for sterilization). Other fibroid tumors often caused menometrorrhagia. One year after her mother died from breast cancer, the patient was discovered to have an ovarian mass. When the patient's surgeon casually said, "We might as well take out your uterus while we're in there," she first panicked and then became severely depressed. As she free-associated to her strange reaction, she said, sobbing, "It would be like losing my mother all over again." She was encouraged to tell her gynecologist that her uterus was important to her, and he agreed not to remove it unless he found an absolute medical indication. She recovered uneventfully.

* * *

A recently menopausal woman who had been advised to have a hysterectomy and salpingo-oophorectomy panicked about the loss of her "childbearing equipment." Associations were to her dying mother and to her fantasy that loss of her reproductive organs would make her weaker and prone to die just like her mother.

For this woman, her uterus represented the internalization of her mother, and, therefore, it made her feel safe and invulnerable, until she was threatened with its loss. We have seen several other women in consultation who, in effect, were seeking permission to keep their uterus even when pregnancy was not contemplated or no longer possible. It was clear in these cases that the uterus symbolized union with their mothers and safety.

Menopausal Exacerbation of Earlier Hysterectomy

A 50-year-old patient sought treatment for panic attacks that had begun to recur despite addiction to large doses of a benzodiazepine with the onset of menopause. (She had had a hysterectomy 14 years earlier without removal of her ovaries.) She was withdrawing from the benzodiazepine during therapy.

Her history was as follows. She had been adopted and was always consciously grateful for this. Dreams and associations around menopause related to her birth mother. During the rocky period of treatment, the patient reminded the therapist repeatedly that she, the patient, had no uterus so that hormones would be safe and that low doses would not cause breakthrough bleeding.

Recently, she has had some return of her anxiety. Her associations are to the increasing frailty of her very aged adoptive mother, who lives with her. The patient can recognize that she is feeling sad and that depression had always been part of her panic attacks. She was always a perfect child who was very fearful of losing her adoptive mother. She has had the same adaptation to her husband and to physicians, agreeing to unwanted surgery and medications. She is afraid to alienate or lose her caregivers.

It is necessary in the course of the treatment of women whether preoperatively or immediately postoperatively many times thereafter to keep in mind the symbolic meaning of genital surgery. Our patients are unconscious of the threat of the symbolic loss of the nurturing mother. It is our task to help them become conscious of this and to develop other strategies which perpetuate a positive identification with a good mother. Once this is accomplished, the reaction to surgery, even when it is mutilating or performed for a potentially lifesaving indication, can be assimilated without profound psychiatric morbidity.

References

1. Budoff PW: Zomepirac sodium in the treatment of primary dysmenorrhea. N Engl J Med 307:714–719, 1982
2. Ylikor Kala O, Dawood MY: New concepts in dysmenorrhea. Am J Obstet Gynecol 130:833–847, 1978

3. Gitlin MJ, Pasnau RO: Psychiatric syndromes linked to reproductive function in women: a review of current knowledge. Am J Psychiatry 146:1413–1422, 1989
4. Green R, Dalton R: Premenstrual syndrome. BMJ 1:1007–1014, 1953
5. Reid RL, Yen SS: Premenstrual syndrome. Am J Obstet Gynecol 139:85–104, 1981
6. Abraham G: Premenstrual tension, in Current Problems in Obstetrics and Gynecology. Chicago, IL, Year Book Medical, 1981, pp 1–39
7. American Psychiatric Association: Diagnostic and Statistical Manual of Mental Disorders, 3rd Edition, Revised. Washington, DC, American Psychiatric Association, 1987
8. Yankauskas E: Primary female syndromes: an update. N Y State J Med, 90 (June):105–301, 1990
9. Keye WR, Hammond DC, Strong C: Medical and psychologic characteristics of women presenting with menstrual symptoms. Obstet Gynecol 68:634–637, 1986
10. London RS, Murphy L, Ktlowski KE, et al: Efficacy of alpha-tocopherol in the treatment of premenstrual syndrome. J Reprod Med 32:400–404, 1987
11. Prior J: Conditioning exercise and premenstrual symptoms. J Reprod Med 32:423–427, 1987
12. Wurthman J: Report presented to the American Society for Psychosomatics in Obstetrics and Gynecology. Clinical Psychiatry News, No 18, 1990, p 16
13. Stone AB: Report at the Annual Meeting of the American Psychiatric Association. Clinical Psychiatry News, No 18, 1990, p 16
14. Frank E, Anderson C, Rubinstein D: Frequency of sexual dysfunction in normal couples. N Engl J Med 299:111–115, 1978
15. Kaplan HS: Disorders of Sexual Desire. New York, Brunner/Mazel, 1979
16. Imboden JP, Urbaitis JC: Practical Psychiatry in Medicine. New York, Appleton-Century-Crofts, 1978
17. Freud S: Female sexuality (1931), in The Standard Edition of the Complete Psychological Works of Sigmund Freud, Vol 21. Translated and edited by Strachey J. London, Hogarth Press, 1961, pp 221–243
18. Freud S: Femininity (1933), in The Standard Edition of the Complete Psychological Works of Sigmund Freud, Vol 22. Translated and edited by Strachey J. London, Hogarth Press, 1964, pp 112–135
19. Masters WH, Johnson JE: Human Sexual Inadequacy. Boston, MA, Little, Brown, 1970
20. Sherffy M: The evolution and nature of female sexuality in relation to psychoanalytic theory. J Am Psychoanal Assoc 14:28–128, 1966

21. Sherffy M: The Nature and Evolution of Female Sexuality. New York, Random/Village, 1973
22. Bernstein AE, Warner GM: Women Treating Women. New York, International Universities Press, 1984b
23. Galenson E, Roiphe H: Some suggested revisions concerning early female development. J Am Psychoanal Assoc 24(suppl):29–57, 1976
24. Becker J: Level of post assault sexual function in post assault and incest victims. Arch Sex Behav 15:37–49, 1986
25. Sherkow SP: Evaluation and diagnosis of sexual abuse of little girls. J Am Psychoanal Assoc 38:347–369, 1990b
26. Schreiner-Engel P: Differential diagnosis of hypoactive sexual desire: reported to the American Society of Psychosomatics in Obstetrics and Gynecology. Clinical Psychiatry News, No 18, 1990, p 30
27. LaFarge L: Emptiness as defense in severe regressive states. J Am Psychoanal Assoc 37:965–995, 1989
28. Isselbacher KJ, Adams RD, Braunwald E, et al: Harrison's Principles of Internal Medicine, 9th Edition, Vol 1. New York, McGraw-Hill, 1980
29. Guinan ME, Hardy A: Epidemiology of AIDS in women in the United States, 1981–1986. JAMA 257:2039–2042, 1987
30. Coolfront report: a PHS plan for prevention and control of AIDS and the AIDS virus. Public Health Rep 101:34–38, 1986
31. Working Group on HIV Testing of Pregnant Women and the Newborn. JAMA 264:2416, 1990
32. Fourcroy J (chairperson): Presentation on the "female condom" at the annual meeting of the American Medical Women's Association, Philadelphia, PA, November 1990
33. Kertzner R: The psychiatric aspects of AIDS and HIV infection. Unpublished manuscript, Psychiatric Medicine, Columbia University College of Physicians and Surgeons, January 1989
34. Tucker S: The role of psychiatry: evaluation and treatment of altered mental status in persons with AIDS, in What to Do About AIDS: Physicians and Health Professionals Discuss the Issues. Edited by McKusichl S. Berkeley, CA, University of California Press, 1986, pp 45–50
35. Cohen SI: Voodoo death, the stress response, and AIDS, in Psychological, Neuropsychiatric, and Substance Abuse Aspects of AIDS (Advances in Biochemical Psychopharmacology, Vol 44). Edited by Bridge TP, Mirsky AF, Goodwin FK. New York, Raven, 1988, pp 95–109
36. Cousins N: Anatomy of an Illness. New York, WW Norton, 1979
37. Cousins N: The Healing Heart. New York, WW Norton, 1983

38. Fullilove MT, Fullilove RE: Intersecting epidemics: black crack use and sexually transmitted disease. J Am Med Wom Assoc 44:146–153, 1989
39. Fullilove MT, Fullilove RE, Haynes K, et al: Black women and AIDS prevention: a view towards understanding the gender roles. Journal of Sex Research 27:47–64, 1990
40. Fullilove RE, Fullilove MT, Bowser BP, et al: Risk of sexually transmitted disease among black adolescent crack users in Oakland and San Francisco, California. JAMA 263:851–856, 1991
41. Lalos A, Lalos O, Jacobson L, et al: A psychosocial characterization of infertile couples before surgical treatment of the female. Journal of Psychosomatic Obstetrics and Gynaecology 4:83–93, 1985
42. Bydlowski M, Dagan-Lintzer M: A psychomedical approach to infertility: "suffering from sterility." Journal of Psychosomatic Obstetrics and Gynaecology 9:139–151, 1988
43. Karahanasoglu A, Barglow P, Grow G: Psychological aspects of infertility. J Reprod Med 9:241–247, 1972
44. Kraft AD, Palombo J, Mitchell D, et al: The psychological dimensions of infertility. Am J Orthopsychiatry 50:618–628, 1980
45. Pennington G, Atlay R: Some surprising results in the investigation of the infertile woman. Journal of Obstetrics and Gynaecology of the British Commonwealth 79:651–653, 1972
46. Wasser S, Isembert D: Reproductive failure among women: pathology or adaptation? Journal of Psychosomatic Obstetrics and Gynaecology 5:153–176, 1986
47. Menninger KA: Emotional factors in organic gynecological conditions. Bull Menninger Clin 7:47-55, 1943
48. Sandler B: Infertility of emotional origin. Journal of Obstetrics and Gynaecology of the British Commonwealth 68:809–815, 1961
49. Benedek T: Infertility is a psychosomatic defense. Fertil Steril 3:527–533, 1952
50. Rubenstein B: An emotional factor in infertility. Fertil Steril 2:80–86, 1951
51. Hall E: The gynaecologist and artificial reproduction. Journal of Psychosomatic Obstetrics and Gynaecology 4:317–320, 1985
52. Sarrel P, DeCherney M: Psychotherapeutic intervention for treatment of couples with secondary infertility. Fertil Steril 43:897–903, 1985
53. Bresnick E, Taymor M: The role of counseling. Fertil Steril 32:154, 1979
54. Downey J, Yingling M, McKinney M, et al: Mood disorders, psychiatric symptoms and distress in women presenting for infertility evaluation. Fertil Steril 52:425–432, 1989

55. Mahlstedt P: The psychological component of infertility. Fertil Steril 43:335–346, 1985
56. Seibel M, Taymor M: Emotional aspects of infertility. Fertil Steril 37:137–141, 1982
57. Platt J, Ficher I, Silver M: Infertile couples: personality traits and self-ideal concept discrepancies. Fertil Steril 24:972–976, 1973
58. Denber H: Psychiatric aspects of infertility. J Reprod Med 20:23–29, 1978
59. Kipper D, Zigler-Shani Z, Sern D: Psychogenic infertility, neuroticism and the female role: a methodological inquiry. J Psychosomat Res 221:353–358, 1977
60. Mai FM, Munday RN, Rump EE: Psychiatric interview comparisons between infertile and fertile couples. Psychosom Med 34:431–440, 1972
61. Menning BE: Infertility: A Guide for Childless Couples. Englewood Cliffs, NJ, Prentice-Hall, 1977
62. Daniluk J: Infertility: intrapersonal and interpersonal impact. Fertil Steril 49:982, 1988
63. Eck Menning B: The emotional needs of infertile couples. Fertil Steril 34:313–319, 1980
64. Jessner L, Welgern E, Farg J: The development of parental attitudes during pregnancy, in Parenthood. Edited by Anthony EJ, Benedek T. Boston, MA, Little, Brown, 1986, pp 209–245
65. McGuire D: Psychological management of infertile women. Postgrad Med 57:173, 1975
66. Berger D: The role of the psychiatrist in a reproductive biology clinic. Fertil Steril 28:41, 1977
67. Walker H: Sexual problems and infertility. Psychosomatics 19:477–484, 1978
68. Lazare C: The adoptive parents' experience, in Infertility: Medical, Emotional, and Social Considerations. Edited by Mazor M, Simons H. New York, Human Sciences Press, 1984, p 108
69. Andrews R: Adoption: the resolution of infertility. Fertil Steril 21:73–76, 1970
70. Forrest JD, Sullivan E, Tietze C: Abortion in the United States. Fam Plann Perspect 11:329–341, 1979
71. Henshaw S, O'Reilly R: Characteristics of abortion patients in the United States, 1979–80. Fam Plann Perspect 15:5–16, 1983
72. Adler NE, David HP, Major BN, et al: Psychological responses after abortion. Science 248:41–44, 1990
73. Ashton J: The psychosocial outcome of induced abortion. Br J Obstet Gynaecol 87:1115–1122, 1980

74. Major B, Mueller P, Hildebrandt K: Attributions, expectations, and coping with abortion. J Pers Soc Psychol 48:585–599, 1985
75. Adler NE: Emotional responses of women following therapeutic abortion. Am J Orthopsychiatry 45:446–454, 1975
76. Belsey EM, Greer HS, Lal S, et al: Predictive factors in emotional response to abortion: King's termination study IV. Soc Sci Med 11:71–82, 1977
77. Bracken MB, Klerman LV, Bracken M: Coping with pregnancy resolution among never-married women. Am J Orthopsychiatry 48:320–334, 1978
78. Shusterman LR: Predicting the psychological consequences of abortion. Soc Sci Med 13A:683–689, 1979
79. Whittington HG: Evaluation of therapeutic abortion as an element of preventive psychiatry. Am J Psychiatry 126:1224–1229, 1970
80. Ford C, Castelnuovo-Teddesco P, Long K: Abortion: is it a therapeutic procedure in psychiatry? JAMA 218:1173–1178, 1971
81. Niswander K, Patterson R: Psychologic response to therapeutic abortion: subjective patient response. Obstet Gynecol 29:702–706, 1967
82. Simon NM, Senturia AG, Rothman D: Psychiatric illness following therapeutic abortion. Am J Psychiatry 124:59–65[97–103], 1967
83. Moseley DT, Follingstad DR, Harley H, et al: Psychological factors that predict reaction to abortion. J Clin Psychol 37:276–279, 1981
84. Patt SL, Rappaport RG, Barglow P: Follow-up of therapeutic abortion. Arch Gen Psychiatry 20:408–414, 1969
85. Payne EC, Kravitz AK, Notman MT, et al: Outcome following therapeutic abortion. Arch Gen Psychiatry 33:725–733, 1976
86. Friedman CM, Greenspan R, Mittleman F: The decision-making process and the outcome of therapeutic abortion. Am J Psychiatry 131:1332–1337, 1974
87. Freeman E, Rickels K, Huggins G, et al: Emotional disorder patterns among women having first or repeat abortions. Obstet Gynecol 55:630–636, 1980
88. Niemela P, Lechtinen P, Rauramo L, et al: The first abortion and the last: a study of the personality factors underlying repeated failure of contraception. Int J Gynaecol Obstet 19:193–200, 1981
89. Franco KN, Tamburrio MB, Campbell NS, et al: Psychological profile of dysphoric women post abortion. J Am Med Wom Assoc 44:113–119, 1989
90. Mueller P, Major B: Self-blame, self-efficacy, and adjustment to abortion. J Pers Soc Psychol 57:1059–1068, 1989

91. Fisch RZ, Tadmor O: Iatrogenic post-traumatic stress disorder. Lancet, December 9, No 8676, 1989, p 1397
92. Alfonso DD, Domino G: Post partum depression: a review. Birth 11:231–235, 1984
93. Cox JL, Connor Y, Kendell RE: Prospective study of the psychiatric disorders of childbirth. Br J Psychiatry 140:111–117, 1982
94. Hopkins J, Marcus N, Campbell S: Post partum depression: a critical review. Psychol Bull 95:498–515, 1984
95. Pitt B: "Maternity blues." Br J Psychiatry 122:431–433, 1973
96. Yalom ID, Lunde DT, Moos RH, et al: "Post partum blues" syndrome: a description and related variables. Arch Gen Psychiatry 18:16–27, 1968
97. Harding JJ: Postpartum psychiatric disorders: a review. Compr Psychiatry 30:109–112, 1989
98. Jamison KR, Wellisch D, Pasnau RO, et al. Psychosocial aspects of mastectomy, I: the woman's perspective. Am J Psychiatry 135:432–436, 1978
99. Kumar R, Robson KM: A prospective study of emotional disorders in childbearing women. Br J Psychiatry 144:35–47, 1984
100. Pitt B: "Atypical" depression following childbirth. Br J Psychiatry 114:1325–1335, 1968
101. O'Hara MW: Social support, life events, and depression during pregnancy and the puerperium. Arch Gen Psychiatry 43:569–573, 1986
102. Paykel ES, Emms EM, Fletcher J, et al: Life events and social support in puerperal depression. Br J Psychiatry 136:339–346, 1980
103. Garvey MJ, Tollefson GD: Post partum depression. J Reprod Med 29:113–116, 1984
104. Kendell RE: Emotional and physical factors in the genesis of puerperal mental disorders. J Psychosom Res 29:3–11, 1985
105. Dean C, Kendell RE: The symptomatology of puerperal illnesses. Br J Psychiatry 139:128–133, 1981
106. Meltzer ES, Kumar R: Puerperal mental illness, clinical features and classification: a study of 142 mother-and-baby admissions. Br J Psychiatry 147:647–654, 1985
107. Oates MR: The treatment of psychiatric disorders in pregnancy and the puerperium. Clin Obstet Gynecol 13:385–395, 1986
108. Cox J: Childbirth as a life event: sociocultural aspects of postnatal depression. Acta Psychiatr Scand Suppl 78 (suppl 344):75–83, 1988
109. Asch S: Crib deaths; their possible relationship to post partum depression and infanticide. Journal of the Mount Sinai Hospital 35:214–220, 1968
110. Cherland E, Matthews PC: Attempted murder of a newborn: a case history. Can J Psychiatry 34:337–339, 1989

111. Resnick PJ: Murder of the newborn: a psychiatric review of neonaticide. Am J Psychiatry 126:1414–1420, 1970
112. D'Orbán PT: Women who kill their children. Br J Psychiatry 134:560–571, 1979
113. Scott PD: Parents who kill their children. Med Sci Law 13:120–126, 1973
114. Egginton J: From Cradle to Grave: The Short Lives and Strange Deaths of Marybeth Tinning's Nine Children. New York, William Morrow, 1989
115. Levan I: Mortality and psychopathology following the death of an adult child: an epidemiologic review. Isr J Psychiatry Relat Sci 119:23–38, 1982
116. Siegel B: A Death in White Bear Lake. New York, Bantam Books, 1990
117. Wilkins AJ: Attempted infanticide. Br J Psychiatry 146:206–208, 1985
118. Post SG: History, infanticide and imperiled newborns. Hastings Cent Rep 18:14–17, 1988
119. Clayton PJ: Bereavement and its management, in Handbook of Affective Disorders. Edited by Paykel ES. New York, Guilford, 1982, pp 403–415
120. Clayton PJ, Desmarais L, Winokur G: A study of normal bereavement. Am J Psychiatry 125:168–178, 1968
121. Sanders HS: A comparison of adult bereavement in the death of a spouse, child and parent. Omega 10:303–322, 1979–1980
122. Schwab JJ, Chalmers J, Conroy S, et al: Studies in grief: a preliminary report, in Bereavement: Its Psychosocial Aspects. Edited by Schoenberg B, Gerber I, Wiener A, et al. New York, Columbia University Press, 1975, pp 78–91
123. Shanfield SB, Swain BJ: Death of adult children in traffic accidents. J Nerv Ment Dis 172:533–538, 1984
124. Shanfield SB, Benjamin GAH, Swain BJ: Parents' reactions to the death of an adult child from cancer. Am J Psychiatry 141:1092–1094, 1984
125. Singh HB, Raphael B: Post-disaster morbidity of the bereaved: a possible role for preventive psychiatry. J Nerv Ment Dis 169:203–212, 1981
126. Osterweiss M, Solomon F, Green M (eds): Bereavement: Reaction, Consequences, and Care. Report by the Committee for the Study of Health Consequences of the Others of Bereavement, Institute of Medicine, National Academy of Sciences. Washington, DC, National Academy Press, 1988
127. Fish WC, Whitney SM: Challenging conventional wisdom about parental bereavement. Forum for Death Education and Counsel Newsletter, No 6, 1983, p 4
128. Rando TA: An investigation of grief and adaptation in parents whose children have died from cancer. J Ped Psychol 8:3–20, 1983

129. Schwartz AM: Comments in section on "The Parents," in Understanding Bereavement and Grief. Edited by Linzer N. New York, Yeshiva University Press, 1977, pp 193–196
130. Worden JW: Grief Counseling and Grief Therapy: A Handbook for the Mental Health Practitioner. New York, Springer, 1982
131. Beckwirth JB: The sudden infant death syndrome (DHEW Publ No HSA 75-5137). Washington, DC, U.S. Government Printing Office, 1975
132. Taylor J, Defrain J, Ernst L: Sudden infant death syndrome, in Parental Loss of a Child. Edited by Rando TA. Champaign, IL, Research Press Co, 1986, pp 159–180
133. Parkes CM, Weiss RS: Recovery From Bereavement. New York, Basic Books, 1983
134. Schiff H: The Bereaved Parent. New York, Crown Publishers, 1977
135. Gunther J: Death Be Not Proud. New York, Harper & Row, 1949
136. Chance S: Left for dead. Psychiatric Times, January 1991, pp 26–27
137. Gorer G: Death, Grief and Mourning. New York, Doubleday, 1965, pp 121–122
138. Fish WC: Differences in grief intensity in bereaved parents, in Parental Loss of a Child. Edited by Rando TA. Champaign, IL, Research Press Co, 1986, pp 415–428
139. Rosenblatt PC: Bitter, Bitter Tears: Nineteenth-Century Diarists and Twentieth-Century Grief Theorists. Minneapolis, MN, University of Minnesota Press, 1983
140. Gurdus L: The Death Train. New York, National Council on Art in Jewish Life, 1978
141. Deutsch H: The Psychology of Women, a Psychoanalytic Interpretation, Vol 1. New York, Grune & Stratton, 1944
142. Deutsch H: The Psychology of Women, a Psychoanalytic Interpretation, Vol 2: Motherhood. New York, Grune & Stratton, 1945
143. Kestenberg JS: Psychoanalytic Studies in Development. New York, Jason Aronson, 1978
144. Breast cancer. P & S Journal, Fall 1989, p 9

Chapter 6

Abuse of Women

In this chapter we discuss the psychodynamic treatment of abused women. This topic covers a wide continuum of related behaviors, including childhood sexual abuse, sexual harassment, rape, battering, and sexual exploitation by therapists and other professionals.

Childhood sexual abuse is defined as "sexual contact that occurs between children and much older persons" and "sexual contact that occurs to a child as a result of force, threat, deceit, while unconscious or through exploitation of an authority relationship no matter what the age of the partner" (Finkelhor and Hotaling 1984,[1] p. 31). *Incest* is a special type of child sexual abuse in which sexual contact occurs between a child and a blood relative or kin (e.g., father, stepfather, uncle, grandfather, sibling, cousin, in-law). Close family friends, mothers' boyfriends, and close family members' lovers may also be included. Most incest involves multiple sexual acts occurring over a period of months to many years. These activities usually begin under the guise of affection, education, or play, and escalate in terms of the intensity of the sexual activity and the amount of threat or coercion employed. Violence may occur but not as often as in adult rapes.

Battering is defined as significant physical aggression directed toward women by men in the context of intimate relationships such as dating, engagement, cohabitation, marriage, divorce, and separation. Victims of this aggression have been called "battered women." The special terms *marital abuse*, *spousal abuse*, or *wife battering* are applied when the couple involved in the battering relationship are either legally married or cohabiting and sexually intimate. *Rape*, which is often considered the endpoint of sexual victimization, involves the physical penetration of the victim and frequently includes exposure to extreme humiliation and degradation, threats to life, and physical assault and injury. In *attempted rape*, the victim is exposed to force or threats of force, including life threats, but no intercourse is achieved. *Sexual harassment* includes a continuum of unwelcome sexual behaviors, ranging from sexual jokes and innuendos to rape, that are perpetrated on the victim via the abuse of the offender's power and authority over the victim's employment or school performance and status. *Sexual exploitation* in professional relationships involves consensual or nonconsensual sexual activity between a woman and man with whom she has a fiduciary relationship. It is the adult counterpart to childhood sexual abuse.

The relationship between childhood sexual abuse and the various forms of adult victimization of women is significant. Women who had been sexually abused as children are at high risk for victimization as adults via mechanisms that will be described in the first section of this chapter. They are also at risk for developing more severe symptomatology in response to adult abuse. In fact, the derepression of memories of childhood abuse is often triggered by adult traumas.

The area of abuse is one in which cultural and societal factors are particularly important. Lack of support for, and even blaming of, the victim, a general lack of support for the complicated multiple roles of women, an indifferent legal system—all complicate and exacerbate a woman's reaction to abuse.

Childhood Sexual Abuse

Bachmann et al. (1988[2]) reported that 15% to 38% of adults had been sexually abused as children. The proportion of women is probably significantly higher. Although Freud (1909b/1955[3]) initially proposed the *seduction theory*, papers about incest are rare in the psychoanalytic literature (Bender and Blau 1937[4]; Bernstein 1989[5]; Ferenczi 1933/1955[6]; Katan 1973[7]; Margolis 1977,[8] 1984[9]; O'Brien 1987[10]; Rascovsky and Rascovsky 1950[11]; Shengold 1980[12]; Steele 1986[13]). Rather, it has been left to psychiatrists, psychologists, social workers, and the victims themselves to describe the experience and treatment of these individuals (Cole 1985[14]; Conte and Schuerman 1987[15]; Donaldson and Gardner 1985[16]; Fraser 1987[17]; Gomes-Schwartz et al. 1985[18]; Goodwin 1988[19]; Herman 1981[20]; Herman et al. 1986[21]; Kluft 1985[22]; Lindberg and Distad 1985[23]; Livingston 1987[24]; Rosenfeld et al. 1977[25]; Wahl 1960[26]).

In this section, data on the effects of incest on the adult woman survivor, as culled from many sources, are organized in the following way. First, we present the symptom clusters that result in damaging behaviors and the symptoms that may be ameliorated by treatments that are not psychodynamic. We then present the symptoms that result from ego function disruption and that require psychodynamic intervention aimed toward reorganization of the personality, integration of the incest experience, and freeing of stunted ego growth.

The least functional defenses against incest trauma include severe dissociation; depression, often accompanied by suicidal attempts and self-mutilation; anxiety leading to alcohol/drug abuse (resulting in an altered state of consciousness) and prostitution; and sadism and identification with the aggressor, especially as they apply to child abuse (Ganzarain and Buchele 1988[27]; Jehu 1988[28]; Kluft et al. 1985[29]; Russell 1986[30]).

Self-help groups and behavioral modification programs ameliorate symptomatic expression of the trauma (Bass and Davis 1988[31]; Persons and Burns 1985[32]). Jehu (1988[28]) has examined the effect of behavioral modification techniques regarding issues of shame, humiliation, self-blame, and self-esteem regulation and reports good results on the basis of replicable psychological testing of a large sample of patients. Bass and Davis (1988[31]) have documented patient histories that illustrate significant adaptational improvement. Certainly self-help groups are more available and affordable and may be the only possible modalities for some survivors. They may, however, become problematic for patients who are already in psychodynamic treatment when these modalities are used as a resistance in defensive splitting. Group therapy for survivors is a better alternative, allowing for collaboration between individual and group therapist regarding problematic defenses and transferences as well as an opportunity for the patient to relieve within the group her sense of isolation, shame, and invalidation.

Incest is one trauma that may cause *posttraumatic stress disorder*. This disorder may occur acutely either during spontaneous derepression or in the course of treatment. Posttraumatic stress disorder may also be chronic. It consists of the following elements:

1. Recurrent and intrusive recollection of the traumatic events
2. Recurrent distressing dreams, nightmares, or night terrors
3. Sudden acting or feeling as if the event were recurring
4. Intense psychological distress in reaction to exposure to events that symbolize or resemble aspects of the trauma
5. Avoidance of thoughts or feelings associated with the trauma and of situations that cause recollections of the trauma, and an inability to recall an important aspect of the trauma

Some individuals experience a generalized sensation of numbness to the environment that reflects the attempt during the trauma to modulate the stimulus input by raising the stimulus barrier (Horowitz 1976[33]). Incest is a repetitive trauma, and the prolongation of numbing is an attempt by the mental apparatus to keep the individual from fully perceiving the assault.

Another reparative attempt that miscarries in terms of later adaptation is the development of *multiple personality disorder* (Coons 1986[34]; Spiegel 1984[35]). Other patients have difficulty falling or staying asleep. These patients may experience affective outbursts of anger or tears, or be generally irritable. They often have trouble concentrating and making decisions, and they may be hypervigilant. They sometimes have flashbacks or untoward startle responses (Ochberg 1988[36]; Ulman and Brothers 1988[37]; Van der Kolk 1987[38]).

Often posttraumatic stress disorder is accompanied by the physiology of panic attack (Ganzarain and Buchele 1988[27]). This results from massive sympathetic nervous system discharge and includes a variety of physical symptoms such as tachycardia (i.e., rapid heart rate); arrhythmia (i.e., palpitations); dyspnea (i.e., shortness of breath); smothering sensation; dizziness; unsteadiness; faintness (or the feeling of faintness); shaking and trembling; sweating; choking; chest, abdominal, or pelvic pain or distress; paresthesia (i.e., numbness or tingling of the extremities); flushes or chills; fear of dying; or fear of going crazy or of doing something uncontrollable (Jehu et al. 1987[39]; Spiegel 1984[35]). In our experience, patients may require pharmacological treatment with antidepressants or antianxiety agents for relief of the intolerable "sympathetic storm."

Other types of physical symptoms also occur secondary to incest trauma. Ganzarain and Buchele (1988[27]) have discussed hypochondriacal anxiety secondary to mind-body splitting. They describe patients with a quasi-delusional system in which the persecution seems to come from a body organ or a body function. In less fragmented patients, somatic symptoms related to the gastrointestinal, urogenital, respiratory, and musculoskeletal systems occur. At certain times no discernible organic pathology can be found. At other times there is a predisposition to recurrent vaginitis, urethritis, bronchitis, gastroenteritis, and spinal disk syndromes. Patients with this predisposition have demonstrable organic pathology, often recurrent and sometimes predictable, in the course of derepression or transference somatic displacements.

Special aspects of the incest trauma include secret keeping (Rush 1980[40]) and feelings of betrayal and deprivation. Some patients will have to mourn for a childhood that never was—for a time of innocence to which they were entitled but was denied them. There is also a disruption in the ego and destruction of the sense of self with concomitant loss of boundaries (Shengold 1979,[41] 1989[42]; Ulman and Brothers 1988[37]).

If incest trauma severely disrupts or interrupts ego functioning (Bernstein 1990[43]; Sherkow 1990a[44]), then residential containment, intermittent or long-term hospitalization, and/or other ancillary modalities may be necessary. We contend that psychodynamic treatment should be instituted in order to effect structural and lasting change. Not only does this modality afford the opportunity for the relief of symptoms and the elimination of less adaptive defenses, but it also allows for the reorganization of the psyche in order to improve the patient's ability to cope with adaptational changes required throughout the life cycle. In each succeeding chapter of this book, we have referred to the obstacles in negotiating adaptational tasks, from adolescence to old age, for the untreated incest victim. We believe that psychodynamic treatment can effect the following:

1. Improve cognitive functioning, self-esteem regulation, and the capacity for self-actualization
2. Allow for committed partnerships and better sexual and reproductive functioning
3. Lead to the experience of satisfaction in career, motherhood, or the combination of both
4. Free the ego to evolve more adaptive coping strategies to deal with later life issues (i.e., menopause, grandmotherhood, widowhood, and aging)

Comfortable and realistic adaptation to these developmental tasks may be impossible for untreated incest survivors. Many patients enter treatment unaware of having been victims. They manifest specific ego deficits. When memories are recovered, they are accompanied by panic and dissociative reactions. The patient's transferences provoke strong countertransference reactions. The range of psychopathology extends from suicidal behavior and self-mutilation to psychosis.

In 1985, the American Psychoanalytic Association held a panel to discuss the constellation of symptoms specific to adult victims of childhood sexual abuse. Among the symptoms identified were the following:

1. Depressive affect
2. Defective sense of ownership or control of self
3. Cognitive deficits
4. An internal gravely disturbed libidinal object (i.e., abuser)
5. Somatizations
6. Doubting of reality, with cognitive confusion
7. Panic associated with recovery of the memories
8. Sleep disorder
9. Identification with the aggressor
10. Compromise of the observing ego

11. Difficulty in establishing basic trust
12. The need for a real relationship with the therapist
13. A transference wish to be seduced.

The last two are major resistances. Depersonalization and derealization can be added to this constellation.

The panel also discussed the role of abandonment, usually by a dysfunctional mother, and the role of confusion of reality in order cognitive areas that is found in some of the abused children. Patients who have been more severely damaged may present with multiple personality disorder, severe borderline personality traits, and, occasionally, acute psychosis. They may require prolonged hospitalization or outpatient care that provides for immediate emergency hospitalization. They also may be unable to tolerate one-to-one care outside of a supportive milieu. These patients may have trouble limiting or stopping substance abuse and handling stress and panic symptoms, thus necessitating the use of ancillary services to sustain the psychodynamic therapy.

The recovery of incestuous and often sadistic material can lead to severe affective storms. During these periods the patients may experience their therapists as abusing and sadistic transference objects. Patients may act out sadistically against their therapists or themselves as manifested in suicide attempts and acts of self-mutilation. Dangerous risk-taking behavior is not uncommon. Severe dissociative reactions may result in injury because of inattention, confusion, and abusive reenactment. These patients may also break off psychodynamic treatment in the midst of a negative transference storm. This may be handled by milieu containment or by the utilization of a treatment team, a supportive consultant, or group therapy.

The countertransference reactions that serve as warning signals are 1) the tendency, at first, to deny the reality of the patient's experiences, 2) the tendency, later, to get caught up in the frightening aspects of the reality endured by the patient, and 3) the experience of the panic as contagious and the wish to stop the painful abreaction. In the case of more seriously ill patients, the countertransference reactions include fear, helplessness, anger, dread, and horror regarding sadistic abuse and torture. Countertransference affects of disgust and shame can occur around episodes of reenactment that are perverse and degrading.

Guilt may be a countertransference reaction to privileged voyeurism. Therapists are also subject to survivor guilt. Countertransference sexualization of the therapeutic relationship may occur. Therapists often endure the feeling of being tortured by the patient because of the patient's successful projective identification. In the midst of a tumultuous countertransference the therapist must be capable of reasonable limit setting, even in periods when the therapeutic alliance seems temporarily lost. It is when the patient cannot or will not listen and loses reality testing that the therapist, not out of a punitive countertransference but as a protective container, may have to implement day programs, hospitalization, residential treatment, or other forms of containment.

In order to demonstrate how the symptom complexes, pathological defenses, and the distortions in ego development that we have described can be treated with psychodynamic psychotherapy, we discuss below cases of incest in both highly functioning and hospitalized patients.

Severe and Prolonged Abuse by Multiple Perpetrators

The patient, a 36-year-old college-educated, married mother of two, worked part time in her husband's furniture business. She was hospitalized for the first time for severe agoraphobia, panic attacks, and depression with escalating suicidal ideation. During her hospitalization, she requested that the consultant find her a new psychotherapist, stating that she had no alliance with her outpatient psychotherapist, with whom she had been trying to work for 3 months prior to the admission. She had no prior psychiatric hospitalizations, although she had attempted "counseling" for several months but discontinued this after she and her counselor shared a hospital room for an appendectomy. After the birth of her second daughter, the patient became agitated and requested counseling but was chastised and told to "settle down and go home with her baby."

The patient, whose mother and father were both severely alcoholic, was often at home alone with her mother while her father was absent from the household for long periods of time engaged in various types of illegal businesses. The patient remembered violent marital quarrels. She stated that her mother was often inebriated and unpleasant. Thus, the patient had to assume responsibility for the care of both her mother and her asthmatic sister. The patient had no memory of events before the age of 10. She became confused about her age when her sister was born: "I can't remember if I was 10 or 11. I seem to have lost a year."

Initially the patient engaged in an angry struggle with the staff and her husband regarding discharge from the hospital, despite marital instability and no aftercare plan. She approached her first therapy session in such an abusive and chaotic manner that her new therapist was prompted to shout above her harangue, "Shut up, you are going to wreck this relationship before it can help you." She calmed herself, agreed to attend sessions regularly, and remarked later that no one had ever told her to do anything before. When asked if, because of her therapist's scheduled maternity leave in 7 months, she would prefer another therapist, the patient replied that it was reassuring to know there would be an out and that she was not sure if she would be able to tolerate sitting with anyone forever.

With her individual psychotherapy and couples therapy arranged, as well as a tentative aftercare program and hospital treatment team backup, the patient was discharged. She quarreled with her husband and impulsively fled her home to live briefly with a series of relatives with whom she also quarreled before returning to her home. At home her situation was complicated by the intrusive and abusive presence of her mother and father, who also worked in her husband's business and were involved in the care of her children. In therapy she both acted out and engaged in multiple provocative struggles over the boundaries of therapy, missing appointments, abusing her psychotropic prescription and alcohol, arriving late, arguing about her billing agreement, bingeing, going on spending sprees, and hoarding money for plane fare to Puerto Rico should she "need to escape all this."

During the fourth month of limit-setting treatment, the patient settled in and began to explore her strong sadomasochistic transference with her therapist in light of her relationship with her mother. As the therapist's maternity leave approached, the patient began to express fears that the therapy was becoming too important to her and the loss would be too great. She resumed her acting-out behaviors and became intermittently suicidal. Her original consultant agreed to be her interim therapist, and her treatment team planned a brief hospitalization to help her contain herself and integrate both her new interim therapist and a new administrator who was joining the team. During her interim therapy the patient derepressed memories of her mother's illness while pregnant with the patient's sister and the emergency hospitalization that was necessary when her mother was near term. The patient also explored a brief period in which she, the patient, physically abused her second daughter. She denied or displaced her rage at her therapist's maternity leave but became provocative and abusive upon her therapist's return, requiring several months of settling.

When her mother actually intruded more in a critical, hostile, and humiliating way, the patient began to engage in intense sadomasochistic transference (i.e., punching herself and smashing her belongings) but was able neither to set limits on her mother's intrusiveness nor to explore her transference with her therapist. Another hospitalization seemed inevitable. However, the patient suddenly disengaged from her intense transference reactions and self-abuse and instead began reporting a flooding of memories of her mother's sadistically abusive behavior. Over the course of the next 8 months, the patient remembered incidents in which her mother, often in an alcoholic state, beat her, deprived her of food, banged her fingers with a hammer, put her finger in a light socket, feigned suicide attempts to frighten her, taunted her regarding a birthmark, and forced her to eat in the basement. The patient's mother also expected her to take full responsibility for her sister's care and encouraged her father's frequent beating and scapegoating of her for "provoking her mother's bad mood and being irresponsible." The patient's injuries were either ignored, treated in an emergency room where the doctors were told she was clumsy and had had an accident, or treated as symbols of shame, requiring that she remain home until the bruises disappeared.

During this period of her therapy, the patient became very focused on having her story heard and maintained a positive transference to her therapist. Acting-out behaviors actually diminished. However, her anxiety and phobic symptoms intermittently escalated, and she developed a severe sleep disorder, necessitating reevaluation of her psychotropic medications. She also had several dissociative episodes that lasted 3 or 4 hours. She often broke out in hives during her sessions, her ulcers were exacerbated, and she appeared occasionally with "accidental bumps and bruises" replicating her earlier injuries. Occasionally she became terrified that she would be punished for disclosing her trauma and often dreamed of being killed by a monstrous and vicious dog who attacked her through a shattered window. Further work uncovered a malignant splitting of her and her sister, with the patient being perceived as bad and undeserving and her sister being perceived as good but fragile, sick, and both deserving of and requiring extreme care.

Between the ages of 11 and 14, the patient had been left at home alone by her parents during the 1-week family vacations, forbidding her to speak to anyone and telling her that the abandonment was a punishment for her bad behavior. Early in her adolescence, the patient's mother began to make critical and humiliating comments in front of her friends and to fondle her breasts and digitally penetrate her vagina to make sure she had not "done anything bad" when she would return from a date. In order to attempt to contain this behavior, she withdrew from any type of peer relationships, gave up temporarily her plans for college, and, during later college years, withdrew and was mute for a period of 3 months. She also placed herself on a schedule different from that of her mother, staying up all night and sleeping during the day to avoid her.

During the earlier parts of her childhood, the patient attempted to contain her abuse by hiding out in the cellar, storing favorite blankets, books, and toys to comfort herself. She sometimes sat against the cellar door to prevent her mother from coming and assaulting her. Recounting these memories, she was able to sustain her alliance with her therapist and either to discuss negative transferential issues or to split them off onto the leader of her group, with whom she engaged in an enraged struggle and then eventually "fired" by quitting the group.

The patient initially rejected behavior therapy but ultimately was able to utilize some relaxation, mood monitoring, and impulse control techniques successfully. A recurring nightmare continued to terrify her and render her incontinent; in this dream she would find herself suspended in the air with her mother in the midst of swirling mist, sometimes with her therapist present and watching and sometimes not. In the context of exploring this dream and tolerating vacation interruptions in her therapy, the patient's therapeutic alli-

ance deteriorated. During her vacation the patient had attempted to set some limits on her mother by refusing to reveal the family's plans to vacation and maintaining telephone sessions with her therapist. When her mother managed to locate them, the patient responded by riding a dirt bike and falling, fracturing her arm.

During her first week back in therapy, her arm was in a sling and multiple bruises were evident; later, her foot was placed in a cast. She rejected her therapist's concern and rationalized explanations for the injuries, with a devaluing indifference. Enraged when her therapist insisted that she needed hospitalization, the patient engaged in a sadistic struggle before resentfully signing herself in. She then quickly split staff and therapist over the issue of her injuries, appearing calm and in control on the unit and presenting rational explanations for her injuries, which her team felt were credible. In therapy she appeared dissociated and engaged in intense sadomasochistic transference.

Although laughing sardonically when her therapist was stung by a bee and had to leave the session to obtain treatment, the patient called an hour later, contrite and terrified that her therapist had died of anaphylactic shock. Only the therapist's firm resolution that she would not accept the patient for outpatient treatment prevented a premature discharge before a therapeutic alliance was reestablished. The patient clearly took pleasure in the team's devaluing of the therapist's input. Just prior to her discharge, the patient revealed that her injuries were indeed self-induced, remarking to her therapist, "I hated to give you the satisfaction of being right, but I guess you deserved it, you were really trying to help."

Shortly after discharge, the patient began having explosive episodes at home during which she broke dishes, punched walls, and screamed at family members, often shouting, "Why doesn't somebody help me?" During brief rehospitalization she revealed that her mother had been slapping and punching her for several months. She had been unable to set limits or reveal this. With help from her husband and the treatment team, she was able to set some limits on her contacts with her mother and to return home. During the next few months she continued to integrate abusive material and attempted to understand the "mist in space" dream that continued to terrify her. She required rehospitalization secondary to escalating self-abuse in the context of finally regaining the memories associated with her terrifying dream:

At one point during her mother's second pregnancy, her mother was being particularly abusive toward her, and the patient, after sustaining a beating, fled to the cellar. While attempting to chase her, the mother fell on the stairs and called for help. Fearing that her mother was just attempting to lure her out of the cellar, the patient did not respond until close to an hour later when she found her mother unconscious and called an ambulance. The family blamed her for the incident, and she was temporarily sent to live with a series of indifferent and hostile relatives who stated that her mother probably would die. When her mother returned with the new baby, the patient, who was now back at home, went upstairs to greet her mother. Her mother lunged at her daughter, screaming "You almost killed me," and then proceeded to hang her out the second story window while threatening to drop her. Neighbors called the police, and the mother was taken to a psychiatric hospital. Several hours later, her father, enraged at her for "provoking her mother," beat the patient and broke her arm in front of several aunts and uncles who were convened to discuss the mother's situation. No one intervened. Later, an aunt secretly took her to an emergency room, again stating that she had slipped and fallen. The patient was then sent to Chicago to live with a series of relatives without knowing the outcome of her mother's status or whether or not she had survived the fall.

During the next 3 years of her therapy following derepression of these memories, the patient was hospitalized four times for containment in the context of exacerbations in self-abuse, falling asleep while driving her car, and falling asleep at home in the middle of conversations. In this context, she derepressed being raped by her father, and by her mother's lover, at age 5, and finding her mother unconscious from a suicide attempt, being taken to the hospital with her mother and later sent home alone without explanation.

The patient's treatment required constant restructuring due to several persistent and serious problems that involved constant splitting between the behavioral orientation of the inpatient treatment hall and the therapist. One striking example of this involved the patient's derepression of her rape by her mother's lover, during which time she was preoccupied with a strange smell that she later identified as her abuser's after-shave lotion. Her splitting was escalated when a new consultant who was invited by the inpatient team reviewed the case and felt that the patient's abuse history was false and manipulative. The couples and behavior therapists became numb and mute.

The patient's therapist became enraged, insisting on a second consultation or on the patient having to decide between a transfer to a more compatible unit or a switch of therapists. With the help of a second consultant, the therapist was offered a liaison administrator who was both respectful of the therapy but also well integrated into the behavioral unit. The patient was informed that if she wished to stay on the unit with which she was most familiar, she would have to tolerate some misunderstanding of her therapy from time to time. It was really not until the last two hospitalizations that the inpatient team fully integrated the abusive elements of the patient's history. It was clear that she sometimes sadistically enjoyed the devaluation of her therapist's input and also that the splits within the team enabled her to continue to dissociate when she could not tolerate the affect she was experiencing.

A second treatment problem involved the patient's enlisting of her husband in collusion with her denial and flights from the hospital. She initially refused to share information regarding the nature of her therapy and later enlisted her husband's support around imposing financial restraints or not fully investigating insurance possibilities. In this way she managed to control her treatment and restrict herself to brief hospitalizations, often leaving prematurely and breaking off working on the derepression of painful memories. During one hospitalization her insurance ran out during a time when she was still experiencing severe flashbacks. The patient had to be transferred to a general hospital. She enlisted her husband and her new treatment team in discharging her over the weekend without consulting with her primary treatment team. Her entire treatment had to be renegotiated, and she spent close to 6 months integrating the renegotiation as a way of containing and binding the therapy as opposed to abandoning it.

She and her husband also engaged in a sadomasochistic relationship, the existence of which he did not fully reveal to her treatment team until much later. Often the patient's husband would be masochistic, take on full home responsibilities, only to retaliate sadistically by withdrawing from her during her hospitalization and criticizing her for her abandonment of him and her children. The patient in turn would vacillate between, at times, pulling away from her own treatment material in order to totally tend to her husband and family and, at other times, abdicating her family responsibilities. Much later she revealed that her husband occasionally was violent toward her. She re-

quired another year's treatment before she could begin to discuss this with him openly in couples sessions and to set limits on his violence. Further intensive work was involved to enable both members of the marital couple to develop the capacity to maintain any level of intimacy and to set limits on abusive relatives in both the patient's family and her husband's family.

A third problem in the treatment involved repeated reenactment of the sadomasochistic bind. The patient constantly denied the significance of her accidents, repeating the position her parents took regarding her injuries and devaluing the therapist's concern for her. She also constantly threatened to withdraw from the therapy and refused hospitalization at times when her self-abuse was most dangerous, reenacting with the treatment team her traumatic separations from home. She was equally chaotic and unreasonable around arranging her discharge. Ultimately these problems were solved. The patient was told that her therapist had set clear and consistent guidelines regarding what symptoms she needed to take seriously and how she might care reasonably for herself, and that she would now be expected to take responsibility for following those standards. She would now be expected to care for herself and to negotiate safety contracts with her administrator as well as negotiate her hospitalizations, saving her therapy as a place for exploration of her self-abuse. With this structure, the patient was ultimately able to contain her own self-abusive behavior and negotiate transitions in and out of the hospital in a far more reasonable manner. During the last year and a half of her treatment she has remained outside of the hospital. She has had no further accidents or self-abusive episodes. She and her husband have continued to work on obtaining a higher level of intimacy.

She feels now that her memories of the past have provided her with a clear picture of what had happened. She has derepressed further memories while exploring the effects her abuse has had on her self-esteem and on her sense of guilt and overresponsibility on the one hand and her lack of responsibility and respect for other people's needs on the other hand. She has begun to make friends and has permitted the evaluation of her children for psychotherapy. She has begun to function socially and has accepted the chairs of several civic committees. As her own daughters approach adolescence, the patient still remains preoccupied with her mother's sexual abuse but now dreams of a miniature poodle with no teeth who cannot penetrate the window that she has repaired.

Patients, such as the one above, who are more severely ill present a challenge by behaving in a manner that leaves the therapist uncertain of the patients' safety or their ability to remain in the therapy without fleeing. Because their dissociations and splitting are so successful, these patients often look healthier to the inpatient team responsible for their crisis management and are often discharged prematurely before integration of therapeutic material. Unidimensional biological models and insurance pressure for rapid discharge often pose additional countertransference problems. The therapist is embattled not only by the patient and/or the patient's family but also by inpatient teams and insurance companies. Patient containment is difficult to secure, and the patient is aided in fleeing from painful material. This often leaves the therapist isolated and doubtful of his or her own reality testing.

Bernstein (1989[45]) has presented the analysis of two adult women who had been victims of incest in childhood. The analytic transference in each patient will be summarized.

In the patient's first analysis she began as a shy adolescent who eventually began to see the analyst as a good mother who would listen to her and help her clear her life and overcome her considerable cognitive limitations. The patient then began an independent analysis outside of her analytic hours and in parallel to them, and interpreted the analyst's failure to interdict this self-analysis as support for independence, undoing a defensive regression that had compromised her capacity for symbolization. Memories were recovered even as the incest trauma remained split off. The analyst in the countertransference felt like the loom upon which the patient rewove the tapestry of her childhood, in a seamless process, as if the analyst provided the structure upon which cognition could be safely built. Only in the context of a maternal transference could the incest be recovered and mourning for the lost good father be transferred to the analyst.

The second analysis proceeded in a different way. Here the initial maternal transference was withholding, cold, and aloof. When the patient's fear of competitive disapproval was explored, she recalled closeness to her father and rage toward her mother, both of which were analyzable. A flood of physical complaints followed along with dreams revealing resistance to the paternal transference. A real event restored the maternal transference with caretaking responses toward a depressed mother. The patient required surgery and being cared for. This was mutative in terms of her ability to introject an involved maternal figure. Again, it seemed as if the introduction of a caring maternal figure was essential to derepression of incest trauma. It allowed for recovery of physical abuse by the mother after which the patient turned to her father for mothering as well as for oedipal needs that led to incest trauma.

In both analytic patients, repair of ego deficits depended on transference analysis of maternal deprivation before the incest trauma could be derepressed.

Sexual Harassment

Since the 1970s, a growing body of literature has documented the significant presence of sexual harassment in the workplace (Gutek 1985[46]; Klein 1988,[47] 1989a[48]; Neugarten and Shafritz 1980[49]; Roy 1974[50]; Russell 1984[51]; Sandroff 1988[52]; Sanford 1981[53]). Broad spectrum studies (see Gutek 1985[46]; Klein 1988[47]; U.S. Merit Systems Protection Board 1987[54]) have repeatedly demonstrated not only that harassment is common but also that the victims are predominantly women. Klein (1989a[48]), in reviewing multiple public sector surveys and proprietary studies for private corporations in the United States, noted that harassment incidence rates ranged from 15% to 21% annually for women, compared with 5% to 7% for men. Large-scale research on federal government employees conducted in 1981 and repeated in 1987 revealed similar proportional rates: about 42% for women compared with 14% for men over a 2-year period (U.S. Merit Systems Protection Board 1987[54]).

In colleges, reports of sexual harassment have ranged from 20% to 30% for female students (Hughes and Sandler 1986[55]). An unpublished survey by (Klein 1989b[56]) encompassing all women in a university system yielded annual rates of harassment at 40% for undergraduates, 28% for graduate students, 6% for faculty, and 13% for staff. Data from specialized studies of female court employees (Klein 1989a[48]) and female medical students and physicians (Lenhart et al. 1991[57]) in Massachusetts further validate high incidence of sexual harassment.

Despite predictions that the rates of sexual harassment would diminish as more women entered the workplace, incidence rates have, in fact, remained rather stable, even with the massive influx of women into the workplace during the 1980s. Both public- and private-sector employment studies have shown that incidence does not decline significantly in a workplace until women constitute over 70% of the workers (Klein 1984[58]). Work units consisting of greater than 75% males not only have significantly higher rates of harassment but also have incidences of greater severity and duration. Young, unmarried women in pioneer positions are at highest risk for harassment, irrespective of educational and economic level (Gutek 1985[46]). The gender balance of the workplace, however, emerges consistently as the greatest predictor of harassment (Klein 1989a[48]). Given the degree of gender blending necessary to stop harassment, and given that women are relatively new in the work force, of which they constitute less than 25% in many jobs and professions, it is easy to conclude that sexual harassment will not diminish in the near future, and thus it needs to be addressed as a serious reality, rather than ignored or dismissed as insignificant.

Almost all of the published reports on sexual harassment cite negative consequences. The bulk of discussion, however, has focused on economic and productivity losses. Relatively little has been written on the psychiatric sequelae of harassment. Most mental health professionals are, in fact, not even acquainted with the legal and phenomenological definitions of harassment. For this reason, readers are referred to Appendix I, in which is presented a brief introduction to the subject of harassment, including legal background, definitions, and dynamic models. A description of the psychiatric sequelae and clinical approaches to treatment are presented below.

For most women the psychiatric sequelae of harassment are related to issues of traumatic stress reactions, narcissistic injury, violation of privacy and physical boundaries, shame, loss of control, depression, and, ultimately, issues of loss and mourning. Women with preexisting histories of rape and childhood sexual abuse constitute a special group for which the psychological consequences of harassment are even more severe. In a study of 262 cases of women who sought professional help for sexual harassment, Crull (1982[59]) reported a 90% incidence of psychological stress symptoms, often accompanied by persistent and obsessive anger and fear. Although adverse changes in physical and psychological health and decreased work performance are frequently cited as negative effects of sexual harassment, there is little in-depth literature on the psychiatric consequences of these experiences. Some of Crull's general observations combined with our own clinical experiences have led to our formulation of a six-step approach to the evaluation and treatment of victims of sexual harassment:

1. Assessment of the severity of the immediate crisis and validation of the seriousness of the experience. Assessment of the nature of the immediate crisis and validation of the serious reality of the patient's experience constitutes an important way to begin the treatment of a woman who has been sexually harassed. Starting out in this context helps the therapist to anticipate areas of stress and to begin to structure an appropriate course of treatment, while encouraging the patient to assess the reality of the external stress and mobilize coping responses rather than internalizing blame and regressing to a devalued, depressed, and helpless state. In order to collaborate with the patient in this initial review of her circumstances, the therapist must be familiar with some relevant economic and cultural factors. Some important guidelines in this area are provided by Crull (1982,[59] p. 542), who emphasizes the following:

1. Most women work out of economic necessity.
2. Most women are in junior- or lower-status jobs, and their harassers are likely to have an authority or advantage over women in the work hierarchy if a confrontation occurs.
3. Cultural norms place women in a no-win situation. If the woman rejects the harasser's advances, she is challenging his masculinity; if she tactfully ignores him, she may be misinterpreted as being coy and he may increase his attentions.

4. Culturally, women are still held responsible for controlling men's sexual behavior and are encouraged to internalize blame for any sexual misconduct.
5. Women are expected to put families before jobs and may interpret sexual harassment as a reminder that they should be at home with their families even if these women are working out of economic necessity.
6. Sexual harassment reinforces the low self-confidence and difficulty in judging one's own abilities that most women bring to the workplace as a result of negative stereotypes they are taught at an early age.

Therapists should also be aware that students and professional women often depend on their harassers for valuable educational and training experiences, verbal and written references, and opportunities for career development and advancement. Because their work is highly specialized, these women have limited opportunities for transfer, job change, and tutorial and mentoring reassignments. In these circumstances, the woman will be forced to continue interacting with her harasser or suffer severe economic, educational, or career development losses.

In instances when the harasser and victim are members of an ethnic or racial minority group, the victim may be inhibited from speaking out to the harasser, requesting assistance, or utilizing formal complaint channels because of a cultural mandate to settle things within the community and not speak out against one of her own. Withdrawal of support from family and informal community sanctions against her could result. This may also be the case regarding sexual orientation. For example, when a gay woman is harassed by another gay woman, the victim may also fear exposure and negative bias toward her due to her sexual preference.

Reviewing the complicated economic, cultural, and personal circumstances in collaboration helps both patient and therapist develop respect for the severity of the challenge and the special areas of stress to be addressed. Appreciating the double-bind nature of the situation is also important at the onset of therapy. This will help both therapist and patient to avoid two common pitfalls: 1) devaluing the patient for any initial inability to take definitive action, and 2) taking immediate but impulsive action, especially toward litigation, that might not be the most effective means of resolving the problem or might not ultimately be in the patient's best interests.

2. Evaluation of the degree of initial depressive, psychosomatic, anxiety, and posttraumatic stress symptoms. Common psychiatric sequelae of harassment that often go undiagnosed and untreated are as follows:

- Poor concentration
- Increased anxiety
- Mood lability
- Sleep disturbance
- Gastrointestinal complaints
- Headaches
- Panic attacks
- Obsessive-compulsive thoughts and actions
- Lethargy
- Muscle spasms
- Depression
- Posttraumatic stress syndrome

Occasionally patients will present with these complaints and make only vague references to work problems. In these instances it is important for the therapist to elicit more detailed history, because the patient may be attempting to deny or minimize the intent of harassment or may simply be unaware of the connection between her physical and psychological symptoms and her harassment experience at work. Severe anxiety, panic, and sleep disturbances can often be treated successfully with psychotropic medication, and it is especially important to offer this modality if the patient's symptoms are interfering with her functioning. The therapist should also elicit a specific history for depressive symptoms in anyone who has been harassed. Mild to moderate depressive symptoms are common, and, again, psychotropic medication may be useful. Severe depression and suicidal behaviors are more rare but have occurred in this context, and depressed victims should be asked specifically about suicidal ideation. Evaluation and relief of stress, depressive, anxiety, and psychosomatic symptoms should be presented in the context of enabling the patient to function at her best possible level so that she can maintain her credibility at work and develop an ultimate strategy to resolve the behavior. Stress and depressive symptoms need to be continually reassessed as the patient progresses through treatment, because traumatic confrontations, prolonged litigation, and so forth may initiate or exacerbate symptoms.

3. Exploration and ventilation of feelings. Intense feelings of anger, guilt, shame, and fear are common to victims of harassment. Obsessional thoughts of retaliation toward the harasser or fears of injury to the victim have also been reported to the present authors. Because direct expression of anger toward the harasser is often not possible, and premature or impulsive expression of anger through litigation is often detrimental, it is advisable to give the victim ample room to express her grievances in detail, explore her anger, and bring it into perspective before she takes any action. True expression of feelings of shame and guilt will assist in clarifying and resolving any concerns regarding her contribution to the harassment as well as doubts and concerns regarding her intrinsic academic, work, and/or professional ability. Additionally, work, home, and/or parenting conflicts, which also tend to be exacerbated by episodes of harassment, often surface around expressions of guilt and shame and need to be put into perspective, or else the woman will be at risk for fleeing the workplace. Fears of physical injury, loss of job, decreased economic stability, derailment from important career or educational pathways, and retaliation should be explored in great detail, not only to reduce anxiety but also to prepare the patient for developing a plan of action that will minimize her losses and protect her from further trauma. Validating the patient's feelings by reviewing the serious reality of her external stress, along with sharing information regarding the large number of other women who have been harassed, will greatly diminish the patient's sense of isolation and narcissistic injury. Referral to a short-term focus discussion/support group for harassment victims can be an excellent adjunct to therapy at this point. (See Hamilton et al. 1988[60] for a report on such a group.)

Because many harassers focus on more than one victim, some patients inadvertently find support among co-workers and fellow students. Patients should, however, be warned regarding the risks of injudiciously speaking to peers in their workplace. Patients can be further traumatized by unsupportive responses as well as expose themselves to later liability for defamation of character. If the patient's emotional responses are extreme or prolonged, or if she is not able to develop a plan of action, a history for more severe underlying pathology should be elicited gently and without implication that the patient is to blame for her harassment. Recommendations for treatment for underlying pathology should be presented in terms of helping her establish her optimal level for coping with the situation, and diminishing and removing any undue anxiety and dysphoria that would interfere with her coping. Patients with a previous history of rape or sexual abuse represent special cases and will be discussed separately later in this chapter.

4. Reestablishment of a sense of control via the development of coping strategies and the formulation of a plan of action. Once the patient's feelings are in perspective, she is ready to develop a plan for action. Her sense of control can be reestablished by stressing her ability to 1) review a variety of options for addressing her situation, 2) choose the option that best suits her needs, 3) proceed with her plan at her own pace, 4) develop protective measures against further harassment or retaliation, and 5) act in a manner that will minimize her ultimate losses. Although therapists cannot hope to be familiar with specific policies and grievance procedures for individual work and academic settings, a general knowledge of the types of options and most common grievance formats is necessary so that the therapist can provide a cognitive basis from which the patient can work out her own personalized plan of action.

5. Assessment of and protection against potential losses or adverse consequences. It is wise at this stage to collaborate with the patient to anticipate all possible losses of adverse consequences so that she may be as protective of herself as possible from the onset. Documenting the quality of her work, maintaining an impeccable attendance record, meeting project deadlines, keeping an accurate record of the harassment episodes and any retaliatory actions, identifying witnesses to the events, collaborating with other students or co-workers who have been harassed, identifying possible transfers to other work areas or to other supervisors/mentors, and identifying and contacting an advocate within the workplace—these are just a few of the many protective devices a woman can employ as she moves toward action. The patient may also build protective support from within her family or via professional and women's organizations.

Other protective steps may become apparent as the patient moves through the process. Four possible routes for addressing sexual harassment have been described (Hughes and Sandler 1986[55]; Rowe 1981[61]). Harassment can be addressed by 1) directly approaching the harasser, 2) utilizing informal channels within the work/educational organization, 3) utilizing formal complaint procedures within the work/educational institution, and 4) taking legal action. Most victims will find one or a combination of approaches reasonable for their situation. Reviewing the patient's primary goals and concerns as weighed against possible risks will usually enable her to select a reasonable approach. When the wish for revenge is the primary motivation, further ventilation of feelings may be necessary before a plan of action is instituted. Total revenge is an unrealistic concept, and attempting to obtain it may lead the victim to impulsive actions that are not ultimately in her best interest or to frustrating obsessional stalemates that make it impossible for her to move on with her life. Focusing abusive and retaliatory measures on a harasser who was genuinely unaware of the difficulties he was creating and is willing to stop his behavior is neither appropriate nor useful to the victim. A brief review of the pros and cons of each approach is given in Appendix J to serve as a guide for therapists and patients.

Whatever course of action the patient selects, it is important for the therapist to encourage her in making the selection that is best for her, to assist her in maintaining control of the process and in proceeding at a pace that is reasonable for her, and to enhance her capacity to anticipate risks and establish appropriate means of protection.

6. Dealing with losses. The final piece of therapeutic work for victims of harassment involves coming to terms with what they have lost. We feel that all women who have been harassed suffer important losses for which they must grieve. Many professionals are unaware of these losses or do not feel they are relevant when a woman handles her harassment well and her plan of action has a positive outcome. As a result, little intervention is made in this area, and the woman is left alone to mourn her loss or to deny it. Asking the patient to talk about what has changed for her as a result of the harassment is an important way to approach the process of grief and mourning. Loss of income, loss of job, loss of important relationships with a teacher and mentor, loss of collegiality with co-workers, loss of belief in her ideals of equality, loss of belief in her institution or superiors, loss of time from personal and career life, sexual dysfunction, marital stress, divorce, withdrawal of family, loss of opportunity for specialized training and education, derailment from career track, diminished confidence, and loss in motivation and love of work are common. Acknowledging the importance of these losses, encouraging the patient to share these losses with other significant and sympathetic people, supporting the patient through the grief process, including management of depressive symptoms, and ultimately helping the patient move on to invest in new work and life situations constitute an essential part of completing treatment. Sometimes, despite supportive help and advice, the victim feels powerless to act. It then becomes imperative to assess the psychodynamic issues that underlie her resistance. What in the past has been reevoked to create the kind of anxiety that paralyzes information gathering, self-assertion, and even cognitive functioning? Sometimes, to take one example, it is the patient's guilt for her own childhood fantasies—wishes about a father or brother who may not have been inappropriately flirtatious that produce paralyzing anxiety or guilt in the situation of harassment. With the analysis of these fantasies and the clarification of then and now, the patient can become capable of working out her own strategy in the present that may be better than any advice or real information we could give them. Generalized fears of childhood aggressive wishes can lead to reaction formations that help shape a very passive adult. Self-esteem issues that interfere with the development of a normal sense of entitlement can also inhibit adult women in developing effective strategies for coping with harassment. These individuals will also report difficulties in other aspects of their work (i.e., salary inequities, overwork, inappropriate work assignments, etc.).

When a victim of harassment has a prior history of rape, incest, or childhood sexual abuse, even the mildest forms of sexual harassment can be extremely damaging and difficult for the victim to address. She may report severe anxiety and depression, poor self-esteem and capacity for self-assertion, and profound confusion regarding boundaries of power, authority, and sexuality. Prior to the harassment, she may demonstrate difficulty in establishing clear work/personal boundaries and may have a history of work-related sexual affairs. These qualities may predispose her to special targeting from harassers. They also make it more difficult for her to cope effectively with harassment and reduce her credibility, sometimes even placing her at risk for being blamed for the harassment. Often the harassment experience will act as a precipitant for the derepression of previously forgotten childhood experiences of abuse. In this instance she may develop a diagnosable posttraumatic stress disorder with flashbacks, nightmares, severe anxiety and panic attacks, severe depression, dissociative episodes, and strong impulses to flee the situation and withdraw. In addition to being compromised in her ability to cope with the harassment situation, she must also deal with a new and serious disorder that is often misunderstood and causes her to be labeled as "oversensitive" or "hysterical." In these instances immediate treatment is needed that focuses on the following:

1. *Short-term stabilization and containment of her posttraumatic stress symptoms.* This can be accomplished with a variety of symptomati-

cally directed psychotropic medications, relaxation training, structured cognitive explanations to help her understand what is happening, and behavioral techniques aimed at containing symptoms and helping the patient control and slow up the process of remembering. The patient may need to defer dealing with her harassment situation until she has stabilized; she may also require time off from work or a plan that minimizes contact with the harasser until she is less symptomatic.

2. *Coping with the harassment situation.* When the patient is stabilized and less flooded, she may be assisted in dealing with her harasser using the format described earlier. Helping her to pace her plan of action so that she does not become overwhelmed and symptomatic will be important. In situations where she does not have to deal repeatedly or directly with the harasser, postponement of action or transfer may be advisable.
3. *Exploration of her previous abuse history and its impact on her current life.* Longer-term treatment for past abuse involving the elucidation of memories and affect should be undertaken only when the patient has stabilized and dealt effectively with the immediate harassment situation and establishes a solid relationship with her therapist.

Various aspects of this treatment approach are exemplified by the psychotherapy of two women who presented for treatment in the context of filing charges for sexual harassment, as summarized below.

Sexual Harassment With Previous Rape History and Posttraumatic Stress Symptoms

Ms. H., a 36-year-old lawyer, was referred for therapy by her attorney for symptoms of anxiety and explosiveness that were exacerbated in the context of court proceedings against her former law partner whom she had charged with sexual harassment. Ms. H. was recruited to the area a year ago to join a midsize firm specializing in her area of expertise. Mr. R., one of the senior partners, was especially helpful to her in negotiating her position and in adjusting to her move to a new city.

Six months after Ms. H. began work, Mr. R. began to pressure her for dates and became irritated when she persistently and firmly declined. He ceased asking and withdrew from contact with her after 3 months. Worried about losing his valuable patronship, she volunteered for extra work, agreed to overtime hours, and in all work areas strived to be conciliatory. She became frustrated and angry when Mr. R. criticized her work in front of the partners and asked for a reevaluation, and when his criticisms were reflected in her evaluation and she did not receive assignment to the type of cases she had been promised at her hiring. Shortly thereafter another senior partner approached her to report vague complaints from secretaries and clients regarding her attitude and department. She was told that she did not fit in and was asked if she would leave the firm quietly. When she refused, she was fired and asked to remove her belongings. Stunned, she began to pack and was interrupted by Mr. R., who entered her office to tell her of his satisfaction at her dismissal and to further devalue her work. Enraged, she attempted to pass by him and out the door. He pushed her back, stating he was not finished talking to her. She retained no memory of the remainder of the conversation. Once at home she was obsessed with Mr. R.'s hands and furious and too anxious to sleep. She invited a friend to stay with her. A legal colleague steered her toward an attorney specializing in discrimination, and she immediately filed suit.

Although active and focused in her sessions with her attorney, Ms. H. began experiencing panic attacks, explosive episodes, and sleep disturbance at home. She became so anxious at the onset of court proceedings that her attorney referred her for therapy. On initial evaluation Ms. H. reported that she was extremely anxious at bedtime and often unable to fall asleep until 2:00 A.M. During the day she experienced panic attacks combined with explosive outbursts of anger directed toward friends and her attorney. Initially she was phobic regarding medication but was ultimately able to control her panic symptoms with antianxiety medications. At the suggestion of her therapist, she instructed her attorney to postpone legal proceedings until she stabilized. Therapy focused on control of her symptomatology, stabilization in her new job, and the creation of a supportive network of friends.

Despite accomplishing these goals, Ms. H. became symptomatic again when her attorney reactivated her case. Her fears at this time focused on the necessity of her having to give testimony. In the context of exploring these fears, she began having nightmares that she ultimately associated to being raped by a date at age 14, an experience that she tried "not to think about." Over a 4-month period she was able to explore this experience in the context of her parents' reaction when she told them about the rape. Her mother had been ashamed and encouraged her to minimize the experience, and her father had accused her of being deliberately seductive and had instituted a stiff curfew. Integration of this material enabled her to testify against her law partner and ultimately to receive a settlement.

Sexual Harassment in the Context of Characterological Issues

Ms. B., a 25-year-old anthropology graduate student, was referred by her student health center for depression occurring in the context of filing a sexual harassment complaint with the EEOC against her institution. At her initial session Ms. B. complained of sleep disturbance, poor concentration, appetite loss, crying spells, loss of interest in her academic work and career goals, and indecisiveness. She declined antidepressant medication, stating that she wanted to talk first.

Over the course of the next four sessions she reviewed the events leading to her referral for treatment. She reported that 1 year ago she had obtained a job as a research assistant with Professor H., who was a national expert in the subspecialty of her field in which she wished to study. She was delighted with the position not only because the salary would help to subsidize her education but also because it solidified an important mentoring relationship and would lead to publications important to her career development. During the course of her daily meetings with Professor H., he began to discuss his personal life with her and to ask her about her boyfriends. Slightly uncomfortable and uncertain of appropriate professional boundaries, she responded with minimal answers but did not directly protest his behavior, as he was otherwise cordial and professional and their work was proceeding well. One afternoon he entered her office, leaned over her shoulder to review her work, and hugged her as he praised her writing. Startled and already late for a class, she abruptly excused herself and left the room. Too anxious to concentrate on the lecture, she returned to her apartment and discussed the incident with her roommate, who encouraged her to speak with the professor.

The following morning she scheduled an appointment with Professor H., during which she explained that the hug had made her uncomfortable and asked him not to repeat the behavior. In a warm, cordial, and slightly condescending tone, Professor H. explained that he meant no harm and considered her a daughter. In the two ensuing months he occasionally patted her and put his arm around her shoulder. Although uncomfortable with the behavior, she felt too confused to pursue it further, as even her friends agreed he was probably just being paternal and her mother frequently reminded her how lucky she was to have landed a job with such an important man.

One afternoon, while reviewing a final manuscript for publication, Professor H. leaned over Ms. B. and kissed her on the neck. She abruptly rose and shouted, "Stop that!" He made no comment and immediately returned to discussing the manuscript, but repeated the behavior 2 days later. Enraged and upset, Ms. B. again asked him to stop, stating that she could not continue on the project unless he could contain his behavior. Professor H. responded that he would continue to kiss her if he wanted and told her to go ahead and report him, because she would end up looking like a fool, not him. Ms. B. was unable to sleep that night but scheduled a meeting with a faculty adviser who, upon hearing of Professor H.'s behavior, referred her to the dean. The dean agreed to speak with Professor H. directly. One week later he reported back to Ms. B. that in his opinion Professor H. had meant no harm. That afternoon Ms. B. experienced a panic attack and was treated in the student health center.

She left school to visit her mother at home for a long weekend and considered dropping out of school. Her mother encouraged her to return and to minimize the episode to save her career, reminding her how proud her father, now dead, would have been of his only child publishing papers with such a prominent man. Ms. B. returned to school but resigned her job as research assistant and began to experience depressive symptoms interspersed with episodes of rage.

During an outburst of anger she impulsively contacted a law student friend, who referred her to a lawyer who specialized in discrimination. Within a day she had met with a lawyer and, upon his suggestion, had filed a complaint with the EEOC against her institution. During the EEOC investigation Ms. B. became increasingly depressed and was referred for therapy. During the course of reviewing her history, Ms. B. reported that she was sleeping better and that her appetite had returned. She continued to feel depressed and uncertain of her career goals.

Despite being reassured by her advisor that another research position would be arranged and that she would not have to deal with Professor H., she continued to experience impulsive thoughts of leaving school. Therapy focused on containment of these symptoms, continued functioning at school, and exploration of the nature of these symptoms. Over time she was able to relate her depressive state to fears and anger regarding never "being heard" by her father. She derepressed memories of his rigid, perfectionistic, and punitively controlling stance regarding her childhood ballet career, and his abrupt, angry withdrawal of funding when at age 14 she did not, at the time of her first audition, gain acceptance to the city ballet theater. Her mother colluded with this behavior and since his death had further idealized him at Ms. B.'s expense.

Validated by an EEOC ruling in her favor, Ms. B. approached her mother and firmly requested financial support for continued psychotherapy to explore "issues important to her." Over the course of her 2-year treatment she was able to explore and resolve the aspects of her relationship with her parents that led to chronic indecisiveness, procrastination, and depression. Although always an honor student, her work became more focused, more creative, and more gratifying to her, and her dating relationships improved, leading ultimately to her engagement to a man who was both warm and respectful. Upon graduation Ms. B. received a highly desirable faculty appointment at a leading university. Her appointment was the result of a successful research project she had completed with the department at that university as part of a fellowship position that she had created and for which she had obtained independent funding the year before.

Sexual harassment can be unwanted sexual attention and behavior or harassment on the basis of fulfilling a role appropriate to one's sex, as in the case of motherhood.

Pregnancy-Based Harassment

A pregnant chief resident in obstetrics and gynecology called one of the authors, who had published some material about maternity leave for female medical residents. Having set up satisfactory arrangements for maternity leave, she discovered, at her amniocentesis in the fifth month of her pregnancy, that she was carrying twins. She applied to her chairman for prematernity leave and was threatened with job loss if she took this leave. She was quite depressed and tearful and experienced a sleep disorder. She felt that she was being made to choose between prematurity and possible nonviability of her twins, and her future in obstetrics and gynecology. This had been a horrendous 5-year training program with a very demanding on-call schedule (i.e., every other night to every third night). She planned her pregnancy to coincide with the end of her program and planned to begin practice after a maternity leave. She was informed that the American College of Obstetrics and Gynecology recommended a 6-week prematernity leave for working women with multiple gestations. It was recommended that she get a copy of this in writing from the board and present it to her department chairman. She did this and her prematernity leave was granted. She gave birth to premature but easily viable twins and received accreditation for her training.

Rape

Rape is the most frequent serious crime in the United States (Kaplan and Sadock 1988,[62] p. 377). In 1984, 84,233 rape offenses were recorded by the Federal Bureau of Investigation (FBI) (Harvey and Koss 1987,[63] p. 1). However, official estimates by the Law Enforcement Assistance Administration (LEAA) (1975[64]) suggest that for every rape reported, 3 to 10 go unreported. Official victimization studies such as the National Crime Survey have yielded higher statistics, but even data from these studies are widely criticized for underrepresenting the scope of the problem. These data are often skewed toward minimization because of a lack of appreciation for the way in which survey questions and interviewing techniques exacerbate the underreporting of acquaintance rapes such as date rape, marital rape, and party rape. These studies are also limited by their utilization of the legal definition of rape that in many states excludes marital rape, which constitutes a large proportion of rape incidences. A series of recent and more clinically focused rape studies (Kilpatrick et al. 1985[65]; Koss 1985[66]; Koss and Oros 1982[67]; Russell 1982,[68] 1983,[69] 1984[70]) have yielded prevalence rates between 5% and 25%.

The FBI defines rape as "carnal knowledge of a female forcibly and against her consent" (Harvey and Koss 1987,[63] p. 1). Most legal definitions of rape have focused on the victim's nonconsent and the perpetrator's use of force. State rape laws vary, however, as to whether or not they specify the sex of the victim and offender, the specific activities that constitute rape, the exclusion of the spouse from culpability, and the use and definition of the terms of force and consent. Considerable debate exists regarding how much victim resistance and what kind of resistance, verbal or physical, constitute nonconsent. Similarly, debate continues on what constitutes force—for example, physical assault, threats of physical assault, deliberate deception, deliberate impairment of judgement with drugs and alcohol, kidnapping threats, threats to hurt or frighten the victim's children, and other forms of psychological coercion, such as threatening the loss of a job. Harvey and Koss (1987)[63] define rape in categories of form, relational context, recognition, spontaneity, and degree of force. Because these definitions are relevant to the psychiatric consequences of victims, they are outlined in detail in Appendix K.

Estrich (1987[71]) provides a detailed discussion of the legal history of rape, including the vicissitudes of its current legal status. She emphasizes that despite the positive effects of the rape reform laws of the 1970s, serious shortcomings still exist. Current laws allow for some consistency in the conviction of aggravated rapes by strangers, but legal redress is problematic for acquaintance rapes such as date rapes, party rapes, and marital rapes, which occur in high numbers and are potentially damaging to the victim. Clinicians need to know their state rape laws and to appreciate that these laws and the conviction rates for rape are not in synchrony with the victim's psychiatric damage. Patients may find legal procedures and outcomes extremely traumatic. Clinicians need to appreciate that their role is not to determine whether their patient's experience meets the legal definition of rape, but rather to

- Clarify the degree to which the experience has been traumatic.
- Assist the patient in handling the immediate crisis in an adaptive way.
- Assess the long-term psychodynamic impact of the rape.
- Determine its effect on developmental functioning and significant relationships.
- Clarify and treat any preexisting factors that diminish the patient's sense of autonomous control and self-protectiveness.
- Target individual stress symptoms, such as anxiety, phobias, and depression, that interfere with the patient's equilibrium and her capacity to process the rape experience.
- Develop a treatment program appropriate to all of these needs as they present over time.

Rape encompasses a wide variety of experiences, some of which have been well-documented and studied and others, such as date rape, party rape, and telephone set-up rapes (Hoyt 1984[72]), that are newly defined, widely unreported, and insufficiently studied.

Rape victims also constitute a multidimensional population with widely differing prerape psychic states, developmental stages, concurrent stresses at the time of the rape, relational networks, and cultural backgrounds. All of these factors contribute to determining the psychiatric sequelae of the rape for each individual.

Prior to the 1970s, rape was not widely studied, and psychodynamic models focused primarily on a narrowly defined spectrum of characteristics that theoretically contributed to the woman's being raped rather than focusing on the psychodynamic impact and sequelae of the rape itself. Rapists were also viewed in a simplistic manner as sexually deviant and unidimensional. This approach was shaped by a lack of real data regarding the diversity of rape experiences and by prevalent sociocultural prejudices.

Beginning in the 1970s, a literature growing out of the women's movement documented the cultural history and myths surrounding rape and questioned the legal management of rape (Brownmiller 1975[73]). Concurrently, clinicians began to study rape victims (Burgess and Holmstrom 1974a,[74] 1974b[75]; Ellis 1983[76]; Hilberman 1976[77]; Notman and Nadelson 1976[78]; Sutherland and Scherl 1970[79]), rape perpetrators (Clark and Lewis 1977[80]; Koss and Leonard 1984[81]), and the prevalence of rape (Kilpatrick et al. 1985[65]; Koss and Oros 1982[67]).

Clinical observations of victims led to documentation of the stages of symptom manifestation and recovery from rape, and eventually the term "rape crisis syndrome" or "rape trauma syndrome" emerged (Burgess and Holmstrom 1974a[74]). This nonofficial but clinically relevant "diagnosis" shifted the treatment orientation of rape. In keeping with classic crisis theory (see, e.g., Lindemann 1944[82]), management of victims was predicated on the assumption that most victims were healthy individuals in the midst of a crisis. Their symptoms were seen as normal responses to their rape and part of a short-term process of coping and reorganization. Short-term crisis intervention approaches that were issue oriented, supportive, and often administered by nonmedical rape counselors became the prevalent treatment of choice (McCombie 1980[83]). Psychotherapy was reserved only for individuals with a past or current history of psychiatric difficulties. Psychodynamically oriented interventions were criticized as pathologizing, blaming, stigmatizing, and unempowering to victims.

As empirical research proliferated, specific postrape symptoms were identified as follows: depression, sexual dysfunction, anxiety and phobic responses, social dysfunction, fatigue, sleep disturbances, poor concentration and intrusive thoughts, poor self-esteem, suicidality, somatic complaints, obsessive-compulsive thoughts, hypervigilance, anger, hostility, diminished capacity for enjoyment, and eating disorders. Specific cognitive, behavioral, and pharmacological approaches targeting these symptoms were added to the basic crisis intervention model of treatment (Ellis 1983[76]; McFarlane et al. 1988[84]; Steketee and Foa 1987[85]).

More recent longitudinal literature (Burgess and Holmstrom 1979[86]; Calhoun et al. 1982[87]; Kilpatrick et al. 1979,[88] 1981[89]; Nadelson et al.

1982[90]; Sales et al. 1984[91]) has documented that a significant number of rape victims do not fit the traditional crisis model because

1. Their symptoms persist over time.
2. Their symptoms occur, reoccur, and remit chronically.
3. Their symptoms are similar to those associated with rape crisis syndrome but occur after a latency period of months or years postrape.
4. The patients do not present with a history of rape, but instead enter therapy for other issues that are not linked to the rape until the patients are well into their therapy.

This more complicated clinical presentation is similar to the presentation of incest and childhood sexual abuse victims, many of whose cases have also been carefully studied for the first time during the 1980s (Courtois 1988[92]; Herman 1981[93]). Other explorations link rape and incest victims with other victims of violence, such as mugging, terrorism, internment, war veterans, and disaster survivors. In this context, a stress trauma model for treatment has emerged (Figley 1985,[94] 1986[95]; Horowitz 1976[33]; Krystal 1988[96]; Ochberg 1988[36]). Most clinicians now formally diagnose rape victims according to official DSM-III-R (American Psychiatric Association 1987[97]) criteria as having either acute or chronic posttraumatic stress disorder rather than character disorders or psychoses.

As described above, the DSM-III-R model stresses a biphasic alternation between numbing and constrictive, versus intrusive, symptoms. In addition to asymptomatic latency periods, one sees long-term side effects—namely, secondary elaboration or chronic character disorder in defense against the recurrence of traumatic memories, as well as posttraumatic decline characterized by impoverishment of activities and role function secondary to ego constriction and phobic avoidance (Krugman 1987[98]). These long-term sequelae are more evident when the trauma has been neither acknowledged nor responded to appropriately, a situation that is quite prevalent among rape victims.

The long-term sequelae to rape elaborated in the posttraumatic stress model dovetail nicely with some more recent psychodynamic explorations of the aftermath of rape (Gise and Paddison 1988[99]; Martin et al.

1986[100]; Renshaw 1989[101]; Rose 1986[102]). In these discussions, the authors do not focus on prerape masochism, provocativeness, or the acting out of unconscious rape fantasies, but rather they emphasize the psychodynamics of the rape itself, including reorganization of character around symptoms, conflicts, and defenses activated by the rape trauma. Rose (1986[102]) noted that the psychological trauma of rape includes threat of death, massive environmental assault, violation of bodily boundaries, narcissistic injury, overwhelming of usual ego function, loss of control, profound regression, disruption of important relationships, and, often, the reorganization of character. Activation and reactivation of unconscious conflicts and fantasies, profound loss and grief reactions, and disruption of important relationships and developmental tasks also play a role. In the material that follows, we discuss a psychodynamic approach to the treatment of rape victims that integrates crisis management and psychopharmacological, behavioral, and cognitive techniques targeted to specific stress symptoms. More detailed elaboration of areas appropriate for psychodynamic intervention is presented as follows:

1. Transference and countertransference reactions both in therapists and in significant others
2. Marital and social discordance
3. Reactivation and activation of unconscious conflicts
4. Interference with developmental life stages
5. Formation of maladaptive defenses such as dissociation and repression, and the resultant vulnerability
6. Characterological reorganization around symptoms and defenses and conflicts activated by the traumata with concomitant dysfunction secondary to ego constriction and phobic avoidance
7. Difficulties in the management of aggression
8. Contributions of the rapist's psychodynamics to the victim's status
9. Issues of loss and grief

Psychodynamically oriented clinicians may encounter rape victims in a variety of situations: 1) as new patients in acute crisis following a rape;

2) as analytic or intensive psychotherapy patients who are raped while undergoing treatment for other issues; 3) as patients in ongoing treatment who, well into the course of the therapy, reveal that they have been raped in the past with or without consciously connecting the rape to any of their current therapy issues; and 4) as new patients who delayed entering treatment after a rape and are currently experiencing symptoms or whose symptoms disappeared and are recurring. In each instance the psychodynamic interventions will be different.

For a healthy woman, well engaged in healthy relationships, it is reasonable to formulate a treatment plan based on 1) crisis therapy administered with due respect to the transference and countertransference issues; 2) couples or family interventions aimed at assisting the patient and significant others to recover adaptively; 3) cognitive, behavioral, or psychopharmacological techniques targeted toward specific stress symptoms; and 4) termination, which includes education regarding possible long-term consequences and the availability of further treatment if indicated, along with observation in widely spaced follow-up appointments over time.

If the rape occurs in the context of ongoing therapy or analysis, an adaptation in the therapy must be made and sufficient time allotted to address the crisis and concomitant stress symptoms in the therapy. Changes in transference and countertransference, and changes in the parameters of the treatment program should be monitored, and the therapist should be prepared to deal with the reactivation of posttraumatic stress symptoms at any point later in the treatment. The return to prerape therapy issues should include monitoring the manner in which the rape may alter previous intrapsychic issues and activate new conflicts as well as the way in which preexisting vulnerabilities may alter and delay recovery from the rape.

In patients who enter therapy long after the rape, or who reveal histories of rape long into a course of therapy, the possibility of characterological reorganization around the rape trauma and the connection between current issues identified for treatment and the past history of rape should be explored. In all cases, transference and countertransference reactions, disruptions in significant relationships, the impact of the rape on current developmental tasks, and the grieving associated with the changes that the rape has caused should be addressed.

Countertransference reactions to rape victims on the part of treating therapists, friends, relatives, and members of the legal system are quite common and very intense. These reactions are the result of cultural myths and biases regarding rape, as well as intense unconscious reactions to the rape itself. Knowledge of these common reactions is necessary not only to provide adequate nonjudgmental, empathic, and respectful care but also to ensure that others support rather than retraumatize the victim. Common *cultural myths* regarding rape include the following (Gise and Paddison 1988,[99] p. 632):

1. The rapist is a sexually unfulfilled man carried away by a sudden uncontrollable urge. **[Most rapes are planned in advance and most offenders are involved in a consensual sexual relationship or have access to nonforcible sexual outlets.]**
2. Rapists are sick. **[Actually rapists often appear psychiatrically normal.]**
3. Rapists are strangers. **[In half of rapes, the victim knows her assailant. If marital rape were to be included, the figure would be even higher.]**
4. Rape occurs on the streets. So long as a woman stays home, she is safe. **[Over half of rapes occur in the victim's residence.]**
5. Most rapes involve black men raping white women. **[In the majority of reported rapes, the rapist and the victim are of the same race.]**
6. Women are raped because they ask for it by dressing seductively or walking provocatively.
7. Only women with bad reputations are raped.
8. Most victims have been in trouble with the law in the past.
9. Only women in the lower social class get raped.
10. Women cannot be raped unless they want to be or enjoy it.

Universal feelings evoked by rape that commonly result in countertransference reactions have been elaborated by many authors (Rose

1986[102]; Silverman and Apfel 1983[103]). These feelings include fear of helplessness and vulnerability, loss of impulse control, identification with the rapist or significant men in the patient's life, identification with the victim, and self and object loss. Female therapists have difficulties with feelings of helplessness and vulnerability. Defenses include questioning the victim's credibility and responsibility for the rape, emphasizing ways in which to avoid the rape, criticizing victim's reactions, and emotional distancing from the victim. Identification with the assailant can lead to countertransference reactions common in male therapists and significant others. Denial that the woman will have any feelings regarding men is one response. Attempting to compensate or provide a corrective experience is another. Lack of ability to focus on the patient's concern is yet another common reaction. For example, the authors are aware of a husband who refused to support his wife's prosecution of her rapist on the grounds that he was "a brother."

Police, lawyers, lawmakers, judges, and so forth often focus on the question of protecting the assailant from false accusations rather than on the damage done to the rape victim. Persistence of the cultural view of women as property or narcissistic objects can lead to a lack of empathy for the victim and to heightened empathy for her father, husband, fiancé, or boyfriend. The woman is seen as devalued, damaged goods. Consequently, she may be abandoned by the significant men in her life, viewed as spoiled or tainted by her mother, and seen as irreparably damaged psychologically by her treaters. Fear of loss of control over impulses can lead to guilt in treaters and family members via identification with the aggressor. This can then be projected onto the victim, leading to beliefs and statements that she "had it coming," that she provoked or wanted it, and/or that she should be punished or put on trial.

When a victim is actively engaged in therapy and neither avoiding, fleeing, nor denying the experience and affects involved with her rape, she commonly develops a transference in which the therapist is seen as the rapist, leading to outbursts of anger, criticism, and needs to overcontrol the therapy. This can happen with both male and female therapists, because the elucidation of the rape experience for psychotherapeutic purposes is painful. Noncritical transference interpretation that is tightly linked to the rape experience and that allows the transference to be used as a tool to help reconstruct the trauma is helpful. Also helpful is when victim and therapist can join in defining and controlling the pace and format of the therapy. Incorrect management of this transference material can result in premature termination, inappropriately formulated referrals to short-term crisis counseling, or avoidance and denial of the rape experience within the therapy.

Regardless of the treatment context, the therapist will be dealing with a life crisis and stress syndrome. The capacity to conceptualize this complex situation and to intervene therapeutically is important and will require some change in the parameters of any ongoing therapy or analysis. Attention to the containment of stress symptoms and support of adaptive responses to the immediate situation must be addressed as well as the psychodynamic implications of the rape and its sequelae. For this reason, a review of the descriptive clinical observations of the phases of response seen in victims of rape, commonly referred to as *rape trauma* or *rape crisis syndrome*, is provided in Appendix L along with relevant clinical interventions based on cognitive, behavioral, psychopharmacological, and crisis intervention models. Several clinicians (Burgess and Holmstrom 1974a[74]; Foreman 1980[104]; Sutherland and Scherl 1970[79]) have contributed to the clinical description of the rape crisis syndrome. Harvey and Koss (1987,[63] pp. 33–37), by integrating these earlier reports, present a three-stage model composed of 1) an *anticipatory* phase, which is when the victim first recognizes danger; 2) an *impact* phase, which includes the attack and its immediate aftermath; and 3) a *reconstitution* phase, which includes the psychological integration of the event and a return to basic living. Notman and Nadelson (1980[105]) and Gise and Paddison (1988[99]) have explored the way in which developmental life factors inhibit resolution and provide secondary focuses for treatment. Remer and Elliot (1988[106]) have summarized the way in which negative responses from significant others impact on the three-phased response (see Appendix L for details).

In their long-term work with victims of rape, Martin et al. (1986[100]) have elaborated three phases. In the first phase, the therapist assesses the actual trauma that the patient has experienced and its subsequent effects on her symptomatology and functioning. This enables the patient to ventilate previously suppressed and probably extremely shameful material. During the second phase, the working alliance phase, therapist and patient work collaboratively to understand how the rape has affected the patient and to help her master her reactions and feelings such as guilt, shame, fear, panic, anger, and loss of control. Assessment of old coping mechanisms, addition of new mechanisms, and the empowerment of the patient's sense of trust in her own perceptions should occur. In the final stage, the patient is helped to mobilize her insights and understandings, return to a prior or even higher level of functional development, and manage any reactions of significant others.

Gise and Paddison (1988[99]) emphasize the themes of loss and of low self-esteem as manifestations of sexual and aggressive fusion turned against the self. These authors identify victims' ambivalence toward men, their fears regarding loss of control over aggressive and sadistic impulses, their maladaptive use of repression and dissociation, and their avoidance of social task performance as major focuses for psychodynamic interventions. In a combined approach to rape and sexual abuse, Gise and Paddison cite goals for therapy as follows:

> (1) Identifying and interrupting any ongoing sexual abuse, (2) understanding the organization of the victim's defensive structure and its relationship to the abuse, (3) modifying the psychological defenses so that the victim can tolerate discussing the abuse, (4) unlinking the trauma at sensory, perceptual, and cognitive levels from dysfunctional behaviors, (5) processing the integrated trauma to past memory, and (6) rebuilding coping behaviors that provide for a positive interaction with the future. Family counseling is also an important feature. (Gise and Paddison 1988,[99] p. 644)

The most detailed account of the psychodynamics of rape was presented by Rose (1986[102]), who wrote the following:

> Loss is the major theme in the psychodynamics and symptomatology of rape victims and in the responses to the victim by significant others and society. Loss is profound and devastating for the rape victim, intrapsychically touching on every stage of psychosexual develop-

> ment, self-concept, and object relations as well as affecting sexuality and relationships with others. The psychodynamics are universal but, in the individual victim, some levels are more profoundly affected than others, this being determined by a combination of the particular nature of each assault, the psychodynamics and past history of the victim, and the response of the environment. However, each level is present to some degree in every rape victim. The psychodynamics of the rape victim can be discerned by examining the nature of the loss, defenses, and characteristic affective responses at each intrapsychic stage of development and in the areas of sexual and social functioning. The impact of the psychodynamics of the rapist must also be considered. (p. 818)

We now summarize Rose's conceptualizations via a review of rape responses encompassing the oral, anal, and phallic stages of development. Rape victims suffer oral annihilation threats via the impact of threats of death experienced during the rape and through the destruction of important parts of the self (Rose 1986,[102] pp. 818–820). Direct threats and acts of violence often accompanied by the use of a weapon are common to most rapes. Additionally, the victim may experience the rapist's murderous rage and need for total control even when no direct threats are made.

A sense of intrapsychic death is experienced via the destruction of basic trust and primitive omnipotence, resulting in an exquisite sense of vulnerability and, later, generalized suspiciousness, especially toward men. A variety of stage-specific defenses may be called into play. Depersonalization and dissociation are often utilized to preserve autonomy and protect ego functioning during the assault. These defenses often persist and are part of the numbing stages described by the posttraumatic stress syndrome model in which a numbed, distant, deadened self exists that represents a mixture of depersonalization, dissociation, depression, and reenactment of the trauma. For example, one victim reported to the authors that she was not herself anymore and that she was gone.

Regression also adds to the sense of the death of the self, as the victims may decline significantly in their level of functioning. According to Rose (1986[102])

> the regression has powerful consequences for the victim's self-concept. The old identity is lost, at least temporarily, as the victim's prior sense of self and level of functioning are superseded by the affects and conflicts activated by the regression. Associated with this is a shift in the predominant defenses to more primitive ones such as projection, introjection, and denial. Consequently, the victim feels "transparent" and that "everyone knows" that she has been raped. She projects massively. As a result, she most often experiences others as critical, unsupportive, voyeuristic, and not wanting to listen. Commonly, others really do respond in these ways, thereby reinforcing the victim's projections. (p. 819)

The characteristic affects at this level are terror, mistrust of self and people, depression, murderous rage, and guilt. Conscious acceptance of the rage is especially well defended, for the victim has already experienced her rapist as losing control of sadistic and aggressive impulses.

Rape disrupts the victim's sense of bodily integrity and psychic identity, functions of key importance during the anal phase:

> Rape disrupts the sense of autonomy, control, and mastery over one's body. The body's boundaries are violated, orifices are penetrated, aversive sensory stimuli cannot be escaped, motor and verbal functions are controlled by the assailant, and, not infrequently, autonomic nervous system responses such as nausea and vomiting, urination, defecation, and syncope occur. Loss of control and mastery over psychic functioning results from the activation of very intense primitive affects, overwhelming of the ego, disruption of stable self and object images, and regression. In addition, the rapist entraps the victim in states when the victim is least able to function optimally, such as when the victim is asleep, is under the influence of drugs or alcohol, is distracted, or is taken by sudden attack. (Rose 1986,[102] p. 820)

The profound sense of shame induced by these violations is most frequently defended by self-blame and attempts to undo the loss of control, competence, and sense of predictability. This defense is often reinforced by sociocultural norms and by the current feminist climate in which short-term rape crisis counseling advocates against self-blame. As a result, these defenses can be prematurely suppressed rather than sufficiently explored and resolved. Abrupt changes in life, via work and living situation, are not always adaptive and are sometimes manifestations of this defense. Such changes should be explored appropriately.

Regressions involving severe shame and control conflicts are common, as are reaction formation and identification with the aggressor. This identification in the victim is manifested by feelings of extreme compassion for the rapist; denial of both rage and sadistic retaliatory functions against the rapist; a sense of feeling dirty and spoiled; and a capacity to make caregivers feel helpless and useless. Under these circumstances, profound feelings of shame, self-disgust, self-blame, sadistic rage, and guilt are common. Victims dread these affective experiences and feel an extreme need to control them. They are particularly disturbed by the intrusive occurrence of symptoms experienced after the assault, and they often experience intense worries and shame about the possibility that they are going crazy.

The sexuality and sexual identity established during the phallic stage are severely disrupted by rage, and many rape victims report permanent changes in their sexual functioning and sexuality (Rose 1986,[102] pp. 821–822). Avoidance, role reversal, and projection are prominent defenses. Victims withdraw from sexual activity and experience their lovers and possible lovers as potential rapists via projection and displacement. Occasional counterphobically premature or forced return to sexual activity in an attempt to deny damage has also been reported. Anger at the rapist and at those persons of the same sex, and guilt over any stimulation or arousal experienced during the assault or any sexual fantasies that were activated, are common following a rape. Confusion, guilt, self-blame, shame, and fear of sexual perversion arise from any arousal occurring during the rape and from any fantasies activated, especially if the rapist has taken sadistic pleasure in arousing the victim. Guilt and denial of rage toward the rapist for destroying sexual pleasure can lead to the establishment of a negative sexual image via unattractive dressing, ungratifying sexual acting out, sexual deprivation, and anorexia and bulimia, which are both self-punitive and unattractive.

The psychodynamics outlined above play a role in the damage and loss to other significant relationships (Rose 1986,[102] p. 822), as mentioned in previous sections. Most of all, the affects, defenses, and conflicts stimulated in the victim as a response to rape interact with and reinforce countertransference responses in significant others (see previous discussion on countertransference). The victim's regressions and affective changes strain relationships. Projection and displacement of affect onto significant others may cause both victims and significant others to mutually withdraw. Intimate relationships will also stimulate flashbacks and other intrusive stress symptoms and may thus be more ambivalently experienced by the victim. The special but not unusual circumstance in which the rapist is a significant other intensifies the issues of trauma and loss for the victim.

The impact of the rapist on the psychodynamics of the victim is a little explored but highly important aspect of treatment. The upsurge of literature documenting the high prevalence and relational significance of situations in which women are raped by husbands (Bidwell and White 1986[107]; Finkelhor and Yllo 1985[108]; Frieze 1983[109]; Hanneke et al. 1986[110]; Weingourt 1985[111]) and by dates and other social peers (Aizenman and Kelley 1988[112]; Koss et al. 1987[113]; Miller 1988[114]; Pirog-Good and Stets 1989[115]; Warshaw 1988[116]) only heightens the importance of exploring the rapist-victim interaction. Harvey and Koss (1987[63]) have noted that rape is unique in that it is an ultimate violation of the self that is perpetrated by another human being who is often trusted by the victim and who leaves the victim stigmatized and blamed. According to Rose (1986,[102] p. 823), the fact that the source of this profound damage is another human being plays a special role in the psychodynamics of the victim, stimulating problems in areas of object relations, identification with the aggressor, introjection, loss of ego boundaries, and projection.

Rose (1986)[102] divides rapists according to the following psychodynamic themes: 1) power reassurance, 2) power assertion, 3) anger retaliation, and 4) anger sadistic excitation. Projection, identification with the aggressor, projective identification, and reenactment are all defenses utilized by rapists to protect against feelings of helplessness, humiliation, pain, rage, guilt, terror, and shame. Introjection of these defenses by the victim can contribute to the psychodynamics of her reaction. If the rapist is someone she knows, cares for, and has contact with, the victim may either strongly identify with the rapist or internalize anger and blame for the event.

Some women, especially those who have been sexually molested or beaten as children, will for a number of complex psychological reasons put themselves in dangerous sexual situations. This may reflect a wish to destroy or punish those aspects of the body that have been imbued with negative characteristics. This behavior usually occurs or is exacerbated prior to the conscious experience of rage toward the original abuser. Some other patients who are generally self-destructive engage in risk-taking behaviors that result in rape. Their conscious and unconscious fantasies have more to do with achieving self-punishment than they do with being specifically raped. There are yet other women who need to prove their omnipotence through counterphobic behaviors. Still others wander about in dissociated depressed states oblivious to risk. We do not state these special examples to blame the victim, but rather to alert therapists so that these possibilities may be explored in the service of preventing trauma or of restoring a rape victim to her full self-protective potential after assault has occurred. Finally, parents may counterphobically encourage sexual promiscuity or risk-taking in their daughters as a defense against rape.

Rape fantasies are not uncommon in women. These are oedipal-stage fantasies in which the girl-woman can have forbidden gratification (with her father) without accepting the responsibility of this symbolically forbidden gratification (Bernstein and Warner 1984b[117]). The most common fantasies involve an already loved man. Other fantasies involve violence and masochism and are punishment for unconscious sexual and aggressive fantasies. They are seldom connected with rape-seeking behavior except in women previously abused. Perhaps it is the recognition and misunderstanding of these fantasies that help maintain the myth that "all women want to be raped."

We now present detailed material from the psychotherapy of victims of rape who presented for treatment months after the rape occurred.

Acquaintance Rape With Prolonged Course and Compromised Functioning

The patient, a 26-year-old mother of three children, worked full time as an executive secretary. She had received a special recognition award that allowed her to have almost completed a college education. The patient had immigrated to this country with part of her immediate family from a culture with a strict religious background and a tradition of arranged marriages. Married in her middle teens to a kind and hard-working laborer, she immediately became pregnant with her first child. She obtained a high school equivalency diploma and went to work, leaving her first and then her second child with family members. Her third child was born 2 years before she began treatment. This child was cared for by his older siblings and left with a neighbor while they were in school. The patient had the sole responsibility for the children and for preparing meals for her husband and cleaning up after him. The patient's sexual relationship with her husband was a matter of quick missionary-position intercourse in the dark. She was anorgasmic but had no complaint. Her husband was gentle and allowed her to avoid him when she chose to in order to prevent unwanted pregnancies. Her first two children were what both considered obligatory pregnancies. She wanted her third child, and her husband had no objection. The family was in a decent financial position and the future looked promising.

On one occasion the patient agreed willingly to work at generous overtime wages on a national holiday. She gratefully accepted her boss's offer to bring her children along and let them play or watch television in his private conference room. She brought the children's lunches and left them in her boss's refrigerator. She was at work at her computer in her office when a man appeared with a knife. He forced her to remain at her desk while he looked around. He told her that if she wanted to spare her baby's life or avoid being raped in front of her children, she would have to "suck him off." She was slow to comprehend the meaning of this, and he responded with verbal abuse and mockery. She remembered being told that she had better make it good or he just might stick the knife into her. From that point on, she remembered being entirely focused on a picture of her own stabbed body and the children coming out to find her dead in a pool of blood. Although he was instructing and criticizing her, she had no way of gauging if she was doing all right. After he ejaculated, he kicked her in the stomach. (She had been forced to kneel in front of him on the floor while he was sitting with the knife to her throat.) The children heard her cry out and fall to the floor. She had the presence of mind to tell them that she had tripped and that she needed to go put cool water on her face. She went to her boss's private bathroom, where she undressed, showered, washed her mouth and hair, and put on fresh makeup, and then, returning, gave the children lunch, finished her work, resigned her position, packed up her belongings, and waited for her husband to pick her and the children up as planned. She went home, made dinner for the family, bathed the children, put them to bed, went to sleep while her husband watched television, saying simply that she was tired, and awakened with a screaming night terror.

Because she was soaked with perspiration, she got up, showered, put on a clean nightgown, and returned to bed. Over the long holiday weekend, she had repeated night terrors. In answer to her husband's few questions, she said that she did not know what was wrong. By Sunday she was quite frantic, knowing that she would have to account for giving up her job. She could not return to the rape scene. She asked her husband's permission to meet privately with his sister, and he readily agreed. This woman, more sophisticated than the patient, insisted on calling a rape hot line and taking the patient for evaluation. The patient received immediate and excellent counseling. She was encouraged to tell her husband, in her sister-in-law's presence, that she had been raped, and she was supported in her reluctance to reveal the details. She was also encouraged to tell her boss in her sister-in-law's presence that she had been raped in the office. He refused to accept her resignation, put her on medical leave, and instituted her disability and compensation benefits, which made it possible for the rape crisis intervention center to refer her for private psychiatric treatment.

Unfortunately, the patient waited several weeks at home before accepting the referral. She became increasingly phobic, began to have flashbacks, and became overtly tearful and depressed. She abandoned a regular community-based activity, withdrew, and became almost incapable of caring for her children. At this point, her husband insisted that she see a doctor. Between the time she made her first appointment for psychiatric treatment, she began interviewing for another job. She also sought legal counsel and was advised of her rights in a civil suit. By the time she was first seen, she had become involved in self-defense class, found a new job, and had enrolled herself in college classes to continue her education. She had, however, gained 40 pounds. She became obsessed with the idea that her baby was unsafe with the baby-sitter, and for a while she made her children stay home on alternate days to watch their brother. She had flashbacks and sudden outbursts of crying, and for the first time she became resentful of her husband's masculine privileges. In a displacement, she took most of her anger out on her eldest son, who responded by beginning to fail in school.

The patient responded to her husband's first sexual advance in panic. He reacted by failing to understand and contributed to her damaged self-image. In all fairness, his concept that rape was immaterial was culturally influenced. However, it contributed to her confusion. On the one hand, her husband did not seem to care about her sexually and, on the other hand, the perpetrator was demanding and demeaning. This was a mixed message from two controlling males. She responded to the rape in terms of intimidation, humiliation, and performance failure. She felt that she had failed her boss, failed to be a desirable sexual object, and was now failing her husband.

She could only be helped to integrate this trauma in her life in terms of her own cultural norms. Treatment had to proceed against the therapist's own egalitarian values and outrage. The patient could only recover by being helped to see the perpetrator as crazy and abnormal in his sexual demands.

The patient had to be encouraged to focus her anger on the intrusion into her life and failure of the security provisions of her job to protect her children. She also had to be helped toward a perception of herself and her own body image independent of external male input. For example, the patient's rapid weight gain prior to treatment was the result of her unconsciously following the suggestion of the perpetrator that she was fat, so she became fat, as much as she had always followed the instructions of her family.

She went to work but stopped using mass transportation. Fortunately, in her culture a basis for female-female validation already existed. (It in fact had determined her choice of turning first to her sister-in-law.)

She became amenorrheic, an unusual complication of her posttraumatic stress disorder. In reality this did not matter because she had undergone a tubal ligation following her last pregnancy. Psychologically it remained the stubborn last vestige of the trauma. Her other problem remained an inability to assert herself with a series of ineffectual male lawyers who failed to take proper charge of her civil suit.

Nevertheless, the patient was gradually able to return to her previous level of functioning. Fortunately, her mother was able to undertake the care of her youngest child until he entered nursery school. The patient felt safe about her daughter, who had entered a special private school program. Her feared aggressive object remained her oldest son. As he entered adolescence he became more, but not abnormally, assertive. The day in therapy when she announced that he had been accepted into high school in a different county, where he would live with members of her extended family, she began not only to menstruate but to hemorrhage in a way that required emergency medical care.

By this time her life was back in place and she was asymptomatic. Over the following 5 years, the therapist has received requests for medical records and testimony from an endless line of law firms. Checking with her, she continues to do well, clearly makes efforts to avoid her own deposition, and is ambivalent about receiving further compensation or reopening the trauma. To this day the specific details have been shared only with the patient's sister-in-law and therapist.

Pair Rape With Prolonged Course

The patient, a very attractive, openly sexual, seductive 25-year-old single female, had graduated from high school and had been functioning independently of her family since she was 18 years old. She had been working as a sales representative in an open glass showroom in one of her city's most prestigious areas. She had complained on several occasions of feeling uncertain about the safety of the electronic lock on the door of the showroom to the street but had been reassured that she would never be left alone and that there would always be members of the management and sales force in the back offices.

One day when the weather was inclement, she invited a female friend to order lunch in with her. The last person left in the back office, who was part owner of the firm, announced his intention to go out for lunch but assured her that he would return in 1 hour. This was the time that she was expected to return to the showroom and when her girlfriend would depart to return to her own desk. The hour having arrived, the girlfriend departed; the man who had promised to reappear, however, failed to return, and the patient remained in the back office. When she heard the front door open she imagined that a member of the back-office staff was returning and began to put her belongings away and return to the showroom. Instead, she was confronted by two men who forced her back into the back offices. The men, who were armed, directed her to show them to the safe and the petty cash. One went to work at the robbery. The other bound her with electrical tape. He also ripped off her gold necklace and bracelet. Because her mouth and part of her nose were bound, she began to feel like she was smothering and was afraid for her life. It did not occur to her that she might be sexually molested. When the robbery was over, she was forced into a back bathroom. Her muffled protests because she could not breathe evidently attracted their attention. One pulled down her panty hose and panties, shoved her against the bathroom sink, and raped her. This was an agonizing experience because she was menstruating and had a tampax in place. She was then raped by the second perpetrator and lost consciousness. She either fell or was thrown into the bathtub and remained unconscious for an indeterminate time, when she was discovered by a fellow employee.

She was hospitalized because of her concussion. It was obvious that she had been molested and was seen by the hospital rape intervention team. Her employer, realizing his potential liability, became alarmed and paid for her private treatment out of pocket. She was referred for private psychiatric care. Her flashbacks were to smothering and a fear of dying rather than to the rape. She was more enraged at the people at her job, whom she perceived to have been responsible, than at the perpetrators.

When she was first seen, her hair pulled back and wearing dark glasses and no makeup, she was bundled in a layer of clothing that made her look like a depressed and paranoid adolescent. Her voice was barely audible, and she complained of insomnia, panic, and aphonia. She was unable to wait in the waiting room despite the fact that she had been identified and buzzed in by the receptionist. Instead she preferred to sit at the receptionist's desk and have the therapist meet her there and escort her to and from the consultation room. The patient was able to remain in her own apartment only as long as a cousin or friend was able to stay with her at night. She was unable to return to work. She bought a dog and a second security system for her apartment. Unable to use her car, she kept it garaged. She paper-trained the dog because she was unable to walk him.

Her family consisted of a divorced working mother who lived in another state with the patient's younger brother, whose employment was undetermined. In addition, she had a father who had been alcoholic and was remarried to a younger woman. The patient was estranged from them. No one wanted to know what had happened to her. Her father sent her an initial sum of money with a letter that indicated that as far as he was concerned, his obligation to her was over. Her brother came to get her car and took it to their home. Her mother called regularly, sent her small sums of money, and "nagged her" to sell her car and get a new job.

The patient was invited to come to her mother's home on weekends. She found her brother to be alcoholic and drug abusive, and a probable drug dealer. Her mother was unable to confront him for fear of his physical violence. The patient, however, confronted him in a rage, which frightened him and he retreated. However, this resulted in her mother's advising her that she had best not come home and insisting that she remove her car from the driveway, where her brother found it to be an annoyance. She responded with a severe retarded depression that required psychotropic medication. It became apparent that the assault and rape were reminiscent of abandonment to violence and that this was redocumented by her mother's abandonment of her in the face of the threat of her brother's violence. She began to remember that her father had been physically and sexually abusive to her mother in her presence, although her mother denied that he had ever abused her. Over the next year she continued to be severely debilitated. She used up much of her finances and wore down the patience of her friends and extended family. She could only work in a local women's clothing store part time during daylight hours with someone else present.

The patient confronted her former boss with her copies of his written complaints about the door locks, and he showed her evidence that he had passed these on to the building landlord. She borrowed money from him to initiate a suit against the landlord. The door lock was repaired, and she was offered her old job back, but she defiantly refused it. She confronted her mother, who then told her to sell her car, move home, and make peace with her brother. Her brother, the patient learned, had been contributing money to enable the mother to remain at home and to continue to at least minimally help the patient, who by now was finding various rooming arrangements. It was apparent that continuing this adaptation would require her to give up her dog. She attempted to confront her estranged father, who in effect told her to forget the past and stop contacting him. Her father's new wife was kinder and tried to offer some help.

The mother volunteered to come and see the therapist, but the patient refused a joint meeting. The mother came to meet with the therapist individually. She was an attractive, nicely dressed woman who appeared younger than her stated age. She, in effect, admitted to blaming her children for her husband's alcoholism and the breakup of her marriage. Clearly, she had never recovered from this loss, had envied her daughter's prior success and male companionship, and was determined not to lose her son. The mother told the therapist that her son was working regularly with a self-help group and was no longer abusing alcohol or drugs. She said that he had a job, gave her money, and had a nice girlfriend whom he was going to marry and bring to live in the house. He was doing construction to covert it to separate apartments. The mother claimed that her son had always been abused by his older sister and her gang of adolescent girlfriends. She admitted to being physically abused by her former husband, who blamed her for not controlling the children's fights. She denied sexual abuse and the possibility that her daughter might have been abused. She did acknowledge, however, a period in which she had been severely depressed and that she could not be certain of what had occurred during that time.

The patient wanted to hear the details of the therapist's meeting with the mother, and plans were made to review those details with her. She appeared metamorphosed in a black leather miniskirt, black stockings and high-heeled boots, a tight sweater, large dangling earrings, and elaborate makeup and hairdo. She looked like a "hooker." Her response to the session with the mother was to take the train out to her mother's home. She sold her car and angrily demanded to be taken in. Her mother agreed but would not let the daughter bring her dog. Her mother was equally startled by her daughter's appearance, which seemed to represent a regression to her adolescence. The patient, enraged, returned to her temporary quarters and refused to meet jointly with her mother and the therapist. She insisted that she would fend for herself. She wrote several months later to say that she had a full-time job and had returned to her old apartment (which had only been sublet). She also said that she had a new boyfriend. Her mother had persistently called and written, but she ignored the calls and returned the letters unopened. The therapist answered her note and encouraged her to stay in touch. The patient now had an unlisted phone number, but she had no further fears or flashbacks. She was occasionally awakened with the feeling of smothering. She wrote brief notes to the therapist about her progress.

The therapist submitted a sworn affidavit in the matter of her civil suit. The patient's mother called twice: the first time to ascertain that her daughter was all right, and the second time to be sure that a letter that she had sent to the therapist had arrived. The letter was sent to tell the therapist that the daughter had won substantial damages and had come "home" on the occasion of her brother's wedding. She seemed fine, brought her boyfriend, and showed off her new car.

One can only speculate about the extent of her childhood abuse or abusiveness. There was something ominous about her session as "hooker," almost as if she were a "bad seed." On reflection, this might have represented a multiple personality, but this possibility did not occur to the therapist at the time. The patient clearly needed to feel protected and yet independent and important. Her boyfriend, her car, and her large financial award clearly helped to repair her narcissistic injury and her ability to magnanimously attend her brother's wedding.

Stranger Rape With Delayed Response and Intergenerational Sequelae

The patient, a 45-year-old married white nurse with four teenage children, presented with panic attacks of several years' duration that were triggered by obsessive fears that her eldest daughter would be kidnapped, raped, and killed. So intense were the patient's fears that she insisted upon either driving her daughter everywhere or having her daughter phone frequently for check-ins, creating great conflict in the relationship. Prior to the designated telephone check-in times she experienced severe anxiety symptoms and often impulsively called the police. Conversely, she was extremely complacent regarding her youngest daughter's whereabouts, tolerating school absenteeism, drug abuse, and "overnights" with a group of friends who were high school dropouts.

Although initially unaware of its relevance, the patient reported that she had been raped as a nursing student by two men of a different ethnic group who attacked her in a parking garage near the hospital where she worked. She was repeatedly threatened and raped for an hour, and was convinced she would have died had she not developed "street smarts" from working with Puerto Rican patients, which allowed her to communicate and bargain with her rapists. Her husband, a jazz musician, met her in the emergency room, where she was examined and consequently found to be 6 weeks pregnant. Although she intellectually realized that the pregnancy was unrelated to the rape, she suffered severe dissociative symptoms during the pregnancy but did not seek treatment. Her husband, a drug abuser, increased his alcohol consumption during this time and did not support her in reporting her rape, stating that he considered the rapists "brothers" (being of an ethnic group similar to his own) and could not blame them.

After the birth of the first child, the patient was relatively unsymptomatic, and the family moved out of the city to an area that she perceived as safer. The patient, whose husband continued to abuse drugs, was marginally functional. As her daughters gradually entered puberty she advised them to be sexually active, reasoning that they would be more likely to survive a rape if they were not virgins. At the encouragement of her therapist, she began to explore her own rape experience in both individual and couples therapy, where her husband was encouraged to enter a drug program. He became severely depressed upon detoxification but remained in treatment, improved, and was eventually able to explore his unsupportive stance toward his wife's rape and to understand his identification with the aggressor as a defense against feelings of helplessness and guilt.

The patient's anxiety symptoms were contained by antidepressants, and with her husband's help she was able to structure a more reasonable schedule with her oldest daughter and allow her to move away to college. A year after her oldest daughter's departure she presented her youngest daughter for treatment for school absenteeism, psychosomatic complaints, and angry outbursts toward her mother. Although initially resistant to treatment, the youngest daughter acknowledged that she was frightened of people, angry with her mother for her erratic behavior, and alternatively proud or guilt ridden at her ability to "hurt" her mother. Three months into her treatment the youngest daughter revealed that she had been gang raped by a group of friends while drunk at a party. Although she denied any significance to this event, she and her mother are currently exploring its impact in individual and family therapy.

These cases demonstrate both the variety of forms in which rape can occur and the variety of psychological sequelae that can result.

Battered Women

In the past decade a growing body of literature has documented the significant degree of physical aggression directed toward women by men in the context of intimate relationships (Dobash and Dobash 1979[118]; Finkelhor and Yllo 1985[108]; Pirog-Good and Stets 1989[115]; Russell 1982[68]; Russell and Van de Ven 1976[119]; Walker 1979,[120] 1984[121]). According to a random nationwide survey (Straus et al. 1980[122]), 3.8% of (or 1.8 million) American women are beaten annually by their marital partners. Almost half of these women were beaten multiple times, with the criteria for beating including behaviors such as punching, biting, kicking, hitting with an object, and threatening with or use of a knife or gun. When the criteria were expanded to include any physically aggressive behavior such as pushing, grabbing, slapping, shoving, and throwing objects, the percentage rose from 3.8% to 12.1%. Additional prevalence studies that took into account all forms of physical aggression found that the incidence for at least one episode of physical violence annually was 16% (Hornung et al. 1981[123]). If engagement, separation, and divorce relationships are included, the numbers are even higher.

Violence toward young women in the context of social and courtship relationships is extremely high and until recently was a neglected area of study. Existing studies examining the prevalence of dating violence have been reviewed and summarized by Pirog-Good and Stets (1989[115]), who reported that these rates ranged from as low as approximately 20% to as high as 58%.

The presence of violence perpetrated by women against men or of mutual violence is also well documented within intimate relationships (Fleming 1979[124]; Gelles 1972[125]; Straus et al. 1980[122]). However, there are few parallels regarding the clinical significance of violence perpetrated by males against females versus that perpetrated by females against males or mutual violence. The negative physical and psychiatric sequelae of violence affect women almost exclusively, and the severest forms of violence, which include repeated batterings, objectification, and forcible isolation from support, are directed almost exclusively against women (Walker 1979,[120] 1984[121]). Death is not a rare occurrence. In fact, 30% of female homicide victims in the United States are killed by husbands or boyfriends (Federal Bureau of Investigation 1982[126]). Also, unlike men, women encounter severe and repeated cultural, legal, economic, and vocational impediments to leaving violent relationships. In some cases, battered women may actually develop psychological sequelae that interfere with their ability to stop the violence (Hilberman 1980[127]; Walker 1979,[120] 1984[121]).

Thus in this chapter we define battered women as *women who receive physically injurious behavior from men in the context of intimate relationships both current and past*.

Despite the serious negative sequelae to women, battering was not widely recognized by the legal system until the late 1970s; in fact, a husband's right to hit his wife was written into United States law until 1874 (D Martin 1976[128]). Prior to the reforms in the 1970s, police were trained to mediate rather than to treat battering behavior as criminal. Batterers were seldom arrested, and even when they were, they were charged with misdemeanors rather than felonies, which would have been the case had they assaulted strangers rather than intimates. This legal approach often led to an escalation of the violence. According to one study, 85% of spouse assault and homicide cases occurred after at least one previous police intervention. In 50% of these cases the police were called to respond five times previous to the actual homicide (The Police Foundation 1977, cited in the Attorney General's Task Force on Domestic Violence 1984[129]). As a result of this inadequate response, few women reported battering incidents, and those who did risked escalating the violence, with little chance of obtaining legal containment.

Fortunately this approach is being systematically revised. In the early 1980s the Attorney General's Task Force on Domestic Violence (1984[129]) issued recommendations that battering be treated as criminal behavior; that arrest, rather than mediation, be the intervention of choice when serious injury or potential danger to the victim was occurring; and that victims receive legal protection from those who have battered them. Currently the majority of states have passed legislation criminalizing wife battering, and there is now a heightened sense of awareness toward all types of battering. The gap between legislation and appropriate intervention, however, remains, and clinicians treating battered women should be familiar with the local laws and be aware that their patients may be further traumatized by inadequate help from the legal system.

Battered women constitute a widely diverse population representing all socioeconomic classes. (Contrary to current myths, black women are not at more risk [Coley and Beckett 1988[130]].) The circumstances of battering are multidimensional. The victims vary in terms of their individual histories and preabuse status; their relationships, including their relationships with their batterers; the type of battering to which they are exposed; their response to the battering; and the resources available to help them end the battering.

It is important to recognize that the definition of "battered" women has evolved, with documented negative psychiatric sequelae, yet there are no solid data that battering constitutes a unitary phenomenon calling for a specific type of dynamic intervention. Multiple etiologic theories and related interventions have developed, and most of these theories have contributed to our understanding of battering and to the development of effective interventions. These same theories are, however, somewhat inconsistent and contradictory and are lacking solid empirical validation. Empirical studies comparing even the most widely accepted etiologic theories are practically nonexistent. In order to contemplate a reasonable clinical intervention with battered women, it is necessary to have a perspective on the current status of these etiologic theories. Margolin et al. (1988[131]) have divided these theories into three categories: 1) intrapersonal, 2) interpersonal, and 3) sociocultural. An adapted summary of their review is presented in Appendix M.

Because battered women represent a highly diverse group affected by a multiplicity of external factors, it is not possible to approach treatment of these women with a unified psychodynamic formulation. Outlining a more general clinical approach to this population is possible and desirable, however, because many of these women seek psychiatric help and encounter damaging misconceptions and clinical mismanagement during the process of treatment.

Battered women may now be diagnosed formally in one of two standard classifications, either as *adult maltreatment syndrome* (ICD-9-CM 995.81[132]) or as *acute or chronic posttraumatic stress syndrome* (DSM-III-R 309.89[97]). Despite the availability of formal means of classifying this syndrome, battered women still remain widely underdiagnosed. Hilberman (1980[127]) has discussed the covert alliance between uninformed clinicians and silent victims that results in the isolated treatment of symptoms related to battering without proper diagnosis and identification of the battering syndrome and appropriate intervention and protection of the abused woman. Shame, self-blame, hopelessness, unrealistic hopes of controlling the problem, denial, fears of retaliation, issues of family loyalty and privacy, fear of misunderstanding, previous negative treatment experiences—all contribute to underreporting by victims. Persistent beliefs in the low incidence of battering result in a low index of suspicion among clinicians. Subscription to patriarchal values and cultural myths regarding battering and the need to deny, minimize, or distance oneself from the overwhelming savagery of violence, combined with fears of malpractice, severe funding cutbacks, and lack of public support for intervention, all move the clinician toward either underdiagnosis or reluctance to intervene.

Clinicians should be aware of common indirect presentations in battered women. Hilberman (1980[127]) has summarized the formats in which these patients present:

1. Frequent visits to emergency rooms for physical injuries
2. Frequent visits to family physicians with complaints of chronic psy-

chosomatic symptoms, anxiety, insomnia, overuse of tranquilizers, and poor treatment compliance
3. Presentations to psychiatrists with chief complaints of severe anxiety, depression, multiple suicide attempts, marital problems (such as spouse alcohol or economic stresses), chronic substance abuse, psychosomatic pain, and children with somatic complaints, school phobias, enuresis, insomnia, disruptive aggressive behavior, and withdrawal
4. Presentations to psychiatric hospitals with acute suicidality, homicidality, or acute reactive psychosis, usually involving a loss of control of aggressive impulses

Patients presenting in any of these formats should increase the clinician's index of suspicion and result in direct but sensitive questioning about whether anyone is hitting, hurting, slapping, or in any other way injuring them at home. Klingbeil and Boyd (1984[133]) present a detailed questionnaire and intervention format to assist clinicians in the detection and treatment of violence in the emergency room. Also, Dickstein (1988b[134]) has provided a checklist of questions that can be used by clinicians to detect battering and that minimize the shame and guilt for the reporting patient.

Negative countertransference reactions to battered women are common. The clinician's difficulties in dealing with either the savagery or the overwhelming scope of the violence, or with his or her own family history of violence, may result in denial, minimization, rationalization, or distancing of the clinician from the victim. Distancing may take the form of disbelief, blaming the victim, or pigeonholing the victim into a different socioeconomic or racial class. Identification with the aggressor can lead to minimizing the patient's suffering, normalizing the abusive behavior, focusing on the woman's pathology, or otherwise blaming her for the situation. Another form of identification with the aggressor involves the clinician's seeing the woman as helpless and incompetent and attempting heroic interventions in order to rescue her. Fear of malpractice and other reprisals, combined with the often accurate history of the patient's multiple unsuccessful attempts to gain help, may result in overidentification with the patient's helplessness. The battered woman's need to control and manipulate everyone and to see even helpful changes as threatening is often not understood as a form of hypervigilance and an attempt to control the violent cycle. Instead, it often triggers angry, retaliative, or distancing responses in the therapist. Similar reactions occur when victims do not accept help; when they repeatedly return to their abusers; or when therapists inappropriately focus the goals of treatment on the victims' leaving the relationship rather than on emotional growth, development of appropriate self-protective mechanisms, and freedom from abuse-related symptoms (Hilberman 1980[127]; Walker 1984[121]).

Multiple authors (Hilberman 1980[127]; Margolin et al. 1988[131]; Walker 1984[121]) have commented on approaches to treating battered women, some authors focusing on target issues such as lack of self-esteem, fragmentation, loss, anxiety, depression, and learned helplessness, and others presenting more general approaches. In what follows, we present a broad overview focusing on issues specifically relevant to dynamically oriented clinicians.

Both victims and therapists have difficulty realistically confronting the real dangers in battering relationships. In the United States, 20% to 50% of all homicides occur within the family (Hilberman 1980[127]). Thirty percent of female homicide victims are killed by husbands, ex-husbands, or boyfriends (Federal Bureau of Investigation 1982[126]). Ten percent of male homicide victims are killed by spouses (Dobash and Dobash 1979[118]) who are often acting in retaliation. Hilberman (1980[127]) reported a subgroup of battered victims who sustained life-threatening injuries such as subdural hematoma or gunshot wounds to the chest. The author then described a variety of other forms of serious assaults and injuries:

> Assault weapons included hands, feet, fists, rocks, bottles, telephones, iron bars, knives and guns. Scratching, slapping, punching with fists, throwing down, and kicking were prevalent, with faces and breasts the most frequently mentioned sights of assault. These assaults led to multiple bruises, black eyes, fractured ribs, subdural hematomas, and detached

> retinas. Some victims also reported having been strangled and choked until consciousness was impaired. Sexual assaults were common, and women described being beaten and raped in front of the children. Guns were available in most of these homes and were constant threats—some men kept guns in bed to intimidate their wives. We know of one woman who slept with her shoes on to permit a "fast getaway."
>
> Most women reported changes in the pattern of violence during pregnancy. There was increasing abuse for some, with the abdomen replacing the face and breasts as targets for battering. This often led to abortions and premature births. (p. 1340)

Walker (1984[121]) and others have reported on the common tendency of the victim to deny the seriousness of her danger or to unrealistically maintain beliefs that she can control or end the violence. It is therefore essential for the clinician to be well informed regarding risk and prevalence and to question the patient specifically on the nature and seriousness of any reported violence as soon as some rapport and trust have been established. Walker (1984[121]) recommends asking the patient to describe in detail her first battering incident, a typical battering incident, and her last battering incident, including information on weapons available, specific life threats, choking and other life-threatening behavior, and examples of psychological abuse.

Children may also be at risk for battering. Gayford (1975a[135]) reported that 54% of wife batterers also beat their children. Hilberman and Munson (1977–1978[136]) report that one out of three children living in homes where the wife is battered are also battered or sexually abused. Typically, older children who attempt to intervene in order to protect their mothers are especially at risk. If either the woman or her children are assessed as in imminent danger, the therapist must actively help them arrange for emergency housing in a shelter, hospital, or other secure protective environment. It is important to review with the woman the need for extra precautions because batterers often seek out their partners when they attempt to separate and escalate their assaults in the context of this separation. A woman entering therapy after a separation from her batterer should be encouraged to have as little contact with the man as possible, to institute strict legal sanctions against violence, and to obtain strict legal limitations on visitations with the children.

Young women are a largely unacknowledged group at risk for violence in dating/courtship relationships and at group social functions such as college fraternity parties or informal gathering at bars. Roark (1987[137]), in a review of violence on college campuses, noted prevalence rates of 19% to 35%. These women tended to deny, minimize, or internalize blame for their situations and may have had trouble realistically assessing the risk of violence and leaving their abusive boyfriends, instead becoming derailed from important work and educational pathways. At the time of the review, these women were just beginning to seek therapy as an option.

Battered women are also at risk for losing control of their own aggressive impulses in the context of being battered themselves. According to Gayford (1975a[135]), about one-third of battered women beat their children. Suicide attempts, self-mutilations, homicidal retaliation toward their batterers, and acute reactive psychosis with active aggressive components also occur regularly and require emergency hospitalization of the battered woman. For women who are not in an emergency state regarding potential danger and who do not wish to leave their relationship with the batterer, it is important to develop an escape plan to be instituted whenever the violence begins to escalate. The plan should include identifying cues for impending violence and specific details necessary to execute the plan for themselves and their children, with specific rehearsal to make the plan automatic in a crisis. Exploring the options of terminating the relationship in a safe manner, including a review of any of the trouble spots, is also important. Insisting that termination of the relationship be a goal of therapy is inappropriate and unworkable for many women. However, assisting these women in identifying and altering the intrapsychic and external barriers to self-protection is an essential ongoing focus for treatment.

Contemporary experts have found few data to support that women remain in abusive relationships because of their own masochistic tendencies. Gelles (1972,[125] cited in Hilberman 1980[127]) notes three major factors that influence a woman's staying in a battered relationship:

1. The less severe and less frequent the violence, the more likely the woman is to stay.
2. The more a woman was struck by her parents as a child, the more likely she is to stay.
3. The fewer her resources and the less her power, the more probable it is she will stay.

We will review these and other impediments to terminating the relationship in more detail later in this chapter.

Concomitant psychiatric illnesses were found in about half of one sample of battered women (Hilberman 1980[127]). Depression was the primary finding, with manic-depressive illness, schizophrenia, alcoholism, substance abuse, and personality disorders also being reported. In addition, as a sequelae to their battering, many victims experience depressions and stress symptoms similar to those described in the previous section for rape victims. In these instances, a diagnosis of posttraumatic stress disorder should be made and treated specifically, as discussed previously for rape victims. Treatment of additional psychopathology should be offered in the spirit of enhancing the woman's ability to cope effectively with the battering.

In prescribing antidepressants, sedatives, and other agents, serious consideration should be taken of the battered woman's significant risk for overdose and the possibility that medication which decreases the woman's vigilance or enhances her sleep when she must be alert to protect herself may result in serious injury. Also, care should be taken to defer secondary psychiatric diagnoses until the symptoms can be clarified as separate from battering characteristics. It has not been uncommon to confuse battering characteristics with characteristics of borderline personality disorder, schizophrenia, and other psychopathological states, only to have the symptoms dissipate when the battering has been contained (Hilberman 1980[127]; Walker 1984[121]).

When acute danger and severe symptoms have been stabilized, the therapist must help the woman assess the intrapsychic and external factors that either inhibit battering or facilitate constructive solutions to being battered. As Gondolf and Fisher (1988[138]) emphasize, many battered women have extraordinary coping and help-seeking skills as well as many intrapsychic strengths that can be mobilized. Talents, education, job skills, conscientious family and friends, and access to legal, educational, vocational and economic supports are also strengths. Conversely, lack of these assets combined with fears regarding homicidal retaliation by the batterer is a realistic inhibitor to the battered woman's moving from the violent relationship. The therapist should help the woman to respect how these impediments have hindered her.

Intrapsychic impediments such as depression, psychotic states, and severe stress reactions are also significant. Some theoretical intrapsychic impediments have been formulated. Lenore Walker's theory of learned helplessness as it applies to battered women involves the postulation that with repeated batterings the woman's cognitive ability to believe in the efficacy of her actions is severely distorted (Walker 1984[121]).

Traumatic regressions, sometimes designated as traumatic psychological infantism, may also impede adequate coping. Another postulation focuses on the principle of traumatic bonding, in which the victim develops a positive and intense attachment to her oppressor in the context of intermittent abuse. Krugman (1987[98]) provides an excellent discussion of how traumatic bonding, anxious attachment, poor self-esteem, and lack of resources trap battered women and how trauma impacts on the entire family structure across generations. Additional intrapsychic focuses for therapy have included the following: 1) poor self-esteem, 2) emotional isolation and mistrust, and 3) fear of loss of control of aggressive impulses.

Combining work on the intrapsychic problem areas with identifying possible life alternatives can help a woman formulate a coping plan. Reviewing the following potential resources can be helpful in this context:

- Medical facilities for reproductive control and medical care
- Social service agencies for financial aid, housing, shelter, and child services
- Criminal justice agencies for obtaining legal sanction against further violence and legal aid for assistance with separation/divorce agreements
- Vocational rehabilitation programs
- Women's groups for support and information

Specific precautions must be taken with women who begin to assume a more assertive life stance, because this behavior may often escalate the abuser's violent behavior. Couples work has also been investigated (Geller and Wasserman 1984[139]; Neidig and Friedman 1984[140]), but there is much disagreement regarding its efficacy. Walker (1984[121]) and others have stated the importance of assuming couples work after the traumatic bonding has been broken and the man and woman can enter the treatment as individuals. A firm understanding of how the violence will be contained during the couples work is also necessary.

Although it is conceivable that some battered women have specific forms of character disorder that should be treated with specific psychodynamic formulations, a single psychodynamic formulation for battered women has not been identified and seems unlikely given the diversity of this population. In a recent review of psychodynamic and psychoanalytic perspectives on family violence, Susan McLeer (1988[141]) has commented on both the usefulness of psychoanalytic constructs in formulating hypotheses regarding family violence and the necessity for obtaining confirmational data. She stresses that the psychoanalytic model provides a valid method of inferences regarding mental functioning when applied to closed systems such as the psychoanalytic situation, but that its validity is reduced when it is applied to open systems such as battering situations. McLeer both praises and cautions with a quotation from Charcot: "The theory is good. It must not be a barrier to the realities of existence" (Charcot, cited in Freud 1893/1953[142]).

We shall now proceed to case material demonstrating a woman at risk for battering and a battered woman who was sexually molested as a child and exhibited self-mutilating behavior as an adult.

Averting of a Potential Battering Situation

A professional woman in her 30s requested a transfer to a branch office when her husband, a free-lance writer, relocated to a full-time position. When she arrived some months after her husband had relocated, she found that he had been enjoying his brief return to single life. He suggested that he preferred that life and that the two should consider separating. Becoming panicky and significantly depressed, the woman sought treatment.

It became clear that while formerly her husband had been much the house husband dependent on her income, now he could be "footloose" and independent. He found himself criticized for his after-hours "fun" with "guys doing the bar scene." This conflict, although in part reflecting the patient's attitudes, was anticipated or projected on the basis of the husband's family history. His father was an alcoholic who was constantly being criticized by his wife, the son's mother. She, in turn, set her son up to be punished for daily misdemeanors by the inebriated and enraged father. The son sowed some wild oats in a rebellious adolescence, and it was repeatedly intimated that he was a bad seed and that no good would come of him.

The patient's mother had been married to an alcoholic who threatened abuse but did not physically harm the family. The patient, however, remembers her sister being chased to her room and the father physically damaging the door. After the patient's parents were divorced, the mother began living with another alcoholic man who did physically abuse her and cause her bodily harm. Nevertheless, she married him after a number of years and lived with him for a considerable time. The patient remembers her hypervigilance and her fear for her mother's safety, sometimes sitting in the stairwell waiting to call the police. With some amount of shame, the patient recalled a relationship with a boyfriend at school in which alcohol was a significant problem for both of them. Although physically abused in that relationship, she feared leaving it and being alone but felt less panicky and dependent than her mother confessed to feeling at the prospect of separating from her second husband. The patient's investment in her school career ultimately led her to leave her abusing relationship. She then met her husband, who dabbled in street drugs and at times became intoxicated with alcohol but was never violent.

During the course of her treatment, the patient recognized that she was often drinking too much with her husband. This behavior stopped in a brief time. Cleared of her intermittent substance abuse, she realized the part she had played in keeping her husband passive and dependent. She also became aware of her own angry, demeaning, demanding behavior, which was like that of both her mother and her mother-in-law. She recognized the contrast of this behavior to her nonassertiveness at work that led to her being overloaded. Later, she took this a step further. She began to be more assertive and less anxious in her business negotiations. At the same time, by getting off her husband's back, he was able to recognize on his own that hangovers and blackouts were no fun for him.

Both partners have now reached a better reconciliation with their families of origin. The patient is able to approach her father in a positive way so that he no longer becomes intoxicated and spoils those holidays they spend together. The couple has started to discuss beginning their own family. The patient's husband has become more open and introspective and has revealed a history of violence toward a younger sibling. Both the patient and her husband are, however, aware of the dangers of repeating victimization and battering in their prospective family.

Battering in a Woman Who Was Sexually Molested During Childhood

A 39-year-old college graduate was married to a prominent politician and worked part time as a publicity agent to keep herself busy since she had no children. Although chronically depressed, she entered treatment because of escalating agoraphobic and depressive episodes consisting of suicidal thoughts and self-mutilating behavior. These episodes occurred in the context of her husband's recent rise from local to state political prominence, which required her to be more "visible" and also to tolerate his absence from home as his career demanded more travel.

The initial approach to therapy was supportive, symptom focused, and psychopharmacological. Couples therapy was also instituted so that the couple could focus on the dual career demands and on helping the husband to understand his wife's problems and to support her treatment. The patient initially improved, but 6 months into treatment she experienced a panic attack in the context of explaining the meaning of her initial self-mutilating symptoms and wondering aloud at her lack of childhood memories. Over the next 2 years of treatment she derepressed memories of severe and persistant sexual and physical abuse by her father occurring in the context of her mother being chronically debilitated and bedridden with Crohn's disease. Although the patient attended sessions with religious regularity, she canceled therapy for two 10-day periods during this time, on each of these occasions maintaining telephone contact with her therapist and reporting severe agoraphobic symptoms that appeared to be related to the derepression of particularly traumatic material.

During her third year of treatment she again reported agoraphobic symptoms and missed two sessions but returned to therapy sooner than in previous episodes. Upon her return her therapist noted a red mark on her cheek and asked her directly what had happened and if she had been self-mutilating. Over the course of several sessions, she reluctantly revealed that in the context of a marital quarrel, her husband had slapped, punched, kicked, and sodomized her and that this behavior had been occurring episodically 1 to 2 times a year since their marriage began. She stated that she did not report this in therapy initially because she did not consider it serious and that, although she never struck back, she assumed she was responsible because she was verbally provocative.

Later, when she realized the significance of this violence in the context of her past history, she opted to cancel sessions, feeling too ashamed to report this "sick situation" to her therapist and also fearful that her husband would withdraw his financial support of her treatment. Reluctantly she agreed to share this information with her couples therapist, who scheduled an extra session to discuss the episode and formulate a safety plan should violence occur again. Her husband's initial response was to be compliant in therapy but angry and abusive at home. This situation necessitated the institution of the safety plan, which the patient was able to carry out with the treatment team's support. Individual sessions with her husband conducted by the couples therapist involved his accepting a referral for individual therapy, and over the next year the couple were able to mutually work together to stop the violence.

These cases demonstrate the variety of situations in which battering can occur, the variety of outcomes that can be accomplished with psychodynamic interventions, and the tragic and lethal potential of uninterrupted battering situations.

Sexual Exploitation in Professional Relationships

Along with recent documentation of the prevalence and serious psychiatric sequelae of incest and other forms of sexual abuse of female children is emerging a parallel documentation and clarification of an adult version of this earlier form of sexual exploitation—namely, sexual exploitation in professional relationships, a phenomenon that has also been documented to affect predominantly women (Akamatsu 1988[143]; Borys and Pope 1989[144]; Gartrell et al. 1986a,[145] 1988[146]; Glaser and Thorpe 1986[147]; Holroyd and Brodsky 1977[148]; Kardener et al. 1973[149]; Pope et al. 1979,[150] 1986,[151] 1987[152]). By this we mean sexual activity, either consensual or nonconsensual, between a woman and a man with whom she has a *fiduciary* relationship, that is, a relationship "where there is a special confidence reposed in one who in equity and good conscience is bound, and in good faith, and with due regard, to the interests of the one reposing the confidence" (Black 1979,[153] pp. 753–754). A wide spectrum of professional relationships fall within this legal definition. Psychiatrists, psychologists, social workers, sex therapists, pastoral and other independent counselors, mental health workers, and nurses who perform psychotherapy and counseling or who work with patients in psychiatric inpatient settings are most widely recognized as being in a position to sexually exploit their patients because of the emotionally intimate nature of their work. Nonpsychiatric physicians, clergymen, chiropractors, attorneys, and dentists are similarly situated, but for slightly different reasons. These latter individuals are in positions where physical and/or emotional intimacy is sanctioned and necessary. They interact with women during vulnerable periods, from a position of power. Other potentially exploitive relationships include teachers, supervisors, professors, advisors, mentors, and bosses. These relationships are potentially exploitive because of the unequal power differential involved, the tendency to idealize these individuals, and the intensity of affect that may develop in intimate work and learning situations.

The degree to which this phenomenon has been explored, documented, and addressed within the professions varies tremendously. Formal research has documented the prevalence of sexual exploitation in the fields of psychiatry (Gartrell et al. 1986a[145]), psychology (Holroyd and Brodsky 1977[148]; Pope et al. 1979,[150] 1986,[151] 1987[152]), and social work (Gechtman and Bouhoutsos 1985[154]), mostly during the past 15 years. A 1984 survey of Wisconsin psychotherapists (Kuchan 1989[155]) included a sampling of clergy, alcohol and drug counselors, nurses, occupational therapists, and nonlicensed mental health aides. However, large-scale definitive studies of these and other relevant professional groups are still lacking. Psychologists, psychiatrists, social workers, and pastoral counselors have ethical codes banning such exploitive behavior and rendering practitioners liable for their acts. Other professionals, such as chiropractors and attorneys, do not. Educational institutions vary widely in their approach. Some provide clear guidelines for faculty regarding professional behavior and well-defined internal complaint procedures to protect students and trainees from exploitation, while others provide just enough information to comply with the Equal Employment Opportunities Commission (EEOC) guidelines. Institutions and corporations employing professionals are in the earlier stages of providing guidelines for professional conduct, and institutional complaint procedures are similarly underdeveloped. The degree to which corporations and institutions may be liable for sexually exploitive behaviors of their professional employees has not yet been well established in the courts despite EEOC guidelines and civil rights laws designed to protect individuals from this more extreme form of sexual harassment.

In this section we will provide information regarding the prevalence and nature of sexual exploitation in professional relationships, the legal implications relevant to professionals treating this type of sexual exploitation, the dynamic formulations that have been proposed to explain these phenomena, the negative psychiatric sequelae of such interactions, and appropriate treatment interventions for victims.

Although data have been collected since the 1960s, professional organizations discouraged the publication of such data, and it has only been in the 1970s and 1980s that prevalence data achieved publication status. Data available in the fields of psychiatry, psychology, and, more recently, social work allow for some comparison. Definitive data for other professions based on large-scale studies have yet to be accumulated.

The most recent study of psychiatrists was performed in 1985 by Gartrell et al. (1986a,[145] 1989[156]), who surveyed 5,574 psychiatrists via mailing and received a 20% response rate. Despite this low response rate, their data were consistent with earlier studies performed by Kardener et al. (1973[149]) and with studies of psychologists (Holroyd and Brodsky 1977[148]; Pope et al. 1979[150]), all of which had considerably higher response rates. The gender distribution in Gartrell et al.'s study was also similar to that of the population of psychiatrists in the United States. Their survey revealed a wide range of information concerning the prevalence and patterns of exploitation and the attitudes and characteristics of the exploiters, some of which is summarized as follows.

Of the respondents, 6.4% "acknowledged having had sexual contact with their own patients" (p. 7). Offenders were more likely to be male, to have completed an accredited residency, and to have undergone personal therapy or psychoanalysis. A small minority of the offenders were residents at the time of their inappropriate behavior. Two-thirds (66.7%) of the offenders were involved with only one patient. The remainder were multiple offenders, with the largest number of patients reported being 12. All offenders who admitted to multiple contacts were male. Only 3.5% of the offenders were female psychiatrists exploiting male patients, and 1.4% were female psychiatrists exploiting female patients. The patients ranged in age from 20 to 48 years, and 87% of the exploited patients were female. In approximately 75% of the cases, the sexual contact included genital contact, and in the remaining cases the sexual contact consisted of kissing, fondling, and undressing. Twenty-five percent of the offenders were pleased to have had the contact, 35% had mixed feelings, and 40% regretted the contact. A larger percentage of female offenders (50%) than of male offenders (38.9%) regretted their sexual contact. One-time offenders did not differ from repeat offenders in their overall assessment of the contact: 18% of the offenders reported sexual contact during therapy sessions, 17% indicated contact outside of therapy but concurrent with the treatment, and 69% stated that the contact occurred after termination. Forty-one percent of the offenders consulted colleagues because of their sexual involvement. Repeat offenders were less likely to seek consultation than one-time offenders. Also, 1.6% of the respondents indicated that they had been sexually involved with their own therapist or analyst. A majority of those exploited by their own therapist were female. Of the psychiatrists who were exploited during their own treatment program, the overwhelming majority reported that the experience was negative. In contrast, the majority of the offenders acknowledged that they engaged in the sexual contact for their own sexual or emotional gratification. They also believed that the patient with whom they were involved had predominantly positive feelings about this contact.

Data for psychologists, as reviewed by Brodsky (1989[157]), are similar in profile to those for psychiatrists. In 1977, Holroyd and Brodsky (1977[148]) surveyed a random sample of 1,000 licensed psychologists and received a 70% response rate. The results indicated that 5.5% of the males and 0.6% of the females admitted to having engaged in sexual intercourse with patients; 10% of males and 1% of females admitted to other types of erotic practices. Eighty percent were repeat offenders, despite frequent comments by offending practitioners that their behaviors were not perceived as beneficial but, rather, harmful. In a later report, Holroyd and Brodsky (1980[158]) correlated nonerotic touching that was selective toward one sex only with actual sexual exploitation in practitioners. In 1979, Pope et al. (1979[150]) surveyed members of the psychotherapy division of the American Psychological Association and found an incidence rate of sex with clients of 7%. In 1986 a mail survey by Pope et al.[151] yielded a 6.5% admission of sexual contact with clients, and a more recent survey of psychologists (Pope et al. 1987[152]) showed a striking decline in prevalence of subjects reporting sexual contact with clients to only 1.9%. The California State Psychological Association (CSPA) polled therapists regarding information the organization had about patients who had had sex with former therapists (Bouhoutsos et al. 1983[159]). Ninety-two percent of the relationships with former therapists were reported to be between male therapists and female patients. The mean age for the practitioner was 42 years and for the patient, 30 years. The CSPA reported the negative sequelae as follows: increased depression, loss of motivation, impaired social adjustment, suicidal intent, increased substance abuse, hospitalizations, decline in intimate relationships, and mistrust of the opposite sex and of therapists (Brodsky 1989, p. 19[157]).

Offender characteristics have been gleaned from the above studies. Offenders are primarily male and primarily middle aged and approximately 16 years older than their patient victims. They are often involved in unsatisfactory love relationships, have predominantly female patients, are likely to be involved with more than one patient at a time, violate other treatment boundaries, and tend to be isolated professionally (Brodsky 1989[157]).

Unlike psychiatrists and psychologists, social workers show a significantly lower prevalence. Gechtman and Bouhoutsos (1985[154]) randomly surveyed social workers and received a 54% response rate. The following findings emerged. The attitudes of social workers were overwhelmingly against erotic contact between therapist and client. However, 2% of the social workers who responded thought that such contact could be beneficial, and 8% were unsure. Erotic contact during the course of therapy was reported by 1.3% of the respondents and by an additional 0.6% after termination of the therapy. Sexual intercourse during the course of therapy was reported by 1.0% and after termination by another 0.1%. All positive responders were male. The overall prevalence of male social workers having erotic contact with clients during the course of therapy or after the termination of therapy was 3.8%. The majority of these contacts were with female clients, and all offenders had at least a master's degree in social work or a more advanced academic degree. Half of the offenders had had their own personal therapy. The majority of offenders expressed a clear opinion that their activities had been destructive. (These findings are adapted from Gechtman 1989,[160] pp. 27–33.)

In all three professions—psychiatry, psychology, and social work—the incidence of reporting of sexual violations and malpractice suits against therapists for sexual exploitation has increased in the past decade.

The treatment of victims of sexual exploitation by professionals occurs in a legal context that directly impacts the therapy. A detailed discussion of the relevent legal issues is presented in Appendix N.

Along with the revelation of the prevalence of sexual exploitation in professional relationships have come both information and controversy regarding the nature of the interaction between the woman and the abusive professional. Some clinicians maintain that any discussion of dynamics immediately shifts blame and responsibility to the woman and away from her exploitive professional partner, while others continue to focus treatment on the woman's psychodynamics and fail to sufficiently validate the trauma and negative psychiatric consequences of the professional's behavior. It is our contention that in order to obtain the maximum benefit from psychodynamic intervention, both of these viewpoints must be understood and integrated into the clinical approach.

First and foremost, sexual exploitation within professional relationships represents a serious boundary violation, and the negative psychological sequelae have been well documented (Apfel and Simon 1985a,[161] 1985b[162]; Barnhouse 1978[163]; Bouhoutsos et al. 1983[159]; Carr and Robinson 1990[164]; Collins et al. 1978[165]; Feldman-Summers and Jones 1984[166]; Kluft 1989[167]; Pope 1988[168]; Schoener et al. 1984[169]). The professional in the dyad is solely and completely responsible for maintaining appropriate boundaries, regardless of the sexual willingness or seductiveness of the female. In the psychotherapy relationship, the therapist has the additional responsibility of assisting the woman in understanding the meaning of any seductive behavior she may be exhibiting and the way in which attempts at seducing her therapist can be destructive to her sexually and to her ultimate growth. These seductive behaviors, when they exist, are not always sadistic or manipulative but instead are often repetitious expressions of old sexual exploitation by fathers or other male authority or parental figures, or attempts to achieve closeness and nurturance via sexual means.

Therapy should both validate and treat any traumatic and negative consequences of the professional's behavior as well as clarify the professional's responsibility in maintaining boundaries. Any psychodynamic issues that either led the woman to encourage sexual boundary violations on the part of a professional or rendered her unable to effectively assert and protect her boundaries must also be explored at some point—not so she can be blamed, but so that these issues can be resolved, leaving her in an empowered position in which she is able to prevent further incidents of violation. By this we do not mean to imply that all women who are exploited must have had some preexisting victim profile. Schoener et al. (1989[170]), in the most comprehensive review of this topic known to us, remind us that exploitation can happen to anyone and that there are no data demonstrating a particular victim profile. If there is contributing psychopathology, however, it should certainly be addressed at the appropriate time in any subsequent therapy rather than ignored in a misguided attempt not to blame the victim.

Furthermore, understanding of the dynamics of the perpetrator is essential to cut through ingrained rationalizations of unprofessional behavior, to prevent focusing psychopathology solely on the victim, and to understand how the perpetrator has impacted on the victim. In this spirit we present both the dynamics of the perpetrator and those of the victim. Useful information regarding the interaction in a sexually exploitive professional relationship has come from a variety of sources. It has focused on various aspects of the relationship and has sprung from differing as well as overlapping theoretical foundations. We summarize below some of the most current clinically oriented material.

Pope and Bouhoutsos (1986[171]) have identified 10 interactional scenarios by which mental health professionals become sexually involved with their patients. Some of these routes may be applicable to other professional relationships as well.

1. In the *role trading scenario* the therapist becomes the patient and his or her needs become the focus of the psychotherapy. Therapists experiencing difficulties in their marriage or in other close relationships, or who are exposed to both developmental life stressors and professional stress, are particularly vulnerable to this scenario.
2. In the *sex therapy scenario* the therapist presents sexual intimacy with the patient as a valid approach to treatment.

3. In the *as if scenario* the patient treats the positive transference as though it were indicative of a real situation rather than a manifestation of transference.
4. In the *Svengali scenario* the therapist creates an exaggerated dependency and then proceeds to exploit this dependency in the therapy.
5. In the *drug scenario*, drugs are used to render the patient more compliant and vulnerable or as a means of blackmailing the patient into being available for sexual favors in return for providing the drugs.
6. In the *rape scenario*, physical force, threats, and intimidation are employed by the therapist.
7. In the *true love scenario* the therapist either rationalizes or truly loses boundaries in such a way that the intensity of emotional interactions overrides the professional nature of the relationship and the professional responsibilities to the woman (see Chapter 4).
8. In the *"It just got out of hand" scenario*, the therapist denies or fails to address in a therapeutic manner an escalating level of emotional intimacy occurring within the therapy situation.
9. In the *time out scenario* the therapist creates an artificial and unreal boundary between the therapy session, what goes on in the treatment, and an outside personal relationship that is treated as though it can run parallel with the therapy. This may also be a common scenario in boss/mentor boundary violations in which the rationalization is that independent personal and professional relationships can run parallel.
10. In the *"Hold me"* scenario the therapist exploits and sexualizes the patient's basic desire for physical contact that is nurturing, not erotic.

Kluft (1989[167]) recently described two additional scenarios:

11. In the *special scenario* the therapist convinces the patient that their relationship is so special that it does not fall under the usual rules of ethical conduct, or the therapist narcissistically places himself as above and beyond conventional mores and constraints.

12. In the *blackmail scenario* the therapist exploits a patient's previous incestuous or molestation history. Using the patient's sense of blame and shame, he attempts to blackmail her into compliance to sexual activity by covertly or overtly threatening to reveal her past and all her badness.

There have been several relatively recent discussions of possible underlying dynamic formulations that can be used to explain these scenarios. The psychodynamic and psychoanalytic literature contains many individual works highlighting aspects of erotic transferences, various boundary violations within therapy, impulsive sexual acting out within therapy, and narcissistic pathology in therapists. Current formulations attempting to illuminate the specific dynamics of sexual exploitation of professional relationships have utilized some of this early material as well as material specific to each of these types of interactions. Several formulations have been proposed in the current literature, none of which are all-encompassing or totally useless, and many of which overlap. Four of the most prominent models are presented below.

Sydney Smith (1989[172]) presents a formulation that involves understanding the historical circumstances from which women and their professional perpetrators come. Smith believes that women who are sexually exploited in a professional context come from one of two circumstances:

1. They have been sexually abused during childhood, usually by the father or a father-substitute, and they have experienced intense sexual feelings toward these figures so that developmental childhood longings become fused with sexual significance.
2. They come from a background of neglect, lack of love and appreciation, obliviousness, isolation, and ostracization, and have grown to believe that they are unlovable and unworthy.

These women enter treatment often with latent depression that is chronic and with intense wishes for a magical cure. Male perpetrators are characterized by strong needs for control and dominance, usually beginning with the need for psychological subjugation and escalating to the need for physical subjugation. If dominance is not the issue for the professional, Smith feels that the therapist is struggling with his own psychological problems and tensions, leaving him vulnerable to confiding personal problems to the patient, role reversal, and mutual nontherapeutic dependence.

Smith further believes that the sexual exploitation occurs in the context of a regressive syndrome in which the woman returns to an infantile state that leaves her with the conviction that she is a helpless figure who cannot assert her strength in the face of her treater or escape his psychological hold. Childhood fears of abandonment reappear and assume monumental proportions in the transference. The therapist has come to represent magical capacities of the early father, both idealized and feared or a source of punishment, who has the power to discard the patient. Concomitant with this regression in the patient, the therapist interacts to move the regression in one of two directions; he either becomes a sexual lover merged with a father figure, which deepens the patient's regression, or he becomes a sadistic punisher who can discard and abandon the patient at will.

Twemlow and Gabbard (1989[173]) view abusing therapists in three broad categories: 1) the psychotic, 2) the antisocial, and 3) the lovesick. The first two categories are self-explanatory. The third, or lovesick therapist, is a broad category subsuming normal individuals through individuals with personality disorders. The authors cite the data of Gartrell et al. (1986a[145]), who reported that many offenders state that they have been in love with their patients and believed it was mutual. Twemlow and Gabbard define *lovesickness* as an altered state of consciousness characterized by an affect-dominated state of mind that contrasts but can coexist with the ordinary language-dominated state of mind. This latter concept explains why many therapists can maintain selfobject differentiation and conduct reasonable psychotherapy during one patient's session and have sex and feel passionately fused during the next patient's session. The authors further elaborate on specific phenomenological features of lovesickness:

1. *Emotional dependence* in which the need for one another is so great that the parties will do anything in each other's presence to evoke eternal images when they are apart, creating a state of intense mutual emotional dependency
2. *Intrusive thinking* that is characterized by constant intrusive thoughts of the love object, often involving extensive fantasies in which the love object is idealized and reality denied
3. *Physical sensations*, such as buoyancy, pounding pulse, dryness in the mouth, and tremulousness, that occur in the physical presence of the partner or when the partner's mental image is created
4. A *sense of incompleteness* in which the lovesick couple feel that they are not whole human beings without each other, each member of the dyad being imbued with only positive and idealized traits
5. *Social proscription* involving excitement and dedication to the relationship heightened by risk-taking behavior and intensified by social taboos or unavailability of the partner
6. *Altered states of consciousness* in which ego functions involving judgment and reality testing are altered in such a way that the partners cannot realistically assess their status and the risks of their relationship

Diverging from earlier psychodynamic formulations of lovesick states based on oedipal issues, Twemlow and Gabbard focus on the dyadic rather than the triadic and competitive nature of these relationships, pointing out that whole object relations are not present in lovesickness as they are in the acting out of oedipal issues. The authors conceive a lovesick relationship as a part self representation connected with a part object representation in which only the idealized aspects of self and object exist.

Although Twemlow and Gabbard focus primarily on the dynamics of the therapist, they imply that the patient can become either equally locked into the lovesick dyad or very uncomfortable with it but unable to extricate herself. Citing the works of Gabbard and Menninger (1988[174]), Vaillant et al. (1972[175]), and Buie (1982–1983[176]), they note that the therapist may be propelled toward lovesickness by long denied yearnings for love and nurturance that are gratified by feeding the patient the same love for which the therapist longs.

Searles (1979[177]) has suggested another etiology of the therapist's thwarted omnipotent strivings: that when ordinary techniques fail to cure, sexual relationships are instituted in desperation. That most sexual activity begins almost immediately in the relationship, however, does not validate this as a common etiology.

Narcissistic problems are posed as another etiology for the lovesick state (Finell 1985[178]). Therapists may long for selfobjects who will mirror them and thereby help them maintain a cohesive sense of self (Claman 1987[179]). Therapeutic interactions in which an immediate attraction is felt may reflect narcissistic experiences through which the therapist feels he is seeing himself in another person. This sense of instant rapport and connection may evolve from some actual mutual life experiences or may occur via projective identification in which the therapist projects aspects of himself into the patient, who may then respond as though she actually is the projected self representation. When therapist and patient are mutually involved in such dyads, there is an unconscious perception that each can satisfy the needs or relieve a conflict in the other. Sometimes the need involves an intense desire to reunite with a split-off aspect of oneself. (Rutter's [1989[180]] elaboration on this type of phenomenon will be presented below.)

Twemlow and Gabbard (1989[173]) conclude their analysis by making a distinction between normal lovesickness and pathological lovesickness. Perverseness is the key element in the differentiation. Drawing on the works of Stoller (1985[181]), the authors define the sexual excitement of the abusing therapist as stemming from an awareness that he is sinning and taking extraordinary risks. His perverse wishes to harm, humiliate, degrade, and be cruel to his patient (and on a deeper level himself) may be conscious or repressed, or split off or disavowed; however, unless he is psychotic or antisocial, there is always some measure of observing ego, by which the therapist is aware that the relationship is incestuous and that he is damaging both his patient and his career.

A third conceptual formulation is offered by Rutter (1989[180]), who combines aspects of cultural stereotyping with the intrapsychic processes of projective identification. He focuses on the notion that both men and women are socialized to split off certain aspects of themselves.

Women are split off from their sense of assertiveness, competitiveness, and power, and men are split off from their feelings of vulnerability and wishes for intimacy. Rutter contends that both men and women are wounded in special unique ways as children and that the sexually exploitative unions that occur in therapy and other professional relationships are often attempts to heal these wounds or to be reunited with the split-off aspects of the self. He groups the patterns of feminine woundedness that put women at risk for sexual exploitation as follows:

1. Overt childhood sexual or psychological intrusion resulting in adult difficulties in maintaining control of physical and psychological boundaries
2. Profound neglect and childhood aloneness resulting in inappropriate and often sexualized adult attention-seeking behavior and difficulty setting limits on abusive attention
3. Exploited compassion in women who were socialized to care for other members of the family and have a highly developed sense of empathy and responsibility toward others, which, when combined with the therapist's vulnerabilities or needs, can result in a role reversal
4. Devalued outer-world potential in women who are restricted by cultural and family stereotypes to focusing on homemaking and nurturing activities. [These women are inhibited in developing a sense of their more assertive, competitive potential for expressing their intellectual, artistic, vocational, and other outer-world focused activities, and become at risk for involving themselves in relationships with men who promise to help them develop these heretofore inhibited aspects of themselves.

Rutter defines the wounds of men as stemming from cultural inhibitions or problematic relationships with fathers and mothers. He believes that men are culturally encouraged to split off feelings of weakness, vulnerability, sensitivity, and intimacy, and are also encouraged to act out aggressive sexual fantasies without necessarily connecting empathically with the woman. Rutter feels that father/son relationships that focus on the establishment of patriarchal authority and nonintimacy only compound these cultural inhibitions. Relationships with mothers and sons involving intrusive merging or deprivation also play a primary role. In merging mother/son relationships, the son may be left with profound feelings of anger toward women for rendering him powerless, or he may have difficulty understanding that women may have different needs from his. Deprivational, uninvolved mothers cause low self-esteem and attempts to recoup through power relationships with women. A variation of this model involves a mother who is injured and emotionally crippled herself and ignores her son's needs but involves him in a caretaking role toward her, leaving the son feeling overwhelmed and exploited. When sons are witness to mothers who are abused by fathers, they may identify with their fathers, or they may model themselves after their fathers via identification with the aggressor and become angry with women for being powerless and unable to protect themselves. Via the mechanism of projective identification, men and women may become involved in professionally exploitive relationships in order to link themselves with split-off, devalued, or bad aspects of themselves, and thus satisfy a deep inner need or resolve a conflict. They may also reenact childhood scenarios of abuse.

Kluft (1989[167]) provides a final model that is based on his emphasis on the number of women who have previous histories of incest or sexual molestation in childhood prior to entering an exploitive professional relationship. According to Kluft, the characteristics of incest victims—namely, their propensity to keep secrets, accept blame, defensively idealize the perpetrator, tolerate abuse and neglect, hang onto the relationship at all costs, and experience themselves as powerless and dependent in relationship with male authorities—make them prime targets for revictimization. He defines four distinct clusters of characteristics:

1. Severe symptoms and problematic traits consisting of overvaluation of attachment to the therapist, regressive dependency, increased vulnerability, dissociative defenses, compromised perceptions and ego strengths, external locus of control, and tendency for misdiagnosis and further misunderstanding

2. Idiosyncratic dynamic determinants leading to sexual seductions in therapy as expressions of repetition compulsion, abusive reenactment attempts to actualize fantasies, resistance to approaching threatening material, reaction formations against anger, hostile acts, attempts at fusing and controlling therapist, and rejection and castration of the therapist
3. Object relations and family dynamics involving anxious attachments in which preoccupation with the state of attachment to others takes precedence over self care and self interest [There is also the need to transform their experiences to meet with the standards imposed by family loyalty and secrecy. Accommodation must be made to a version of reality in which the child, and then woman, must abandon her sense of self and reality in the interests of survival and acceptance.]
4. Deformation of the observing ego and debased cognition in which the trauma disrupts cognitive maturation, leading to cognitive distortions and misperceptions of events, along with preoccupation with anticipating and containing the abuse, which in essence results in the victim's taking responsibility for the abusive behavior

Although the four dynamic formulations for patient/therapist sexual relationships presented do not represent a complete review of current ideology, they are representative of the most prominent conceptual models. Each of the models both overlaps and differs from the other models, and no single model can hope to explain all exploitive pairings. Although sexual exploitation in nontherapy professional relationships has not been as well studied, descriptive scenarios of exploitive professors (Dziech and Weiner 1984[182]) and clergy (Rassieur 1976[183]) can be fit into these formulations.

Negative consequences of sexual exploitation in professional relationships have been documented both by surveys of victims who report negative consequences and by descriptions from clinicians who have treated these victims (Apfel and Simon 1985a[161], 1985b[162]; Barnhouse 1978[163]; Bouhoutsos et al. 1983[159]; Carr and Robinson 1990[164]; Collins et al. 1978[165]; Dahlberg 1970[184]; Feldman-Summers and Jones 1984[166]; Kluft 1989[167]; Pope 1988[168]; Schoener et al. 1984[169]).

Pope (1988[168]) has proposed 10 major damaging aspects:

1. Unresolvable ambivalence toward the abusive therapist
2. Guilt and responsibility for the sexual involvement
3. Negative impact on the sense of self and the self in relation to others, leading to feelings of emptiness and isolation
4. Sexual confusion
5. Inability to trust
6. Identity, boundary, and role confusion
7. Emotional lability or dyscontrol characterized by episodic anxiety and rage, depression, and panic
8. Suppressed rage
9. Increased suicide risk
10. Cognitive dysfunction characterized by disturbances of concentration and attention, intrusive thoughts, nightmares, and flashbacks

Apfel and Simon (1985a[161]) provide a similar listing of negative sequelae, including the following:

1. Ambivalence toward treaters and treatments, leading to difficulty in accepting help
2. Impaired confidence of reality testing and sanity
3. Repetition of pathological childhood situations
4. Bondage to a therapist
5. Exacerbation of original symptoms, including sexual dysfunction
6. Difficulties with intimacy
7. Rage and desire for revenge toward men
8. Excessive guilt and shame
9. Constricted use of imagination
10. Disorganization and crisis secondary to abrupt terminations in therapy

Schoener et al. (1984[169]) provide a final listing of negative responses:

1. Guilt and shame
2. Grief and mourning

3. Anger/rage
4. Depression and lowered self-esteem
5. Ambivalence and confusion
6. Fear
7. Serious problems with trust

The degree to which women exploited in professional relationships exhibit posttraumatic stress symptomatology, particularly those women with previous histories of incest, has been well documented (Kluft 1989[167]; Pope 1988[168]). Psychic numbing, dissociation, and withdrawal interspersed with periods of intrusive flashbacks, intensive affective episodes, and high anxiety states are common. This relatively current information suggests that we will soon be called upon to treat various individuals demonstrating a variety of symptomatology in psychodynamic treatment.

The role of therapy in exploitive situations is to provide a safe atmosphere in which the patient can 1) clarify and resolve the exploitive interaction in the previous therapy, including clarification of boundaries of responsibility for the event and what the patient wishes to do about it; 2) explore any dynamics that would lead the patient toward vulnerability for repeated victimization; and 3) resolve the original problems that initially led the patient into therapy. Luepker (1989a[185]) suggests a treatment model based on a series of increasingly larger concentric circles. The patient's early experiences and original presenting problems are in the inner circles, the abusive therapy is in the middle ring, and the negative sequelae of the abusive therapy and the current problems are in the outer rings. Treatment must address all of the issues represented by the circular areas at the appropriate time.

Pope and Bouhoutsos (1986)[171] have presented issues for the initial phase of treatment, as follows:

1. The therapist must listen with an open mind.
2. The patient must be able to proceed at his or her own pace, feeling in control and not affectively flooded.
3. The legal context of the therapy must be openly discussed.

4. Adequate records must be kept.
5. Fee arrangements must be clarified.
6. Prejudices and countertransference must be processed.
7. Concerns about trust must be respected and explored.
8. The patient must be allowed to reconstruct the events without the therapist attempting to fill in the gaps.
9. Suicidal risks must be evaluated.
10. A comprehensive assessment must be completed.
11. The therapist must avoid giving legal advice.
12. Education and cognitive information about the therapist/patient sexual intimacy must be provided.
13. It must be made clear that the patient's autonomy is respected, especially with regard to actions against the abusing therapist.
14. A treatment plan must be evolved and mutually contracted.
15. Roles and communications must be clarified between multiple treaters.

Pope and Bouhoutsos list additional issues that become important as therapy gets underway: ambivalence, anger, guilt, depression and suicide risk, isolation, sexual confusion, and cognitive dysfunction.

Kluft (1989,[167] pp. 490–499) provides an extensive discussion of the treatment process, which we will summarize. The author notes that patients exploited by previous therapists usually enter subsequent therapy with either blind, unrealistic, magical optimism or overt or covert mistrust, misgivings, and testing. Symptomatic decompensations are frequent at the onset of treatment and reoccur in the context of discussing the previous exploitation. Kluft recommends that the therapy be conducted according to eight basic principles:

1. Therapy requires clear limits and definitions of roles so that it does not replicate earlier boundary violations.
2. Therapy should be conducted with the utmost sense of responsibility so that the therapist provides a model for the rational assignment of responsibility. The patient should be helped toward taking responsibility for her life and her decisions and for setting her own life and treatment goals.

3. Therapy should proceed in a way that allows the patient to take control.
4. The collaborative nature and need for the patient's active input should be stressed to counterbalance the sense of helplessness.
5. The therapist should understand the patient's sense of isolation and confusion and be prepared to actively build bridges via an empathic and supportive collaborative stance.
6. Therapy should allow for the abreaction of the trauma and full resolution of associated affect rather than encourage a premature moving on.
7. Therapy should be consistent, reality based, and grounded in a reasonable and ethical world view that explains but does not minimize or rationalize the exploitation.
8. Therapists should beware of their narcissistic investments in the therapy. They should maintain an empathic link to the material that is important to the patient and a pace that will not overwhelm the patient's ego strengths or toleration of anxiety.

Kluft (1989, pp. 495–499[167]) also comments on the process of therapy, which, in his view, must address issues of helplessness by empowering the patient. Clarification of the therapy process and the responsibilities of both the patient and the therapist must occur. The therapist must recognize when the patient is too upset and confused to be assertive as well as when she is capable, and in the latter case encourage and support her in taking control of the process. A full discussion of ambivalent feelings toward the previous therapist must occur, allowing for prolonged periods of working through issues of grief and betrayal, as well as periods during which the patient will need to retain the old therapist as positive, magical, and powerful. The therapist must be able to tolerate powerful, angry feelings and assist the patient in the transition from self-directed anger. Slow and careful work must be done with the patient's sense of shame, guilt, and self-blame and the tendency of patients to keep these secret and prematurely seal over in a positive mode. Depression, suicidal concerns, pressures toward self-mutilation, and the way in which dissociative symptomatology may exacerbate the risks must be monitored at all times, with hospitalization or safety plans enacted when necessary. The patient's sense of isolation and withdrawal must be counteracted through empathic connections or by group therapy and activities. When the patient is feeling better, her notion of sexuality should be clarified in an atmosphere of safety, candor, and openness, with the understanding that premature or forced exploration of this issue may result in revictimization. Pacing of the treatment in a way that cognitive dysfunctions do not overwhelm the patient, and careful attention paid to lapses in concentration and intrusive flashbacks, are essential. Reworking of the traumatic experience, both in the therapy and in any earlier childhood exploitive experiences, is similarly essential. Important in this process is the concept of the patient's difficulty in communicating and her difficulty both in putting events into words and in understanding the events through what gets recreated in the transference. Therapists must be tolerant of a patient's need to express issues in an indirect manner and, at other times, interpret them as real resistance.

Both Kluft (1989[167]) and Pope and Bouhoutsos (1986[171]) caution that therapy may proceed in a variety of fashions, either long term or in bits and pieces. The patient may withdraw or change focus, or return to unfinished work later. These authors also note the danger of abrupt and traumatic terminations in which patients flee from treatment. In this instance, ancillary treatments such as groups and milieus may help to contain patients from such flight.

Countertransference and transference reactions are highly problematic. Therapists may be aroused via the mechanism of projective identification or because of their own vulnerabilities and may react by distancing themselves from the patient or by becoming punitive. They may become guilty, anxious, or confused in the face of their sexual feelings, causing the patient to withdraw from the topic. Therapists may be unsettled by the actions of the exploiting colleague, leading them to question their own professional identity and treatment models and to either attack or defend the abusive therapist. They may see their patient as hopelessly sick or dangerous and withdraw, or as extremely vulnerable and thus overreact with nurturing or advocacy stances. They may try to be perfect to make up for their patient's previous bad experience. Therapists may react coutertransferentially by stereotyping and simplifying the exploitive situation. In addition to these reactions, some of the common transference and countertransference mechanisms already cited in the previous sections on childhood sexual abuse and rape apply.

Many individual therapies have been facilitated by conjoint group treatment of either time-limited or open-ended nature. Groups can help relieve the patient's sense of isolation, assist in containing the therapy during periods of intense transference reactions, and provide valuable information and support regarding methods of redress. Luepker (1989b)[186] has provided a descriptive outline for such time-limited groups. The use of antidepressant and antianxiety medication in patients whose previous abuse was not facilitated by drugs, who do not feel overwhelmed or controlled by these substances, and who are able to contain tendencies to abuse them can also be extremely helpful. One-day workshops may help patients who are too anxious to enter individual therapy or too geographically separated to form a group. Kluft (1989[167]) summarizes a proper overall treatment perspective as follows: "The treatment of such [sexually exploited] patients is facilitated by arranging the therapy in a way that maximizes safety and clear communication. The importance of hearing the patient'[s] own reconstructions, pacing the treatment to the patient's tolerance, and respecting the patient's agenda cannot be overemphasized" (p. 499).

As in the case of rape, there are also secondary victims when a women is exploited in a therapy relationship. The spouse, children, friends, and parents of the victim, as well as the spouse, family, friends, colleagues, patients, and the institution/practice of the abusing therapist, are also adversely affected to a greater or lesser degree. Spouses may respond with anger, hurt, shame, and confusion and may become overly involved in the decisions regarding possible redress or may have difficulty sustaining their commitment to the marriage.

Parents and siblings may be the first to notice the patient's symptoms and may be supportive during recovery, or they may have become isolated from the patient during the exploitive relationship. Multiple family members may have been seeing the exploitive therapist, which can then cause complex reactions. Family and spouse, who may be called upon to support the patient during regressive periods, will need help for themselves and help in clarifying the limits of support they can offer the patient. Children are affected by the woman's preoccupation, mood lability, and, at times, inability to care for them. Adolescents are sometimes embarrassed and confused by the sexual nature of the issue. Friends may be supportive or frustrated by the patient's inability to leave the therapist. They may become estranged by the patient's isolation. Other patients of the abusive therapist are often traumatized and derailed from their treatment.

A final note is needed regarding the issue of traumatization of the profession. Although recognition and potential treatment and support for these secondary victims are receiving some attention in the literature, discussion on the trauma these issues create for mental health professionals has only just begun. We are aware of numerous negative sequelae:

1. Disillusionment with mentors and teachers
2. Anxiety regarding which colleagues are trustworthy and how to respond if a colleague is accused
3. Anxiety and uncertainty regarding the efficacy of treatment modalities
4. Public erosion of trust in psychotherapy
5. Global undifferentiated devaluation of professionals and of established theoretical models for their failure to illuminate these problems earlier
6. Inappropriate and potentially destructive rejection of a professional's training and of the helpful aspects of established models
7. Polarization of professional attitudes toward the problem, ranging from reluctance to explore the patient's dynamic contributions to exploitive relationships, at the expense of complete treatment, or punitive attempts to blame the patient or to rationalize the therapist's behavior in an inappropriately protective way
8. Increased competitiveness and splitting off of blame among professional groups and by the public [For example, a recent newspaper advice column suggested that patients only see psychologists be-

cause psychiatrists abuse their patients. Several months later advice in the column directed the public toward treatment from outside all conventional forms of therapy as being the only safe way to avoid abuse.]

9. Erratic and extreme reactions by licensing boards and professional organizations
10. Professionals' experience of intense feelings of guilt and shame engendered by the unprofessional behavior of colleagues, alternating with periods of rage at the accusations and devaluation directed toward ethical practitioners
11. Defensive inhibition of appropriate contact with patients

It is our hope that these issues will be discussed more openly among colleagues in professional organizations and across professional groups. All mental health professionals need to actively reestablish a sense of pride and integrity in their work while they integrate the need for concern regarding unethical practices and attain the kind of theoretical and clinical perspective that will enable them best to help the victims of such abuse.

Sexual Involvement With a Psychiatrist

The patient, a divorced mother of two latency-age sons, came for treatment because of anxiety, emotional lability, and the use of marijuana for sleep. Since the divorce she had been involved in emotionally exploitive relationships with several boyfriends. The only daughter of a family who had several sons, the patient had also been emotionally exploited by her brothers. She was very hungry for their love, approval, and attention. When asked specifically about incest, she denied it. She did, however, reveal that she had once been involved sexually with a therapist, but she refused to discuss this further. Two years later she saw the abusing therapist on a television talk show discussing the treatment of masochistic women. He had written a book on the subject. She felt fearful for other patients and felt willing to at least share her story in therapy.

She had begun treatment with this male therapist while in the throes of divorce negotiations. She enjoyed her sexual relationship with him and stated that it had helped her to regain her self-esteem. Her major regret was that her treatment hours were used for sex rather than to help her negotiate a better settlement in terms of custody for her sons. She had very nicely consented to a joint custody arrangement that involved the week being split between two parents, on an ongoing basis. She stated that the boys always seemed more unhappy and unruly upon their return and that indeed her youngest son was unwilling to go to his father's home. She could have, with help for herself, negotiated custody and visitation because she had proof of her ex-husband's infidelity. Arrangements were always hectic and often arbitrary, and the patient felt enslaved by her sons' schedules and their unhappiness.

Indeed, when their father, whom she guessed had only wanted them for narcissistic gratification and not out of love, took his life, her life became settled; her boys were better and less angry and did extraordinarily well at school. She would not reveal the name of her former therapist and felt that filing any kind of charges would be disruptive to her life. She said ruefully, "Just chalk it up to a few thousand dollars I paid for sex."

Abuse by a Physician-Employer

One patient was seen in middle age because of a severe retarded depression secondary to the breaking up of a first homosexual relationship. She was a married mother who had never enjoyed sex with her husband. Her history was one of growing up like a tomboy, determined to avoid men and get an education. (Two sisters had their lives derailed by out-of-wedlock pregnancies.) Her family was poor. There is some suggestion that she may have been sexually abused by her father, but this is still split off from the patient's consciousness.

The patient's family was unwilling for her to attend college, but she determined to work her way through. She found a job in the office of a married physician with two young children. The two established an intimate relationship in the course of late working hours. They then established a sexual relationship that stopped short of intercourse. Her involvement with him kept her away from her studies, and she barely graduated. He was instrumental in getting her to agree to marry her husband because he said that it looked like her best chance (in economic terms). Their sexual involvement stopped except for his furtive attempts to touch and squeeze her surreptitiously.

He remained her family physician and referred her to one of the authors, swearing her to secrecy about their relationship. Asked directly at one point if they were only friends, the patient lied to confirm this. Her derepression improved. She lost weight and began to be desirable to men. At this point, she suddenly reverted to her sleep disorder and began overeating and feeling depressed. In desperation, she revealed that she had had further sexual contact with her physician and former employer. Only by being helped to see that he had taken advantage of her in the past, derailing her career plans then and now, did she become angry. She decided to return for the professional education she had missed. Finances were a problem. Convinced that this man owed her, she approached him for partial funding, to which he agreed.

Employer-Employee Sex

A young woman took a job at a small advertising agency upon graduation from college. The only girl and youngest child in a large family, she had been pampered and infantilized. Even though she was very intellectually gifted and adept at several endeavors, little was expected of her intellectually. She was expected simply to get married and the sooner the better. At work her boss appreciated her creativity and ardor to become successful. A married father, he began a love affair with her, although he refused intercourse with her. She performed fellatio, and he masturbated her manually. She worked overtime to help him out and never knew when he could stay late or find time to spend with her outside of work.

She had the fantasy that she was both beloved and essential to the man and that eventually he would leave his marriage for her. Her hopes were dashed when he announced the imminent birth of a second child. She broke off the relationship and changed jobs, secretly hoping that he would not be able to give her up and would pursue her. In fact, he did not and she became seriously depressed. This is a case of a young woman who allowed herself to be abused and used in her work situation because she so desperately needed a father. The working through of the oedipal dynamics enabled her to attend graduate school.

Avoidance of Workplace Abuse

The patient, a senior associate at a prestigious law firm, fell in love with a partner in the same firm who was not her direct superior. He was, however, on the committee that decided on partnership. After the two began a clandestine affair, he recommended that she make a lateral move and offered to help her so that her chances for partnership would not be jeopardized. He felt wisely that if he supported her partnership at their common firm and their relationship became public, she would not be credited for earning it on her merits. She then changed law firms, became a partner in her own right, married her lover, and made a substantially better income because of her lateral move.

Abuse by a Clergyman

The patient, a 21-year-old college student, was engaged in long-term psychodynamic therapy for prolonged and perverse childhood incest. During the first 2 years of treatment, she had derepressed memories of abuse by her father and brother and, with the help of several hospitalizations, had contained her suicidal and self-mutilating urges. Although uncertain and plagued by vague memories of abuse by her uncle and brother, she took a therapeutic "breather" and refocused the work on therapy to emphasize returning to college, stabilizing herself as an outpatient, and reestablishing ties with people. She was able to return to college successfully, arrange an appropriate cooperative apartment situation, join an outpatient incest support group, and reestablish contact with her oldest girlfriend.

She joined a church and volunteered to work 6 hours a week in the church office. Although she performed well academically and appeared to be doing well socially, she became increasingly depressed and anxious in a manner that seemed difficult for the therapist to understand, especially since she was not engaged in the derepression of earlier material and there was no evidence of intrusive flashbacks. In the course of a month's gentle exploration of these symptoms, the patient revealed that while working at the church office the minister had been extremely friendly and solicitous, and complimentary about her work. After the Thanksgiving service he had invited her and another young woman to join him at a parishioner's home for dinner. During the dinner he had become both patronizing and physically intrusive to them both, putting his arm around them solicitously and hugging them. After dropping off the other young woman, he had attempted to rape the patient in his car, threatening to reveal her sinfulness if she spoke up. Her prior therapy had made her aware of the potential for revictimization, and she felt especially shamed and humiliated at being "so stupid again." She felt she had failed at her therapy and that her therapist would be disappointed in her, and so she had been unable to disclose the incident in therapy.

Exploration of this material alleviated her symptomatology and allowed her to reconnect in therapy. She was able to take steps to protect herself from further advances, but she did not wish to take any action against the clergyman. Her therapy continued, and she was able to derepress memories of abuse by her uncle and brother while maintaining her outpatient status and finishing college. She now supports herself and has developed a better sense of her own capabilities. In this context she is beginning to discuss possible action against the clergyman.

These cases illustrate the multiplicity of situations, symptoms, and resolutions associated with sexual abuse and exploitation.

Notes

1. Finkelhor D, Hotaling GT: Sexual abuse in the national incidence study of child abuse and neglect: an appraisal. Child Abuse Negl 8:23–32, 1984
2. Bachmann GA, Moeller T, Bennet J: Childhood and sexual abuse and the consequences in adult women. Obstet Gynecol 71:636–638, 1988
3. Freud S: Notes upon a case of obsessional neurosis (1909b), in The Standard Edition of the Complete Psychological Works of Sigmund Freud, Vol 10. Translated and edited by Strachey J. London, Hogarth Press, 1955, pp 151–320; see pp 206–207
4. Bender L, Blau A: The reaction of children to sexual relations with adults. Am J Orthopsychiatry 7:500–518, 1937
5. Bernstein AE: Analysis of two adult female patients who had been victims of incest in childhood. J Am Acad Psychoanal 17:207–221, 1989

6. Ferenczi S: Confusion of tongues between adults and children (1933), in Final Contribution to Psychoanalysis. New York, Basic Books, 1955, pp 156–174
7. Katan A: Children who were raped. Psychoanal Study Child 28:208–224, 1973
8. Margolis M: A preliminary report of a case of consummated mother/son incest. Annual of Psychoanalysis 5:267–293, 1977
9. Margolis M: A case of mother–adolescent son incest: a follow-up study. Psychoanal Q 53:355–385, 1984
10. O'Brien JD: The effects of incest on female adolescent development. J Am Acad Psychoanal 15:83–92, 1987
11. Rascovsky MW de, Rascovsky A: On consummated incest. Int J Psychoanal 31:42–47, 1950
12. Shengold L: Some reflections on a case of mother/adolescent son incest. Int J Psychoanal 61:461–475, 1980
13. Steele D: Child abuse, in The Reconstruction of Trauma. Edited by Rothstein A (Workshop Series of the American Psychoanalytic Association). NJ, American Psychoanalytic Press, 1986, pp 59–72
14. Cole C: A group design for adult female survivors of childhood incest. Woman and Therapy 4:71–82, 1985
15. Conte J, Schuerman J: Factor associated with an increased impact of child sexual abuse. Child Abuse Negl 11:201–211, 1987
16. Donaldson M, Gardner R: Diagnosis and treatment of post-traumatic stress among women after childhood incest, in Trauma and Its Wake: The Study and Treatment of Post Traumatic Stress Disorder. Edited by Figley CR. New York, Brunner/Mazel, 1985, pp 356–377
17. Fraser S: My Father's House: A Memoir of Incest and of Healing. Toronto, Ticknor & Fields, 1987
18. Gomes-Schwartz B, Horowitz JM, Sauzier M: Severity of emotional distress among sexually abused preschool, school-age, and adolescent children. Hosp Community Psychiatry 36:503–508, 1985
19. Goodwin J: Evaluation and treatment of incest victims and their families: a problem-oriented approach, in Modern Perspectives in Psychosocial Pathology. Edited by Howells J. New York, Brunner/Mazel, 1988, pp 43–57
20. Herman JL (with Hirschman L): Father-Daughter Incest. Cambridge, MA, Harvard University Press, 1981
21. Herman JL, Russell D, Trocki K: Long-term effects of incestuous abuse in childhood. Am J Psychiatry 143:1293–1296, 1986
22. Kluft R: Childhood Antecedents of Multiple Personality. Washington, DC, American Psychiatric Press, 1985

23. Lindberg F, Distad L: Post-traumatic stress disorder in women who experienced childhood incest. Child Abuse Negl 9:329–334, 1985
24. Livingston R: Sexually and physically abused children. Journal of the American Academy of Child Psychiatry 26:413–415, 1987
25. Rosenfeld A, Nadelson CC, Krieger M, et al: Incest and sexual abuse of children. Journal of the American Academy of Child Psychiatry 16:327–339, 1977
26. Wahl CW: The psychodynamics of consummated maternal incest: a report of two cases. Arch Gen Psychiatry 3:96–101[188–193], 1960
27. Ganzarain R, Buchele BJ: Fugitives of Incest: A Perspective From Psychoanalysis and Groups. Madison, CT, International Universities Press, 1988
28. Jehu D: Beyond Sexual Abuse: Therapy With Women Who Were Childhood Victims. Chichester, UK, Wiley, 1988
29. Kluft RP, Braun B, Sachs R: Multiple personality intrafamilial abuse and family psychiatry. Int J Fam Psychiatry 5:283–301, 1985
30. Russell DEH: The Secret Trauma: Incest in the Lives of Girls and Women. New York, Basic Books, 1986
31. Bass E, Davis L: The Courage to Heal: A Guide for Women Survivors of Child Sexual Abuse. New York, Harper & Row, 1988
32. Persons J, Burns D: Mechanisms of action of cognitive therapy: the relative contribution of technical and interpersonal interventions. Cognitive Therapy and Research 9:539–551, 1985
33. Horowitz MJ: Stress Response Syndromes. New York, Jason Aronson, 1976
34. Coons P: Child abuse and multiple personality disorder: review of the literature and suggestions for treatment. Child Abuse Negl 10:455–462, 1986
35. Spiegel D: Multiple personality in a post-traumatic stress disorder. Psychiatr Clin North Am 7:101–110, 1984
36. Ochberg F (ed): Post-Traumatic Therapy and Victims of Violence. New York, Brunner/Mazel, 1988
37. Ulman RB, Brothers D: The Shattered Self: A Psychoanalytic Study of Trauma. Hillsdale, NJ, Analytic Press, 1988
38. Van der Kolk BA: Psychological Trauma. Washington, DC, American Psychiatric Press, 1987
39. Jehu D, Gazan M, Klassen C: Therapy With Women Who Were Sexually Abused in Childhood, Part 8: Stress Disorders. Winnipeg, University of Manitoba, Psychological Services Center, 1987
40. Rush F: The Best Kept Secret: Sexual Abuse of Children. Englewood Cliffs, NJ, Prentice-Hall, 1980

41. Shengold L: Child abuse and deprivation: soul murder. J Am Psychoanal Assoc 27:533–559, 1979
42. Shengold L: Soul Murder: The Effects of Childhood Abuse and Deprivation. New Haven, CT, Yale University Press, 1989
43. Bernstein AE: The impact of incest trauma on ego development, in Adult Analysis and Childhood Sexual Abuse. Edited by Levine H. Hillsdale, NJ, Analytic Press, 1990, pp 65–93
44. Sherkow S: Consequences of childhood sexual abuse on the development of ego structure: a comparison of child and adult abuse cases, in Adult Analysis and Childhood Sexual Abuse. Edited by Levine H. Hillsdale, NJ, Analytic Press, 1990a, pp 93–116
45. Bernstein AE: Analysis of two adult female patients who had been victims of incest in childhood. J Am Acad Psychoanal 17:207–221, 1989
46. Gutek B: Sex and the Workplace. San Francisco, CA, Jossey-Bass, 1985
47. Klein F: The 1988 Working Women Sexual Harassment Report Executive Report. Cambridge, MA, Klein Associates, 1988
48. Klein F: Sexual harassment in Massachusetts trial courts and the legal profession: implications from the gender bias study. Boston Bar Journal, July/August 1989a, pp 17–19
49. Neugarten DA, Shafritz JM (eds): Sexuality in Organizations: Romantic and Coercive Behaviors at Work. Oak Park, IL, Moore Publishing, 1980
50. Roy P: Sex in the factory: informal heterosexual relations between supervisors and work groups, in Deviant Behavior: Occupational and Organizational Bases. Edited by Bryant C. Chicago, IL, Rand-McNally, 1974
51. Russell DEH: Sexual Exploitation: Rape, Child Sexual Abuse, and Workplace Harassment. Beverly Hills, CA, Sage, 1984
52 Sandroff R: Sexual harassment in the Fortune 500. Working Woman Magazine 13 (December):69–73, 1988
53. Sanford W (ed): Fighting Sexual Harassment: An Advocacy Handbook. Boston, MA, Allyson Publication/The Alliance Against Sexual Coercion, 1981
54. U.S. Merit Systems Protection Board: Sexual Harassment in the Federal Workplace: Is It a Problem? Washington, DC, U.S. Government Printing Office, 1987
55. Hughes JO, Sandler BR: In Case of Sexual Harassment: A Guide for Women Students. Washington, DC, Project on the Status and Education of Women, Association of American Colleges, 1986
56. Klein F: Unpublished survey of sexual harassment in a university system. Cambridge, MA, Klein Associates, 1989b

57. Lenhart SA, Klein F, Falcao P, et al: Gender bias against and sexual harassment of AMWA members in Massachusetts. J Am Med Wom Assoc 46:121–125, 1991
58. Klein F: Sexual harassment in employment: factors affecting incidence, severity, duration and relationship to production. Doctoral dissertation, Brandeis University, Waltham, MA, 1984
59. Crull P: Stress effects of sexual harassment on the job: implications for counseling. Am J Orthopsychiatry 52:539–544, 1982
60. Hamilton JA, Alagna SW, King LS, et al: The emotional consequences of gender-based abuse in the workplace: new counseling programs for sex discrimination, in Women, Power, and Therapy: Issues for Women. Edited by Braude M. New York, Haworth Press, 1988, pp 155–182
61. Rowe MP: Dealing with sexual harassment. Harvard Business Review, May/June 1981, pp 42–48
62. Kaplan H, Sadock B: Synopsis of Psychiatry: Behavioral Sciences, Clinical Psychiatry, 5th Edition. Baltimore, MD, Williams & Wilkins, 1988
63. Harvey M, Koss MP: The Rape Victim: Clinical and Community Approaches to Treatment. Lexington, MA, Greene Press, 1987
64. Law Enforcement Assistance Administration: Criminal Victimization Surveys in 13 American Cities. Washington DC, U.S. Government Printing Office, 1975
65. Kilpatrick DG, Best CL, Veronen LJ, et al: Mental health correlates of criminal victimization: a random community survey. J Consult Clin Psychol 53:866–873, 1985
66. Koss MP: The hidden rape victim: personality, attitudinal and situational characteristics. Psychology of Women Quarterly 9(2):193–212, 1985
67. Koss MP, Oros CJ: Sexual Experiences Survey: a research instrument investigating sexual aggression and victimization. J Consult Clin Psychol 50:455–457, 1982
68. Russell DEH: Rape in Marriage. New York, Macmillan, 1982
69. Russell DEH: The incidence and prevalence of intrafamilial and extrafamilial sexual abuse of female children. Child Abuse Negl 7:133–146, 1983
70. Russell DEH: Sexual Exploitation: Rape, Child Sexual Abuse, and Workplace Harassment. Beverly Hills, CA, Sage, 1984
71. Estrich S: Real Rape. Cambridge, MA, Harvard University Press, 1987
72. Hoyt JR: The telephone rape: crisis intervention for an obscene phone call. Issues in Health Care of Women 4:107–113, 1984
73. Brownmiller S: Against Our Will: Men, Women & Rape. New York, Simon & Schuster, 1975

74. Burgess AW, Holmstrom LL: Rape trauma syndrome. Am J Psychiatry 131:981–986, 1974a
75. Burgess AW, Holmstrom LL: Rape: Victims of Crisis. Bowie, MD, Robert J Brady Company, 1974b
76. Ellis EM: A review of empirical rape research: victim reactions and response to treatment. Clinical Psychology Review 3:473–490, 1983
77. Hilberman [Carmen] EH: The Rape Victim. Washington, DC, American Psychiatric Association, 1976
78. Notman MT, Nadelson CC: The rape victim: psychodynamic considerations. Am J Psychiatry 133:408–413, 1976
79. Sutherland S, Scherl DJ: Patterns of response among victims of rape. Am J Orthopsychiatry 40:503–511, 1970
80. Clark L, Lewis D: Rape: The Price of Coercive Sexuality. Toronto, Women's Press, 1977
81. Koss MP, Leonard KE: Sexually aggressive men: a review of empirical findings, in Pornography and Sexual Aggression. Edited by Malamuth NM, Donnerstein E. Orlando, FL, Academic, 1984, pp 213–232
82. Lindemann E: Symptomatology and management of acute grief. Am J Psychiatry 101:141–148, 1944
83. McCombie SL (ed): The Rape Crisis Intervention Handbook: A Guide for Victim Care. New York, Plenum, 1980
84. McFarlane AC, McFarlane CM, Gilchrist PN: Posttraumatic bulimia and anorexia nervosa. International Journal of Eating Disorders 7:705–708, 1988
85. Steketee G, Foa EB: Rape victims: post traumatic stress responses and their treatment: a review of the literature. Journal of Anxiety Disorders 1:69–86, 1987
86. Burgess AW, Holmstrom LL: Adaptive strategies and recovery from rape. Am J Psychiatry 136:1278–1282, 1979
87. Calhoun KS, Atkeson BM, Resick PA: A longitudinal examination of fear reactions in victims of rape. Journal of Counseling Psychology 29:655–661, 1982
88. Kilpatrick DG, Veronen LJ, Resick PA: The aftermath of rape: recent empirical findings. Am J Orthopsychiatry 49:658–669, 1979
89. Kilpatrick DG, Veronen LJ, Resick PA: Effects of a rape experience: a longitudinal study. Journal of Social Issues 37(4):105–122, 1981
90. Nadelson CC, Notman MT, Zackson H, et al: A follow-up study of rape victims. Am J Psychiatry 139:1266–1270, 1982
91. Sales E, Baum M, Shore B: Victim readjustment following assault. Journal of Social Issues 40(1):117–136, 1984

92. Courtois CA: Healing the Incest Wound: Adult Survivors in Therapy. New York, WW Norton, 1988
93. Herman JL (with Hirschman L): Father-Daughter Incest. Cambridge, MA, Harvard University Press, 1981
94. Figley CR (ed): Trauma and Its Wake: The Study and Treatment of Post Traumatic Stress Disorder, New York, Brunner/Mazel, 1985
95. Figley CR (ed): Trauma and Its Wake, Vol 2: Traumatic Stress Theory, Research and Intervention. New York, Brunner/Mazel, 1986
96. Krystal H: Integration and Self-Healing: Affect, Trauma, Alexithymia. Hillsdale, NJ, Analytic Press, 1988
97. American Psychiatric Association: Diagnostic and Statistical Manual of Mental Disorders, 3rd Edition, Revised. Washington, DC, American Psychiatric Association, 1987
98. Krugman S: Trauma in the family: perspectives on the intergenerational transmission of violence, in Psychological Trauma. Edited by van der Kolk BA. Washington, DC, American Psychiatric Press, 1987, pp 127–151
99. Gise LH, Paddison P: Rape, sexual abuse, and its victims. Psychiatr Clin North Am 11:629–648, 1988
100. Martin CA, Warfield MC, Braen GR: Psychotherapy of rape. Current Psychiatric Therapies 23:65–73, 1986
101. Renshaw DC: Treatment of sexual exploitation: rape and incest. Psychiatr Clin North Am 12:257–277, 1989
102. Rose DS: "Worse than death": psychodynamics of rape victims and the need for psychotherapy. Am J Psychiatry 143:817–824, 1986
103. Silverman DC, Apfel RJ: Caring for victims of rape, in Treatment Interventions in Human Sexuality. Edited by Nadelson CC, Marcotte DB. New York, Plenum, 1983, pp 195–213
104. Foreman BD: Psychotherapy with rape victims. Psychotherapy: Theory, Research and Practice 17:304–311, 1980
105. Notman MT, Nadelson CC: Psychodynamic and life-stage considerations in the response to rape, in The Rape Crisis Intervention Handbook: A Guide for Victim Care. Edited by McCombie SL. New York, Plenum, 1980, pp 131–142
106. Remer R, Elliot JE: Characteristics of secondary victims of sexual assault. International Journal of Family Psychiatry 9:373–387, 1988
107. Bidwell L, White P: The family context of marital rape. Journal of Family Violence 1:277–287, 1986
108. Finkelhor D, Yllo K: License to Rape: Sexual Abuse of Wives. New York, Free Press, 1985

109. Frieze IH: Investigating the causes and consequences of marital rape. Signs 8:532–553, 1983
110. Hanneke CR, Shields NM, McCall GJ: Assessing the prevalence of marital rape. Journal of Interpersonal Violence 1:350–361, 1986
111. Weingourt R: Wife rape: barriers to identification and treatment. Am J Psychother 39:187–192, 1985
112. Aizenman M, Kelley G: The incidence of violence and acquaintance rape in dating relationships among college men and women. Journal of College Student Development 29:305–311, 1988
113. Koss MP, Gidycz CA, Wisniewski N: The scope of rape: incidence and prevalence of sexual aggression and victimization in a national sample of higher education students. J Consult Clin Psychol 55:162–170, 1987
114. Miller JB: Date rape: time for a new look at prevention. Journal of College Student Development 29:553–555, 1988
115. Pirog-Good MA, Stets JE: Violence in Dating Relationships: Emerging Social Issues. New York, Praeger, 1989
116. Warshaw R: I Never Called It Rape. New York, Harper & Row, 1988
117. Bernstein AE, Warner GM: Women Treating Women. New York, International Universities Press, 1984b
118. Dobash RE, Dobash RP: Violence Against Wives: A Case Against the Patriarchy. New York, Free Press, 1979
119. Russell DEH, Van de Ven L: Crimes Against Women: Proceedings of the International Tribunal. Millbrae, CA, Les Femmes, 1976
120. Walker LE: The Battered Woman. New York, Harper & Row, 1979
121. Walker LE: The Battered Woman Syndrome. New York, Springer, 1984
122. Straus MA, Gelles RJ, Steinmetz SK: Behind Closed Doors: Violence in the American Family. Garden City, NY, Anchor Books, 1980
123. Hornung CA, McCullough BC, Sugimoto T: Status relationships in marriage: risk factors in spouse abuse. Journal of Marriage and the Family 43:675–692, 1981
124. Fleming JB: Stopping Wife Abuse. Garden City, NY, Anchor, 1979
125. Gelles RJ: The Violent Home: A Study of Physical Aggression Between Husbands and Wives. Beverly Hills, CA, Sage, 1972
126. Federal Bureau of Investigation: Uniform Crime Reports, Washington, DC, U.S. Department of Justice, 1982
127. Hilberman E: Overview: the "Wife-Beater's Wife" reconsidered. Am J Psychiatry 137:1336–1347, 1980 [Reprinted in The Gender Gap in Psychotherapy: Social Realities and Psychological Processes. Edited by Rieker P, Hilberman E. New York, Plenum, 1984, pp 213–236]

128. Martin D: Battered Wives. San Francisco, CA, Glide, 1976
129. Attorney General's Task Force on Domestic Violence. Washington, DC, U.S. Government Printing Office, 1984
130. Coley SM, Beckett JO: Black battered women: a review of empirical literature. Journal of Counseling and Development 6:266–270, 1988
131. Margolin G, Sibner LG, Gleberman L: Wife battering, in Handbook of Family Violence. Edited by Van Hasselt VB, Morrison RL, Bellack AS, et al. New York, Plenum, 1988, pp 89–117
132. World Health Organization: Ninth Revision of the International Classification of Diseases—Clinical Modification (ICD-9-CM). Geneva, World Health Organization, 1977
133. Klingbeil KS, Boyd VD: Emergency room intervention: detection, assessment, and treatment, in Battered Women and Their Families: Intervention Strategies and Treatment Programs. Edited by Roberts AR. New York, Springer, 1984, pp 7–32
134. Dickstein LJ: Spouse abuse and other domestic violence. Psychiatr Clin North Am 11:611–628, 1988b
135. Gayford JJ: Battered wives. Med Sci Law 15:237–245, 1975a
136. Hilberman E, Munson K: Sixty battered women. Victimology: An International Journal 2:460–470, 1977–1978
137. Roark ML: Preventing violence on college campuses. Journal of Counseling and Development 65:367–371, 1987
138. Gondolf EW, Fisher ER: Battered Women as Survivors. Lexington, MA, DC Heath, 1988
139. Geller JA, Wasserman J: Conjoint therapy for the treatment of domestic violence, in Battered Women and Their Families. Edited by Roberts AR. New York, Springer, 1984, pp 33–49
140. Neidig PH, Friedman DH: Spouse Abuse: A Treatment Program for Couples. Champaign, IL, Research Press Company, 1984
141. McLeer SV: Psychoanalytic perspectives on family violence, in Handbook of Family Violence. Edited by Van Hasselt VB, Morrison RL, Bellack AS, et al. New York, Plenum, 1988, pp 11–30
142. Freud S: Charçot (1893), in Sigmund Freud Collected Papers, Vol 1. Edited by Jones E. New York, Basic Books, 1953, pp 9–23
143. Akamatsu TJ: Intimate relationships with former clients: national survey of attitudes and behavior among practitioners. Professional Psychology: Research and Practice 19:454–458, 1988
144. Borys DS, Pope KS: Dual relationships between therapist and client: a national study of psychologists, psychiatrists and social workers. Professional Psychology: Research and Practice 20:283–293, 1989

145. Gartrell N, Herman J, Olarte S, et al: Psychiatrist-patient sexual contact: results of a national survey, I: prevalence. Am J Psychiatry 143:1126–1131, 1986a
146. Gartrell N, Herman J, Olarte S, et al: Psychiatric residents' sexual contact with educators and patients: results of a national survey. Am J Psychiatry 145:690–694, 1988
147. Glaser RD, Thorpe JS: Unethical intimacy: a survey of sexual contact and advances between psychology educators and female graduate students. Am Psychol 41:43–51, 1986
148. Holroyd JC, Brodsky AM: Psychologists' attitudes and practices regarding erotic and non-erotic physical contact with patients. Am Psychol 32:843–849, 1977
149. Kardener SH, Fuller M, Mensh IN: A survey of physicians' attitudes and practices regarding erotic and nonerotic contact with patients. Am J Psychiatry 130:1077–1081, 1973
150. Pope KS, Levenson H, Schover LR: Sexual intimacy in psychology training: results and implications of a national survey. Am Psychol 34:682–689, 1979
151. Pope KS, Keith-Spiegel P, Tabachnick BG: Sexual attraction to clients: the human therapist and the (sometimes) inhuman training system. Am Psychol 41:147–158, 1986
152. Pope KS, Tabachnick BG, Keith-Spiegel P: Ethics of practice: the beliefs and behaviors of psychologists as therapists. Am Psychol 42:993–1006, 1987
153. Black HC: Black's Law Dictionary, Revised 5th Edition. Edited by Nolan JR, Connolly MJ. St Paul, MN, West Publishing, 1979
154. Gechtman L, Bouhoutsos JC: Social workers' attitudes and practices regarding erotic and nonerotic physical contact with their clients. Paper presented at the Annual Conference of the California Society for Clinical Social Work and The National Federation of Societies for Clinical Social Work, Universal City, CA, October 1985
155. Kuchan A: Survey of incidence of psychotherapists' sexual contact with clients in Wisconsin, in Psychotherapists' Sexual Involvement With Clients: Intervention and Prevention. Edited by Schoener GR, Milgrom JH, Gonsiorek JC, et al. Minneapolis, MN, Walk-In Counseling Center, 1989, pp 51–64
156. Gartrell N, Herman J, Olarte S, et al: Prevalence of psychiatrist-patient sexual contact, in Sexual Exploitation in Professional Relationships. Edited by Gabbard GO. Washington, DC, American Psychiatric Press, 1989, pp 3–13

157. Brodsky AM: Sex between patient and therapist: psychology's data and response, in Sexual Exploitation in Professional Relationships. Edited by Gabbard GO. Washington, DC, American Psychiatric Press, 1989, pp 15–25
158. Holroyd JC, Brodsky AM: Does touching patients lead to sexual intercourse? Professional Psychology: Research and Practice 11:807–811, 1980
159. Bouhoutsos J, Holroyd J, Lerman H, et al: Sexual intimacy between psychotherapists and patients. Professional Psychology: Research and Practice 14:185–196, 1983
160. Gechtman L: Sexual contact between social workers and their clients, in Sexual Exploitation in Professional Relationships. Edited by Gabbard GO. Washington, DC, American Psychiatric Press, 1989, pp 27–38
161. Apfel RJ, Simon B: Patient-therapist sexual contact: psychodynamic perspectives on the causes and the results. Psychother Psychosom 43:57–62, 1985a
162. Apfel RJ, Simon B: Patient-therapist sexual contact: problems of subsequent psychotherapy. Psychother Psychosom 43:63–68, 1985b
163. Barnhouse RT: Sex between patient and therapist. J Am Acad Psychoanal 6:533–546, 1978
164. Carr M, Robinson GE: Fatal attraction: the ethical and clinical dilemma of patient-therapist sex. Can J Psychiatry 35:122–127, 1990
165. Collins DT, Mebed AAK, Mortimer RL: Patient-therapist sex: consequences for subsequent treatment. McLean Hospital Journal 3:24–36, 1978
166. Feldman-Summers S, Jones G: Psychological impacts of sexual contact between therapists or other health care practitioners and their clients. J Consult Clin Psychol 52:1054–1061, 1984
167. Kluft RP: Treating the patient who has been sexually exploited by a previous therapist. Psychiatr Clin North Am 12:483–500, 1989
168. Pope KS: How clients are harmed by sexual contact with mental health professionals: the syndrome and its prevalence. Journal of Counseling and Development 67:222–226, 1988
169. Schoener GR, Milgrom JH, Gonsiorek J: Sexual exploitation of clients by therapists, in Women and Mental Health: New Directions for Change. Edited by Mowbray CT, Lanir S, Hulce M. New York, Haworth Press, 1984, pp 345–358
170. Schoener GT, Milgrom JH, Gonsiorek JC, et al (eds): Psychotherapists' Sexual Involvement With Clients: Intervention and Prevention. Minneapolis, MN, Walk-In Counseling Center, 1989
171. Pope KS, Bouhoutsos JC: Sexual Intimacy Between Therapists and Patients. New York, Praeger, 1986

172. Smith S: The seduction of the female patient, in Sexual Exploitation in Professional Relationships. Edited by Gabbard GO. Washington, DC, American Psychiatric Press, 1989, pp 57–69
173. Twemlow SW, Gabbard GO: The lovesick therapist, in Sexual Exploitation in Professional Relationships. Edited by Gabbard GO. Washington, DC, American Psychiatric Press, 1989, pp 71–87
174. Gabbard GO, Menninger RW: The psychology of the physician, in Medical Marriages. Edited by Gabbard GO, Menninger RW. Washington, DC, American Psychiatric Press, 1988, pp 23–38
175. Vaillant G, Sobowale N, McArthur C: Some psychologic vulnerabilities of physicians. N Engl J Med 287:372–375, 1972
176. Buie DH: The abandoned therapist. International Journal of Psychoanalytic Psychotherapy 9:227–231, 1982–1983
177. Searles HF: Countertransference and Related Subjects: Selected Papers. New York, International Universities Press, 1979
178. Finell JS: Narcissistic problems in analysis. Int J Psychoanal 66:433–445, 1985
179. Claman JM: Mirror hunger in the psychodynamics of sexually abusing therapists. Am J Psychoanal 47:35–40, 1987
180. Rutter P: Sex in the Forbidden Zone. Los Angeles, CA, Jeremy Tarcher, 1989
181. Stoller RJ: Observing the Erotic Imagination. New Haven, CT, Yale University Press, 1985
182. Dziech BW, Weiner L: The Lecherous Professor: Sexual Harassment on Campus. Boston, MA, Beacon Press, 1984
183. Rassieur CL: The Problem Clergymen Don't Talk About. Philadelphia, PA, Westminster Press, 1976
184. Dahlberg CC: Sexual contact between patient and therapist. Contemporary Psychoanalysis 6:107–124, 1970
185. Luepker ET: Clinical assessment of clients who have been sexually exploited by their therapists and development of differential treatment plans, in Psychotherapists' Sexual Involvement With Clients: Intervention and Prevention. Edited by Schoener GR, Milgrom JH, Gonsiorek JC, et al. Minneapolis, MN, Walk-In Counseling Center, 1989a, pp 159–176
186. Luepker ET: Time-limited treatment/support groups for clients who have been sexually exploited by therapists: a nine-year perspective, in Psychotherapists' Sexual Involvement With Clients: Intervention and Prevention. Edited by Schoener GR, Milgrom JH, Gonsiorek JC, et al. Minneapolis, MN, Walk-In Counseling Center, 1989b, pp 181–194

Chapter 7

Later Life Issues

Grandmotherhood

Grandparenthood, a unique developmental stage in life, has received little attention in the psychiatric literature. It is sometimes difficult to separate the tasks of this phase of development from the concomitant adaptation to aging, changing health status, and the inevitable need to confront the finiteness of life. Erikson (1959[1]), who first wrote about developmental stages from the perspective of tasks, states that the ego moves from the stage of generativity, which includes bearing one's own children, to the stage of ego integrity versus despair. In this eighth and final stage, Erikson's focus is on the need to make inner peace with one's own parents, one's own conflicts, and one's own life's achievements. Erikson, however, overlooks the generative possibilities of grandparenthood and great-grandparenthood.

Grandparenthood offers the opportunity for a second chance at parenting (Robinson 1989[2]), the opportunity to rework unresolved conflicts, and the opportunity to be a child again and thus to play in ways that were perhaps not possible during one's own childhood. By way of play, sports, and activities with children, grandparenthood may be a way of positively reattaching to the parents of one's childhood (Myers 1989[3]).

Grandparenthood, however, may also be a conflictual experience, reevoking loss and conflict. Psychotherapeutic intervention to resolve problematic issues in this phase of development may free the individual to find pleasure and enhanced self-esteem.

The authors wish to thank Cassandra Klyman, M.D., of the Detroit Psychoanalytic Institute for supplying clinical material for cases appearing on pp. 481–484.

There seem to be two major determinants of the individual's ability to adapt to grandparenting. The first concerns a broad array of sociological issues. The population is not homogeneous in terms of economic and social class, culture, race and ethnicity, religion, and age of both the grandparent(s) and parent(s). Individuals may come from nuclear, extended, fractured, and recombined families. Sometimes step-grandparenthood is a pivotal issue. Given women's greater longevity, grandparenthood spans a greater period of the life history of a grandmother, her child or children, her grandchildren, and even her great-grandchildren.

The second major determinant affecting adaptation to grandmotherhood includes intrapsychic and often unconscious issues. The ability to resolve these issues in psychodynamic psychotherapy is almost exclusive to middle-class or affluent patients. There are some hospital or community-based sliding-scale clinics, but these are the exception rather than the rule for geriatric patients. This group of patients tend to be treated for depression with brief cognitive therapies or psychotropic medications. Later in this chapter we will document the effectiveness of even brief, economically feasible psychodynamically oriented interventions accomplished through psychiatric consultation-liaison services or via short-term inpatient individual psychotherapy. Most of our data on intrapsychic issues will, however, be drawn from a limited segment of the population.

Before moving into this area, however, let us return briefly to social issues to see how these may impinge on or even determine the general styles of interaction between grandparents and their progeny. Neugarten and Weinstein (1964[4]) were the first investigators to explore interactional styles. They studied varied groups of individuals and defined five general styles of grandparental interaction:

1. *Formal grandparent* (i.e., maintaining clearly demarcated lines between parent and grandparent)
2. *Funseeker* (i.e., leisure orientation characterized by self-indulgence and mutuality of pleasure)
3. *Surrogate parent*

4. *Reservoir of family wisdom*
5. *Distant grandparent* (i.e., ritualistically and fleetingly involved)

A clear example of the way one social variable affects interactional style was reported by Claven (1978[5]), who found that in lower socioeconomic groups, grandparents are more integrated into the ongoing family life than in middle-class families, in which the author found little evidence of grandparents being an integral part of the family unit. Recently, there has been an even sharper shift in family patterns in these two groups and their various subdivisions. In poverty-level families, the occurrence of teenage pregnancy is the norm. Also included in the norm is the pattern of grandchild or grandchildren and their mother physically residing with an oftentimes single grandmother in her 40s. On the other end of the socioeconomic spectrum are career-oriented parents who begin a family in their late 30s and are geographically and often culturally separated from more elderly grandparents. The abundance of retirement communities and stratified-care nursing home facilities often effectively separates grandparents from their grandchildren. On the other hand, a more recent pattern is the bringing of the elderly frail great-grandparents into the home of the great-grandchildren. Shifts of caregiving help are often available but are beyond the budget of all but the most affluent. We mention these issues because they are many times a significant part of our patients' real world. Eventually cognitive and national choices need to be made in relation to a multiplicity of social issues.

Our task, however, is to understand and be able to treat intrapsychic issues related to grandparenting in order to make a conflict-free sphere of the ego available for the cognitive choice of alternatives. Abraham (1913/1955[6]) noted that in many of his cases, grandchildren used their grandparents defensively against emotions directed toward the parents, thus leading the author to hypothesize that the special emphasis often given to grandparents might be "rooted in a violent rejection of the parents" (p. 44). Death wishes, wishes for a different parent, and wishes to overpower the father could be expressed by substituting another more remote object. Abraham did not, however, discuss whether the grandparents experienced themselves positively as containers for their grandchildren's emotions and facilitators of their maturation, or negatively as the receptacles for their grandchildren's hostile projections.

Deutsch (1945[7]) speculated about what constituted a "good" grandmother. She defined a good grandmother as one who promotes family peace by once again assuming the role of mother, for the purpose of need fulfillment, by identifying with the parent as an assistant mother or helpmate. Grandmothers who are not able to identify in this way often experience regressions, with ambivalence and aggression manifested by depressive mood, paranoid traits, and a cognitive focus on what they perceive to be the shortcomings and deficits, rather than the assets and achievements, of their grandchildren.

Benedek (1959b[8]) discussed positive potential of the role of grandmother. She noted the ease with which some postmenopausal women accept the role of grandmotherhood, and underlined the value to the grandmother of the displacement from self-interest to interest in a new love object. Implied in this displacement is the capacity to identify with the reproductive capacity of one's daughter(s) and the ability to enhance one's own self-esteem by investing in others. Cath (1982[9]) observed that at some point an aging person must cope with loss and depletion of certain aspects of the self. Repletion could then come from positive objects in the environment. Anthony and Benedek (1970[10]) pointed out the capacity of the grandmother to experience a new lease on life because of the love and need of grandchildren. The authors described the analysis of a would-be grandmother who experienced a reactive depression after her daughter experienced multiple miscarriages. The somatic correlates of the older woman's depression revealed the depth of identification with her daughter and her wish to survive through her grandchildren.

Severino et al. (1986[11]) reported on a 40-year-old mother of five children who sought a second analysis because of an increasing depression coincident with her children leaving home. As this second analysis unfolded, the pivotal conflicts centered around the patient's relationship with her maternal grandmother, with whom she had lived since the age of 6 following her father's accidental death. Her grandmother represented the "bad" mother, and her mother a rivalrous sister. The patient both hated and depended on her grandmother, who was the source of stability for her weak mother. To the extent that she identified with the capable grandmother, she also internalized and directed her hostility onto her own self representation. Obviously until this could be analyzed, the prospect of grandparenthood could not be helpful in replacing the loss of her children.

In the 1980s Gloria Warner had the opportunity of treating six grandmothers who developed reactive depressions on the occasion of the birth of a grandchild (G. Warner, personal communication, 1984). The source of the depression involved an identification with a daughter or daughter-in-law and a regression to a period when the patient herself had sustained a postpartum depression due to either object loss, loss of the baby often equated with the penis, or loss of the narcissistic gratification of special treatment during pregnancy. Those women who had had reparative mothering during their own pregnancies ultimately identified with their daughters as the recipients of this mothering. Some others treated their daughters as narcissistic extensions of themselves and experienced difficulties not from grandparenting but rather from the threatened loss of the daughter as gratifying object and the fantasies that the daughter would turn to her own child and abandon her mother.

We are aware of cases of grandmothers who could not tolerate the impact of grandchildren on their own internal object worlds for a variety of reasons. On several occasions the choice of the grandchild's name identified that child with either a beloved or a hated family member. In another instance the birth of the second female grandchild reevoked the grandmother's own negative feelings about not having given birth to a son, and she began to subtly denigrate her daughter and physically moved away without telling her daughter of her moving date. Another grandmother, a divorced and remarried woman in her 50s with a successful career, two grown stepdaughters, and three step-grandchildren, experienced rage and narcissistic injury related to her envy of her husband's indulgence of her stepdaughters and step-grandchildren, which she found painful to witness given her own deprived childhood and premature self-sufficiency as a young adult.

Another woman had herself hospitalized for a cancer workup the day before her son's wedding to a wife who was from a different religious background, claiming her son and his wife would "kill her" if they dared raise the expected grandchild in the wife's religion. Fortuitously, based on a sonogram, the child was found to be the sex that the parents had preagreed to bring up in the father's religion. The son responded to this news by contemplating the use of his mother's family name for the child, thus exposing the grandchild to the threat of the same kind of attempt at symbiosis that the son had been attempting to understand and undo.

A highly narcissistic great-grandmother in her eighth decade was remarkably unenthusiastic about the birth of her first great-grandchild, allocating a large sum of money to the child but no personal gift. This detached behavior was similar to the pattern she had established with her grandchildren, whom she seldom referred to by name and whose ages she frequently forgot or whose names she misspelled on ritually mailed birthday cards. To her children she referred to her grandchildren as "your children," "your daughter," "your son," and so forth. She clearly saw them from the beginning as evidence of her aging but remained serenely unaware of her lack of involvement.

Another type of problem we have seen is when the grandmother allies herself with her grandchildren against the parents. This can be especially destructive during an adolescent grandchild's struggle for separation and individuation. In one case, an adopted adolescent, against the wishes of her adoptive family and with the surreptitious financial aid of her grandmother, went far away to college and later was successful in the quest for and reunion with her birth parents. This common hostility thus allowed for a positive collaboration between grandmother and granddaughter at the expense of the adoptive mother. In another case, a grandmother reported sensing her daughter's dyscontrol in the face of provocation by the granddaughter. The granddaughter, a young academic, would appear at family occasions with mismatched clothing or clearly needing a haircut or styling. The grandmother would ask her what she planned to wear, offering to treat her to evening shoes or to an appointment at the beauty parlor, and would use the expression, "Let's not aggravate your mother—you know how she is." Thus in this case there was a secret collusion that both expressed and affirmed the hostility but also allowed for a positive outcome. The mother approved of her daughter, and the daughter and her grandmother would share knowing glances.

A Grandmother "Reincarnated" in Her Grandchild

A woman had a grandmother who was deeply beloved by her, her husband, and their three children. The couple agreed to try and conceive a daughter to be named for her. When indeed this happened and the child was born, the family had an almost delusional "folle en famille" that she was not only the symbolic but the physical incarnation of this grandmother. Indeed, the daughter was especially and uniquely beautiful and good natured. The family could image Grandma Kathy smiling at all their achievements with approval but especially at little Kathy. When "little Kathy" was 10, she said, "I am my Great-Grandma Kathy and that's why my Grandma E. loves me so much because I remind her of her mother."

Grandmothers as Surrogate Parents

The supervision of a resident, working twice a week in a clinic with a young black teenage woman who had become depressed, gave one of us the opportunity to see the family dynamics of a grandmother acting as a surrogate parent. This young woman had gotten a job in a bar, dropped out of school, and looked forward to a pregnancy as a way of solving her feelings of hopelessness and loneliness. She lived with a young single mother and was herself the result of an out-of-wedlock pregnancy. She assured her therapist that her mother was looking forward to taking care of a "grandbaby." The would-be grandmother had made it clear to this teenager that a baby of her very own was valuable but a man was not.

* * *

The above case is in contrast to a white middle-class mother's reaction to her daughter's best friend's refusal to have an abortion and the latter's insis-

tence on leaving college and moving back in with her family. This woman felt that the about-to-be grandparents were put out and unfairly burdened and that they gave in only because of their fear that to do differently would forever estrange them from their daughter. Another motivation the patient projected onto the mother of her daughter's best friend was to get this girl back into college so that she could meet an eligible husband and not have her life ruined forever. This projection was later confirmed.

* * *

The husband of another patient, a 55-year-old obese diabetic mother of five adult children, had died in a work-related accident 12 years before. He left the family able to manage financially. The patient's older son, 30 years old, was severely retarded, and the patient had to ready him for his developmental center program each day. Her eldest daughter, a nurse, also a mother of five, returned to work, leaving her children with the patient. The patient initially said that she had raised five of her own, so she could raise another five. The patient was hospitalized a few weeks later with chest pain. There was no electrical or enzyme evidence of a heart attack. She was seen in consultation with attention to how burdened she really felt. This resulted in the return of the three school-age grandchildren to their parents. The patient felt that she could now manage the preschoolers without difficulty.

A Matriarchal Grandmother

One of the present authors treated a patient who was able, when it became necessary, to relinquish to others her matriarchal role to her grandchildren. She was treated with short-term psychodynamic intervention through a geriatric consultation-liaison service. The patient, a 72-year-old black college-educated woman, was admitted for evaluation of memory loss, poor concentration, and agitation. Initially she refused psychiatric consultation, stating angrily that there was nothing wrong with her head. Upon a return visit, however, she did agree to regular meetings, acknowledging her declining mental status, her confusion and concern about the meaning of her symptoms, and her worry about her grandchildren.

She was the widow of a successful businessman and prominent politician, the mother of three, and the grandmother of five adult grandchildren ranging from ages 25 to 32. Since her husband's death 10 years ago she had served as the head of her family, maintaining various business enterprises and the family's position of civic leadership within the black community. As her neuropsychiatric workup progressed, it became clear that she had compensated for a significant loss of organizational skills with an elaborate system of bookkeeping and that her family members, although bright and accomplished, were unaware of her deficits and looked to her for leadership. She held weekly family caucuses in the hospital during which she dispensed political, financial, and business advice with relish. She spoke warmly, enthusiastically, and shrewdly about the individual skills and shortcomings of her children and grandchildren.

Eventually grasping the extent and significance of her symptoms, the grandmother alternated between angry denial, imperious control, and assertive reality-based questioning regarding her differential diagnoses and their implications. She was deeply sobered when a diagnosis of Alzheimer's disease was made, but insisted that her family not be told. She became very depressed and expressed concerns that she would shame her family and her community with her deteriorating status. She also ruminated about how her family would manage their various civic and economic concerns, while either refusing family visits or fighting with family members.

During the fifth week of her hospitalization, she requested that her therapist schedule a meeting with her entire family and that the therapist be present in the meeting to hear "what I'm going to tell them." At the meeting she seated her therapist beside her and announced that she had important news to share with everyone. She stated that she would be unable to carry on as head of the family. She outlined her symptoms and how she had disguised them. She revealed her diagnosis and its implications and how she had struggled with her mourning. She then proceeded to delegate responsibilities to each of her five grandchildren, negotiating roles and responsibilities as would a CEO. She utilized the remainder of the hospitalization to organize care for herself, utilizing her therapist to consider options and to help her manage her family's reactions. After discharge she opted out of follow-up visits but wrote her therapist a year later to report on her progress and on the establishment of a scholarship fund in her honor by her grandchildren.

A Deceased Mother's Impact on Her Daughter's Ability to Become a Mother

A young pregnant professional woman sought treatment because of the severe phobia of becoming poisoned that began when the office next door to hers was being painted, shortly after she had finally conceived a child after years of treatment for infertility. The phobia escalated to include the "rays" from an office computer, the home microwave, and even gasoline fumes from the car and camphor fumes from a locked storage closet. Meanwhile, she exhibited anorexic behavior. She was advised to gain weight, which she could not seem to do. She had a severe iron-deficiency anemia that required treatment. She seemed not to care that her anemia might be more harmful to the fetus than would the things she feared. Her husband's anger forced her to eat better and gain weight.

The patient was the second daughter of a mother who returned to professional school shortly after the patient's birth. The patient was cared for early on predominantly by her father and an older sibling. In latency she was already a latchkey child responsible for her own food shopping and preparation. Her mother was very beautiful and narcissistically self-involved. Her father was hardworking but financially unsuccessful. The patient was very successful academically but spitefully uncaring of her looks or her social life. She met her husband after her father's sudden death

Her mother had a very late recurrence of what the patient later found out was a cancer operated on when the patient had been a teenager. At the time she had been told merely that her mother was away for a while. She had guessed correctly that she was not to ask questions, and so she had not. She was not informed of the cancer's recurrence until it was almost too late to visit her mother in a nearby hospital. She and her husband rushed to her mother's side and visited briefly. The woman did not wish to see her again. While the patient waited in the waiting room, her mother died. She felt vaguely sad, confused, and disbelieving but never mourned.

The daughter was embroiled in the settling of her mother's complicated estate when she first sought treatment. She categorically denied any fantasies or associations that would link her unborn child to either of her deceased parents. Many of her dreams and the interweaving of her associations revealed a defensive connection to her mother. Yet aside from the initial bold outlines of her childhood history, she was amnestic for her childhood early experiences. It occurred to the therapist to ask what she would name this unborn child. She immediately furnished a single female name, a variant of her mother's first name. The patient was confronted with the fact that she had fantasized that she was pregnant with a daughter who would bear her mother's name. She responded naively by asking, "She should have her grandmother's name, don't you think?" The therapist said that she was not sure why the patient thought so, because she did not have very many memories of her mother and those she did have seemed to make her sad.

The patient then arranged to call her sibling and visit in an attempt to reconstruct and remember her early life. She confirmed an unhappy, isolated childhood. The patient adored her attentive father. She remembered that her mother had often locked herself away in her room to study or to primp or sleep. It was interpreted that the patient's mother had treated her as if she were poison and wanted no part of her. The patient confirmed this with a bizarre story of abandonment. For the first time, she cried and reminded her therapist that the anniversary of her mother's death was approaching. She began the work of mourning, which involved the expression of anger as well as the feeling of loss. She subsequently became less fearful about most things. She started to get angry at her husband's mother, who, when she visited, reinforced the patient's fear of lead in water and led to compulsive clean-up behavior.

When a sonogram confirmed that her baby would be a little girl, the patient and her husband decided on a quite lovely first name for the baby—one that was neutral and that they had found in a book. At her mother-in-law's insistence that the baby be named for someone, the patient planned to give her daughter the approximation of her mother's name as a middle name. The baby was small but healthy and was placed in a regular nursery. The therapist visited the hospital as the baby was brought to be breast-fed. The patient did not have the vaguest notion of how to do this, nor did she ask anyone for instruction. She vaguely assumed that someone would show her.

Initially she seemed happy, if clumsy, with the baby. The patient became severely depressed when her daughter required evaluation for two remediable complaints. She became able to further work out some of the details of the fantasy of being poisoned.

Another element that led to the uncovering of the paucity of her relationship with her mother was her total puzzlement about every aspect of mothering. As she brought her questions and doubts to therapy, the details of her own deficits became apparent, and she was helped to correct these.

The patient was enabled to acknowledge her jealousy and sadness for what she lacked in her own life. Once in a while she still has irrational fears for the safety of her daughter. A second pregnancy with a fetus known to be a male is causing far less anxiety.

This last case illustrates how a daughter's resolution of issues concerning her own mother is essential to her achieving satisfaction in a parental role later in her life.

Those patients who are unable to accomplish the task of achieving satisfaction in grandparenting have problems that fall into the following categories:

1. Identification with the daughter and the wish to use the daughter to fill the patient's own narcissistic needs
2. Perceived loss of the daughter as a gratifying object
3. Rejection of grandchildren because they are evidence of aging
4. Reflection of a grandchild as a reincarnation of a dead great-grandparent
5. A sense of being overburdened and angry
6. The realization of the loss of one's own abilities and the subsequent failure of the fantasy of reunion with one's own childhood and parents

We feel that preventive psychodynamic work can be done with female patients at any time in the life cycle. This would ensure that grandparenthood would be a time of not only ego integrity (Erikson 1959[1]) but also satisfaction and continuing pleasure through positive identifications with successors.

Menopause and Midlife

Menopause is defined retrospectively as the cessation of menstrual periods for 1 year. The median age for menopause in industrialized countries is 50 years (McKinlay et al. 1972[12]). A wide range of individual age variation encompassing the late 30s through the late 50s exists. *Perimenopause* is a term used to define the menopausal transition period of varying duration in which ovarian function is diminished and hormonal status is changing, yielding noticeable changes in the menstrual period as evidenced by alterations in flow, duration, regularity, and cycle intervals, and by the presence of anovulatory cycles.

The biology of menopause and the perimenopausal period was recently reviewed by Cumming (1990,[13] pp. 172–174), whose discussion is summarized in Appendix O.

Menopause has been associated with a wide variety of psychological, psychosomatic, and physical complaints. There has been a tendency to automatically and indiscriminately ascribe any psychosomatic or distressing physical, psychological, and behavioral experiences of midlife women to their menopausal status, and much controversy has developed over two highly polarized views of menopause. In the first view, menopause is considered a normal developmental phase. In the second view, menopause is defined as an endocrinopathy, a pathological syndrome. No doubt, the ambiguity and variability of the perimenopausal period, and the retrospective and thus vague nature of the definition of menopause combined with the pervasiveness of social and cultural stereotypes and the concomitant processes of aging, developmental, and environmental issues, help to create this atmosphere of controversy and lack of clarity in the minds of women, clinicians, and researchers. As Notman (1984[14]) has stated:

> An assessment of a menopausal woman's entire life situation is crucial if appropriate treatment is to be undertaken. The extent and amount of discomfort created by symptoms must be evaluated for each woman and a thorough history with attention to the stresses and supports in her life, her family situation and her patterns of adaptation must be taken. Separation of midlife concerns from endocrine menopausal effects makes it possible to offer help for both. (p. 453)

In this section we discuss 1) the historically changing perspectives of menopause; 2) the female midlife developmental and intrapsychic issues relevant to menopause, including the way in which life-style concerns, individual adjustment patterns, and the individual psychological meaning of menopause influence a woman's experience of menopause; 3) the impact of social and cultural factors on the menopausal experience; 4) the biological processes of menopause as differentiated from the aging process; and 5) the symptoms commonly associated with menopause, with emphasis on those that have been documented to have a direct correlation to the menopausal process or that have important ramifications for psychodynamic therapists.

Historical Perspectives†

Menopause can best be understood in its historical perspective as outlined recently by Utian (1990[15]). Known references to menopause date back to biblical and prebiblical times. With each new scientific advance in the early stages of medicine came a related theory for the etiology of menopause. Medical literature of the 1700s and 1800s documented the emergence of negative attitudes toward menopause, which continue into contemporary times. As recent as the 1960s menopause was referred to as a "tragedy or catastrophic attack" (Rhoades 1967[16]), and postmenopausal women were described as "cow-like, dull, unattractive" (Wilson and Wilson 1963[17]). Early remedies included administration of crude ovaries and ovarian juices and powders. Isolation of the hormone estrone in 1929 by Butenandt ushered in the modern era of research on menopause.

Schwartzman and Leiblum (1987[18]) have reviewed the literature and provide a historical account of menopause during the last 50 years. During the period 1945 through 1965 psychoanalytic and epidemiological works prevailed. Deutsch (1945[7]) and Benedek (1950[19]) formulated the early psychoanalytic view of menopause, conceptualizing the psychological sequelae as constituting a grief reaction to the loss of menstruation and its ties to reproduction and femininity. This format was in keeping with the then prevalent defensive view of female psychology in

†The material in this section has been adapted from Schwartzman and Leiblum 1987,[18] pp. 12–22.

which feminine identity is seen as developing in the context of compensating for something that is missing, different, or deficient. Benedek postulated a healthy outcome, in that menopause provided an opportunity for mastery and potential growth by emancipating women from sexual competition and fears of rejection, and by releasing talents and qualities previously suppressed. She differed with Deutsch, who viewed the expansion of interpersonal relationships and pursuits outside the home as a defense against narcissistic mortification and decline. Both women based their writings on their experience with problematic clinical populations. Their views were reinforced by the DSM-I diagnosis of "involutional melancholia" (American Psychiatric Association 1952[20]). In contrast, epidemiological studies with nonpatient populations (Neugarten and Kraines 1965[21]; Neugarten et al. 1963[22]) indicated that 1) despite a high incidence of somatic and psychosomatic symptoms, only a small number of women experienced psychiatric difficulties at menopause, and 2) older women regarded menopause more positively than their younger cohorts. Of those who viewed menopause with anticipatory negativism, not knowing what to expect was cited more often than loss of enjoyment of sexuality or childbearing potential as the primary factor.

During the period 1966 through 1974, the works of Robert Wilson (1966[23]) dominated views on menopause. Wilson regarded menopause as a deficiency disease. He recommended estrogen replacement therapy (ERT) for the alleviation of psychological and physiological conditions of global proportion, and promised that women could remain "feminine forever." Joining the analysts in ignoring epidemiological studies which showed that menopause presented problems for only a small percentage of women, Wilson (1966[23]) insisted that untreated postmenopausal women would "see the world through a gray veil and live as docile, harmless creatures, missing most of life's values" (pp. 352–353). He minimized the risks of cancer due to estrogen. Due to the popularity of Wilson's theories, the drug Premarin ranked as the fifth most widely prescribed medication from 1970 through 1974. In 1975 Premarin ranked second behind Valium (National Prescription Audit 1972–1975[24]; also see Chapter 1).

The period 1975 through 1979 was dominated by investigations linking estrogen replacement with endometrial cancer (Gray et al. 1977[25]; Mack et al. 1976[26]; McDonald et al. 1977[27]; Smith et al. 1975[28]; Ziel and Finkle 1975[29]). While the medical community struggled to find a balance between a clear need for more carefully designed long-term studies and a clear need not to be alarmists, the feminists formulated their viewpoint. They responded with a broad concern about the use of all sex hormones, pointing to comparable difficulties with contraceptive pills and diethylstilbestrol (DES). They also rejected ERT, viewing its use as a political issue based on political concerns that 1) the medical profession had pathologized a natural female condition, 2) women were not treated respectfully by their physicians, and 3) financial gain by physicians and the pharmaceutical industry was taking precedence over women's health. The feminists encouraged women to join menopause self-help groups to share and validate their own perceptions, and they emphasized the use of alternative remedies, many of which were not validated as efficacious.

The period 1979 to the present has brought a return to ERT and the use of estrogen/progestin combinations, based on the discoveries that progestin could counteract the carcinogenic impact of unopposed estrogen on the endometrium and that these regimens were also beneficial in preventing atherosclerotic disease and osteoporosis (Aitken 1976[30]; Bush et al. 1983[31]; Christiansen et al. 1981[32]; Corson 1984[33]; Lindsay and Cosman 1990[34]; Lindsay et al. 1978[35]; Lobo 1990[36]; Recker et al. 1977[37]; Studd et al. 1980[38]; Whitehead et al. 1981[39]). The multidimensional nature of the menopausal event and the tendency to confuse menopausal symptoms with developmental issues of midlife have been illuminated (Notman 1978,[40] 1979,[41] 1984,[14] 1990[42]). Feminist positions have altered to some degree, sanctioning the use of hormonal replacements when appropriate but providing other alternatives as well. Possible links of hormonal replacement therapy to breast cancer have been reported (Brinton 1990[43]), stimulating continued confusion in the minds of women and practitioners regarding the use of estrogen and progestin replacement therapy. Lock (1982[44]) documented that a variety of practice models exist with regard to treatment of menopause.

Kaufert and Gilbert (1986[45]) note that, currently, women are exercising control over the determination of whether they wish to treat menopause with medical intervention or as a normal adaptation. Finally, and most optimistically, there has been a growth in the literature documenting the need for multidisciplinary approaches to menopause. Posner (1976[46]) illustrated the way in which the highly polarized viewpoints of the medical model and feminist model can lead to the conclusion that menopausal distress is characterized by expressions such as "Its all in your head." A more scholarly commentary on this issue is offered by Parlee (1990[47]), who comments on how the integration of biological and social scientific research on menopause can be realized. A recent North American Menopause Society symposium represents the largest multidisciplinary presentation on the subject of menopause known to us, and its proceedings were recently published in the *Annals of the New York Academy of Sciences* (Flint et al. 1990[48]).

Midlife Issues

The developmental and intrapsychic issues of women at midlife influence the psychological impact of the menopause itself, as well as create independent psychological problems that are often erroneously ascribed to the menopause. Although persons ages 40 to 65 are commonly referred to as "middle-aged," variations of the definition ranging from 35 to 70 years have occurred in the literature. Chronological age has been shown to be less useful in defining midlife than the illumination of specific tasks and issues. Chiriboga (1981,[49] p. 3) notes that we have begun to accumulate data that substantiate the need to define midlife as a developmental phase—namely, that 1) major definable changes do occur, 2) these changes are directional, and 3) individuals have similar psychological characteristics during this phase of life. Havighurst (1948[50]) defined specific developmental tasks for midlife as 1) development of adult civic and social responsibility, 2) establishment of economic standard of living, 3) parenting of children into healthy adulthood, 4) development of leisure activities, 5) relating to spouse as a person, 6) acceptance and adaptation to aging, and 7) adjustment to aging parents. Erikson (1950[51]) defined midlife in terms of the crisis of generativity versus rejectivity, or, simply stated, the capacity to nurture and guide the next generation versus the capacity for self-absorption, alienation, and stagnation.

In 1968, Rossi[52] defined midlife as beginning when children leave home. But given the variability of life options for women and the fact that many are having their first babies at age 40, this definition is outdated. Neugarten (1968a[53]) presented a more appropriate concept that stresses a shift in the perspective of time from a sense of limitless future to the sense of time "left to live." In this context, introspective reflection and self-evaluation become more prominent. Chiriboga (1981[49]) has documented themes of mastery, competence, and social responsibility in midlife men and women, noting that these occur via different processes and time sequences for men and women, respectively. He notes that assumptive worlds based on examples such as the dedication to work or to child rearing may be shaken by changes or setbacks, resulting in disruptions and disequilibrium. These "midlife crises" result in the emergence of new or more appropriate assumptions.

Concomitant with these types of shifts, several authors have noted the midlife balancing of feminine and masculine styles, with men becoming more affiliative and nurturant and women becoming more comfortable with assertiveness, autonomous mastery, and egocentric pursuits (Cameron 1976[54]; Monge 1975[55]; Neugarten 1968a[53]; Terman and Oden 1959[56]). Pollock (1977,[57] 1981[58]) elaborates midlife themes of loss, mourning, and diminished function but emphasizes the option for new development, new organization, and creativity, perhaps explaining why many women feel released and energized by menopause. Chiriboga (1981[49]) and Neugarten (1968a[53]) have pointed out that biological age-guided events have less impact and salience in midlife than in childhood and adolescence, while non-normative, unexpected events have more salience. This may account for the recent empirical findings of Lennon (1982[59]), who found that when menopause occurs during the expected time frame, it is not associated with psychological stress, but if it occurs at either earlier or later stages in the life course, it is apt to be a source of psychological distress. Reports that the majority of menopausal women do not find the menopause a highly disruptive event corroborate this notion (Neugarten and Kraines 1965[21]; Neugarten et al. 1963[22]).

The Experience of Menopause

Notman (1978,[40] 1979,[41] 1984,[14] 1985,[60] 1990[42]) has explored the impact of midlife psychological and developmental issues on the experience of menopause. She notes that midlife male and female development differ regarding key issues. Male development is organized around the themes of separation and individuation and autonomous achievement, proceeding linearly through a series of sequential stages. Female development, on the other hand, proceeds in the context of relationships, affiliations, and attachments that remain important throughout the life cycle and are closely connected with a woman's sense of self-esteem and self-confidence, and with issues of anxiety and conflict. Midlife women may therefore be less affected by menopause than by changes or losses in key relationships with maturing children, aging parents, spouses, late-life babies, or the babies they wish they had had. The development of women in midlife is more variable, with different patterns and stages occurring simultaneously. These differences for women have a central relationship to the time-limited nature of female reproduction and menopause and to how women integrate this aspect of their life into their overall life cycle. Women may combine family with schooling and work or sequence these life events in a variety of ways. They may enter menopause with different developmental issues resolved or unresolved and different sources of gratification and stress. Drawing from the work of Barnett and Baruch (1978[61]), Notman (1990,[42] pp. 151–153) points out that the working through of issues of autonomy and identity prevalent in young adulthood may be interrupted by the experience of pregnancy and motherhood, which, according to Benedek (1959a[62]) and Bibring et al. (1961[63]), is a developmental experience of its own, changing the woman's relationship with her mother, herself, and her child's father and consolidating her identifications with parents and the adult role, and her personal sense of femininity. For example, Notman notes that a woman may return to school as a grandmother at age 40 to refocus on earlier issues of autonomy and achievement. Conversely, a career woman may be pregnant for the first time at age 40. She may have resolved many issues of autonomy and achievement, but her concept of femininity and her relationship with her mother remain unsolidified. The former woman may have no children at home at the time of menopause and may either miss them or feel exhilarated and restored to herself in their absence. The latter woman may still be rearing latency-age and teenage children at the time of her menopause and feel either extremely fulfilled or envious and competitive toward her children's youthful potential.

Focusing on the continued central importance of relationships and connectedness for women, Notman (1979[41] [pp. 1272–1273], 1990[42] [pp. 153–154]) has explored the relationship between the individual psychological meaning of menopause and the impact of midlife shifts or losses in important relationships. She notes that contrary to popular beliefs, the women reporting the greatest psychological distress in menopause are not childless women but rather women who have invested tremendously in their mothering roles. They lose both status and a sense of usefulness when their childbearing capacity ceases (Bart and Grossman 1978[64]). Childless women may respond with sadness at the opportunities now closed to them. These women may have adapted to and sublimated the issues associated with their childless state, or they may have always felt deep ambivalence regarding children and relief that the current cultural norms allow them to opt out. Grown children may exit from the family at midlife, leaving those women who have found child rearing gratifying with a sense of profound sadness, especially if their opportunities are limited, or with a combination of sadness and an exhilarating sense of being freed up to pursue other interests, if they have multiple options available to them. Other women are able to successfully adapt their relationships with grown children to allow for an expanded, continued, and vital relationship with their adult children and/or grandchildren and their worlds.

Notman points out that women who have not been gratified in their roles as mothers, who have experienced major conflicts with their children, or who have been burdened with too many children, may feel a great sense of relief at menopause. Children who fail in their efforts to separate and who either return home or have continued difficulties as young adults may create major stresses for their mothers. The separation issues experienced with young adult children may reactivate old issues of separations in these midlife mothers. Shifts regarding marriage and relationships with spouse are concomitant with menopause. Unmarried women may equate menopause with the end of their ability to create a family network for themselves and thus may respond negatively, not because of hormonal changes or sense of loss of femininity or attractiveness but rather because of loss of the potential for creating these important relationships. For married women, the independence of children and the retirement of their spouse may place stress on the marriage and require a new equilibrium in the marital relationship. Loss of husbands via illness, death, or divorce has severe repercussions on midlife women, independent of their menopausal status. Changes in male arousability and sexual performance and in male midlife concerns are sometimes expressed by a decrease in the male's sexual interest or by his turning toward younger women. This may impact negatively on a woman's sexuality independently of, or conjointly with, her own psychological and physical midlife changes. The relative unavailability of suitable male sexual partners for divorcees and widows in midlife may further diminish these women's sense of controlling gratification in their heterosexual activities. In addition, a domino effect, beginning with dyspareunia secondary to hormonal changes, may lead to a decline in arousability and an avoidance of sex. Parents may die during a woman's midlife years, or more commonly they become ill and physically dependent, necessitating increased levels of care from the woman. These parental needs often run parallel to child-rearing responsibilities. This special state of stress is described as the problem of the "sandwich generation" (see Chapter 4).

Throughout her writings, Notman emphasizes the current tendency to confuse midlife developmental issues and disruptions with menopausal symptoms and to look for uniform psychological meanings for menopause rather than to tackle the highly individualized impact of menopause that she has documented. Formanek (1988[65]) supports this approach, noting the interplay of life-style, life experience, life stressors, relationships, and culture in a woman's experience of menopause.

In addition to elaborating the developmental and relational issues, Notman also cites works by Deutsch (1945[7]), Bibring et al. (1961[63]), and Benedek (1950[19]), whose findings support the notion that psychological responses to menopause may activate repetitions of behaviors and self concepts present at the onset of menstruation or at the time of the first pregnancy. Notman notes that at each of these points in a woman's life, somatic and biological changes interweave with complex psychological and cultural effects. The following factors may be more relevant in understanding menopausal women who present with psychological complaints than the menopause itself (Notman 1985[66]): 1) individual patterns of adaptation or maladaptation to life transitions, 2) individual personality traits, 3) preexisting psychopathology, and 4) identification with their own mother's menopause. Schindler (1987[67]), reporting on midlife psychiatric illnesses, includes menopause as only one of many potential etiological factors. McKinlay and McKinlay (1973[68]) and Parlee (1976[69]), in reviewing the menopause literature, criticize the methodology of the research, noting that in the more reliable studies by McKinlay et al. (1972[12]), psychosomatic and psychological complaints were not recorded more frequently by so-called menopausal women than by younger women.

Social and cultural factors also play an important role in a woman's experience of menopause. Preliminary studies by Goodman (1977,[70] 1978[71]) indicate that there is biological homogeneity across ethnic groups regarding the age at onset of menopause; however, interesting ethnic and cultural differences are found in 1) the occurrence and experience of menopausal symptoms, 2) attitudes toward menopause, and 3) the status and role accorded to postmenopausal women. These differences modify the psychological experience of menopause and menopausal symptoms. In cultures where menopause is considered normal and does not result in a decline in status, one would presume fewer menopausal symptoms and less distress than in cultures that define menopause as a negative event, provide no roles for postmenopausal women, and pathologize menopause via the elaboration of a constellation of symptomatology. Despite a general lack of data and the occurrence of some methodological problems and contradictory reports, there is evidence to support this premise (Flint 1975[72]; Mead 1968[73]). A high incidence of menopausal symptomatology is reported in North American and European women who come from cultures that are oriented toward youth and beauty and that do not provide specific roles for postmenopausal women.

Studies exploring attitudes toward menopause in the context of cultural expectations have yielded some validation for the hypothesis that the culture's definition of menopause as a positive or negative event affects the women's experience of this event (Lock 1982[44]; McPherson 1980–1981[74]; Severne 1982[75]; Woods 1982[76]). Kaufert (1982[77]) has documented the way in which menopausal symptoms as universal as hot flashes are not attributed to menopause in cultures that define menopause as symptom free. Perlmutter (1978[78]) has noted the lack of correlation between endocrine status and symptomatology, and both she and Notman (1978,[40] 1979,[41] 1984,[14] 1990[42]) have noted the way in which symptoms are indiscriminately attributed to menopause in cultures like the United States where there has been a tradition of defining menopause in pathological terms.

Socioeconomic level also has been shown to have relevance to the menopausal experience in Western cultures. Studies have noted that middle- and upper-class women report less anxiety, fewer symptoms, and more positive reactions to menopause than do lower-class women (Bart and Grossman 1978[64]; Neugarten and Kraines 1965[21]; Van Keep and Kellerhals 1974[79]). Dege and Gretzinger (1982[80]) report a similar trend in upper-middle versus lower-class families' attitudes toward menopause. Polit and LaRocco (1980[81]) have noted increased incidence of menopausal symptomatology in women who were not well educated and not employed full time. Class differences in values, in expectations, and in options for gratifying life-styles beyond childrearing could account for these differences. Goldstein (1987[82]), in her report of the psychotherapy of two menopausal Italian-American women, documents the need for awareness of social and cultural factors.

Clinical symptoms associated with menopause have been discussed by Utian (1990[15]), who summarizes four relevant factors in the biology of menopause:

1. Morphological changes in the ovary (fibrosis versus hyperplasia versus hypertrophy)
2. Alteration in hormonal status, with a decrease in sex steroids, especially estrogenic ones, and elevated follicle-stimulating hormone (FSH) and luteinizing hormone (LH) levels
3. Changes in reactive tissue, most notably in the urogenital system, but also in the skin and peripheral and central nervous systems
4. Clinical signs and symptoms of estrogen deficiency

This formulation is helpful for understanding why many investigators have chosen to call menopause an endocrine deficiency disease. It does not explain, however, why large numbers of women report few symptoms or negative sequelae to menopause, nor does it account for the concomitant process of aging.

In proceeding to discussion of the predominate clinical symptoms associated with menopause and relevant to psychodynamic clinicians, it is important to note again what we have documented earlier: namely, that the majority of women are not significantly affected by adverse physical or psychological symptoms of menopause. Many women report positive reactions. A multitude of developmental/relational issues rather than menopause dominate female midlife psychology. For many the anticipatory anxiety and negative cultural implications of menopause are worse than the actual event. Some women at midlife, however, present with serious, authentic complaints that are treatable with medical and psychiatric interventions. We are therefore choosing to discuss the predominant symptoms associated with menopause, not to contribute to the notion of menopause as a vague, undifferentiated syndrome, but instead to 1) clarify what is known regarding each symptom and its etiology, 2) to debunk myths associated with certain symptoms, and 3) to discourage clinicians from either minimizing and dismissing treatable menopausal physical and psychiatric problems or overemphasizing the menopause and indiscriminately associating symptoms that are unrelated to the menopause but attributable to other treatable causes.

A wide variety of physical, psychosomatic, and psychological complaints have been reported as menopausal. Physical complaints include hot flushes, cold sweats, sleep disturbances, headaches, weight gain, cold hands and feet, numbness and tingling, breast pain, constipation, diarrhea, skin crawls, back and neck aches, dry skin, joint pain, osteoporosis, atherosclerotic cardiovascular disease, dyspareunia, and other complaints related to urogenital atrophy. Psychosomatic complaints have included fatigue, headache, palpitations, dizziness, and blind spots. Psychological complaints include irritability, mood lability, depression, "blue" moods, forgetfulness, poor concentration, excitability, crying spells, panic, feelings of suffocation, worries about the body, nervousness, and anxiety. Despite this multitude of symptoms, little documentation exists to actually link these symptoms with physiological menopause; in fact, numerous studies have demonstrated a lack of correlation for most of these symptoms (Greene and Cook 1980[83]; McKinlay and Jefferys 1974[84]). Only those symptoms most directly relevent to psychodynamic issues in menopause will be discussed in detail. Expanded discussions of primarily biological functions in menopause are available in Appendixes O and P.

Hot "Flashes" (Flushes) and Vasomotor Instability

According to a recent review by Raunikar (1990,[85] pp. 13–17), the symptoms of hot flushes and other vasomotor instability include nausea, dizziness, headaches, palpitations, diaphoresis, insomnia, night sweats, and probable associated sleep disorders. A prodromal episode, the hot flush (or "hot flash") is pathognomonic of vasomotor instability. It consists of the patient's subjective experience of feeling different immediately before the vasomotor episode and the physical experience of vasodilitation (usually in the upper body), increased sweating and peripheral skin temperature, and increased heart rate. A summary of the current theory and biological treatment of hot flushes is available in Appendix P.

Hot flashes may vary in severity and frequency from individual to individual and with regard to the subjective experience based on psychological variables. Feelings of shame, vulnerability, exposure, and lack of control have been triggered by these events and may require psychodynamic intervention.

Menopause and Depression

Depression as a second significant clinical entity of midlife has been reported by Winokur (1973[86]) and more recently by Schindler (1987[67]), who noted the occurrence of reactive depressions, dysthymic disorders, panic disorder, and major depression in midlife women. These disturbances, however, appear to be related to psychosocial variables other than the menopausal hormonal status. Weissman and Klerman (1977[87]; see also Weissman 1979[88]) dispute the correlation between menopausal hormonal status and clinical depressions and note the lack of increase in depression rates with menopause.

More current reviews of this issue (Coulam 1981[89]; Gitlin and Pasnau 1989[90]; Osborn 1984[91]; Roy et al. 1986[92]) continue to show no significant correlation between menopausal hormonal status and the various forms of depression. Indiscriminate linking of subjective complaints of depression and vegetative symptoms of depression with menopause can lead to a lack of exploration of the various psychodynamic issues surrounding those midlife stressors, losses, and shifts in relationships already discussed. It can also lead to minimization of the well-known constellation of symptoms constituting panic disorder, major depression, and other forms of affective illness, with the resultant failure to administer appropriate psychotropic medication. Current studies of the psychobiology of midlife depression are reviewed in Appendix Q.

Menopause and Cardiovascular Disease

Cardiovascular disease accounts for 53% of deaths in women over age 50 and is also a leading cause of disability in this age group (Bush 1990[93]). The relationship between estrogen deficiency and cardiovascular disease has received much attention in the current literature (Corson 1984[33]; Lobo 1990[36]; Sitruk-Ware and Iberra de Palacios 1989[94]; Stampfer et al. 1990[95]). There is general agreement that the estrogen decreases associated with menopause expose women to a greater risk of atherosclerosis and coronary heart disease (see Appendix R for details).

Menopause and Sleep Disorders

A variety of menopause studies (Ballinger 1976[96]; Jaszmann et al. 1969[97]; McKinlay and Jefferys 1974[84]) have reported significant increases in sleep complaints during the perimenopausal and immediate postmenopausal periods. Sleep disturbances directly related to menopause as differentiated from age-related sleep disturbances and disturbances related to psychiatric morbidity have not been fully elaborated, but differential patterns are emerging (Fry 1987[98]) (see Appendix S).

Menopause and Decline in Sexual Functioning

In a review of the literature on perimenopausal and postmenopausal sexuality, Morokoff (1988[99]) concludes that 1) most women continue to enjoy and engage in sexual activity during and after menopause, and the majority of these women are nondysfunctional; 2) menopause is associated with a decline in female sexual functioning in a smaller percentage of women during the perimenopausal period and in a larger percentage of women postmenopausally; and 3) estrogen may be relevant to reversing some aspects of this decline in sexual functioning. Young (1990[100]) further emphasizes the inappropriateness of assuming inevitable or precipitous decline in sexual activity related to menopause in women with suitable opportunities for expressing their sexuality.

Of those women experiencing sexual dysfunction associated with menopause, complaints generally occur in the following categories (Sarrel 1987[101]):

1. Diminished sexual responsiveness
2. Dyspareunia
3. Decreased sexual activity
4. Decline in sexual desire
5. Dysfunctional male partner

These complaints stem from a various etiologies, including menopausal hormonal factors, aging, chronic diseases and their treatment, psychological factors, sexual partners, and combinations of the above.

Bachmann (1990[102]) provides a detailed discussion of the negative impact of various situations:

1. Cervical cancer, with concomitant surgical/radiation changes in the vaginal vault
2. Hysterectomy, with concomitant changes in vaginal vault, decreased genital sensation, loss of the speculated cervical trigger to orgasm, and psychological impact
3. Coronary artery disease, hypertension, and strokes, with related psychological inhibition of sex
4. Physiologically based decline in libido, in achievement of orgasm, and in vaginal lubrication
5. Pharmacological treatment which has side effects that negatively impact sexual functioning
6. Breast cancer, with psychological inhibitions of sexuality

The author also notes that age-related progressions in chronic diseases such as arthritis and diabetes, lack of physical fitness, surgical procedures, death of partner, or age-related decline in sexual function of partner all have a negative impact on sexual functioning.

The problems stemming from changes in an older woman's sexual partner are as follows (Bachmann 1990[102]):

1. Emotional issues following death of spouse
2. Lack of availability of appropriate sexual partners for older women
3. Midlife marital stresses and role changes
4. Midlife conflicts in partner
5. Age-related sexual dysfunction in partner
6. Partner's social and cultural inhibitions to late-life sexuality
7. Partner's focus on coitus and failure to consider alternate strategies when coitus becomes problematic
8. Poor communication with partner resulting in lack of understanding and resolution or age- or menopause-related sexual symptoms

Bachmann (1990[102]) has reviewed in detail the direct impact of the menopausal hormonal states on sexual functioning. A declining estrogen level results in changes in vaginal anatomy and physiology as follows:

1. Thinning of the vaginal epithelium
2. Decreases in vaginal blood flow
3. Decreases in vaginal secretions and lubrication
4. Vaginal atrophy, with decline in vaginal elasticity and support to pelvic structures

Estrogen decline can also result in vulval atrophy, increased urinary frequency and urgency, predisposition to vulvovaginitis, and diminished neurological perception and skin sensitivity. All of these estrogen-related factors can diminish sexual responsiveness and increase dyspareunia, which can secondarily lead to a decline in sexual desire and activity and occasionally even to a dysfunction in the male partner, who may become inhibited by his concerns that coitus is hurting his partner. In addition, Bachmann (1990[102]) notes that sexual gratification, desire, arousal, and fantasy may be linked to testosterone levels, which are affected by menopause. She also notes that women who remain sexually active maintain better genital health than do their inactive counterparts. Sarrel (1990[103]) reports that many of these estrogen-related symptoms occur when estradiol levels are below 50 pg/ml. For those who wish more detailed information, Walling et al. (1990[104]) provide a comparative review of sexual outcomes for a variety of hormonal replacement therapies involving estrogen, including estrogen/progesterone combinations and estrogen/androgen combinations.

The interplay of menopausal hormonal changes and psychodynamic factors is complicated in the case of menopause-related changes in sexual functioning. Thus, we have presented more detail in this section to enable therapists to acquaint themselves with the variety of factors that must be considered in the formulation of a treatment program. Iddenden (1987,[105] p. 93) suggests asking the following questions during preliminary evaluations for sexual complaints:

1. Are you sexually active?
2. Has there been a change in your level of desire?
3. Is intercourse satisfactory?
4. Is there any discomfort during intercourse?
5. Have you noticed any change in lubrication when you become aroused?
6. Do you reach orgasm satisfactorily?
7. Do you have a partner at the present time?
8. Are there any sex-related problems with your partner?

Osteoporosis and Menopause

Bone mass loss proceeds rapidly following menopause, leading to the development of osteoporosis and related bone weakness fractures (Lindsay and Cosman 1990[34]; Melton 1990[106]; see Appendix T). The concomitant process of aging and lack of exercise on osteoporosis and its relationship to menopausal change is not well documented.

Nondepressive Psychiatric Disturbances Associated With Menopause

At present there are no well-documented psychiatric disturbances associated with menopause. Schindler (1987[67]) has reported the prevalence of depression (see subsection on menopause and depression above) as well as phobic anxiety disorder and somatoform disorders, psychogenic pain, psychosomatic complaints, and conversion reactions in this age group. He also notes, however, that menopause is only one of many possible etiologies. Many of the vague psychosomatic and psychological complaints commonly associated with menopause have not stood the test of empirical validation, and midlife psychiatric complaints may be more related to life events, psychosocial changes, and psychosocial risk factors than to biological events. Psychotropic drug use is associated with menopausal women but does not correlate well to their menopausal status (Kaufert and Gilbert 1986[45]). In short, clinicians evaluating psychiatric complaints in menopausal women should look beyond menopause for their etiologies.

Having reviewed the complex developmental issues of midlife women, as well as the specific symptoms related to the menopausal hormonal status, we provide as a transition to the presentation of patient material the discussion of a recent study of menopausal women in psychoanalytic treatment by Mendell (1988[107]). She characterizes current psychoanalytic views regarding depressive reactions to menopause as somewhat polarized, with Lampl–de Groot (1983[108]) contending that coping well is the norm, and Lax (1982[109]) insisting that a menopausal crisis accompanied by a depressive reaction with a period of sadness and mourning is inevitable and in fact necessary for ultimate adaptation. Stressing the current psychoanalytic trend to view menopause within an adaptive developmental framework, Mendell reviewed the results of open-ended interviews with the analysts of 13 menopausal women. Several dominant themes emerged:

1. Menopause is experienced as a signal of aging that stimulates a reevaluation of the past and of its limitation, and an active formulation of the future.
2. Sexual fulfillment, sexual competition, and childbearing are reviewed in terms of lost capacities and opportunities, and accompanying regrets. This sense of regret was independent of whether the women in this sample actually had children.
3. Body awareness is heightened concomitant with the reexperiencing of earlier developmental phases.
4. The meaning of menopause is unique to each individual and related to her own life experience and adaptive and defensive structures.

The women in the study worked through menopause positively and creatively. They did not suffer clinical depression, but they did manifest the fears of change and sense of loss of former identity common to transitions in developmental stages. These findings, although based on a limited, uncontrolled patient sample, are consistent with, on the one hand, the adult developmental model consisting of a series of stages and specific tasks and a transitional period characterized by regressions, and with, on the other hand, the notion that menopause is a unique, highly individualized experience rather than a universal undifferentiated phenomenon.

We now turn to clinical patient material, advising therapists treating patients during the perimenopause and postmenopausal periods to be guided by several clinical principles:

1. Therapists should be familiar with treatment modalities and research data regarding etiologies beyond the scope of their field of specialty so that biological and psychological components can be appropriately separated and treated.
2. Psychological and developmental issues are especially relevant during midlife and must be considered in any symptom reports associated with menopause.
3. Global references to an undifferentiated menopausal syndrome are unwarranted and undermine good clinical treatment. Individual symptoms should be pursued carefully without presuming relationships and with the possibility of multiple etiologies kept in mind.
4. Although many midlife complaints have been thoughtlessly ascribed to the menopausal syndrome and most women proceed through menopause without major distress, some women do experience authentic and serious symptomatology amenable to both biological and psychiatric intervention if the symptomatology is properly diagnosed.
5. The lifespan of women will most likely continue to increase, making the postmenopausal period a predominant phase of life and of increasing importance to clinicians and patients.

Menopausal-Like Symptoms Unrelated to Physiology

A 49-year-old perimenopausal woman was referred by her internist for psychiatric evaluation of symptoms of night sweats, dizziness, and facial tingling and tinnitus. Initially these symptoms were associated with her reports of diminished menstrual periods; however, they did not correspond to decreased estrogen levels and did not respond to ERT. An ear-nose-and-throat workup was also negative. Meanwhile, the patient's symptoms were worsening.

The patient was a competent, successful professional woman who was childless but reportedly happily adjusted to a second marriage with a compatible partner with whom she was experiencing no sexual or interpersonal difficulties. She reported some minor professional difficulties related to inhibited creative aspirations but was otherwise happy with her professional and personal life. Past psychiatric history was negative except for a panic attack prior to a hysterectomy performed in her late 30s for fibroids. She related no regrets at being childless, stating this had always been her wish and that she felt relieved to be able to put her energy into her work and her marriage. Social and recreational adaptations were good.

About her impending menopausal state, the patient again reiterated that she had no regrets regarding children; in fact, she felt it was "safer" without them. Exploration of this interesting choice of words left the patient anxious, confused, and inarticulate. Over the next 3 months she became aware that she was having nightmares accompanied by sweating. Images of children of various ages overwhelmed by dark shadows terrified her. Over the course of her 2-year treatment she was able to derepress episodes of childhood sexual abuse related to three separate abusers. Her symptoms of tinnitus, facial tingling, and dizziness disappeared with the memory of a family friend who abused her and intimidated her into silence by clapping his hands sharply across her cheeks and ears.

Physiological-Like Symptoms Relieved With Estrogen Replacement Therapy

A 45-year-old married mother of two adult children came to analysis because of difficulty in achieving her professional goals. She was a masochistic and depressed woman as a result of her identification with a mother who had similar problems. As the patient began to become more successful and to build her self-esteem, she became menopausal. She had no immediate other problems in her life and was in fact doing well. She had vascular instability with flushing and sweating, both during the day, of sufficient severity to disrupt her sleep at night. She was referred for evaluation for ERT, which was begun. Her symptoms improved within 3 weeks and her analysis continued to progress. After a year she was encouraged to try a "hormone holiday," and her symptoms returned. ERT was reinstituted, and she remains well.

A Patient for Whom Estrogen Replacement Therapy Affected a Physical Disorder and Bolstered Her Self-Esteem

A patient in her mid-50s who was the divorced mother of two adult children sought therapy because of a threatened breakup with a recent boyfriend, a relationship that she thought was unsuitable to her socioeconomic or interest level. After the relationship broke off, the patient embarked on making a new life for herself. She got a new hairstyle and coloring, bought some updated clothing, moved to a more suitable location for a single woman, and became involved in new social activities. Her skin was marred by a series of wrinkles that seemed to her therapist more characteristic of estrogen depletion than of aging. She was referred for ERT despite the absence of other menopausal symptoms. Within weeks her dry skin plumped up and her hair, which she had not complained about, was noted by her hairdresser to be less dry and brittle. Her appearance so changed that people she had known at a previous job hardly recognized her. She felt increased self-esteem with her changed appearance. She felt less like an old lady and developed a more realistic appraisal of being at midlife, with a view to the opportunities that midlife holds.

Menopausal Symptoms That Were Unrelieved With Estrogen Replacement Therapy but Relieved in Analytic Treatment

The patient, a married woman in her early 40s who had one daughter, came to treatment because of a writer's block. A great deal of analysis was accomplished around the issue of being intellectually discouraged and being treated as a second-class citizen in contrast to her brother. Her father had been a violent and irascible individual who cowed her mother into submission. Her husband had always appreciated and encouraged her intellectual interests. For the patient, completing her work and becoming successful meant surpassing her mother and symbolically killing her father. She had resumed writing, lost weight, and looked generally brighter when she began to experience menopausal symptoms. In addition to hot flushes and sweating she had a sleep disturbance, became bulimic, and was generally more depressed. She was referred for ERT. Although this helped the symptoms of vascular instability, it did not ameliorate the sleep and eating disorders.

The problems generated by menopause were not easily elucidated. Initially the patient reflected on the fact that she had had only one child and that perhaps menopause had dashed her hope of having another. Upon closer reflection the patient was able to discuss a symbiotic relationship between her husband and her daughter. Furthermore, she discussed her husband's potency problems, always a source of frustration. With the occurrence of menopause she revealed that she had always tolerated her asexual marriage by a series of love affairs. Her entrance to midlife, she felt, endangered her attractiveness and cemented her into her marriage, which she had sometimes thought of abandoning. As her anger and disappointment came into focus, she began to sleep better, brightened in her affect, and resumed her investment in her career.

Widowhood

According to Holmes and Rahe (1967–1968[110]), the death of a spouse ranks as life's most stressful event, not only in terms of the intensity and duration of the mourning process but also in terms of the complexities of readjustment. The importance of this event is further heightened by Barrett (1977[111]), who documents its high prevalence among women. He notes that in the United States there are over 10 million widows, who tend to remain unmarried for an average of 18 years following the deaths of their husbands. Given the greater life expectancy for women, Barrett also predicts that 75% of married women living today will experience widowhood. As the current population ages, these figures will obviously increase significantly. The mean age for widows in the United States is 66 years, and among women 65 years and over, 51% are widows (Hansson and Remondet 1988[112]).

Psychiatric literature has emphasized the seriousness of grief reactions and documented various forms of pathological grief. Developmental and sociological literature has documented that the majority of women adapt quite successfully to this major life change, and a significant number even report positive growth following the death of their spouse, particularly in areas of competence and independence. Psychodynamic and developmental writers focusing on geriatrics have illuminated a series of complex life tasks and adult developmental lines, making clear that there are a multitude of life events that evolve during the time many women spend as widows and that go well beyond adjustment to the death of their spouses.

Our purpose in this section will be to provide a broad overview of this important phase of women's lives. We focus not only on the most current information regarding pathological grief reactions and psychodynamic interventions, but also on the multitude of life events occurring during this time frame and the ways in which psychodynamic interventions, when focused on some of these other areas, may make a positive contribution not only to successful grieving but also to the ultimate potential for growth during this period.

The Normal Course of Widowhood

The loss and mourning aspects of widowhood—that is, the negative sequelae and psychiatric interventions directed toward depression and pathological bereavement—has been emphasized in the psychiatric literature. Although numerous authors (Blackburn et al. 1987[113]; Ferraro 1984b[114]; McCrae and Costa 1988[115]; Thomas et al. 1988[116]) have documented the resiliency and adaptivity of most widows, much of this acquired information on the normal progression of widowhood remains in the gerontology and sociology literature, leaving mental health professionals either uninformed or focused on a primarily pathological model. To correct this lack of perspective, we begin with a selective overview of information regarding the normal course of widowhood. From this perspective we then examine the psychodynamics and styles of bereavement, pathological grief reactions, dynamically oriented treatment interventions for pathological grief, and psychodynamic issues and interventions during widowhood that are unrelated to grief reactions.

Heinemann and Evans (1990[117]) provide an excellent structure for the review of recent literature on the normal process of widowhood. They place widowhood in the context of a model encompassing loss, change, and adaptation. Their loss-and-change model is defined in terms of three flexible, broad and overlapping phases: 1) preparation and anticipatory grief, 2) grief and mourning, and 3) adaptation. They emphasize the highly individualized variations and time frames of these phases as well as the fluctuations in the nature of the losses and changes throughout the process. Some of the losses and changes are intrapsychic and some are external. Some occur early in the process, some later. Some are transient and some enduring. We will summarize their model and literature review and integrate additional relevant information.

Preparation and Anticipatory Grief

The preparation phase (Heinemann and Evans 1990[117]) begins with the recognition of impending loss and ends with the actual death of the spouse. This phase includes learning adaptive behaviors, acquiring life skills and resources necessary for coping with widowhood, planning for widowhood, and anticipatory grieving. Although not yet well investigated, this phase has an important impact on the final adjustment to widowhood and is prominent in the experiences of women whose husbands are in poor health or terminally ill or who are well advanced in age and for whom death is anticipated.

Rehearsal and anticipatory planning for widowhood can occur on many levels: conscious, subconscious, behavioral, social, emotional, or cognitive. Provided the rehearsal takes the form of adaptive coping rather than negative rumination, it is associated with successful adaptation. (See Appendix U for a comprehensive review.)

Anticipatory grieving is the final component of the first (i.e., preparation) phase of adjustment. Fulton and Fulton (1971[118]) define anticipatory grieving as follows: 1) depression, 2) heightened concern for the terminally ill person, 3) rehearsal of the death, and 4) attempts to adjust to the consequences of the death. Futterman et al. (1972[119]) have identified a number of related tasks of anticipatory grieving: 1) acknowledging the death as inevitable, 2) experiencing and expressing the emotional impact of the anticipated loss, 3) reconciling oneself to the anticipated loss, 4) detaching oneself emotionally from the dying person, and 5) memorializing the dying person.

The current literature reports both positive and negative aspects of anticipatory grief. Sudden, unanticipated traumatic deaths are associated with prolonged grieving and inhibited coping, whereas some warning time and anticipatory grief facilitates adaptation (Bumagin and Hirn 1982[120]; Glick et al. 1974[121]; Schwab et al. 1975[122]; Vachon et al. 1982a[123]). If, however, the period of anticipatory grief is prolonged, as it is in some chronic, terminally ill patients, the grieving is associated with difficulties such as premature detachment, ambivalence, guilt, inhibited mourning, stress, and compromised health status (Clayton et al. 1973[124]; Rando 1984[125]). In addition, some age-related variables seem to be at play. For widows under 50, sudden death of spouse is associated with negative outcome (Ball 1976–1977[126]; Glick et al. 1974[121]; Parkes 1975[127]; Parkes and Brown 1972[128]; Rando 1984[125]). In older widows, this does not appear to be the case, perhaps because these individuals have prepared for widowhood as a life-stage task. Elderly widows are more seriously affected by prolonged chronic anticipatory situations (Ball 1976–1977[126]; Gerber et al. 1975[129]; Schwab et al. 1975[122]), perhaps because they have fewer resources to deal with the burden of care required during this period.

Grief and Mourning

The second phase, the grief and mourning period, begins with the death of the spouse and ends with the widow's acceptance of the loss and her ability to rebuild a new life (Heinemann and Evans 1990[117]). Most researchers describe this period as lasting from 1 to 3 years, but there is a great deal of individual variability as well as evidence to support the view that for some women, this period is extremely prolonged and enduring. During this period of time, the widow's patterns of daily living, her relationships, and her self-image are disrupted. After a short protective period of shock, numbness, and denial, most widows experience a variable time of intense emotional pain and yearning for their husbands, often accompanied by physical symptomatology. Common complaints are sadness, anxiety, tearfulness, anergia, guilt, anger, weight loss, sleep disturbances, gastrointestinal complaints, and listlessness (Parkes 1970[130]).

Socialization with others during this period is in the service of making the loss real, both internally and externally. If the widow's social network permits and supports the expression of grief and the clarification of the meaning of her loss, she will progress. If it does not, her grieving may become prolonged or maladaptive. The role of support is important but complicated. It can be harmful, helpful, or inconsequential, depending on where the widow is in the process, the type of support given, and who provides the support (Bankoff 1981,[131] 1983b[132]). Types of support include psychological, task, service, and advice. Psychological support is most often provided by women, and advice is often given by men. During grieving, socioemotional support is the most valued (Warner 1987[133]).

As Ben-Sita (1983[134]) has documented, grieving and catharsis require people such as relatives and long-standing friends who are capable of listening, nurturing, and expressing intense feelings. Bankoff (1983a[135]) has documented the crucial importance of elderly mothers to their newly widowed daughters, providing both empathy as well as role models for these younger women. In addition to Bankoff's study, Warner (1987[133]) and Lopata (1979[136]) identify women as being most supportive, especially daughters, daughters-in-law, and mothers. Availability of service and task supports during periods of "numbness" or emergencies is also helpful. Married friends and family close to the deceased allow the widow an important link to her deceased spouse as she attempts to clarify the meaning of her loss.

Late in the process the support network should become more diverse and provide more social and information networks as well as more encouragement to move beyond the deceased. Walker et al. (1977[137]) have documented how overly supportive task-service help can be regressive at this point. Morgan (1986[138]) has shown that the initially positive commitment and obligatory ties of families may later become conflict ridden and inflexible during the adaptation phase.

Support groups led by professionals or peers for widows have been documented as being helpful (Farrell and Wilner 1986[139]; Lieberman and Videka-Sherman 1986[140]; Redburn and Juretich 1989[141]), as long as the widow does not become overly reliant or rigid in conforming to the grief models discussed in the group (Wambach 1985–1986[142]). Professionally led groups focusing on emotional support, socializing, and education have also been documented as being helpful, especially for women with limited social contact or those women with few personal resources; widows focused on self-reliance may, however, find these groups regressive (Barrett 1978[143]; Ben-Sita 1983[134]; Constantino 1981[144]; Debor et al. 1983[145]).

Cultural and religious traditions of grieving are a crucial part in the social network at this time. They provide a valuable supportive structure for grieving. When these traditions are misunderstood or inhibited, an additional stress is created. Doka (1986[146]) has documented the intensity of the divorced widow's grief as well as the complications of bereavement that are due not only to her ambivalent feelings but also to her ambiguous disenfranchised social role.

Under positive conditions, a widow's symptoms prominent during the first year of bereavement will decrease with time (Clayton et al. 1973[124]; Parkes and Brown 1972[128]; Blanchard et al. 1976[147]). Vachon and associates (1982a[123]) identified three predominant patterns that occur during the first year of widowhood: 1) 30% of the patients had no high psychological distress level, 2) 14% had an initial high level of distress with a gradual tapering off, and 3) 29% had an initial high level of distress sustained over a 2-year period. For young widows, 25% experienced deleterious psychological symptoms, and some of these women resorted to sedative and tranquilizer use (Maddison and Viola 1968[148]; Parkes 1964,[149] 1970[130]). Young widows' bereavement does not seem to influence major diseases, physical status, or psychiatric conditions (Heinemann and Evans 1990[117]). Elderly widows, in contrast, perceive an immediate decline in their health status and experience significant psychological symptoms when compared with same-age control subjects (Breckenridge et al. 1986[150]; Ferraro 1985–1986[151]). Heyman and Gianturco (1973[152]) found no actual relationship between grief and physical health status in the geriatric population. Despite the psychological symptoms reported by most widows, and the increase in alcohol, tobacco, and tranquilizer use by some widows, mental health scores, on average, indicate no serious pathology (Breckenridge et al. 1986[150]), and widows seldom require psychiatric hospitalization (Clayton 1973[153]).

Cain (1974[154]) and Gates (1990[155]) provide both detailed descriptions of the mourning period and various coping strategies that are important and that go beyond the social networks we have already described.

Numerous authors (Akiyama et al. 1986–1987[156]; Clark et al. 1986[157]; Folkman and Lazarus 1980[158]; Gass 1987[159]; Moss and Moss 1984[160]; Schuchter and Zisook 1988[161]; Wambach 1985–1986[142]) have illuminated various coping strategies, including using protective denial, keeping busy, increasing participation in social groups, doing leisure and religious activities, learning new skills, maintaining spiritual and emotional ties to the deceased, exercising, keeping well groomed, keeping journals, participating in family outings, caring for pets, and attending support groups. Avoidance, denial, prolonged use of fantasies, prolonged use of psychotropic medication, alcohol and excessive use of tranquilizers, and bargaining with the self and God, were identified as unhelpful strategies (Gass 1987[159]). There is general agreement that coping strategies change as grief progresses and may vary in helpfulness according to the individual and what stage of mourning is represented. For example, although, early on, denial can be helpful and provide for gradual adjustment to loss, over the long term it can inhibit grief and recovery. Maintaining an emotional tie with a deceased spouse may be a help over the short term in cushioning the shock, and also over the long term, especially in elderly women with few other coping methods available or in women who maintain the tie with the deceased but do not let this interfere with developing other ties and activities. It can also, however, be associated with an inability to move toward a more functional adaptation in widows who have a multitude of options available but whose flexibility is limited by this tie.

Adaptation

According to Heinemann and Evans (1990[117]), the third and final phase of adjustment to widowhood, adaptation, involves the struggle to develop new relationships, the restructuring of old relationships, and the acquisition of new skills and abilities or the resurrection of dormant ones in order to create a life that has meaning for the widow and that enables her to integrate into a coherent social system. They caution, appropriately, to be cognizant of the wide variety of possible outcomes in this period, noting that while the majority of widows adapt well and go on to fruitful lives, some just get by, and a minority never recover. A surprisingly large number of widows exhibit positive growth in terms of independence, competence, and freedom as well as relief from negative or burdensome relationships to which they feel obligated and for which they feel themselves responsible for maintaining. Thomas et al. (1988[116]) documented 45% of their study sample reporting this type of healthy development.

Heinemann and Evans (1990[117]), again, provide an excellent review of how this generally positive outcome unfolds. For many widows the process of rebuilding is evident after the first year of bereavement, concomitant with the establishment of periods of emotional equilibrium (Glick et al. 1974[121]). Ferraro (1984b[114]) has documented that the death of a spouse intensifies rather than attenuates social relationships. Adaptive shifts in relationships occur as the importance of couple-oriented relationships diminishes, new friends or old friends supportive of the widow's new identity become more important, and family roles are renegotiated (Lopata 1973,[162] 1979[136]; Brock and O'Sullivan 1985[163]; Reinhardt and Fisher 1989[164]). Lewittes (1989[165]) has documented the importance of continued intimate and reciprocal relationships for older women and the maintenance of a relational identity. Family ties and roles that are based on obligation remain the most stable, and those that are based on mutual interests, such as with siblings and extended kin, are more subject to change (Anderson 1984[166]).

Contrary to popular opinion, widowed mothers are not deserted by their children. Even those children who are working and are geographically distant remain responsible and involved. Remnet (1987[167]) has documented the complexity of the response of adult children to their widowed mothers. In addition, several authors (Brody and Schoonover 1986[168]; Schoonover et al. 1988[169]) have focused on the patterns of care, intersibling tensions, strain, and guilt of daughters who feel responsible for their mothers' care.

The mother/daughter relationship has been documented by various authors (Bankoff 1983a[135]; Brody and Schoonover 1986[168]; Lopata 1979[136]; Warner 1987[133]) as being especially important, not only to older widows who depend on their daughters for emotional support and ongoing relationships but also to young widows who look to their older widowed mothers as both empathic supports and role models. For some, reentry into the work force is a source of personal satisfaction (Strugnell 1974[170]) or an economic necessity, stimulating a variety of organizational and institutional efforts to empower these women who are reentering (Towns and Gentzler 1986[171]). Others become involved in religious or social organizations and hobbies and leisure activities (Cain 1974[154]; Gates 1990[155]). Younger widows may find a sense of purpose in their children along with inhibitions to other social options, especially with men; older widows are more likely to focus on children or grandchildren, with special emphasis on their daughters (Glick et al. 1974[121]; Lopata 1979[136]).

Lopata (1988[172]) has noted the great heterogeneity of life-styles and supports that widows organize for themselves and relates this to the existence of great social change, concomitant with the perseverance of traditional life patterns. Glick and associates (1974[121]) have identified four life-styles that emerge in widows over time, centering around 1) remarriage, 2) a commitment to a man in a nonmarital relationship, 3) close supportive relationships with kin, or 4) being independent of close relationships except for children. Although most successfully adapted widows tend to become more competent and autonomous, they also continue to define themselves in the context of important relationships, even following the death of their spouses, as has been documented by Thomas et al. (1988[116]), who suspect that widowhood impacts identity and intimacy in a combined fashion rather than in a focused identity fashion as previously described. This hypothesis is in keeping with Gilligan's (1982)[173] notion that for women these tasks of intimacy and identity are fused and the woman comes to know herself as she is known through her relationship with others.

Regarding sexuality and remarriage, young widows are more responsive than older widows to resumption of an active heterosexual life and to remarriage. Spanier and Glick (1980[174]) have noted that remarriage is more probable for women who married young and who lost their husbands early in marriage. Younger widows also tend to be more concerned about age-related body changes, which they feel will inhibit sexuality. Older widows report missing more nonsexual heterosexual activities, such as talking or going out with a man, more than they miss the sexual activity. Older widows, according to one study (Malatesta et al. 1988[175]), find ways in which to express various aspects of their sexuality through attractive clothing, grooming, spirituality, and child care. Kansky (1986[176]) has studied sexual adjustment and activity in widows during the first year of bereavement. Her results show that younger widows who anticipated their husband's death had sexual experience outside the marital relationship, did not have a strong intimate marital bond or were beginning to detach from one, and were more likely to experience sexual desire and engage in coitus during the first 14 months of bereavement.

Several studies (Gentry and Schulman 1988[177]; Gentry et al. 1987[178]) have noted that remarriage can be a means of coping with problems of economics, loneliness, and child care. The authors document the success of these marriages as well as the failure of another group of widows who are interested in remarrying for relational needs.

Most widows are not remarried and spend, on average, 18 years of their lives as widows (Barrett 1977[111]; Cleveland and Gianturco (1976[179]) report that beyond age 55, 14% of women will remarry. For women over 65, the probability of remarriage is low (i.e., .004). Many widows choose not to remarry because of the lack of partners, the number of which continues to diminish over the life-span due to differing mortalities in women and men. However, they also may make this choice for their own particular reasons, including that 1) no one measures up to their spouse, 2) they wish to remain autonomous and free, and 3) they do not wish to be a caregiver again (Arschault 1986[180]; Gentry et al. 1987[178]; Lopata 1979[136]). A significant number of widows experience loneliness but find this preferable to being considered a burden (Lopata 1979,[136] 1987[181]).

The role of social networks in providing respite from this significant loneliness and in contributing to the overall morale, well-being, and positive adaptation has been explored by many investigators. Daughters, nuclear family, siblings, extended family, married friends, single friends, old friends, new friends, neighbors, social and religious organizations—all play a role and vary in their helpfulness based on where the widow is in the process of adaptation. Relationships previously mentioned as helpful during the grieving period may actually become negative or regressive during the adaptation phase, unless the participants are able to make a shift and encourage the widow toward a new and competent life-style. New friends, daughters, and kin who encourage new skills, provide information, and help shape new identities, as well as institutions that perform the same functions, are most important in this adaptation phase. Schoonover et al. (1988[169]) and Brody and Schoonover (1986[168]) note that, despite common perceptions of abandonment by family, family members continue to remain involved with widows regardless of geographic distance and involvement of many of the daughters in the work force.

Heinemann and Evans (1990[117]) cite some additional information regarding the social support of widows during the adaptation phase:

1. Widowed elderly women receive more help from children and friends than do their married counterparts (Roberto and Scott 1986[182]).
2. Family members continue to be supportive and friendships increase between the first and fourth years of bereavement (Ferraro et al. 1984[183]).
3. Neighbors tend to be most supportive of elderly widows with children living outside the area and are less involved with widows having children living close by or those who are childless (O'Bryant 1985[184]).
4. A childless elderly widow's friends are more supportive than relatives, although relatives, especially siblings, play a somewhat important role in the widow's support systems (Goldberg et al. 1986[185]).
5. Race and ethnicity are not factors in predicting informal networks of the elderly widow. However, the use of formal support does vary among subculture groups; it is higher for blacks and whites than for Hispanics and Asians (Pelham and Clark 1987[186]).

6. Reciprocal relationships among friends and neighbors, perceived good health, and adequate economic resources are determinants of well-being and morale among widowed persons (Arens 1982[187]; Arling 1976b[188]; Scott and Kivelt 1985[189]). Older widows tend to be happier than younger widows (Arens 1982[187]). Financial problems lead to greater negative feelings in widows than in their married counterparts (Arens 1982[187]).

Pathological Grief

Despite the generally positive adaptation we have just documented for most widows, the severity of grief problems for those who do encounter them has generated much theoretical and empirical research, as well as treatment interventions, focused on the pathological grief syndromes. (For a review of the psychoanalytic literature on mourning, refer to Appendix V.) Several theoretically different psychodynamic formulations for pathologic grief have evolved. These models have proven invaluable to clinicians and are deeply ingrained in the thinking of most psychiatric professionals. They have served as the genesis for much of the more rigorous empirical research done in recent years.

Despite this abundance of both theoretical and empirical work, both Rynearson (1990[190]) and Raphael and Middleton (1990[191]) point to the significant heterogeneity of both normal and pathological bereavement processes and warn against an attitude of certitude in the precise defining of normal and pathological grief as well as in the treatment of grief reactions. Rynearson (1990[190]), in particular, refers to the current clash between the realistic complexities of the grieving process and those traditional theoretically based clinical axioms that are assumed to be representative of all grief, such as

- the world is despised with mourning—the self is despised with grief,
- mourning is inevitable and necessary and resolves in months,
- mourning follows a sequence of discrete stages,
- grief is a denial or aberrant fixation of mourning,
- ambivalent cathexis is the sine qua non of grief,
- ambivalent cathexis is developmentally determined, and
- cathexis and active mourning promise recovery. (p. 298)

Rynearson (1990[190]) notes that rigorous empirical studies cannot verify these axioms and states:

> It is at this intersection—when extreme and parsimonious theory is confronted by rigorous and precise empiricism—that we witness a head-on accident with no survivors.
>
> What is required in studying so subjective and diverse a referent as pathologic grief is a tentative approach tolerant of multiple hypotheses and that the demand for empirical validation be softened until precise and specific measurements have been developed. (p. 298)

It is in this spirit, using outlines developed by Raphael and Middleton (1990[191]) and Rynearson (1990[190]), that we will present the psychodynamic models of pathological grief and a descriptive typology of pathological grief reactions.

The earliest model of pathological grief was developed by Freud (1917/1961[192]) and later elaborated by Lindemann (1944[193]). Freud proposed that ambivalent feelings toward the lost object account for the primary difference between normal mourning and melancholia, its pathological variation. Such ambivalence toward the lost object results in difficulties in relinquishing bonds, and much of the negative affect surrounding the lost figure falls upon the ego of the bereaved (its internalized symbol), resulting in low self-esteem and a sense of guilt and defectiveness—in short, melancholia. Any intense anger toward the lost object is directed at the self. The unconscious denial of this ambivalence results in a depression in which the self is seen as bad and worthless rather than the external world appearing depleted and impoverished, as in normal mourning. This psychodynamic equation of pathological grief with depression led to the works of Clayton et al. (1968,[194] 1971,[195] 1972,[196] 1974[197]), Raphael (1977,[198] 1978[199]), Parkes and Weiss (1983[200]), Jacobs and Kim (1990[201]), and others who viewed bereavement as a reactive depression and pathological bereavement as an extensive, severe, and intense variation of this depression. Works by Parkes (1990[202]), Bruce et al. (1990[203]), and Freedman and Blumenfield (1987[204]) further explore links between depression and bereavement.

Interestingly, Byrne (1989[205]) has reported on depression in the elderly that is distinct from the mourning process. Ultimately, however, despite this voluminous work, solid empirical links between depression and bereavement remain to be established.

Bowlby (1973,[206] 1980[207]) described bereavement in terms of attachment and loss. He noted phases of grief that include 1) an initial shock and denial, 2) a separation reaction (including anxiety, protest, pining, sadness, despair, depression, and disorganization), and 3) a reorganization. Prominent in this theory is the particular dimension of grief, which involves the act of pining for the lost person. Such pining reflects an intermittent and intrusive wish to recover the lost person as an integral part of the separation reaction. Bowlby was the first to suggest the notion that the impact of loss can be lessened by forming substitute attachments, therefore offering a theoretical basis for understanding the healing function of other people.

Bowlby also explained the adaptive function associated with grief in suggesting that all behavior patterns need to be broken down before they can be adapted to new objects and goals. He defined two forms of pathological grief: absence of grief, and chronic mourning. With the denial of loss comes the prolonged absence of conscious mourning and failure to let go of the lost person. Works by Deutsch (1937[208]) and Volkan (1970[209]) corroborate this perception, as does the work of Parkes (1965[210]) on inhibited or delayed grief reactions. Maddison and Walker (1967[211]) provide some empirical evidence that absence or inhibition of the grieving process leads to poor outcome. Singh and Raphael (1981[212]) have documented no pathological outcomes associated with a small group of individuals who demonstrated no grief reactions following loss of loved ones. The solid empirical validation of this concept remains to be determined.

Bowlby's concepts of pathological and chronic mourning suggest a pattern of continued pining for, focusing on, and idealization of the lost person as predominant, along with feelings of intense bitterness. Such prolonged patterns may be recurrent or continuous. Although widely accepted, this type of pathological reaction also requires further empirical studies to define and investigate this syndrome as well as to differentiate it from posttraumatic stress reactions.

Another pathological model of grief stems from the work of Horowitz (1990[213]) and Krystal (1987[214]). These authors view bereavement as a posttraumatic stress reaction, with periods of intrusive images of the bereaved and intrusive affects related to bereavement alternating with periods of numbness and withdrawal, and pathological grief. These writers envision a posttraumatic stress reaction that is interrupted, interminable, or of abnormally high intensity. The bereaved may become overwhelmed or rigidly fixed in states of rage, fear, and/or shame, or debilitated by withdrawal reactions associated with images of helplessness, vulnerability, weakness, abandonment, or badness. These latter negative images can be postulated to be latent self-images from earlier in development that are reactivated by the loss. This model also requires further scientific validation as well as some differentiation from depression.

A final model of pathological grief having no direct psychodynamic etiology but multiple psychodynamic implications is based on numerous statistical studies that assess risk factors associated with overall morbid outcome from bereavement, rather than a specific pathological pattern of grief. Morbidity has been defined in terms of health impairment, increased symptomatic complaints, negative immune changes, increases in alcohol and substance abuse, increase in medical care needed, and development of psychiatric problems. According to Raphael and Middleton (1990[191]), the following factors have been documented by multiple investigators as predisposing an individual to poor bereavement outcomes:

1. Sudden, unexpected, untimely bereavements
2. Highly ambivalent, dependent, or conflicted relationships with the deceased
3. Lack of support of the social network and primary group in facilitating the expression of grief and other relevant interventions
4. The concurrence of multiple life events such as multiple losses at the same time
5. Preexisting vulnerabilities in the bereaved related to earlier experiences or sociodemographic factors
6. Intensely high distress early after the loss

Parkes (1990[202]), in a recent general review of bereavement risks, adds some additional specific factors:

1. Previous psychiatric problems
2. Low self-trust, leading to intense grief
3. Diminished trust in others, predisposing to avoidance and minimal grief
4. Anxious and conflicted parents, predisposing children to insecurity in adulthood and to anxious and conflicted grief patterns
5. Absent or rejecting parents, predisposing children to depressions after bereavement in adult life
6. Compulsive self-reliant traits, resulting in delayed grief after bereavement
7. Marriages in which more than two areas of conflict exist, yielding conflicted grief (characterized by initial denial), followed by delayed grief in which feelings of anger and guilt complicate the mourning

Parkes also reviews and summarizes the risk factors studied by other researchers and organizes them according to 1) mode of death, 2) social supports, 3) bereaved's relationship to the deceased, and 4) predisposing factors in the bereaved.

Those additional factors most relevant to widowhood are as follows:

1. Young age of bereaved (Maddison and Walker 1967[211]; Van Rooijen 1978[215])
2. Poverty of bereaved (Vachon et al. 1982b[216])
3. Low self-esteem of bereaved (Stroebe and Stroebe 1987[217])
4. Bereaved unaware of diagnosis or prognosis of deceased (Duke 1980[218])
5. Bereaved remote from deceased (Duke 1980[218])
6. Deceased died by suicide (Cain 1966[219])
7. Deceased died by murder or manslaughter (Danto 1982[220])
8. Deceased died by long terminal illness (Gerber et al. 1975[221])
9. Deceased overtly dependent on bereaved (Parkes and Weiss 1983[200])

10. No family or children near bereaved (Parkes and Weiss 1983[200])
11. Family seen as unhelpful by bereaved (Maddison and Walker 1967[211])

Certain personality factors may also lend themselves to morbid outcome. Middleton (1989[222]) is currently exploring these issues but they remain to be empirically validated. Traits that are under consideration are 1) neuroticism and age at detachment, yielding extreme separation reactions; 2) intensely dependent personality, yielding absent grief syndromes; 3) narcissistic individuals who experience minimal grief; 4) avoidant personalities or schizoid personalities who are unable to obtain intimacy to permit grief; and 5) borderline personalities presenting with bizarre reactions related to narcissism, poor impulse control, and poor self concept.

Premorbid characterological traits such as apprehensiveness, worry anxiety, and low locus of control, yielding vulnerability to depression or high distress during bereavement, were noted by Parkes and Weiss (1983[200]), Stroebe and Stroebe (1987[217]), and Sanders (1988[223]). Sanders (1988[223]) also linked personality traits with specific types of bereavement outcomes, including 1) disturbed and depressed, 2) denying, and 3) normal. In summary of these statistical phenomena, Parkes (1990[203]) remarks rightly:

> In short, statistical studies confirm what common sense leads one to suspect, that secure people whose experience of life has led to a reasonable trust in themselves and others will cope well with anticipated bereavement provided they are well supported by a family who respects their need to grieve. However, multiple or unexpected and untimely losses of people on whom one depends or who depended on the survivor can overwhelm the most secure person and lack of security and support can undermine a person's capacity to cope with all types of bereavement. (p. 309)

To bridge the gap between the theoretical and psychodynamic models of pathological grief that we have just elaborated, and to facilitate the practical clinical treatment of disorders of bereavement, Parkes and

Weiss (1983[200]) and Raphael (1983[224]) have undertaken long-term prospective studies to monitor dysfunctional responses or pathological grief syndromes. They have attempted to link descriptive syndromes of dysfunctional bereavement with premorbid individual risk factors in specific forms of death, thus enabling the clinician to predict the outcome of the bereavement as well as the appropriateness of the variety of treatment interventions now available.

Rynearson (1990[190]) recently reviewed these syndromes and their relationship to the psychodynamic models we have discussed. He elaborates three specific syndromes but also emphasizes that the individual nature of grief imposes the probability of combinations and interactions among these syndromes. Rynearson (1990[190]) describes the three syndromes as follows:

> **1. *Dependent (chronic) grief syndrome.*** Dependent grief syndrome links clinging or over-reliant attachment to responses of immediate pining and chronic grief. Dependence in this instance refers to a relationship of relative nondifferentiation in which ones's image of self is contingent upon the availability of another. This dependence demands continuing interchange as a requisite in maintaining an image of the self as whole and acceptable. The death of the dependent figure initiates a pathogenic shift in the self-image of being weak, uncaring, and incompetent. These pathologic self-images are potent and compelling organizers of perception, and they independently deform the thoughts, feelings, and behavior of the pathologic grief syndrome. Horowitz and associates, in specifically applying this model with pathologic grief, found:
>
>> that the recent internalization of ambivalent attitudes toward attributes of the lost person is not the major reason for states of pathologic grief. Although these new identifications and attitude formations are important processes, a major cause of pathologic grief appears to be the emergence of earlier self-images and role relationship models.
>
> The pathogenic self-images in individuals predisposed to dependent grief syndrome may have been evident during early developmental phases of self-differentiation, and the lost relationship may have offered a buffer-

ing effect that prevented their emergence. Authors have identified these pathogenic self-images with character disorders (i.e., dependent, borderline, and narcissistic) that have been associated with dependent grief syndrome, but these findings are based on retrospective case reports.

2. ***Unexpected loss (distorted) grief syndrome.*** This syndrome links unexpected loss to responses of immediate disbelief, avoidance, and anxiety, leading to chronic anxious withdrawal. The explanatory model for this syndrome proposes that the mode and onset of the dying itself has pathogenic effects. In assuming this focus, the model does not disregard the pathogenicity of premorbid ambivalence or dependency, but cites the specific effects of sudden and often unnatural dying. Unexpected loss commonly qualifies as a traumatic stressor that "would evoke signs and symptoms of distress in almost anyone."

The model of psychologic trauma applied under circumstances of unexpected loss would propose that the event of dying is so fearful and overwhelming as to preclude assimilation and accommodation. In this circumstance of unexpected loss accompanied by overwhelming affect, the image of self is perceived as fragmented or annihilated. Even though the actual death rarely is witnessed, the close identification with the lost person may commit the bereaved to the task of adjusting to a highly traumatized, internalized percept. A dysfunctional syndrome follows that reflects the incomplete and fragmentary resolution: the posttraumatic stress syndrome of hyperreactivity (startle reactions, explosive outbursts of anger) and recurrent intrusive recollections of the dying (flashbacks and nightmares) alternating with compensatory psychic numbing, constriction of affect and social functioning, and the loss of sense of control over one's destiny. Posttraumatic stress phenomena (identified as stages of shock or numbness) are commonly observed with initial adjustment to death from any cause. However, these phenomena are intensely preoccupying and enduring following unexpected loss.

When unexpected loss is associated with an unnatural cause (such as accidents, suicide, or homicide), the bereaved is further traumatized by the obligatory involvement in the investigation and media coverage of the dying. With accidental and homicidal dying, a continuing obligation of trial and punishment of dying bears the social stigma of transgression. Violence, violation, and volition are elements of unnatural dying that catalyze a prolonged traumatic bereavement. Preliminary studies of subjects bereaved by unnatural dying have suggested specific syndromal effects associated with these "three Vs": violence with posttraumatic stress, violation with victimization, and volition with compulsive inquiry to establish blame and punish the perpetrator.

3. Conflicted (delayed) grief syndrome. Conflicted grief syndrome links conflicted ambivalent attachment to minimal immediate response with delayed responses of anxiety and pining. This syndrome follows the death of an ambivalently valued figure in which ambivalence cannot be psychologically tolerated. This model is based on the autoplastic distortions of unconscious drives. The ambivalent investment toward the lost figure is turned back on its internalized symbol, and the self is experienced as guilty and defective. Intense anger for the lost figure is directed at the self.

Freud originally identified this dynamic as the basis of depression in which the self is viewed as bad and worthless, rather than in mourning in which the external world seems impoverished. This has become a central paradigm in the psychoanalytic understanding of depression that is conceptually synonymous with pathologic grief.

Subsequent amplification of this intriguing speculation has introduced more convoluted theory, but little that would enhance or revise the clinical prediction or management of complicated grief. Bowlby has written an extensive review and critique of the application of psychoanalytic concepts of pathologic grief. The concepts of object relations and individuation are central to psychoanalytic theorists who use loss of a valued object as a metaphoric model for pathology and corrective treatment.

The conceptual error inherent in this model is the reductive imperative that pathologic grief is an epiphenomenon of early developmental parental rejection or loss. This reductive explanation has not been validated by prospective studies of children who subsequently develop pathologic grief. Although there are limitations of this model as an explanatory principle for conflicted grief syndrome, the unconscious denial of ambivalence might be operative when the grief appears after an inordinate delay. (pp. 299–300)

Rynearson's (1990[190]) elaboration of dysfunctional grief syndromes follows with some discussion of psychotherapy for grief reactions. He presents initial recommendations that proceed from a unifying formulation based on pathological grief as an "enduring emotion that draws us toward something or someone who is missing, whose absence is accompanied by a dysfunctional revision of assumptions of self and future" (p. 300). He further emphasizes the importance of engaging patients around their presenting self concept and their presenting concept of the meaning of the death. Focus on the presenting distortion of self concept can lead to the diagnosis of a specific syndrome of bereavement and, therefore, to the type of therapeutic intervention that would be most appropriate.

Exploring the initial meaning of the death may help identify distortions regarding the hopelessness and purposelessness of the future that, if left unaddressed, would actually prevent engagement with a therapist. In addition, such exploration may lead to the delineation of areas that have been meaningful to the patient in the past and toward which she can be refocused. The patient can also be encouraged to find some adaptive meaning for the death.

As indicated by Rynearson, different types of therapeutic approaches are indicated for different types of grief syndromes. Cognitive-behavioral models focusing on the clarification and restructuring of negative self-images and gradual exploration of these images within the transference reaction would be appropriate for dependent grief syndrome. Abreactive techniques focusing on conscious recovery and expression of ambivalent affects would be appropriate for inhibited or complicated grief reaction. On the other hand, traumatic sudden loss or distorted grief reaction would respond well to supportive and anxiolytic therapy.

Schuchter and Zisook (1990[225]) suggest a more longitudinal approach to treatment interventions with widows, utilizing the specific syndrome-related strategies defined by Rynearson, but also focusing on 1) the long-term adaptive tasks, 2) the painful, dysfunctional, and healthy aspects of even normative grief processes, and 3) exacerbations of grief precipitated by other life events—all of which can benefit from psychodynamic interventions. The authors view bereavement of a series of experiences that affect every aspect of the widow's life, including reactions to the loss, efforts to cope, continued relationships with the dead spouse, changes in health functioning, identity changes, and changes in relationships. Schuchter and Zisook have also documented in empirical fashion a more longitudinal bereavement process than has been thus far defined. They utilize the term "hovering over the bereaved" to communicate the need for the therapist to remain open and available to the bereaved person over a long period of time to help her deal with pathological grief syndromes, difficult aspects of normative grief, and intensification of grief around specific precipitants not related to pathological syndromes. Some examples include the following: 1) a later unrelated depression may unleash negative self-images associated with the initial grieving reaction; 2) anxiety around resuming sexual relationships may emerge as one makes the final adjustment to the loss; and 3) family conflicts may be exacerbated in the absence of the deceased. Schuchter and Zisook note that a variety of interventions can be performed in piecemeal fashion over time, depending on the issues that emerge. This model expands the realm of psychodynamic intervention for widows beyond a scope that includes pathological grief reactions that are only encountered by a minority of widows.

Working within this broader framework, numerous clinicians have elaborated specific techniques or particular aspects of psychodynamic interventions appropriate for widows, particularly those who are elderly. Schuchter and Zisook (1988[161]), in writing on the widow's continued relationship with the dead spouse, recommend a shift from, on the one hand, Freud's emphasis on decathexis of the lost object toward, on the other hand, an adaptive reintegration of the relationship with the deceased spouse. The authors emphasize the importance of this continuing relationship with the deceased spouse both in accepting what has been lost and in obtaining comfort by remembering what was positive and holding on to it in the relationship.

Myers (1987[226]) and Schuchter and Zisook (1988[161]) have reviewed the ways in which dreams may be used by patients to document specific issues in the grieving process. Common dreams include initial wish-fulfilling dreams in which people are reunited with their husbands; dreams of alternate leave-taking and returning; and dreams related to conflicts surrounding the death, such as guilt regarding the marriage. Also,

Polivka (1987[227]) has described the use of cartoon humor in helping to engage a 55-year-old widow in accessing fully the affects necessary for grief work.

Van der Hart and Goossens (1987[228]) have elaborated specific therapeutic leave-taking rituals for patients suffering conflicted grief. This directive approach consists of three phases: 1) *preparation*, in which the therapist explains how performing a ritual might help in taking leave of the deceased; 2) *reorganization*, in which the patient carries out certain tasks related to the deceased; and 3) *finalization*, which consists of a leave-taking ceremony, cleansing rite, and a reunion ritual that symbolically express the patient's most important relationships in his or her new stage of life.

Jacobs et al. (1987[229]) have discussed the use of tricyclic antidepressants as ancillary to psychotherapy and bereavement-related depression, especially that which persists more than a few months or beyond the first year after death. They report specifically on 10 cases with positive responses, primarily in the areas of sleep disorder, in addition to disturbances in appetite and mood and cognition.

Psychotherapy groups for widows focusing on the facilitation of grief work and education, as well as mutual help groups that tend to focus on social support, acquirement of adaptive knowledge and skills, and a cognitive understanding of grief, are commonly offered in addition to or instead of individual psychotherapy. Some research has been conducted on these formats (Barrett 1978[143]; Marmar et al. 1988[230]). However, differential documentation of their efficacy in elaboration of specific models remains.

For those clinicians attempting to differentiate pathological grief reactions from other types of older adult psychopathology, Whanger and Myers (1984[231]) provide a comprehensive guide to evaluation, diagnosis, and treatment interventions for this population.

Positive Adaptations to Widowhood

Although the bulk of psychiatric writing, both psychodynamic and otherwise, has focused on pathological grief reaction, we would like to return once again to the more positive adaptations documented earlier in this chapter for the majority of widows. Given that the average widow lives 18 years beyond the death of her spouse, that the majority make positive adaptations to their widowhood, and that a significant number even report higher levels of competence and well-being after widowhood, it is more reasonable to consider this a life stage with potential for growth rather than just a crisis event leading to pathological grief. Widowhood is also a gender issue, as females who become widows greatly outnumber the men who become widowers, in part because of the difference in life span between men and women, and in part because most widowers remarry and most widows do not. Also, men tend to marry women younger than themselves and do not live as long as widowers as do their peer group of widows (Windholz et al. 1985[232]; Heinemann and Evans 1990[117]).

Baltes et al. (1980[233]) generated a life-span developmental orientation toward widowhood that holds that growth and adaptation are possible at any stage of life, and specifically that there are opportunities for change and personal control at any time during the later years. In this same context, Hansson and Remondet (1988[112]) suggest a career orientation toward widowhood that encourages widows not to consider themselves at the end of a productive life but rather at the beginning of a major segment of a life course; this segment should be pursued vigorously in order for it to be successful and fulfilling, much like midlife career changes requiring the individual to recognize the implications of her new situation, assess strengths and limitations, and find a way to rise to the occasion. This more problem-oriented, rather than affect-oriented, approach and appraisal of widowhood was also associated with higher morale (Gass and Chang 1989[234]).

Further, Hansson and Remondet (1988[112]) suggest stages in a typical widow's future, including

- Recovering emotionally from bereavement
- Taking stock of one's current real-life situation
- Reestablishing or restructuring supportive relationships

- Formulating personal directions for the future
- Discovering a comfortable and satisfying independent life-style
- Determining an approach to maintaining economic, psychological, and social functioning
- Undergoing personal growth and change
- Reasoning and considering one's last years and asserting a degree of control over the arrangements surrounding one's own decline and death

Taken in combination with Schuchter and Zisook's (1990[225]) notion of hovering over the bereaved, a therapist might intervene at various crisis or conflicted points in this time frame rather than focus on and continually return to pathological grief.

A recent collection of psychoanalytically oriented therapy interventions conducted during the second half of life and compiled in a volume by Nemiroff and Colarusso (1985[235]) provides further evidence for the notion that positive growth is possible during this period and that psychodynamic intervention can be useful in a variety of ways. The authors conceptualize the notion of adult developmental lines that continue throughout life well into the phase in which most women are to become widows. Specific age-related tasks during middle adulthood (ages 40 to 60 years) and late adulthood (ages 60 years and above) make it infinitely clear that different psychological factors may be at work beyond the episode of bereavement and may serve as focuses for positive psychodynamic intervention.

These developmental tasks are identified by Nemiroff and Colarusso (1985,[235] pp. 48–49) as related to middle adulthood (ages 40 to 60) and late adulthood (ages 60 and above). Prominent in middle adulthood are adjustments to physical and sexual changes regarding the finiteness of life; deepening of relationships with children and grandchildren; adjustments to illnesses and deaths of parents and contemporaries; acceptance of social and financial responsibilities; appropriate alteration of work identity; identification with persons of all ages; and transmittal of values and skills to the younger generation. Late adulthood tasks focus on health maintenance; adjustment to impairments and infirmities in ways that allow for continued sexual and life gratification and a sense of identity; adaptation to loss of spouse and friends, and role reversals with children; orientation to present and future as well as past; continuance of meaningful work and play; openness to new emotional ties; and productive allocation of financial resources.

We would suggest to clinicians that they consider interventions not only around pathological grief reactions, which are indeed significant and necessary to treat, but also around 1) developmental tasks, 2) adaptations to widowhood, 3) intensification or reactivations of the bereavement precipitated by separate events, 4) conflicts reactivated by changes in the nature of relationships, and 5) the development of new relationships and the merging of intimacy and identity issues for widows.

The following patient material will therefore not be limited to pathological bereavement. Parkes (1990[202]) points out that "people vary enormously in their response to bereavement. Some suffer lasting damage to their physical, mental, social, and spiritual status. Some take bereavement in their stride, and others become more mature, effective, and well-balanced than they were before they were bereaved" (p. 308).

Widowhood Resulting in Positive Growth

Ms. A., a 50-year-old woman, had been in more or less constant psychiatric treatment since early childhood for irritability, fright and withdrawal, and, questionably, autism. She was the daughter of a beautiful, somewhat narcissistic and critical mother and a very smart, sadistically sarcastic father. She negotiated a regular private school and married a dull but caring man, who was taken into her father's business. Her first child was hyperactive and beyond her control even with constant household help. Her second child was normal except for the coping mechanism of overeating.

With her husband's collusion, this self-educated woman (who had an enormous and varied library) avoided most social contact. Her mother had been dead for several years and her father had died suddenly. Her son was estranged from the family and at times could not be located. Her daughter, a college graduate, worked and had an apartment in a nearby city.

After only a few months of retirement, when the patient was 53, her husband, at age 55, died of a sudden myocardial infarction. She seemed to be in a state of shock, and both her sister and her daughter despaired for her ability to live alone and manage her life day to day. She joined a widow's group, began to accept family invitations, and met a man with whom she lived for a while. She asked him to leave because of his work failure and was soon dating again. She soon found a steady boyfriend, a widower, who moved in with her. After negotiating a prenuptial agreement, the two were married. She, who had never before made a party, arranged a lovely wedding. Despite phobic feelings, she was willing to accompany her new husband on a vacation abroad. She now accepts social invitations for them and for the first time entertains at home.

The above case is an instance when widowhood seems to have jolted a patient out of severe passivity, overwhelming dependency, regression, and failure to function interpersonally and socially.

Anticipatory Grief Complicated by Unresolved Issues

Ms. R., a 52-year-old history professor and mother of two adolescents, entered therapy for anxiety and depressive symptoms, including problems with concentration and decision making. The history revealed that her symptoms had appeared 2 years ago when her husband approached age 60, the age at which his father had died of a heart attack. Mr. R. subsequently suffered a severe heart attack and was in the ninth month of recovery at the time Ms. R. presented for treatment.

Ms. R. was vague and affectively detached in reporting on her husband's current health status and thus could provide little information on the nature and treatment of his myocardial infarction. Her children, she stated, were more involved with "all that" but seldom spoke of it and had, she noted, become strangely distant from her over the past year. The concentration and decision-making problems of which she complained were focused on her current work situation in which she had been presented with several options for promotion but found herself unable to "think about my future." When the therapist suggested that there might be a connection between these events and her symptomatology, she initially denied the possibility but became increasingly sad and anxious. Ms. R. reported bursting into tears when a friend reported on a funeral she had attended. She also became panicky when her husband went on a business trip and she awoke in bed alone.

Although motivated in treatment and grasping the therapist's explanation of anticipatory grief, she was nonetheless unable to move toward the recommended steps of learning the exact nature of her husband's status and prognosis, discussing this with him and the children, sharing feelings within the family, and making appropriate plans together. Instead, she decompensated and became immobilized by her depression. Antidepressant medication was instituted along with supportive therapy aimed at helping her remain functional at work and at home. When her functioning was stable, exploration revealed that Ms. R.'s mother had been diagnosed with a terminal illness when Ms. R. was 12 and died when her daughter was 14, the same ages as Ms. R.'s children were now. There was little family sharing or preparation during her mother's illness, and shortly after her mother's death her father abandoned her to remarry, relegating her to a boarding school in a neighboring state.

After a period of therapy during which Ms. R. reexperienced her previous traumatic loss, she was able to approach her husband and attend a joint session with him and his cardiologist. Communication with the children improved, and together the family made some life-style alterations to support Mr. R.'s recovery as well as plan how the family would carry on should he deteriorate or die.

Pathological Grief

Ms. W. was a 79-year-old mother and grandmother who was still working full time in her own business. Looking 15 years younger, she would never tell her age. When her husband cut down to part-time employment and announced his planned retirement, she experienced insomnia and anorexic symptoms, as well as phobic symptoms about driving to work. She was treated with a tricyclic antidepressant, which resulted in phobic symptom removal. She continued to feel generally depressed and hopeless. Ms. W. seemed already to be mourning her husband's death. She felt that after retiring he would become a vegetable, even though she knew he enjoyed working and reading and intended to enroll in adult education classes. Yet she continued to feel that she was all alone in the world. Clinically she looked like she was having a pathological mourning reaction even though her husband was in reality very much alive and her life had not changed. She became paranoid in anticipation that her daughters would try to take away everything she had and send her to an old-age home. In reality, she had always been the breadwinner and in control of the family finances.

Treatment for pathological mourning and melancholic reaction led to the uncovering of her very angry feelings about her husband. She had worked hard all her life and raised her children, whereas he had not worked hard. Now he was retiring, and she felt unable to retire for unrealistic financial reasons. In reality, she had nothing in common with her husband and dreaded leaving her work to be with him. In addition, she was angry at her daughters to whom she had "given everything," because they preferred their father, probably because he was more kind and laid back.

She had a horror story about their escape from Germany that she had had the responsibility of engineering. She had never stopped resenting the rescue that had been her agony and her responsibility. Catharsis and the sharing of this story with her daughters resulted in improvement in her depression and in her decision to retire. This was the first time her children appreciated her, and she felt less threatened that they would "take her money and put her away." Their appreciation of her allowed her to resent her husband less.

Initial Denial of Loss

Ms. G., a 70-year-old mother and grandmother, was brought to one of the authors as an emergency case 24 hours after the death of her husband. Her husband had been diabetic for many years and had had severely deteriorating health with multiple hospitalizations over the past 18 months. On the afternoon of his sudden death he had been in the park in a wheelchair with the family's housekeeper of 30 years. Ms. G. had been out at a usual afternoon card game. Returning home she saw the housekeeper, her husband, and the paramedics and was told that her husband was dead. She and her housekeeper returned home. Ms. G. went to sleep while the housekeeper called her children. When they arrived at the house she awakened surprised to see them, apparently unaware of her husband's death. When they told her, she said, "Oh no. You must be mistaken," but did not attempt to look for him. While her sons went to the hospital, Ms. G. was taken by a daughter-in-law to one of her son's home. After seeing her grandchildren, she bathed and went to sleep for the night.

The next day, while being told about the funeral arrangements, she showed no emotion. She attended the funeral, showed no visible signs of grief, and indeed seemed somewhat confused and disoriented. Her family feared that she had had a stroke or was in some kind of psychiatric shock. A neurological examination was normal. A mental status examination revealed intact sensorium and cognition along with denial of her husband's death. She confabulated the reason for being at her daughter-in-law's home and denied that she had been to a funeral. She stated that she felt very tired but restless and not sleepy. The decision was made to sedate her and follow her closely.

The next day she was willing to believe that her husband had died, but she had no emotional response and wondered why she had not been permitted to attend the funeral. As time progressed she remembered having gone to play cards while her husband had been in the park with the housekeeper. She continued to have both anterograde and retrograde amnesia. She noted that he had died while she was playing cards and regretted not having been with him. The therapist anticipated that there might be a severe grief reaction upon her return home. This, however, did not happen. She said that she and her husband had realized that he would not recover, but she imagined that his death must have been a shock to her.

Thereafter she spoke very affectionately about him but did not mourn. Her children had never recalled seeing her cry at any time in her life. After an episode of severe dissociation, she recovered with no sequelae.

Aging

Erikson (1959[1]), in his description of the life cycle, discussed the last phase life task as the triumph of integrity over despair. A report of an American Psychoanalytic Association Panel on Aging (Zinberg

1964[236]) acknowledges that the psychological response to aging depends on several factors, including what has transpired in one's life, the integration of the individual, and the impact of disease processes. Despite Abraham's (1927[237]) recognition that elderly patients (i.e., in their late 40s or 50s) could be treated psychoanalytically, it is only in the last 20 years that analytic institutes have accepted applicants of this age for control or training cases, or even as candidates. The publication of books in psychiatric medicine devoted to the treatment of the elderly began in the 1960s. By the early 1970s, the definition of the elderly population, aside from those prematurely aged, began to include individuals in their 70s and 80s. This trend directly parallels the increased life expectancy and the increased population of those persons over 70 years of age.

There is no universally accepted definition of aging. Busse and Blazer (1980[238]) offered a definition that separates what he calls "primary aging" from "secondary aging." *Primary aging* is defined as that decline in functioning uniform to the organism, determined by inherent and hereditary influences. *Secondary aging* is the appearance of defects and disabilities that are caused by environmental factors, including trauma and acquired disease. Because aging is a complicated phenomenon, with many afflictions falling into what are still gray areas of our medical knowledge, there is no agreement about primary and secondary aging. For example, diabetes mellitus is a hereditary disease with complex genetics that are not yet understood. Yet it is not inevitable to the organism. Rather its clinical manifestation is often determined by other factors such as obesity, lack of exercise, or intercurrent infections.

The gender skew toward women in the elderly population is also not understood. The American Association of Retired Persons reported in 1987[239] that a 65-year-old female could be expected to live another 18.5 years but a male of the same age could be expected to live only 14 more years. Busse (1989[240]) points out that the sex imbalance in the elderly population has many social and medical implications. Most older men are married, whereas most older women are single. Also, single older men tend to marry or be remarried to younger women, contributing further to the preponderance of older women living without a spouse. Ironically, in one recent exhaustive review of geriatric psychiatry (Busse and Blazer 1989[241]), the authors do not mention the special problems of the geriatric woman except that she is likely to be single. Parenthetically, there is one slender volume about elderly men who must live alone (Rubinstein 1986[242]).

Aside from the medical and psychiatric problems related to menopause, which we have discussed, there are other specifically gender-related problems. These are often a function of a woman's chosen or designated role through life—namely, generativity, caregiving, homemaking, and the emphasis, internal and external, on appearance and youthfulness. Also, experiences around managing menstrual flow earlier in life impinge on the problems of aging related to bladder and bowel control.

Except for the profound reaction to mutilating surgery, discussed previously, the literature reveals no substantial gender difference in depression and anxiety secondary to physical disease. There is also no gender difference in the affective reaction to the initial realization of the loss of cognitive capacity secondary to Alzheimer's disease, multiinfarct dementia, or the loss of gray matter due to the aging process. Men's lives and identities often revolve around their breadwinning abilities and their sexual and physical prowess. There is some decrement in both erectile and ejaculatory capacity in men with age. Aside from loss of vaginal lubrication due to decreased estrogen, which can be remedied medically, women can maintain an active sexual life longer, if they wish.

Women do grieve hair loss and skin wrinkling more than men. Anecdotal stories inform us of how much women in nursing homes look forward to beauty services such as hair dressing and manicures. For all the reasons we have discussed in Chapter 3, the threatened or real loss of youth and beauty is more painful to women than to men. Some elderly women are coping with this problem and also attempting to remain healthy by embarking on active exercise programs. Idiculla and Goldberg (1987[243]) and Notelovitz (1990[244]) discuss the benefits and structure of a vigorous exercise program for postmenopausal women, noting significant positive results in cardiovascular fitness, weight control, flexibility, and the prevention of osteoporosis. Cultural norms are changing, making exercise an acceptable activity for women as well as men.

The loss of independence and the development of increasing dependency needs affect both sexes. Surveys of women who work full time show us that even when husbands help in child care, shopping, laundry, and food preparation, most women consider themselves in charge of those functions (see Chapter 4). The truly egalitarian marriage is much more rare than the traditional or semi-traditional one. Men often expect to be fed, have their laundry done for them, and so forth, and have less trouble accepting this help from caregivers. Although some women experience relief at being cared for, others are uncomfortable relinquishing these functions. Elderly women more frequently attempt to boss and control their caregivers. Women who are helped by daughters or daughter-age caregivers often get back into the old rivalries they had had with their own mothers or their daughters. This regression makes it difficult for all concerned. It is problematic for women to move in with their daughters without trying to take over the management of kitchen or children, at least verbally, from their daughters.

The problem of bladder or bowel incontinence causes regression to anal-stage conflicts as well as shame and loss of self-esteem in elderly persons of both sexes. For women there may be the added dimension of shame and loss of control over menstrual flow. Memories of cleaning up in early adolescence also evoke yearning for lost generativity and sexuality. Prevalence rates of 11.6% for urinary incontinence in women over 65 provide further indication of the significance of this problem for elderly women (Jolleys 1988[245]).

Geriatric psychiatry is now a highly skilled subspecialty requiring training in medicine, neurology, and an understanding of the pharmacology of psychotropic medications. Psychotropic drug administration requires knowledge of metabolism in the elderly, including the understanding of paradoxical reactions in which sedatives may act as stimulants, and stimulants as sedatives. Also, the understanding of degradation sites for medications informs the choice of medication. For example, in the presence of decreased liver function one would use a drug primarily excreted by the kidney, while with damaged renal function a drug degraded by the liver would be the drug of choice. Drug interactions must be understood because many elderly patients will be taking medications for hypertension, myocardial lung, vascular disease, arthritis, and diabetes, to name only the most common.

Preventive work needs to be done with younger patients to prepare them to cope with aging. The better the job we do overall in psychodynamic treatment, the more integrated and flexible our patients will be. Most patients do have fantasies of retirement or old age, and these will come to be examined and understood only if the therapist asks about or attends to what might be said in passing. The patient who states that she would rather die than get old, or die than need her family's help, is warning us of terrible trouble ahead.

As dynamic therapists it is our duty to work out these problems while a patient is in our care. Fewer elderly women commit suicide than elderly men (Blazer et al. 1986[246]). Because there are more women than men in the geriatric population, it is the former who may burden their caregivers, which in turn may lead to neglect and even maltreatment of these patients. The psychiatric literature on battering has just begun to include discussion on elderly victims. Three categories of abuse have been commonly found: overt physical abuse, deliberate neglect, and verbal abuse (Pillemer and Finkelhor 1989[247]). Pillemer and associates have studied both the problems of maltreatment of patients in nursing homes (Pillemer 1988[248]) and the problems of abuse that occur when children and elderly parents live together (Sutton and Pillemer 1986[249]). These investigators found no correlation between the state of parents' health and conflict with adult children serving as caregivers. Also, Pillemer (1985[250]) found no difference in the level of impairment between abused elders and control cases. Doty and Sullivan (1983[251]) documented numerous incidents of abuse of elderly persons reported to state and federal agencies. Although we have no direct experiences with elderly patients who have been abused either by their families or in nursing homes, we would speculate that the psychodynamics involved would be similar to those reported in child abuse and the battering of women (see Chapter 4).

Because there seems to be no difference between men and women who face dying and death in any phase of the life cycle, we include no discussion of these issues specific to the psychodynamic treatment of women. The patient material presented below includes female-specific issues—that is, those related to unresolved early life conflicts, generativity and caregiving, appearance, youthfulness and sexuality, and incontinence.

Elderly Woman With Caregiving Issues

The patient was a married mother of two married children who in her 70s was still operating a small neighborhood shop. She had always been successful and in charge of the family finances and had funded her children's college and graduate educations. Her husband of over 50 years was a passive, mild-mannered man, retired from a modest middle managerial-level job in a company he had worked for all of his life but without advancement. The couple retained a full-time live-in housekeeper.

The patient had managed the chronic health problems of these two adults all of her life. She came to treatment because of the development of a phobia that threatened her ability to work. The precipitating episode was the threat that one of two long-term employees who had recently moved out of the neighborhood would leave. The patient was furious at this woman with whom she had always been generous and who was in reality trying to blackmail her now for a large salary increase.

Therapy dealt with a chronic unconscious rage toward the variety of people whom she felt she had carried on her back all these years.

Her husband took suddenly ill with a severe headache and high fever and was admitted to the hospital for meningitis. In the course of this admission, a tumor was found in his chest for which exploratory surgery was required. The patient traveled a great distance to see her husband every day and continued to run her business. Fortunately, the tumor was benign, but her husband had a small stroke that compromised his ability to walk. At the same time, her housekeeper developed congestive heart failure and expressed the desire to retire to a nursing home. The patient arranged three shifts of help at home and also shopped, cooked, and continued to run her business.

A short time later the patient fell, fracturing her leg, which required internal fixation. She became severely depressed. The specter of leaving her shop and retiring was unacceptable to her. She developed the delusion that her daughters would declare her and her husband incompetent and have them admitted to a nursing home. In reality, they were attempting to help her to accept the reality of retirement.

The patient's grandchildren, widely dispersed in the United States and Canada, expressed their wishes to have their grandparents visit. They were willing to visit with their grandmother and help her organize a life of retirement. She had two grandchildren for whose education she had paid, and they were grateful and loving. She criticized and rejected holiday gifts that they sent, feeling that they should have paid her back more substantially than they did.

She could not accept relinquishing her dominant role in the family or her own dependency needs. Despite continuing therapy, she became more and more embittered and prayed every night to die so as not to face what she regarded as her horrible life. She left treatment when the therapist refused to give her enough medication to kill herself.

Mourning and Caregiving Issues

A 65-year-old widowed woman who had been living with her daughter and cheerfully caring for two school-age grandchildren was admitted to the hospital with a sudden severe retarded depression marked by somnolence, significant weight loss, and dehydration. She was placed on hyperalimentation and a tricyclic antidepressant.

It was not until the patient recovered from the medical consequences of her depression that the precipitating episode could be pinpointed. Her son-in-law, whom she adored, had been 2 hours late for dinner and had not called. This was quite unusual for him. Despite her daughter's reassurance, the patient remembered the deep conviction that her son-in-law had gotten killed. This made no conscious sense to her even as she reported it.

It took several months of outpatient psychotherapy to discover that she had grown up in a village in Poland, as an only child in an orthodox Jewish family. Her father earned his living as a traveling teacher. When he was at home, the two enjoyed a very special relationship. Clearly she was a beloved child. She was eager to learn, and he taught her, delighting in her achievements. His comings and goings were erratic. When the patient was 6 years old and her father had been gone for an inordinate length of time, her mother, with the aid of the community and itinerant travelers, was able to trace her father's journey. He had been killed in a pogrom in a distant village. Her mother, on the one hand, refused to believe that her husband was dead and, on the other hand, began a continuous mourning process. This in effect deprived the patient of her mother as well as her father. In the prodrome of World War II, relatives who had emigrated to America sent for the patient and her mother. Her mother refused to leave but was willing to send her daughter to America.

The patient came to the United States in the custody of other villagers and was warmly accepted into the home of her distant relatives as their own daughter. This was a very happy home, and the patient consciously considered that her life had begun at this juncture. She never mourned the loss of either parent. In New York she was schooled and married by arrangement to a man whom she came to love. When he died, she mourned appropriately. Clearly her son-in-law had conjured her feelings about her father, and the dread and conviction of his loss precipitated a pathological mourning reaction.

In therapy the patient remembered both of her parents. She had never tried to ascertain the fate of her mother, assuming that she was a victim of the Holocaust. The determinants of her failure to seek out facts about her mother's fate were oedipal. After analysis of her oedipal conflict, she began to try to trace her mother's fate. Indeed, it was established that all the inhabitants of her village had been taken to a concentration camp. At this time the patient began to mourn the loss of her mother. Her daughter, son-in-law, and grandchildren stood by her during this process and guaranteed a permanent home for her with them.

Over time she was able to divest her son-in-law of the adoration she had had for her father and to love him on his own merits. In the transference she brought the therapist gifts of homemade food and a handmade crocheted apron. She made the therapist a "good and feeding mother." As this transference was explored, the therapist discovered that the patient's own mother, in her confusion and grief, had frequently forgotten to feed her daughter. Through the defense of undoing, the patient had always fed her grandchildren wonderfully, and they adored her for this quality. She had been unconsciously worried about losing their love at a time when she could no longer perform this function. She was able to be less active in regard to feeding her grandchildren and they still adored her. She continued to handmake special articles of clothing for them (the crocheted apron in the transference), a skill that she had learned from her adoptive mother who had made beautiful clothing for her. The patient began to accept that she need not feel threatened about losing her daughter, her son-in-law, or her grandchildren, and that they loved her and would care for her as long as she lived.

Issues of Youth and Physical Aging

A patient in her late 60s who did not appear to be younger was brought to the hospital by her niece because of an agitated depression. The patient, who had lost 10 pounds, had insomnia and was unable to sit still. Her niece said that she had had brief episodes in the past like this one, always related to "the same business." The patient was unmarried, had her own apartment near her niece, and worked as an infant nurse living with various families for 2 weeks after the birth of an infant and taking time off between cases. Her agitation, insomnia, and anorexia responded quickly to a tricyclic antidepressant.

She was initially unable to talk about "that business," but gave her other history. She had lived in Germany during World War II. Her sister had given birth to an illegitimate child whose lineage was suspect. The patient became a member of the Nazi party and got a civilian job. Her motive was to become trusted enough to take her niece, whose care she had undertaken, to Switzerland and thereafter to the United States.

Indeed, sewing valuables into her clothing she crossed the border with this young girl and brought her to the United States. The girl called her "mother." The patient never married, worked hard, and gave her niece a higher education. Having confided her activities to a Jewish therapist who managed the countertransference, she was able to talk about her "little businesses." She had refused to accept aging and had had plastic surgery on her face. Having "missed her youth," she would periodically become involved with very young men who inevitably abandoned her. Her last lover, to whom she had given a great deal of money, also abandoned her. She located and confronted him, and he called her an "old bag." So grave was the narcissistic injury that she would have commited suicide if not for her obligation to her niece. The patient had developed an agitated depression.

She was seen as an outpatient twice over the next 15 years. After retiring to Germany to live, she had become involved with young men. The second time she was so ill that her niece had flown over to bring her back to the therapist. Her appearance was truly remarkable. She had had plastic surgery on her face and breasts and looked younger than the first time she had ever been seen by the therapist. Her niece, married herself, said, "Madi refuses to grow old. She rejects older gentlemen and behaves with all the foolishness of a young girl." The patient pointed out to us both that she had never had the opportunity to be a young girl. She had become a responsible mother while still a teenager, and she would have her foolish "little businesses" or die. The patient knew that her therapist would always be there to get her well. Again she recovered rapidly on medication.

Incontinence

Ms. F. was a 60-year-old housewife and volunteer worker diagnosed as having a bipolar disorder who first came to treatment following recovery from a hysterectomy. During the convalescence from that surgery, her husband had temporarily left her, and she felt abandoned by her previous psychiatrist, who was dealing with his terminally ill wife and unavailable to meet her demands. She complained of fecal incontinence that she said had worsened after her last surgery but had begun after earlier hemorrhoidal surgery. The incontinence was complicated with her gastrointestinal problems of irritable bowel. With flatus there was often leakage, and following constipation she would often dig out stool with her fingers. She complained of sores over her perianal and inguinal areas and had infected nail beds. Interestingly, she had a fastidious standard of care for her housekeepers.

It was apparent to the therapist that the patient's infections were connected with a lack of personal hygiene. In confronting her with this, the therapist stepped into the role of the patient's latency-age mother who, stuffing the patient with a breakfast of prunes and hot water, would not let her go off to school until she had a bowel movement. The patient recovered memories of adolescent conflicts over insisting on vacuuming the living room before her date arrived on Saturday nights, risking the wrath of her Jewish-Orthodox parents who wanted her to keep the Sabbath. Their hollering and screaming was dreaded and often heard by the patient's date when ringing the doorbell.

Her loud, abrupt, explosive manner continued into adulthood and was now alienating her family members, whom she longed to have close now that she was feeling older and less capable. As the patient's life was in disarray because of her husband's stroke, which occurred following his return to the marital home, her "mess" in her pants became both an expression of her lack of control and an additional burden. It also served an interesting gratification. No longer having a uterus, the patient had a reason to carry sanitary napkins with her and many pads and pay attention to her genital area and the act of cleansing, which seemed less embarrassing and humiliating than the masturbation with an enema tip that she would shamefacedly admit to. Sphincter mastery improved as she was able to isolate and compartmentalize issues in her life and work on them individually to some resolution. She was able to conduct a successful media campaign against war toys, produce a film festival, and start a cousin's club with her grandchildren. As she initiated, fashioned, and completed "projects" she was like the toddler who moved from bodily concerns to those concerns of the external world. In the transference the therapist became the new mother who was more interested in the activities outside of the home than those on the commode. The patient felt less shame and therefore less readiness to be sensitive to criticism, and her interactions with family members improved.

* * *

Ms. K. was a 48-year-old Dutch émigrée whose father had been a landowner, a military officer, and a resistance leader in World War II. Her mother gave over the care of her children to nursemaids. The brother of one nursemaid molested Ms. K. in a stable, covering her face with a dog. Subsequently, the patient lived in silence or superficial banter. She was terrified to speak of sexual matters in general, of any physical pain, or of the actual trauma. She endured endometriosis and severe metrorrhagia, leading to anemia and fainting spells.

She came to therapy on the advice of a pulmonary specialist who thought that her chronic respiratory illness, which had required multiple hospitalizations, might have a psychogenic component. Ultimately, her gasping for breath did lead back to memories of childhood sexual abuse, secrets of double ceilings, and hidden Jews. Her gradual willingness to speak up and find a sympathetic, compassionate listener led her to the acceptance of pelvic exams and the determination that she had huge fibroids. After the hysterectomy she was most delighted, not so much at the absence of pain or regained strength but at her ability to control her bladder capacity and function. Even with the therapist, her first confidant, she had been unable earlier to talk about her urinary incontinence. The incontinence had prevented her from going out. Her shame about it was enormous, and of course it "borrowed" the shame from her earlier experience as the sexually abused child. Working through this final self representation of being the smelly, dirty, guilty, shameful child improved the patient's overall mental and physical health. She had the words to speak, and the asthmatic gasping became a lesser mode of communication.

* * *

Ms. S., *a 54-year-old homemaker married to a hearing-impaired pharmacist, was the mother of three hearing-impaired sons—a psychiatrist, a cook, and a college student (the latter still living at home).* Ms. S. *was referred to therapy for pain management of right nasolabial pain. She was severely overweight and her bladder capacity was diminished. She had to urinate frequently or else she became incontinent. Her pain, which essentially remained undiagnosed and untreatable, seemed to follow upon some dental work.*

Following her second pregnancy the patient had suffered a postpartum depression connected with her shame and disbelief that she had borne a second handicapped child. Although the family had known the hearing deficit was genetic, they were told that they had a 50/50 chance of having a child born with a hearing impairment. But her second son was also disabled.

The patient had many realistic worries. Her overriding thought associations had to do with her inability to control the mess in her home. She talked about the overflowing closets and desks, complaining that if only her mother had not died or if her mother had taught her instead of just criticizing her or taking over, her life would be more in order. The patient's need to urinate before and after each session ended was both an interference in the "time" spent and a major nonverbal communication. The remark "I can't control myself" reflected her inability to have a healthy child and to have a clean house, keeping her tied to her maternal object. She benefitted some from the administration of Elavil for pain diminution, but because the desire for mastery and control seemed real (not the wish to prolong suffering), the therapist encouraged her seeking neurological or dental relief. Ultimately, the pain was diagnosed and treated. With that resolved, she had one less urgent sensation to deal with, and she could cope better with her oral- and anal-phase conflicts.

As we have tried to show, aging affects everyone. However, the negative sequelae of aging afflict women more than they do men. In addition, there is a "double standard" of aging (Sontag 1972[252]) in that American society is more permissive regarding aging in men and offers fewer rewards for aging women. These conditions occur in Western society because of the emphasis on physical beauty and youthfulness. Furthermore, there is a differential in the ability of older women to remarry, which we have discussed earlier in this chapter. Last, we must emphasize that femininity in our society is often equated with passivity, incompetence, helplessness, and noncompetitiveness, which are characteristics of elderly persons (Sontag 1972,[252] p. 31). Although there may be rewards for women at all stages of the life cycle, the potential for abuse, derision, and devaluation sadly exists even in old age.

Notes

1. Erikson EH: Identity and the Life Cycle. New York, International Universities Press, 1959
2. Robinson LH: Grandparenting: intergenerational love and hate. J Am Acad Psychoanal 17:483–492, 1989
3. Myers W: I can't play ball anymore. J Geriatr Psychiatry 21:121–139, 1989
4. Neugarten B, Weinstein K: The changing American grandparent. Journal of Marriage and the Family 26:204, 1964
5. Claven S: The impact of social class and social trends on the role of grandparent. The Family Coordinator 27:355–357, 1978
6. Abraham K: Some remarks on the role of grandparents in the psychology of neurosis (1913), in Selected Papers of Karl Abraham, Vol 2: Clinical Papers on Psycho-Analysis. Edited by Abraham HC. New York, Basic Books, 1955, pp 44–48

7. Deutsch H: The Psychology of Women, A Psychoanalytic Interpretation, Vol 2: Motherhood. New York, Grune & Stratton, 1945, pp 483–486
8. Benedek T: Sexual functions in women and their disturbances, in American Handbook of Psychiatry. Edited by Arieti S. New York, Basic Books, 1959b, pp 727–748
9. Cath SH: Vicissitudes of grandfatherhood: a miracle of revitalization, in Father and Child. Edited by Cath SH, Gurwitt AR, Ross JM. Boston, MA, Little, Brown, 1982, pp 329–337
10. Anthony E, Benedek T (eds): Parenthood and Its Psychology. Boston, MA, Little, Brown, 1970, pp 197–206
11. Severino K, Teusink J, Pender V, et al: Overview: the psychology of grandparenthood. J Geriatr Psychiatry 19:13–17, 1986
12. McKinlay S, Jefferys SM, Thompson B: An investigation of the age at menopause. J Biosoc Sci 4:161–173, 1972
13. Cumming DC: Menarche, menses and menopause: a brief review. Cleve Clin J Med 57:169–175, 1990
14. Notman MT: Psychiatric disorder of menopause. Psychiatric Annals 14:448–453, 1984
15. Utian WH: The menopause in perspective: from potions to patches. Ann N Y Acad Sci 592:1–8, 1990
16. Rhoades FP: Minimizing the menopause. J Am Geriatr Soc 15:346–354, 1967
17. Wilson RA, Wilson TA: The fate of the nontreated postmenopausal woman. J Am Geriatr Soc 11:347–362, 1963
18. Schwartzman LC, Leiblum SR: Changing perspectives on the menopause. Journal of Psychosomatic Obstetrics and Gynecology 6:11–24, 1987
19. Benedek T: Climacterium: a developmental phase. Psychoanal Q 19:1–27, 1950
20. American Psychiatric Association: Diagnostic and Statistical Manual of Mental Disorders (DSM-I). Washington, DC, American Psychiatric Association, 1952
21. Neugarten BL, Kraines RJ: "Menopausal symptoms" in women of various ages. Psychosom Med 27:266–273, 1965
22. Neugarten BL, Wood V, Kraines RJ, et al: Women's attitudes towards the menopause. Vita Humana 6:140–151, 1963
23. Wilson RA: Feminine Forever. New York, Evans, 1966
24. National Prescription Audit (NPA): The top 20 drugs. Pharmacy Times, April 1972–1975
25. Gray LA, Christopherson WM, Hoover RN: Estrogens and endometrial carcinoma. Obstet Gynecol 49:385–389, 1977

26. Mack TM, Pike MC, Henderson BE, et al: Estrogens and endometrial cancer in a retirement community. N Engl J Med 294:1262–1267, 1976
27. McDonald TW, Annegers JF, O'Fallon WM: Exogenous estrogen and endometrial carcinoma; case control and incidence study. Am J Obstet Gynecol 127:572–580, 1977
28. Smith DC, Prentice R, Thompson DJ, et al: Association of exogenous estrogen and endometrial carcinoma. N Engl J Med 293:1164–1167, 1975
29. Ziel HK, Finkle WD: Increased risk of endometrial carcinoma among users of conjugated estrogens. N Engl J Med 293:1167-1170, 1975
30. Aitken JM: Osteoporosis and its relation to estrogen deficiency, in The Management of the Menopause and Postmenopausal Years. Edited by Campbell S. Lancaster, UK, MTP Press, 1976, pp 225–236
31. Bush TL, Cowan LD, Barrett-Connor E, et al: Estrogen use and all-cause mortality. JAMA 249:903–906, 1983
32. Christiansen C, Christiansen MS, Transbol I: Bone mass in postmenopausal women after withdrawal of oestrogen/progestin replacement therapy. Lancet 1:459–461, 1981
33. Corson SL: Impact of estrogen replacement therapy on cardiovascular risk. J Reprod Med 34:729–746, 1984
34. Lindsay R, Cosman F: Estrogen in prevention and treatment of osteoporosis. Ann N Y Acad Sci 592:326–337, 1990
35. Lindsay R, Hart DM, MacLean A, et al: Bone response to termination of oestrogen treatment. Lancet 1:1325–1327, 1978
36. Lobo RA: Cardiovascular implications of estrogen replacement therapy. Obstet Gynecol 75:18S–35S, 1990
37. Recker RR, Saville PD, Heany RP: Effect of estrogen and calcium carbonate on bone loss in postmenopausal women. Ann Intern Med 87:649–655, 1977
38. Studd JW, Thom MH, Paterson MEL, et al: The prevention and treatment of endometrial pathology in postmenopausal women receiving exogenous estrogens, in The Menopause and Postmenopause. Edited by Pasetto R, Paoletti R, Ambrus JL. Lancaster, UK, MTP Press, 1980, pp 127–139
39. Whitehead MI, Townsend PT, Pryse-Davies J, et al: Effects of estrogens and progestins on the biochemistry and morphology of the postmenopausal endometrium. N Engl J Med 305:1599–1605, 1981
40. Notman MT: Women and midlife: a different perspective. Psychiatric Opinion 15:15–25, 1978
41. Notman MT: Midlife concerns of women: implications of the menopause. Am J Psychiatry 136:1270–1274, 1979

42. Notman MT: Menopause and adult development. Ann N Y Acad Sci 592:149–155, 1990
43. Brinton LA: Menopause and the risk of breast cancer. Ann N Y Acad Sci 592:357–362, 1990
44. Lock M: Models and practice in medicine: menopause as syndrome or life transition. Cult Med Psychiatry 7:261–280, 1982
45. Kaufert PA, Gilbert P: Women, menopause and medicalization. Cult Med Psychiatry 10:7–21, 1986
46. Posner J: It's all in your head: feminist and medical models of menopause (strange bedfellows). Sex Roles 5:179–191, 1976
47. Parlee MB: Integrating biological and social science research on menopause. Ann N Y Acad Sci 592:379–389, 1990
48. Flint M, Kronenberg F, Utian W (eds): Multidisciplinary Perspectives on Menopause. Annals of the New York Academy of Sciences, Vol 592. New York, New York Academy of Sciences, 1990
49. Chiriboga DA: The developmental psychology of middle age, in Modern Perspectives in the Psychiatry of Middle Age. Edited by Howell JG. New York, Brunner/Mazel, 1981, pp 3–25
50. Havighurst RJ: Developmental Tasks and Education. New York, Longmans Green, 1948
51. Erikson EH: Childhood and Society. New York, WW Norton, 1950, pp 247–274
52. Rossi A: Transition to parenthood. Journal of Marriage and the Family 38:26–39, 1968
53. Neugarten BL: Adult personality: toward a psychology of the life cycle, in Middle Age & Aging. Chicago, IL, University of Chicago Press, 1968a, pp 137–147
54. Cameron P: Masculinity/femininity of the generations: as self-reported as stereotypically appraised. Int J Aging Hum Dev 7:143–151, 1976
55. Monge RH: Structure of the self-concept from adolescence through old age. Exp Aging Res 1:281–291, 1975
56. Terman LM, Oden MH: Genetic Studies of Genius V5: The Gifted Group at Midlife. Stanford, CA, Stanford University Press, 1959
57. Pollock G: The mourning process and creative organizational change. J Am Psychoanal Assoc 25:3–34, 1977
58. Pollock G: Aging or aged: development or pathology, in The Course of Life: Psychoanalytic Contributions Toward Understanding Personality Development, Vol 3. Edited by Greenspan SI, Pollock GH. Washington, DC, National Institute of Mental Health, 1981, pp 549–585

59. Lennon MC: The psychological consequences of menopause: the importance of timing of a strange life event. J Health Soc Behav 23:353–366, 1982
60. Notman MT: The menopause, in The Psychiatric Implications of Menstruation. Edited by Gold JH. Washington, DC, American Psychiatric Press, 1985, pp 87–102
61. Barnett R, Baruch G: Women in the middle years: a critique of research and theory. Psychology of Women Quarterly 3:187–197, 1978
62. Benedek T: Parenthood as a developmental phase. J Am Psychoanal Assoc 7:389–417, 1959a
63. Bibring GV, Dwyer TF, Huntington DS, et al: A study of the psychological processes in pregnancy and of the earliest mother-child relationship. Psychoanal Study Child 16:9–72, 1961
64. Bart P, Grossman M: Menopause, in The Woman Patient: Medical and Psychological Interfaces VI. Edited by Notman M, Nadelson C. New York, Plenum, 1978, pp 337–354
65. Formanek R: Menopause: myth and reality, in Critical Psychophysical Passages in the Life of a Woman: A Psychodynamic Perspective. Edited by Offerman-Zuckerberg J. New York, Plenum, 1988, pp 199–214
66. Notman MT: The menopause, in The Psychiatric Implications of Menstruation. Edited by Gold JH. Washington, DC, American Psychiatric Press, 1985, pp 87–102
67. Schindler B: The psychiatric disorders of midlife. Med Clin North Am 71:71–85, 1987
68. McKinlay S, McKinlay J: Selected studies on the menopause. J Biosoc Sci 5:533–555, 1973
69. Parlee M: Social factors in the psychology of menstruation, birth and menopause. Prim Care 3:477–490, 1976
70. Goodman MJ: Patterns of menopause: a study of certain medical and physiological variables among Caucasian and Japanese women living in Hawaii. J Gerontol 32:291–298, 1977
71. Goodman MJ: Age at menopause in relation to reproductive history in Japanese, Caucasian, Chinese and Hawaiian women living in Hawaii. J Gerontol 33:688–694, 1978
72. Flint M: The menopause: reward or punishment. Psychosomatics 16:161–163, 1975
73. Mead M: Male and Female: A Study of the Sexes in a Changing World. New York, Dell, 1968
74. McPherson K: Menopause as disease: the social construction of a metaphor. ANS 3:95–113, 1980–1981

75. Severne L: Psychosocial aspects of the menopause, in Changing Perspectives on Menopause. Edited by Voda AM, Dinnerstein M, O'Donnell SR. Austin, TX, University of Texas Press, 1982, pp 239–247
76. Woods N: Menopausal distress: a model for epidemiological investigation, in Changing Perspectives on Menopause. Edited by Voda AM, Dinnerstein M, O'Donnell SR. Austin, TX, University of Texas Press, 1982, pp 220–238
77. Kaufert P: Myth and the menopause. Sociology of Health and Illness 4:141–166, 1982
78. Perlmutter J: A gynecological approach to menopause, in The Woman Patient VI: Medical and Psychological Interfaces. Edited by Notman M, Nadelson C. New York, Plenum, 1978, pp 323–336
79. Van Keep PA, Kellerhals JM: The impact of socio-cultural factors on symptom formation: some results of a study on aging women in Switzerland. Psychother Psychosom 23:251–263, 1974
80. Dege K, Gretzinger J: Attitudes of families towards menopause, in Changing Perspectives on Menopause. Edited by Voda AM, Dinnerstein M, O'Donnell SR. Austin, TX, University of Texas Press, 1982, pp 60–69
81. Polit DF, LaRocco SA: Social and psychological correlates of menopausal symptoms. Psychosom Med 42:335–345, 1980
82. Goldstein MZ: Aspects of gender and ethnic identity in menopause: two Italian-American women. J Am Acad Psychoanal 15:383–394, 1987
83. Greene JG, Cook DJ: Life stress and symptoms at the climacterium. Br J Psychiatry 136:486–491, 1980
84. McKinlay S, Jefferys M: The menopausal syndrome. British Journal of Preventive and Social Medicine 28:108–115, 1974
85. Raunikar V: Physiology and treatment of hot flushes. Obstet Gynecol 75:35–175, 1990
86. Winokur G: Depression in the menopause. Am J Psychiatry 130:92–93, 1973
87. Weissman MM, Klerman GL: Sex differences and the epidemiology of depression. Arch Gen Psychiatry 34:98–111, 1977
88. Weissman MM: The myth of involutional melancholia. JAMA 42:742–744, 1979
89. Coulam CB: Age estrogens and the psyche. Clin Obstet Gynecol 24:219–229, 1981
90. Gitlin MJ, Pasnau RO: Psychiatric syndromes linked to reproductive function in women: a review of current knowledge. Am J Psychiatry 146:1413–1422, 1989
91. Osborn M: Depression at the menopause. Br J Hosp Med 32:128–129, 1984

92. Roy A, Markku L, Jimerson DC, et al: Pre-menopausal and post-menopausal depressed women. Aust N Z J Psychiatry 20:464–469, 1986
93. Bush TL: The epidemiology of cardiovascular disease in postmenopausal women. Ann N Y Acad Sci 592:263–345, 1990
94. Sitruk-Ware R, Iberra de Palacios P: Oestrogen replacement therapy and cardiovascular disease in postmenopausal women: a review. Maturitas 11:259–274, 1989
95. Stampfer MJ, Colditz GH, Willett WC: Menopause and heart disease. Ann N Y Acad Sci 592:193–263, 1990
96. Ballinger CB: Subjective sleep disturbance at the menopause. J Psychosom Res 20:509–513, 1976
97. Jaszmann L, Van Lith WP, Zaat JLA: The perimenopausal symptoms; the statistical analysis of a survey. Med Gynaecol Sociol 4:268, 1969
98. Fry JM: Sleep disorders. Med Clin North Am 71:95–111, 1987
99. Morokoff PJ: Sexuality in perimenopausal and postmenopausal women. Psychology of Women Quarterly 12:489–511, 1988
100. Young DD: Some misconceptions concerning the menopause. Obstet Gynecol 75:881–883, 1990
101. Sarrel PM: Sexuality in the middle years. Obstet Gynecol Clin North Am 14:49–62, 1987
102. Bachmann GA: Sexual issues at menopause. Ann N Y Acad Sci 592:87–94, 1990
103. Sarrel PM: Sexuality and menopause. Obstet Gynecol 75:26S-30S, 1990
104. Walling M, Anderson BL, Johnson SR: Hormonal replacement therapy for postmenopausal women: a review of sexual outcomes and related gynecologic effects. Arch Sex Behav 2:119–137, 1990
105. Iddenden DA: Sexuality during the menopause. Med Clin North Am 71:87–94, 1987
106. Melton LJ: Epidemiology of osteoporosis; predicting who is at risk. Ann N Y Acad Sci 592:295–306, 1990
107. Mendell D: A study of menopausal women in analytic treatment, in Critical Psychophysical Passages in the Life of a Woman: A Psychodynamic Perspective. Edited by Offerman-Zuckerberg J. New York, Plenum, 1988, pp 183–197
108. Lampl–de Groot J: On the process of mourning. Psychoanal Study Child 38:9–13, 1983
109. Lax R: The expectable depressive climacteric reaction. Bull Menninger Clin 46:151–167, 1982
110. Holmes TH, Rahe RH: The social readjustment rating scale. J Psychosom Res 11:213–218, 1967–1968

111. Barrett CJ: Women in widowhood. Signs 2:856–868, 1977
112. Hansson RO, Remondet JH: Old age and widowhood: issues of personal control and independence. Journal of Social Issues 44:159–174, 1988
113. Blackburn JA, Greenberg JS, Boss PG: Coping with normative stress from loss and change: a longitudinal study of rural widows. Journal of Gerontological Social Work 11:59–70, 1987
114. Ferraro K: Widowhood and social participation in later life. Res Aging 6:451–468, 1984b
115. McCrae RR, Costa Jr PT: Psychological resilience among widowed men and women: a 10-year follow-up of a national sample. Journal of Social Issues 44:129–142, 1988
116. Thomas LE, DiGiulio RC, Sheehan WW: Identity loss and psychological crisis in widowhood: a re-evaluation. Int J Aging Hum Dev 26:225–239, 1988
117. Heinemann GD, Evans PL: Widowhood: loss, change, and adaptation, in Family Relationships in Later Life, 2nd Edition. Edited by Brubaker TH. Newbury Park, CA, Sage, 1990, pp 142–168
118. Fulton R, Fulton JA: A psychosocial aspect of terminal care: anticipatory grief. Omega 2:91–99, 1971
119. Futterman EH, Hoffman I, Sabshin M: Parental anticipatory mourning, in Psychosocial Aspects of Terminal Care. Edited by Schoenberg B, Carr AC, Peretz D, et al. New York, Columbia University Press, 1972, pp 243–272
120. Bumagin VE, Hirn KF: Observations on changing relationships for older married women. Am J Psychoanal 42:133–142, 1982
121. Glick IO, Weiss RS, Parkes CM: The First Year of Bereavement. New York, Wiley, 1974
122. Schwab JJ, Farris PB, Conroy SJ, et al: Funeral behavior and unresolved grief, in Acute Grief and the Funeral. Edited by Pine VR, Kutscher A, Peretz D, et al. Springfield, IL, Charles C Thomas, 1975, pp 241–249
123. Vachon ML, Rogers J, Lyall WA, et al: Predictors and correlates of adaptation to conjugal bereavement. Am J Psychiatry 139:998–1002, 1982a
124. Clayton PJ, Halikas J, Maurice W, et al: Anticipatory grief and widowhood. Br J Psychiatry 122:47–51, 1973
125. Rando TA: Grief, Dying and Death: Clinical Interventions for Caregivers. Champaign, IL, Research Press Company, 1984
126. Ball JF: Widows' grief: the impact of age and mode of death. Omega 7:307–333, 1976–1977
127. Parkes CM: Determinants of outcome following bereavement. Omega 6:303–323, 1975

128. Parkes CM, Brown RJ: Health after bereavement: a controlled study of young Boston widows and widowers. Psychosom Med 34:449–461, 1972
129. Gerber I, Rusalem W, Hannon N, et al: Anticipatory grief and aged widows and widowers. J Gerontol 30:225–229, 1975
130. Parkes CM: The first year of bereavement: a longitudinal study of the reaction of London widows to the death of their husbands. Psychiatry 33:444–467, 1970
131. Bankoff EA: Effects of friendship support on the psychological well-being of widows. Research in the Interweave of Social Roles 2:109–113, 1981
132. Bankoff EA: Social support and adaptation to widowhood. Journal of Marriage and the Family 45:827–839, 1983b
133. Warner SL: A comparative study of widows' and widowers' perceived social support during the first year of bereavement. Arch Psychiatr Nurs 1:241–250, 1987
134. Ben-Sita Z: Loss, stress and readjustment: the structure of coping with bereavement and disability. Soc Sci Med 17:1619–1632, 1983
135. Bankoff EA: Aged parents and their widowed daughters: a support relationship. J Gerontol 38:226–230, 1983a
136. Lopata HZ: Women as Widows: Support Systems. New York, Elsevier, 1979
137. Walker K, McBride A, Vachon M: Social support and the crisis of bereavement. Soc Sci Med 11:34-41, 1977
138. Morgan LA: The financial experience of widowed women: evidence from the LRHS. Gerontologist 26:663–668, 1986
139. Farrell D, Wilner N: Mutual help groups for widows: a study of the process. Isr J Psychiatry Relat Sci 23:297–305, 1986
140. Lieberman MA, Videka-Sherman L: The impact of self-help groups on the mental health of widows and widowers. Am J Orthopsychiatry 56:435–449, 1986
141. Redburn DE, Juretich M: Some considerations for using widowed self help group leaders. Gerontology and Geriatrics Education 9(3):89–98, 1989
142. Wambach JA: The grief process as a social construct. Omega 16:201–211, 1985–1986
143. Barrett CJ: Effectiveness of widows' groups in facilitating change. J Consult Clin Psychol 46:20–31, 1978
144. Constantino RE: Bereavement crisis intervention for widows in grief and mourning. Nurs Res 30:351–353, 1981
145. Debor L, Gallagher D, Lesher E: Group counseling with bereaving elderly. Clinical Gerontologist 1:81–90, 1983
146. Doka KJ: Loss upon loss: the impact of death after divorce. Death Studies 10:441–449, 1986

147. Blanchard CG, Blanchard EB, Becker JV: The young widow: depressive symptomatology throughout the grief process. Psychiatry 39:394–399, 1976
148. Maddison D, Viola A: The health of widows in the year following bereavement. J Psychosom Res 12:297–306, 1968
149. Parkes CM: Recent bereavement as a cause of mental illness. Br J Psychiatry 110:198–204, 1964
150. Breckenridge JN, Gallagher D, Thompson LW, et al: Characteristic depressive symptoms of bereaved elders. J Gerontol 41:163–168, 1986
151. Ferraro KF: The effect of widowhood on the health status of older people. Int J Aging Hum Dev 21:9–25, 1985–1986
152. Heyman DK, Gianturco DT: Long-term adaptation by the elderly to bereavement. J Gerontol 28:359–363, 1973
153. Clayton PJ: The clinical morbidity of the first year of bereavement: a review. Compr Psychiatry 14:151-157, 1973
154. Cain L: Widow. New York, William Morrow, 1974
155. Gates PA: Suddenly Alone: A Woman's Guide to Widowhood. New York, Harper & Row, 1990
156. Akiyama H, Holtzman JM, Britz WE: Pet ownership and health status during bereavement. Omega 17:187–193, 1986–1987
157. Clark PG, Siviski RW, Weiner R: Coping strategies of widowers in the first year. Family Relations 35:425–430, 1986
158. Folkman S, Lazarus RS: An analysis of coping in a middle age community sample. J Health Soc Behav 21:219–239, 1980
159. Gass KA: Coping Strategies of Widows. Journal of Gerontological Nursing 13:29–33, 1987
160. Moss MS, Moss SZ: Some aspects of the elder widow(er)'s persistent tie with the deceased spouse. Omega 15:195–206, 1984
161. Schuchter SSR, Zisook S: Widowhood: the continuing relationship with the dead spouse. Bull Menninger Clin 52:269–279, 1988
162. Lopata HZ: Widowhood in an American City. Cambridge, MA, Schenkman, 1973
163. Brock AM, O'Sullivan P: From wife to widow: role transition in the elderly. J Psychosoc Nurs Ment Health Serv 23:6–12, 1985
164. Reinhardt JP, Fisher CB: Kinship versus friendship: social adaptation in married and widowed elderly women. Unpublished doctoral dissertation, Fordham University, New York, 1989
165. Lewittes HJ: Just being friendly means a lot—women, friendship and aging, in Women in the Later Years. Edited by Gray L. New York, Haworth Press, 1989, pp 139–159

166. Anderson TB: Widowhood as a life transition: its impact on kinship ties. Journal of Marriage and the Family 46:105–114, 1984
167. Remnet VL: How adult children respond to role transitions in the lives of their aging parents. Educational Gerontology 13:341–355, 1987
168. Brody EM, Schoonover MA: Patterns of parent-care when adult daughters work and when they do not. Gerontologist 26:372–381, 1986
169. Schoonover CB, Brody EM, Hoffman C, et al: Parent care and geographically distant children. Res Aging 10:472–492, 1988
170. Strugnell C: Who the widow-to-widow program served, in Helping Each Other in Widowhood. Edited by Silverman P, MacKenzie MP, Wilson E. New York, Health Sciences Publishing, 1974, pp 31–56
171. Towns K, Gentzler R: Empowering re-entry women: an organizational case study, in The Dynamics of Feminist Therapy. New York, Haworth Press, 1986, pp 159–166
172. Lopata HZ: Support systems of American urban widowhood. Journal of Social Issues 44:113–128, 1988
173. Gilligan C: In a Different Voice. Cambridge, MA, Harvard University Press, 1982
174. Spanier GB, Glick PC: Paths to remarriage. Journal of Divorce 3:283–298, 1980
175. Malatesta UJ, Chambless DL, Pollack M, et al: Widowhood, sexuality and aging: a life span analysis. J Sex Marital Ther 14:49–62, 1988
176. Kansky J: Sexuality of widows: a study of the sexual practices of widows during the first fourteen months of bereavement. J Sex Marital Ther 12:307–321, 1986
177. Gentry M, Schulman A: Remarriage as a coping response for widowhood. Psychol Aging 3:191–196, 1988
178. Gentry M, Rosenman L, Schulman AD: Comparison of needs and support systems of remarried and non-remarried widows, in Widows, Vol 2: North America. Edited by Lopata HZ. Durham, NC, Duke University Press, 1987, pp 158–170
179. Cleveland WP, Gianturco DT: Remarriage probability after widowhood; a retrospective method. J Gerontol 31:99–103, 1976
180. Arschault AM: Sources of support of elderly Acadian widows. Health Care of Women International 7:203–219, 1986
181. Lopata HZ: Widows: North America, in Widows, Vol 2: North America. Edited by Lopata HZ. Durham, NC, Duke University Press, 1987, pp 3–31
182. Roberto KA, Scott JP: Confronting widowhood: the influence of informal support. American Behavioral Scientist 29:497–511, 1986

183. Ferraro KF, Mutran E, Barresi CM: Widowhood, health and friendship support in later life. J Health Soc Behav 25:246–259, 1984
184. O'Bryant SL: Neighbors' support of older widows who live alone in their own homes. Gerontologist 25:305–310, 1985
185. Goldberg GS, Kantrow R, Kremen E, et al: Spouseless, childless elderly women and their social supports. Social Work 31:104–112, 1986
186. Pelham AO, Clark WF: Widowhood among low income racial and ethnic groups in California, in Widows, Vol 2: North America. Edited by Lopata HZ. Durham, NC, Duke University Press, 1987, pp 191–222
187. Arens DA: Widowhood and well-being: an examination of sex differences within a casual model. Int J Aging Hum Dev 15:27–40, 1982
188. Arling G: Resistance to isolation among elderly widows. Int J Aging Hum Dev 7:67–86, 1976b
189. Scott JP, Kivelt VR: Differences in the morale of older rural widows and widowers. Int J Aging Hum Dev 21:121–136, 1985
190. Rynearson EK: Pathologic grief: the queen's croquet ground. Psychiatric Annals 20:295–304, 1990
191. Raphael B, Middleton W: What is pathologic grief? Psychiatric Annals 6:304–308, 1990
192. Freud S: Mourning and melancholia (1917), in The Standard Edition of the Complete Psychological Works of Sigmund Freud, Vol 14. Translated and edited by Strachey J. London, Hogarth Press, 1961, pp 237–258
193. Lindemann E: Symptomatology and management of acute grief. Am J Psychiatry 101:141–148, 1944
194. Clayton P, Desmarais L, Winokur G: A study of normal bereavement. Am J Psychiatry 125:168–178, 1968
195. Clayton PJ, Halikas JA, Maurice WL: The bereavement of the widowed. Diseases of the Nervous System 32:592–604, 1971
196. Clayton PJ, Halikas JA, Maurice WL: The depression of widowhood. Br J Psychiatry 120:71–78, 1972
197. Clayton PJ, Herjanic M, Murphy G: Mourning and depression: their similarities and differences. Can J Psychiatry 19:309–312, 1974
198. Raphael B: Preventive intervention with the recently bereaved. Arch Gen Psychiatry 34:1450–1454, 1977
199. Raphael B: Mourning and the prevention of melancholia. Br J Med Psychol 51:303–310, 1978
200. Parkes CM, Weiss RS: Recovery From Bereavement. New York, Basic Books, 1983
201. Jacobs S, Kim K: Psychiatric complications of bereavement. Psychiatric Annals 20:314–317, 1990

202. Parkes CM: Risk factors in bereavement: implications for the prevention and treatment of pathologic grief. Psychiatric Annals 20:308–313, 1990
203. Bruce ML, Kim K, Leaf P, et al: Depressive episodes and dysphoria resulting from conjugal bereavement in a prospective community sample. Am J Psychiatry 147:608–611, 1990
204. Freedman AM, Blumenfield M: Recognizing the role of bereavement and reactive depression in modern psychiatry. Psychopathology 19:37–46, 1987
205. Byrne GJA: Studies on the Impact of Recent Spouse's Bereavement on Elderly Men. Herston Queensland, University of Queensland, 1989
206. Bowlby J: Attachment and Loss, Vol 2: Separation. New York, Basic Books, 1973
207. Bowlby J: Attachment and Loss, Vol 3: Loss: Sadness and Depression. New York, Basic Books, 1980
208. Deutsch H: Absence of grief. Psychoanal Q 6:12–22, 1937
209. Volkan V: Typical findings in pathological grief. Psychiatr Q 44:231–250, 1970
210. Parkes CM: Bereavement and mental illness. Br J Med Psychol 38:1–26, 1965
211. Maddison D, Walker WL: Factors affecting the outcome of conjugal bereavement. Br J Psychiatry 113:1057–1067, 1967
212. Singh B, Raphael B: Postdisaster morbidity of the bereaved. J Nerv Ment Dis 169:203–212, 1981
213. Horowitz MJ: A model of mourning: change in schemas of self and other. J Am Psychoanal Assoc 38:297–324, 1990
214. Krystal H: The impact of massive psychic trauma and the capacity to grieve effectively, in Treating the Elderly With Psychotherapy. Edited by Sadavoy J, Leszcz M. Madison, CT, International Universities Press, 1987, pp 95–156
215. Van Rooijen L: Widows' bereavement stress and depression after one and a half years. Paper presented at the Advanced Study Institute in Environmental Stress, Cambridge, UK, 1978
216. Vachon MLS, Sheldon AR, Lanacee WJ, et al: Correlates of enduring distress patterns following bereavement: social network, life situation and personality. Psychol Med 12:783–788, 1982b
217. Stroebe W, Stroebe MS: Bereavement and Health: The Psychological and Physical Consequences of Partner Loss. London, UK, Cambridge University Press, 1987
218. Duke D: A study of the effects of bereavement. Unpublished doctoral thesis, Newcastle Polytechnic, Newcastle, UK, 1980

219. Cain AC: The legacy of suicide; observations on the pathogenic impact of suicide upon marital partners. Psychiatry 29:406–411, 1966
220. Danto BL: Survivors of homicide, in The Human Side of Homicide. Edited by Danto BL, Bruhns J, Kutscher AH. New York, Columbia University Press, 1982, p 147
221. Gerber I, Rusalem R, Hannon N: Anticipatory grief and aged widows and widowers. J Gerontol 30:225–229, 1975
222. Middleton W: Studies in the Phenomenology of Grief. Herston Queensland, University of Queensland, 1989
223. Sanders CM: Risk factors in bereavement outcome. Journal of Social Issues 44:97–111, 1988
224. Raphael B: The Anatomy of Bereavement. New York, Basic Books, 1983
225. Schuchter SR, Zisook S: Hovering over the bereaved. Psychiatric Annals 20:327–333, 1990
226. Myers WA: Dreams of mourning and separation in older individuals, in The Interpretations of Dreams in Clinical Work. Edited by Rothstein A (Workshop Monograph 3). New York, American Psychoanalytic Association, 1987, pp 125–144
227. Polivka J: Cartoon humor as an aid in therapy. Clinical Gerontologist 7:63–67, 1987
228. Van der Hart O, Goossens FA: Leavetaking rituals in mourning therapy. Isr J Psychiatry Relat Sci 24:87–98, 1987
229. Jacobs SC, Nelson JC, Zisook S: Treating depressions of bereavement with antidepressants; a pilot study. Psychiatr Clin North Am 10:501–511, 1987
230. Marmar CR, Horowitz MJ, Weiss DS, et al: A controlled trial of brief psychotherapy and mutual help group treatment of conjugal bereavement. Am J Psychiatry 145:203–209, 1988
231. Whanger AD, Myers AC (eds): Mental Health Assessment and Therapeutic Intervention With Older Adults. Rockville, MD, Aspen, 1984
232. Windholz MJ, Marmar CR, Horowitz MJ: A review of research on conjugal bereavement: impact on health and efficacy of intervention. Compr Psychiatry 26:433–447, 1985
233. Baltes PB, Reese HW, Lipsett LP: Life-span developmental psychology. Annu Rev Psychol 31:65–110, 1980
234. Gass KA, Chang AS: Appraisals of bereavement, coping, resources, and psychosocial health dysfunction in widows and widowers. Nurs Res 38:31–36, 1989
235. Nemiroff RA, Colarusso CA: The Race Against Time: Psychotherapy and Psychoanalysis in the Second Half of Life. New York, Plenum, 1985

236. Zinberg NE: Psychoanalytic consideration of aging. J Am Psychoanal Assoc 12:151–159, 1964
237. Abraham K: The applicability of psychoanalytic treatment to patients at an advanced age, in Selected Papers of Karl Abraham, M.D. London, Brunner/Mazel, 1927, pp 312–317
238. Busse EW, Blazer DG: The theory and processes of aging, in Handbook of Geriatric Psychiatry. Edited by Busse EW, Blazer DG. New York, Van Nostrand Reinhold, 1980, pp 3–27
239. American Association of Retired Persons: A Profile of Older Americans. Washington, DC, American Association of Retired Persons, 1987
240. Busse EW: The myth, history, and science of aging, in Geriatric Psychiatry. Edited by Busse EW, Blazer DG. Washington, DC, American Psychiatric Press, 1989, pp 3–34
241. Busse EW, Blazer DG (eds): Geriatric Psychiatry. Washington, DC, American Psychiatric Press, 1989
242. Rubinstein RL: Singular Paths: Old Men Living Alone. New York, Columbia University Press, 1986
243. Idiculla AA, Goldberg G: Physical fitness for the mature woman. Med Clin North Am 71:135–143, 1987
244. Notelovitz M: Exercise and health maintenance in menopausal women. Ann N Y Acad Sci 592:204–262, 1990
245. Jolleys JV: Reported prevalence of urinary incontinence in women in a general practice. BMJ 296:1300–1302, 1988
246. Blazer DG, Bachar JR, Marston KG: Suicide in late life: review and commentary. J Am Geriatr Soc 34:519–525, 1986
247. Pillemer K, Finkelhor D: Causes of elder abuse: caregiver stress versus problem relatives. Am J Orthopsychiatry 59:179–187, 1989
248. Pillemer K: Maltreatment of patients in nursing homes: overview and research agenda. J Health Soc Behav 29:227–238, 1988
249. Sutton JJ, Pillemer K: Explaining conflict when adult children and elderly parents live together. Journal of Marriage and the Family 50:1037–1047, 1986
250. Pillemer K: The dangers of dependency: new findings on domestic violence against the elderly. Social Problems 33:146–158, 1985
251. Doty P, Sullivan E: Community involvement in combating abuse, neglect and maltreatment in nursing homes. Milbank Q 61:222–251, 1983
252. Sontag S: The double standard of aging. Saturday Review of the Society, September 1972, pp 29–38

Appendix A

Differences in the Structure of the Brain in Men and Women

There are several ways in which the brains of women differ from those of men (Erwin et al. 1989[1]; Gur et al. 1982,[2] 1992[3]). Women have a larger corpus callosum, a structure known to provide connections between the right and left hemispheres of the brain. On psychological tests, women consistently score higher in subjects thought to be dependent on right-hemisphere function, such as verbal skills, emotion, and empathy. Men score higher on abstract reasoning, mapping, and spatial relations, functions that are believed to be mediated by the left hemisphere of the brain. Women have more branches on their dendrites (i.e., the structures that receive chemical messages and transmit them to other neurons). Men have more spines on their dendritic branches. The functions of these spines are not yet elucidated. We do not yet know when this anatomical difference in the neurological substate occurs. Is it genetic, intrauterine, hormone responsive, or secondary to use or disuse?

Neuroreceptor sites in the chemical transmitter systems believed to be important in anxiety and depression are not known to differ in males and females.

Notes

1. Erwin RJ, Mawhinney-Hee M, Gur RC, et al: Effects of task and gender on EEG indices of hemisphere activation: similarities to previous CBF findings. Neuropsychiatry Neuropsychology Behav Neurol 2:248–260, 1989
2. Gur RC, Gur RE, Obrist WD, et al: Sex and handedness differences in cerebral blood flow during rest and cognitive activity. Science 217:256–261, 1982
3. Gur RC, Erwin RJ, Gur RE: Neurobehavioral probes for physiological neuroimaging studies. Arch Gen Psychiatry 49:409–414, 1992

Appendix B

Neurochemical Systems That Affect Appetite

Fava et al. (1989[1]) have reviewed the neurochemical systems that affect appetite. These include the serotonergic, adrenergic, noradrenergic, dopaminergic, and opioid systems, as well as those systems involving corticotropin-releasing hormone or factor (CRH or CRF), vasopressin, and cholecystokinin.

The noradrenergic system provides 117 important neural substrates for anxiety (Charney and Heninger 1985[2]) and depression (Price et al. 19863). These affective states are often observed in patients with anorexia or bulimia nervosa. After reviewing studies of anorexic women and women in the refeeding state, Fava et al. (1989[1]) feel that a pervasive defect in epinephrine metabolism may be a "trait" marker of anorexia nervosa. The complicated mechanisms of noradrenergic mediation in the central nervous system and the linkage in the locus coeruleus are in the process of elucidation.

Animal studies of the role of serotonergic systems involved in satiety have been reviewed (Hoefel and Liebowitz 1981[4]). Studies in humans with anorexia are still unclear. Observations in bulimic patients are consistent with the hypothesis that increased brain serotonin turnover contributes to satiety (Kaye et al. 1988[5]; Wurthman 1982[6]). CRH has been shown to be at higher levels in the cerebrospinal fluid of anorexic patients (Hotta et al. 1986[7]; Kaye et al. 1987[8]). Study of a small number of anorexic patients has implicated a defect in vasopressin (Gold et al. 1983[9]). Systemic cholecystokinin, a polypeptide that is released from the small intestine after eating and plays a role in appetite suppression, is found in lower concentrations in bulimic women (Geracioti and Liddle 1988[10]).

It is clear that the neurochemical mediation of satiety and of its disturbances is as complicated as the psychological determinants.

Notes

1. Fava M, Copeland PM, Schweiger V, et al: Neurochemical abnormalities of anorexia nervosa and bulimia nervosa. Am J Psychiatry 146:963–971, 1989
2. Charney DS, Heninger GR: Noradrenergic function and the mechanism of action of antianxiety treatment. Arch Gen Psychiatry 42:473–481, 1985
3. Price LH, Charney DS, Robin AL, et al: Alpha2 adrenergic receptor function in depression. Arch Gen Psychiatry 43:849–858, 1986
4. Hoefel BG, Liebowitz SF: Brain monoamines in the modulation of self stimulation, feeding, and body weight. Res Publ Assoc Res Nerv Ment Dis 59:103–147, 1981
5. Kaye WH, Gwirtsman HE, Breweston FD, et al: Binging behavior and plasma amino acids: a possible involvement of brain serotonin in bulimia nervosa. Psychiatry Res 23:31–43, 1988
6. Wurthman RS: Nutrients that modify brain function. Sci Am 246:50–59, 1982
7. Hotta M, Shibasaki T, Masuda A, et al: The responses of plasma adrenocorticotropin and cortisol to corticotropin-releasing hormone and cerebrospinal immunoreactive CRH in anorexia nervosa patients. J Clin Endocrinol Metab 62:319–324, 1986
8. Kaye WH, Gwirtsman HE, George DT, et al: Elevated cerebrospinal fluid levels of immunoreactive corticotropin-releasing hormone in anorexia nervosa: relation to state of nutrition, adrenal function, and intensity of depression. J Clin Endocrinol Metab 64:203–208, 1987
9. Gold PW, Kaye WH, Robertson RL, et al: Abnormalities in plasma and cerebrospinal fluid arginine vasopressin in patients with anorexia nervosa. N Engl J Med 308:1117–1123, 1983
10. Geracioti TD, Liddle RA: Impaired cholecystokinin in bulimia nervosa. N Engl J Med 319:683–688, 1988

Appendix C

Drug Use in Adolescence

As of 1981, an estimated 10% of 14-year-olds were heavy consumers of alcohol, and 7% of high school students reported daily use of marijuana. Barbiturate tranquilizers and amphetamines have also been abused. However, less than 7% of high school seniors in 1980 reported use of barbiturates in the previous 12 months as reported in a study by Johnston et al. (1979[1]). Methaqualone, also known as quaalude or "lude," is a nonbarbiturate sedative-hypnotic that produces a dissociative high and ultimately leads to a compelling addiction. In 1981 less than 7.6% of high school seniors reported having used quaaludes in the previous 12 months. Yet this was an increase from 1977 according to a study done by Pascarelli (1973[2]).

Amphetamines belong to a class of drugs known as *sympathomimetics*. The most common amphetamine is dextroamphetamine sulfate (Dexedrine), which is commonly prescribed to suppress appetite, restore energy, and elevate mood. This drug gives the sensation of speeding, thus the street name "speed." Amphetamines are usually used in low doses and infrequently (Blum 1979[3]).

Use of LSD and other hallucinogens reached a plateau in the early 1970s and then declined (Peterson and Stillman 1979[4]).

Phencyclidine, or PCP (also known as "angel dust"), is a dangerous drug that may lead to paranoia, psychotic states, and assaultive behavior. The use of this drug is associated with both homocide and suicide (Peterson and Stillman 1979[4]). Fortunately, its use seems to be declining.

Use of cocaine (also known as "coke," and "snow")—and its most dangerous, most addictive form, "crack" cocaine (also known as "ice")—has been dramatically increasing: an estimated 5% to 8% of high school students are users (Kleber 1988[5]).

The consequences of drug abuse for adolescent women, especially those of color, have been dramatic and tragic because, in part, of the "toss-up" phenomenon (i.e., the trading of sex for drugs) (Fullilove et al. 1990[6]). Although these patients cannot be neglected, their treatment goes beyond the scope of individual psychodynamic psychotherapy. For those readers interested in neighborhood programs, day treatment, therapeutic communities, and the treatment of committed adolescents who abuse drugs, we refer you to Friedman and Bechner (1985[7]).

Notes

1. Johnston GD, Bachman JF, O'Malley PM: Highlights from student drug use in America, 1975–78 (DHHS Publ No ADM-82-1208). Rockville, MD, National Institute on Drug Abuse, 1979
2. Pascarelli EF: Methaqualone: the quiet epidemic, in Drug Use in America: Problem in Perspective, Second Report of the National Commission on Marijuana and Drug Abuse, Vol 1. Edited by Shafer RP. Washington, DC, U.S. Government Printing Office, No 5266-00004, 1973, pp 102–105
3. Blum EH: Youthful drug use, in Handbook on Drug Abuse. Edited by Dupont RI, Goldstein A, O'Donnell J. Washington, DC, U.S. Government Printing Office, 1979, pp 257–269
4. Peterson RC, Stillman RC: Phencyclidine (PCP) Abuse: An Appraisal (GPO No 017-024-00785-04). Washington, DC, U.S. Government Printing Office, 1979, p 231
5. Kleber H: Cocaine abuse: historical, epidemiological, and psychological perspectives. J Clin Psychiatry 49:3–7, 1988
6. Fullilove MT, Fullilove RE, Haynes K, et al: Black women and AIDS prevention: a view towards understanding the gender roles. Journal of Sex Research 27:47–69, 1990
7. Friedman AS, Bechner GM (eds): Treatment Services for Adolescent Substance Abusers (DHHS Publ No 87-1342). Rockville, MD, National Institute on Drug Abuse, 1985

Appendix D

Neurochemistry of Panic Disorder

1. *Catecholamine theory*. This theory proposes that panic attacks are the manifestation of massive discharge from the beta-adrenergic neurotransmitter system, accompanied by palpitations, tremulousness, sweating, and decreased blood pressure. However, despite claims for the efficacy of specific beta-adrenergic blockers such as propranolol, no studies have shown that these inhibitors are specifically effective in blocking panic attacks (Gorman et al. 1983[1]).

2. *Locus coeruleus theory*. The locus coeruleus contains 50% of all noradrenergic neurons in the central nervous system (CNS) and has projections to many other CNS areas. Yohimbine, which increases locus coeruleus discharge, has been shown to provoke anxiety when administered to humans. Clonidine, propranolol, benzodiazepines, morphine, endorphin, and tricyclic antidepressants curtail locus coeruleus firing. As we have noted, however, not all of these substances are effective in blocking panic attacks in humans.

3. *Carbon dioxide sensitivity*. Gorman et al. (1984[2]) have found that controlled hyperventilation does not routinely provoke panic attack in most patients with panic disorder.

4. *Lactate theory*. Pitts and McClune (1967[3]) administered intravenous infusions of sodium lactate to patients who seemed to have anxiety disorders and found that most of these patients suffered anxiety attacks during the infusion. Repeated studies confirm this finding, but the mechanism is not yet understood.

5. *Gamma-aminobutyric acid–benzodiazepine theory*. GABA agents administered to animals block benzodiazepine receptors and produce acute anxiety (Skolnick and Paul 1982[4]).

Notes

1. Gorman JM, Levy GF, Liebowitz MR, et al: Effect of acute beta-adrenergic blockade on lactate-induced panic. Arch Gen Psychiatry 40:1079–1083, 1983
2. Gorman JM, Askanazi J, Liebowitz MR, et al: Response to hyperventilation in a group of patients with panic disorder. Am J Psychiatry 141:857–861, 1984
3. Pitts FN, McClune JN: Lactate metabolism in anxiety neurosis. N Engl J Med 277:1329–1336, 1967
4. Skolnick P, Paul SM: Benzodiazepine receptors in the central nervous system. Int Rev Neurobiol 23:103–140, 1982

Appendix E

Women Who Compete With Women

A. The "queen bee": Having an "out to kill you off" strategy.

Strategy 1: Withdraw from confrontation.
Strategy 2: Be gracious and look for support from others. There is strength in numbers.

B. The "token woman": "I've done fine; there are no problems."

Strategy 1: Pull her into the problem, ask her advice, or invite her to chair a committee or run a group on problem solving.
Strategy 2: Let her know that you are looking for advice about how to handle "your problem."
Strategy 3: If it is clear that she is protecting her "token woman" status, leave.

C. Angry survivor: "I've suffered, so should you."

Strategy 1: Confront her directly with the fallacy of having each person reinvent the wheel.
Strategy 2: Empathize with her difficult experiences, and ask her to share those experiences and how she survived.
Strategy 3: Diffuse anger by asking her if she would not have felt better with help or if she would not feel better helping others to turn the tables.

D. Denier: "I don't see what the problem is."

Strategy 1: Show person how she is really like you but does not let herself know it.
Strategy 2: If the individual who denies problems persists and cannot see her denial, work around her.

E. Uninformed: "I didn't realize that there are ways to cope."

Strategy 1: Provide logical information.
Strategy 2: Ask for advice.

F. Peer/sibling rivalry between women of the same age or level of accomplishment

Strategy 1: Determine how you dealt with this earlier in life and use the same strategies.

G. Unempowered groups—housekeepers, baby sitters, au pairs, nurses, clerks, junior administrators, cleaning women, hostesses, cooks, etc.

Strategy 1: Share power by sharing authority, decision making, etc.
Strategy 2: Ask for help and support.
Strategy 3: Empower them by letting them know that they are an important element in your success.

H. Reciprocal networking

Strategy 1: Do not approach a mentor/advisor in an infantile and needy way. She can help and encourage but she is not a "quick fix." Remember that senior colleagues or friends need the active support of junior or younger women.
Strategy 2: Do not approach a mentor/advisor in a spirit of entitlement.
Strategy 3: Think of, or ask, in what ways you can help your mentor/advisor.
Strategy 4: Do not displace your anger onto your mentor/advisor.

Appendix F

Premenstrual Syndrome

The salient points of the premenstrual syndrome (PMS) are as follows. Autonomic control of the reproductive system involves all organs and their processes. The major sympathetic neurotransmitter is norepinephrine. Dopamine, epinephrine, acetylcholine, and the prostaglandins are all also involved.

Stress is related to catecholamine excess. For example, an excess of catecholamine affects the smooth-muscle functioning of the oviduct. Steroids are known to influence neuroreceptor properties.

A norepinephrine surge normally accompanies luteinizing hormone release during estrus. Serotonin stimulates prolactin. Melatonin concentrations are highest in the 12 days before ovulation and lowest at ovulation. The connections between serotonin, melatonin, and depression have been under investigation for a number of years.

Stress affects adrenal steroidogenesis. The resultant excess androgens can upset the balance between luteinizing hormone and progesterone, and result in an ovulation.

A full discussion of the limbic pituitary interaction and the consequences for thyroid and adrenal function is beyond the scope of this appendix but must be mentioned. A very fine and precise homeostatic balance and rhythm must exist for ovulation, fertilization, implantation, and fetal retention to take place.

Appendix G

Lesions of Reproductive Organs

The most common organisms involved lesions of reproductive organs are bacteria, yeast, and protozoa. The most common yeast infection is *Candida albicans*, which can be diagnosed by microscopic examination of a vaginal smear. This infection is treated either locally or systemically with one of several antiyeast agents. *Trichomonas vaginalis* is a protozoal infection easily diagnosed in a wet-mount slide. This infection is treated systemically, and both sexual partners must be treated to avoid reinfection. Among the bacterial infections found are those caused by *E. coli* and *Pseudomonas*, usually due to fecal contamination. These infections are diagnosed microscopically with gram stain and are then treated systemically with antibiotics that are specific for gram-negative organisms.

Neisseria gonorrhoeae is a gram-positive bacterium capable of infecting and permanently damaging the entire genital tract. In the early stages it is diagnosed by microscopic examination of a gram-stained cervical smear. The infection is treated by a systemic antibacterial medication. The treatment of this infection has become complicated because of the occurrence of resistant strains of the bacterium.

If the initial gonorrheal infection has been missed, it can present later as abdominal pain and may not be diagnosed on physical examination. Diagnosis may require an extensive medical evaluation along with sonography, X ray, and other imaging techniques. Once the diagnosis of pelvic inflammatory disease (PID) has been made, an invasive surgical technique such as abdominal laparoscopy may be required to obtain a culture for identification and to determine antibiotic sensitivity. PID is most commonly associated with gonococcal infection, but one of the present authors has recently seen a patient diagnosed with a staphylococcal infection secondary to sexual activity.

The differential diagnosis of these ulcerative lesions includes syphilis, herpes, and, in rare cases, chancroid and granuloma inguinale. Clinical examination is often diagnostic. Dark field examination often reveals the spirochete responsible for syphilis. The Treponema pallidum immobilization test (TPI) is a highly accurate blood test for syphilis. The herpesvirus requires cytological examination, because it is often seen inside the cell. It is initially a vesicular and painful lesion. It is sometimes accompanied by system effects, tiredness, lethargy, and anorexia, which also characterize other systemic viral infections. Herpes can be treated with specific systemic antiviral medication. *Hemophilus ducreyi*, the cause of chancroid, can be detected via culture on specially enriched media. This disease is treated systemically. Other viral infections, which are primarily systemic, such as Epstein-Barr virus, cytomegalic inclusion disease, and hepatitis B, require blood tests, and the treatment of these infections is nonspecific and supportive.

Appendix H

Medical Infertility: Evaluation and Treatment

For the male partner

Medical history and general examination
- Laboratory examination of blood and urine samples

Sexual history
- Treatment of sexual dysfunction (e.g., premature ejaculation)
- Sperm sample for count, motility, and viability
- Correction of anatomical defects (e.g., varicocele)
- Correction of hormonal abnormalities (e.g., androgen)
- Guinea pig test to determine if the sperm can penetrate an ovum
- Sexual abstinence prior to intercourse scheduled to coincide with ovulation
- Sperm samples for artificial insemination or in vitro fertilization

For the female partner

Medical history and physical examination
- Laboratory examination of blood and urine samples

Sexual history
- Treatment for disordered sexual functioning (e.g., vaginismus)
- Instruction on positioning to keep semen in prolonged contact with the cervix
- Gynecological examination for gross pathology or infection and examination of mucus at ovulation

For the female partner (continued)

Sexual history (continued)
- Establishing time of ovulation by daily basal body temperature, urine test kit, or blood samples of hormones

Undergoing a postcoital test (i.e., patient is seen after intercourse for examination of reaction of husband's sperm to her vaginal mucus)

Establishing patency of female genital tract

Sonography with or without air insufflation X-ray examination after introduction of contrast media into the cervix

Possible direct visualization or correction via laparoscopy or abdominal surgery

Artificial insemination with partner's sperm

Treatment with hormones that cause multiple ovulation (e.g., Clomid, Pergonal [the latter is given by daily injection])

Injections of progesterone are added to hyperovulatory drugs. Ovum retrieval and replacement in the uterus after fertilization are then required.

Appendix I

Legal and Dynamic Models of Sexual Harassment

The legal history of sexual harassment began over 25 years ago with Title VII of the Civil Rights Act of 1964, which prohibited sexual discrimination. Despite widespread publicity from women's groups in the 1970s, another 15 years passed before the sexual harassment aspects of this law were clearly delineated by the Equal Employment Opportunity Commission (EEOC). In 1972, Title IX was passed, prohibiting sexual discrimination of students in any program of a higher educational institution that was receiving federal funds. The law was later narrowed to include only those parts of programs receiving federal funds, and then restored again to its original form via the Civil Rights Restoration Act of 1987.

In 1980, the EEOC (the federal agency responsible for overseeing Title VII) published a historic set of guidelines designed to assist employers in understanding that sexual harassment is a specific form of sex discrimination, as covered by the 1964 law. The EEOC guidelines state that

> unwelcome sexual advances, requests for sexual favors and other verbal or physical conduct of a sexual nature constitute sexual harassment when 1) submission to such conduct is made either explicitly or implicitly a term or condition of an individual's employment, 2) submission to or rejection of such conduct by an individual is used as the basis for employment decisions affecting such individual, or 3) such conduct has the purpose or effect of unreasonably interfering with an individual's work performance or creating an intimidating, hostile or offensive work environment." (Equal Employment Opportunity Commission 1980,[1] p. 15)

Researchers have elaborated a continuum of behaviors that constitute harassment, as follows:

1. Sexual remarks, jokes, teasing, questions
2. Suggestive looks, gestures
3. Pressure for dates
4. Deliberate touching, leaning over, caressing
5. Pressure for sexual favors
6. Letters, phone calls, written material, pictures
7. Actual or attempted sexual assault

The EEOC guidelines created a clear and strong mandate for employers to prevent and eliminate sexual harassment in their workplaces. In response, many businesses and institutions began to develop sexual harassment policies, and a number of states passed legislation prohibiting harassment. Between 1980 and 1988 over 38,500 cases were filed with the federal government (Klein 1988[2]). In the first sexual harassment case to be heard by the U.S. Supreme Court, *Meritor Savings Bank v. Vinson*, the Court unanimously upheld the EEOC guidelines, finding that sexual harassment is in violation of the law if it is pervasive and severe enough to create a hostile and abusive work environment. This decision set a precedent for further lawsuits, with settlements in 1987 as high as 3.2 million dollars (Klein 1988[2]). Despite this evolving legal support, the process of filing a complaint or instituting legal action can be a traumatic, prolonged, and frustrating experience for victims, and it is often, as we will discuss later, a necessary focus for treatment.

In addition to the significantly lower prevalence rates of sexual harassment for men than for women, there is also a significant difference in the interactional process and outcome for men in comparison with women. Understanding these dynamics further highlights why this phenomenon affects women more adversely than men, and serves as a useful orientation to the psychiatric sequelae of harassment.[†]

[†]Homosexual harassment has been reported in low numbers but will not be included in this discussion because the primary problem for women is heterosexual harassment.

In her book *Sex and the Workplace*, Barbara Gutek (1985,[3] pp. 63–66) studied the characteristics of harassment and the victim's reactions. She found that, in general, male harassers were 1) older, 2) predominantly married, 3) less physically attractive, 4) in supervisory positions or having some power to affect their victims' work status, and 5) likely to harass multiple victims. Female harassers tended to 1) be young, 2) be attractive, 3) be unmarried, 4) hold nonsupervisory positions in which they usually did not have the power to influence their victims' work state, and 5) focus their harassment behavior on only one victim whom they could usually not influence in regard to work performance status or promotion.

Gutek found that the experience of victims also varied greatly with gender. Male victims usually perceived a mutuality in the interaction and stressed the genuine sexual attraction and relationship between them and their female harassers. They often felt they were responsible for initiating or encouraging the harassment behaviors and often described a positive outcome in the form of enhanced self-esteem or a personal relationship. In the minority of incidences when the male victims did not perceive any genuine interest on the part of their female harasser, they often cited attempts to gain privileges, have their work noticed, or gain inside information as inferred motivations. In either case, it was significant that the male victims reported that the harassment had few if any detrimental effects on their work.

Female victims of male harassers described entirely different and more negative experiences in Gutek's survey. These women did not, as a group, experience feelings of mutuality or personal enhancement, nor did they feel responsible for encouraging the harasser, except in a minority of cases when they perceived him as attractive. Instead, they stressed that their harasser targeted many women or that certain impersonal work conditions such as office parties, conferences, and evening work hours stimulated the behavior, making the interaction more dehumanizing and embarrassing than enhancing. The female victims also reported negative work outcomes in the form of fear of or actual experiences of 1) punitive retaliations, 2) loss of job, 3) punitive transfers, 4) negative work assignments, 5) poor recommendations, and

6) decreased opportunity for promotion and career advancement. As a group the female victims described the experience as intrusive and an abuse of power that had negative work consequences; in contrast, the male victims, as noted above, described a more positive and mutual sexual experience having little impact on their work.

Notes

1. Equal Employment Opportunity Commission, Federal Register 45(219):14–15, 1980
2. Klein F: The 1988 Working Women Sexual Harassment Report. Executive Report, Klein Associates, Cambridge, MA, 1988
3. Gutek BA: Sex and the Workplace: The Impact of Sexual Behavior and Harassment on Women, Men and Organizations. San Francisco, CA, Jossey-Bass, 1985

Appendix J

Approaches to Sexual Harassment

Direct approach (verbal and written)

Experts often recommend direct action by the victim (i.e., the offended person) toward the harasser even if further steps are ultimately necessary. Despite the double bind that it places on the offended person, Dr. Mary Rowe, a labor economist and ombudsperson with extensive experience in sexual harassment, recommends approaching the harasser directly because it is effective, it focuses the anger outside the person, and it lays a foundation of favorable evidence for any later legal or institutional actions. According to Rowe (1981,[1] p. 43), the aims of individual action are as follows:

> To give the offended and offender a chance, usually for the first time, to see things the same way. Since neither person may have any understanding of how the other sees the problem, discussion may help. Entry of a third party at this stage usually further polarizes the views of the opposing persons.
>
> To give those who are wrongly accused the chance to defend themselves.
>
> To give those who are correctly, or to some extent correctly, accused the chance to make amends. (This may not be possible in serious cases.)
>
> To provide some evidence of the offense, since usually there is no substantive evidence at all. This step is vital if management or the courts must later take action.
>
> To give aggressors who do not understand what they were doing a fair warning, if this is appropriate.
>
> To provide the offended employee a chance to get the harassment stopped without provoking public counterattack, experiencing public embarrassment, harming third parties, damaging the company's reputation, or causing the aggressor to lose face. In my experience, these points are almost always considered important by the aggrieved person.
>
> To provide offended persons a way to demonstrate that they tried all reasonable means to get the offender to stop. This step may be convincing later to supervisors, spouses, and others who become involved.

> To encourage ambivalent complainants, as well as those who have inadvertently given misunderstood signals, to present a consistent and clear message
>
> To encourage those who exaggerate to be more responsible.

Whether the individual action should be taken in verbal or written form should also be considered. Informing the harasser that his attentions are not wanted is very empowering for some women, and it is often the quickest and most effective means of stopping a harasser who is unaware that his behavior is affecting women adversely. The message should be delivered in a polite, calm, firm, unsmiling, and explicit manner. The offended woman should be prepared to quickly terminate the interaction if the harasser responds negatively or escalates the behavior. The victim should document her verbal objection in case she decides to file charges at a later date. Writing a letter to the harasser can also be valuable to the victim both as a way of preparing to address him directly or as an alternative to verbal interaction. Rowe (1981,[1] p. 43) suggests the following format:

> Writing a letter: One method that works quite consistently, even when many verbal requests have failed, is for the offended person to write a letter to the accused. I usually recommend a polite, low-key letter (which may necessitate many drafts).
>
> The letter I recommend has three parts. The first part should be a detailed statement of facts as the writer sees them: "This is what I think happened . . ." I encourage a precise rendition of all facts and dates relevant to the alleged harassment. This section is sometimes very long.
>
> In the second part of the letter, writers should describe their feelings and what damage they think has been done. This is where opinions belong. "Your action made me feel terrible"; "I am deeply embarrassed and worried that my parents will hear about this"; "You have caused me to ask for a transfer (change my career objectives; drop out of the training course; take excessive time off; or whatever)." The writer should mention any perceived or actual costs and damages, along with feelings of dismay, distrust, revulsion, misery, and so on.
>
> Finally, I recommend a short statement of what the accuser would like to have happen next. Since most persons only want the harassment

to end, the letter might finish by saying so; "I ask that our relationship from now on be on a purely professional basis." Someone who knows that he or she contributed to the problem does well to say so: "Although we once were happy dating, it is important to me that we now reestablish a formal and professional relationship, and I ask you to do so."

If the letter writer believes some remedy or recompense is in order, this is the place to say so: "Please withdraw my last evaluation until we can work out a fair one"; "I will need a written answer as to the reference you will provide from now on"; and statements of that type.

Even if the victim decides not to send the letter it can be a valuable cognitive exercise for the therapist to give to the patient, because it helps the victim organize her thinking and express her feelings in a responsible manner as well as focus on her goals for resolution. The present authors often recommend and collaborate with the patient in writing a letter as preparation for considering other options.

Informal Grievance Procedures Within the Work Organization (adapted from Hughes and Sandler 1986,[2] p. 5)

Informal procedures involve the intervention of a third party or parties who have authority over the harasser and who are perceived to be sympathetic and supportive of the victim (e.g., student deans, senior partners, supervisors, department heads, etc.). Informal procedures concentrate on confidentiality and conciliation rather than sanctions. The victim does not have to face the harasser directly and can maintain more control over the entire process. The victim may identify an appropriate third party and request that this person specifically ask the harasser to stop, or that the third party locate the appropriate person in the work hierarchy and then confront the harasser. Alternatively, the victim may ask the third party to send out a general memo/letter reminding the entire department of the institution's policy against sexual harassment. Copies of the policy, along with specific examples, can be included. Informal channels may also be used to help the victim discover whether others have complained about their harasser and what his status/vulnerability is within the organization. In less severe harassment situations when the victim wishes to maximize confidentiality, avoid direct confrontation, and obtain isolation without significant time investment, informal procedures can be very effective.

Victims should be counseled to check their specific policy to ascertain what level of confidentiality is guaranteed, to make clear to the third party why they find it inadvisable to confront their harasser directly, and to inform the third party what steps they would like him or her to take and what steps they would be uncomfortable with. The victims should be made aware of possible disadvantages: they can be less sure of the outcome, their satisfaction is dependent on the objectivity and fairness of the person handling the complaint, and they cannot be completely assured of confidentiality or control of the procedure. They should be prepared to deal with an unsympathetic response and be able to move directly on to another potential advocate. If the person they initially contact agrees to help, they should ask specifically how and when they will approach the harasser, when they can meet and learn the outcome, and what other approaches are possible.

Formal Complaint Procedures Within the Work Organization (adapted from Hughes and Sandler 1986,[2] pp. 5–6)

Formal grievance procedures involve several prescribed steps and have time deadlines for filing complaints. The victim files a complaint (usually written), an investigation or hearing is held within the institution, a decision is made regarding what sanctions, if any, will be taken against the harasser, and an appeals process may be instituted if either party finds the decision unacceptable.

Advantages to the formal complaint system are that by filing the complaint 1) the victim usually gains legal protection from retaliation and 2) she may know ahead of time what she is getting into. She should ask in advance whether she and any witnesses are protected from retaliation, and whether she can maintain control of the process and exercise other options for redress or is committed to the formal complaint procedure once she speaks with a representative of her institution. She can ask directly who conducts the investigation, what the time frame is, under what circumstances lawyers and cross-examiners are involved, what sanctions are possible and whether she will be informed, and what the outcome and duration of previous grievance procedures have been. Many victims feel empowered by taking definitive action against the harasser, and the real possibility of sanctions may be more effective in stopping more serious incidents of harassment.

The disadvantages of the procedure are 1) it is public and may lead to labeling the victim as a "troublemaker" or "whistle blower" and result in informal blackballing and ostracizing; 2) the victim must compile substantial evidence; 3) the procedure is time consuming and sometimes intimidating and traumatic; 4) institutions sometimes stall the procedure if they do not wish to act; 5) sanctions may be minimal, especially if the perpetrator is valuable to the institution.

Legal Action (adapted from Hughes and Sandler 1986,[2] pp. 7–8)

If the harassment behavior violates Title IX or Title VII as previously described, it is in violation of federal law. Information regarding Title VII may be obtained from the Equal Employment Opportunity Commission, 2401 E Street, N.W., Washington, D.C. 20507. Title IX information may be obtained from the Office for Civil Rights, U.S. Department of Education, Mary Switzer Bldg., 330 C St., S.W., Washington, D.C. 20202. In addition, many states have laws prohibiting sexual discrimination and harassment. Women may obtain information about these laws via several routes: 1) state civil rights commissions, 2) state women's commissions, 3) state Fair Employment Practices Commissions, 4) local Office for Civil Rights under the Department of Education, 5) state bar associations, 6) local chapters of the National Organization for Women, and 7) local chapters of the American Civil Liberties Union.

In some instances or circumstances civil suits may also be brought against both the harasser (e.g., assault and battery, intentional infliction of emotional distress, interference with a contract, defamation) and the institution/employer (e.g., breach of contract, negligent retention). In civil suits, however, the victim exposes herself to countersuit. Criminal suits may be brought if physical assault or sexual abuse has taken place.

Legal action can be effective if financial restitution is important to the victim or if she feels empowered by taking legal action, or if she has lost something of value that cannot be restored by other means (e.g., job positions, training opportunities, promotions, salary increases, recommendations, etc.). Many lawyers are willing to work on a contingency basis, and many women feel empowered by facing their harasser in court, where the laws against harassment are firmly established and treatment is likely to be more objective.

There are, however, many disadvantages to taking legal action of which the patient and therapist should be aware. Suits are often costly, extraordinarily time consuming and traumatic, and uncertain in outcome. Some suits take as long as 6 to 8 years to bring to completion, and the present authors are aware of many victims who have been retraumatized rather than empowered by courtroom appearances. Lengthy legal proceedings can significantly delay the woman's ability to move on in her life, and when negative outcomes occur, they often precipitate a severe sense of loss with intense and complicated mourning reactions. Professional women who file suits are sometimes permanently blackballed from their fields via informal networks. Patients should be cautioned not to move impulsively and unrealistically toward legal action. The therapist should be aware of the ongoing need for support and possible reevaluation of symptoms that may occur during the proceedings. Patients should also be encouraged to have a separate "forensic evaluator" to testify in any legal proceeding.

Notes

1. Rowe MP: Dealing with sexual harassment. Harvard Business Review, May/June 1981, pp 42–48
2. Hughes JO, Sandler BR: In Case of Sexual Harassment: A Guide for Women Students. Washington, DC, Project on the Status and Education of Women, Association of American Colleges, 1986

Appendix K

Subcategories of Rape

Rapes can appear in a variety of forms. An *individual rape* involves one perpetrator. A *pair rape* involves two perpetrators collaborating and raping the same victim. *Multiple rape* involves three or more perpetrators who either have sexual relationships with the victim or assist in threatening or forcing her to submit. In addition, cases have been reported of husbands, boyfriends, acquaintances, or even telephoning strangers (Hott 1983[2]) setting up victims for rape but not participating in the actual incident. More than one perpetrator can compound the victim's sense of violation, as well as her feelings of being overwhelmed and powerless. In the case of multiple rapes such as fraternity rapes and party rapes, the victim must also contend with continued interactions with the offenders and the betrayal of valued relationships.

Rapes can occur in a variety of relational contexts that are psychologically relevant to the victim. *Acquaintance rape* is the term used when the parties knew each other prior to the assault and includes perpetrators such as relatives, neighbors, family, friends, classmates, social or work acquaintances, dates, co-workers, and teachers. Acquaintance rapes are those that occur in the context of a relationship (excluding relationships with family, co-workers, or teachers) in which the expression of some sexual behavior would be appropriate but where the force, threat, coercion, and nonconsensual status of the woman are apparent. The special terminology of *date rape*, *party rape*, and *marital rape* have been given to subtypes of acquaintance rape that are occurring in rapid numbers and are notable for not being reported as well as for often not being recognized by the victim as rape. The incidence of rape is also

---

The information in this appendix is adapted from Harvey and Koss 1987,[1] pp. 10–13.

significant among cohabiting couples who are not married, but the authors are not aware of any special terminology for this situation.

Stranger rape is the term used to describe a situation in which the victim and offender have never met. They are often called "blitz rapes" because of the high degree of violence and surprise to the victim. They are very damaging to the victim's sense of control, autonomy, and physical integrity. Victims of stranger rapes, however, tend to receive more support from families and friends and are less likely to be blamed for their assault. These victims are also viewed more sympathetically by the legal system and are associated with a higher success rate of convictions against the rapist. All of these factors can contribute to a speedier and more positive resolution of the immediate crisis.

Victims of acquaintance rape receive less sympathy and support from family and friends, are held more responsible for the assault, and tend to be more self-blaming. Victims of acquaintance rape must often deal with a significant loss of boyfriend, spouse, or fiancé as a secondary result of the rape. They are not well regarded by the legal system, and they seldom obtain successful convictions against the rapist. They must deal with the betrayal of trust in an ongoing relationship. They sometimes must cope with continued interaction with their assailants and, in the case of child incest or abuse, must often depend on their assailants for a prolonged period of time. In the instance of marital rape the victim must cope with economic dependence, involvement of children in any decision-making process, lack of legal redress in most states, and conflicts regarding family loyalty.

Rapes also vary regarding the degree of spontaneity, violence, and public recognition. *Planned rapes* involve the deliberate selection of a site and victim and elaborate plans to entrap her. *Partially planned rapes* involve an offender who meets the victim spontaneously and then proceeds to make plans to rape her. *Unplanned rapes* are impulsive and often committed under the influence of drugs or alcohol. Violence and coercion range from urging with candy or money to intimidation with guns or knives, to actual physical assault. *Reported rapes* are rapes in which the victim acknowledges she has been raped and reports the incident to the police. A reported rape may or may not meet the legal definition of rape (e.g., marital rapes in many states). An *unreported rape* is an incident that meets the legal definition of rape but is not reported to the police, either because the victim knows she has been raped but does not wish to report it because of fear, shame, etc. (i.e., *acknowledged rape*), or because the victim does not realize her experience constitutes rape (i.e., *unacknowledged rape* [e.g., date rape]).

Notes

1. Harvey M, Koss MP: The Rape Victim: Clinical and Community Approaches to Treatment. Lexington, MA, Greene Press, 1987
2. Hott JR: The telephone rape: crisis intervention for an obscene phone call. Issues in Health Care of Women 4:107–113, 1983

Appendix L

The Rape Crisis/Trauma Syndrome

Clinical observations of rape victims led to documentation of the stages of symptom manifestation and recovery, and, eventually, the term *rape crisis/trauma syndrome* emerged. Harvey and Koss (1987[1]) have integrated this literature to present a three-stage model of this syndrome composed of an anticipatory phase, an impact phase, and a recovery phase.

During the *anticipatory phase*, the victim first begins to recognize that her situation has potential for danger. Defenses such as dissociation, suppression, and rationalization are common and used to preserve the illusion of invulnerability.

The *impact phase* encompasses the actual assault and its immediate aftermath. Commonly reported is an intense fear for personal safety and life, resulting in varying degrees of disintegration and disorganization. Shock, numbness, and disbelief are major psychological reactions along with coping behaviors such as verbal tactics, physical actions, attempts to minimize provoking the attacker, memorizing details, and so forth. Victims typically interact in either a controlled style characterized by calm, subdued affect and demeanor, or in an expressive style characterized by intense expressions of anxiety, confusion, helplessness, and worry (often expressed verbally or through crying), as well as motoric restlessness and tremulousness. Traumatic reactions commonly encountered during this phase include skeletal muscle tension, soreness, fatigue, sleep disturbance, exaggerated startle response, stomach pain, nausea, decreased appetite and taste, vaginal discharge, dysuria, rectal bleeding and pain, and tremulousness. In compounded impact reactions, women

The information in this appendix is adapted from Harvey and Koss 1987,[1] pp. 33–37.

describe and react not only to the immediate rape but to previously repressed or unresolved sexual traumas or to other previous life traumas. More severe symptoms such as psychotic behavior, suicidality, debilitating depression, alcohol and drug abuse, and maladaptive sexual behavior are commonly associated with compound reactions.

During the *recovery phase*, the patient begins to attend to and to sustain functional and basic living considerations while psychologically assimilating the experience of the rape. Three subphases are often described: denial, symptom formation, and resolution. The *denial subphase* is characterized by superficial, mechanical outward appearances of adjustment, along with disregard for the importance of the rape, and frequent rejection or unmotivated responses to treatment interventions. Weeks to months later a *decompensation* or *symptom formation subphase* appears. This period can be brief, with minimal disruptive effects, or prolonged, chronically intermittent, and severely debilitating. It encompasses many symptoms commonly noted during the impact phase and corresponds in many ways to the symptoms described in the intrusive phase of the posttraumatic stress model. Intense, nonspecific anxiety, nightmares, fears, phobias, catastrophic fantasies, sleep disturbances, intense feelings of vulnerability and helplessness, increased startle response, and hyperresponsiveness are common. Depression, guilt, shame, isolation, and a sense of alienation have also been reported as well as sexual dysfunction, social dysfunction, and somatic complaints. Periods of numbness, withdrawal, and constriction and increased anxiety corresponding to the numbing phase of the posttraumatic stress model have also occurred. During this subphase many patients are receptive to treatment. However, they may, because of their severe symptomatology, be unable to attend to life functions or to the psychodynamic issues of the rape because of specific symptoms including 1) anxiety, fears, and phobias; 2) depression; 3) sexual dysfunction, especially desire response inhibition; and 4) social dysfunction.

As an outgrowth of both the crisis intervention model, which stresses a return to equilibrium, and of the posttraumatic stress syndrome model, which emphasizes biphasic symptoms of intrusion and numbing, specific debilitating symptoms have been targeted for special kinds of treatment interventions. Depression, anxiety, and phobic symptoms have been treated with various cognitive, behavioral, and psychopharmacological interactions. Sexual dysfunctions have been treated with behavioral and adapted conventional sex therapies. Crisis intervention techniques are also offered at this stage and include provision of adequate time for ventilation, providing concrete reassurance and active support of adaptive behaviors, and education of the patient and significant others. Therapists must be sensitive to the reality that a woman cannot work effectively with a therapist on dynamic issues unless she has achieved some containment over specific intense and debilitating stress symptoms and restored some sense of equilibrium to her life. The primary therapist must be able to utilize a variety of appropriate therapeutic interventions or to refer the patient to appropriate collaborating clinicians. The symptom formation subphase may be prolonged and the resolution phase (see below) inhibited by traumatic legal proceedings involving the prosecution of the rapist, past traumas, developmental life crises precipitated by the rape, and the loss of significant others secondary to the rape.

Notman and Nadelson (1980[2]) explored the way in which developmental life-cycle factors inhibit resolution and form secondary focuses for treatment. Gise and Paddison (1988[3]) recently listed these life-cycle factors as follows:

> 1) If the rape is the first sexual experience for a single young woman, confusion about the relationship between sexuality, violence, and humiliation may be prominent. She may also view herself as tainted or may be devalued and viewed in that way by significant others. 2) For a young woman in the process of separating from her family, the rape may lead her to feeling she cannot take care of herself and may trigger protective responses from her family that only exacerbate a regression. 3) A college student living away from home may not tell her parents for fear that they will insist that she return. 4) A woman in a sexual relationship may choose not to tell her partner, fearing the disclosure will disrupt their relationship, but the relationship may suffer anyway because of her anxiety, guilt, and withdrawal. 5) A divorced or separated woman experiences the stress of her life-style, character, and

> morality being questioned. 6) A woman with children must decide what to tell her children and when, as the event may be known in the community or at school. 7) The middle-age or older woman will have concerns about her ability to take care of herself, and she may already be in a turmoil over changing roles and relationships and other losses at this stage of her life. 8) In the case of the rape of an elderly woman, anxieties and fears of death can be exacerbated, and an intense decline in sense of autonomy and independence is not uncommon, disputing the myth that older women have less to lose by a rape. (p. 637)

Negative responses of significant others such as spouses, children, extended family, friends, colleagues, and caregivers are also problematic and require therapeutic intervention (Harvey and Koss 1987[1]; Remer and Elliot 1988[4]). These responses include divorce, separation, emotional withdrawal, sexual withdrawal, assigning of blame, patronization, overprotection, encouragement of regression, minimization of the impact of the rape, devaluation, stigmatization, withdrawal of support, identification with the rapist and lack of sympathy for the victim, impatience or pessimism regarding the length of recovery required by the victim, and severe and symptomatic secondary trauma reactions among significant others that strain the relationship and minimize the significant others' capacity to support the victim.

The *resolution subphase* is the third and final stage of the recovery phase. At this point the rape experience is assimilated and integrated with other life experiences, and the woman is able to discuss the rape with appropriate affect but without an upsurge of intense feeling or the return of stress-related symptomatology. Healthy reappraisal regarding the meaning and direction of one's life, a sense of ability to maintain competence under extreme stress, the development of strong convictions, and the heightened sensitivity to dehumanization and horror without a constant sense of vigilance or vulnerability are often reported. Personality is organized around healthy adaptive defenses as opposed to symptoms, conflicts, and defenses activated by the trauma or attempts to ward off traumatic memories. Any preexisting difficulties interfering with healthy self-assertion and self-protectiveness have been mastered. Secondary crises around life developmental tasks, changes in significant relationships, or old unresolved conflicts reactivated by the trauma have been adequately addressed. Initially, this resolution was hypothesized to occur within 1 year, but the longitudinal studies previously mentioned have shown that only a small portion of victims feel fully recovered in that time period, about half recover in several years, and one-quarter require 4 to 6 years or state that they have never fully recovered.

Appropriate psychodynamic interventions for the prevention and treatment of long-term sequelae to rape should focus on several issues (Krugman 1987[5]; Rose 1986[6]):

1. Traumatic activation of old unconscious and unresolved conflicts unrelated to the rape via the weakening of normal psychological defenses and heightened cognitive and affective awareness of material previously well defended and inaccessible
2. Activation of conflicts specific to the rape itself, such as conflicts over autonomy, trust, and sexuality
3. Attempts to ward off the rape defensively via maladaptive dissociation and repression
4. Reorganization of the personality around symptoms, conflicts, and defenses activated by the rape, resulting in a maladaptive rigid structure that actually interferes with recovery
5. Impact of the psychodynamics of the rapist
6. Grief regarding the changes that have occurred as a result of the rape

Notes

1. Harvey M, Koss MP: The Rape Victim: Clinical and Community Approaches to Treatment. Lexington, MA, Greene Press, 1987
2. Notman MT, Nadelson CC: Psychodynamic and life stage considerations in response to rape, in The Rape Crisis Intervention Handbook: A Guide for Victim Care. Edited by McCombie SL. New York, Plenum, 1980, pp 131–142
3. Gise LH, Paddison P: Rape, sexual abuse, and its victims. Psychiatr Clin North Am 11:629–649, 1988

4. Remer R, Elliot JE: Characteristics of secondary victims of sexual assault. International Journal of Family Psychiatry 9:373–387, 1988
5. Krugman S: Trauma in the family: perspectives on the intergenerational transmission of violence, in Psychological Trauma. Edited by Van der Kolk BA. Washington, DC, American Psychiatric Press, 1987, pp 127–151
6. Rose DS: Worse than death: psychodynamics of rape victims and the need for psychotherapy. Am J Psychiatry 143:817–824, 1986

Appendix M

Theories of Battering

Intrapersonal theories of battered women proliferated in the 1960s and 1970s when battering was felt to be a relatively rare phenomenon and investigators looked for pathological conditions in both victims and batterers. Early literature was based on extreme samples and was poorly controlled. Pathological characteristics such as masochism, aggressiveness, and immaturity were assigned to battered women (Scott 1974[2]; Shainess 1977[3]; Snell et al. 1964[4]). These characteristics were later criticized as being too narrow in scope and as placing too much blame on the victims.

More recent literature has refuted these traits (Kuhl 1984[5]). More current studies have focused on men's responsibility for their abusive behavior and women's developing pathological symptoms such as depression, anxiety, substance abuse, and posttraumatic stress syndrome as sequelae to being battered (Douglas and Der Ovanesian 1983[6]; Hughes and Rav 1984[7]; Rosewater 1984[8]; Telch and Lindquist 1984[9]; Walker 1984[10]). Less pathological attitudes and behaviors such as attitudinal acceptance of violence, the pairing of traditional sex role husbands with nontraditional wives, low self-esteem, difficulties with assertiveness, and expression of affect in the batterers have been highlighted but not tightly and empirically linked to violent versus discordant relationships.

Battered women vary greatly regarding their functional and coping capabilities. Some of these women have past psychiatric histories; some abuse drugs or medications; some have severe deficits in ego strength, self-esteem, and coping behaviors; and some exhibit severe stress-related symptoms such as anxiety, psychosomatic complaints, depression,

---

The information in this appendix is adapted from Margolin et al. 1988,[1] pp. 93–99.

hypervigilance, conversion reactions, and dissociation (Hilberman 1980[11]; Margolin et al. 1988[1]). Some do not vary greatly from the nonbattered population. Still others have reported unusually high perceptions of internal strength and sensitivity (Walker 1984[10]) and extraordinary survival and coping skills (Gondolf and Fisher 1988[12]).

Interpersonal theories attempt to explain the phenomenon of battered women by examining the interaction between the batterer and the victim as well as their prior interactional histories. Margolin et al. (1988,[1] pp. 95–97) reviewed three major interactional theories that have been applied to battered women: 1) social learning theories, 2) systems theories, and 3) Walker's cyclic theory of violence.

Social learning theories are based on the premise that individual behaviors are influenced by the person's social environment, especially his or her family of origin. This influence is achieved via the mechanisms of modeling, reinforcement, and coercion. Numerous studies (Gayford 1975b[13]; Rosenbaum and O'Leary 1981[14]; Roy 1977[15]; Straus et al. 1980[16]) have shown that batterers and their victims often come from families in which they were either victims or witnesses of violence. Batterers may therefore be modeling the batterers in their own families, and battered women may be modeling the passive and avoidant responses to violence that they observed in their families. If battering produces the desired outcome of compliance or submission on the part of the woman, the battering behavior may be positively reinforcing and thus repeated. If the woman's compliance or placating or self-blaming behavior precedes the termination of the violence, she may be negatively reinforced in her belief that her behavior will stop the aversive stimuli (i.e., the beating). In coercion mechanisms, intimates learn to control others via the use of aversive stimuli. Women may learn via their own battering experience how violence controls and become violent themselves in an attempt to take control, or the battering (i.e., the aversive event) may be so frequent and repeated that the woman's normal control mechanisms fail her (chaining and fogging effect as described by Walker 1979,[17] 1984[10]).

Systems theories explain battering as a product of the couple or family system rather than on the basis of individual psychopathology

(Margolin et al. 1988,[1] pp. 96–97). Actions on the part of one member of the relationship stimulate reactions in the other member, and these reactions in turn stimulate further action in a continuing causal cycle culminating in patterns of interaction specifically conducive to maintaining the violent cycle (Giles-Sims 1983[18]). Special characteristics of families or intimates, such as the amount of time they spend together, the intensity of their involvement, any impinging and conflicting needs, and the right to influence, have been postulated as making these families or individuals conducive to violence (Gelles and Straus 1979[19]). In addition, specific characteristics of wife-beating systems have been suggested such as poor communication, tight boundaries between perpetrators and the outside world, inflexible family rules, rules of secrecy, difficulty with maintaining limits, and status incompatibilities (Hornung et al. 1981[20]; Traicoff 1982[21]). Some systems theorists postulate that when a critical incident occurs and the wife makes a decision to seek feedback from outside the closed family system, this breaks the cycle and makes it possible for the woman to consider leaving the system.

Walker's cyclic theory of violence elaborates three phases to the battering interaction (Walker 1979,[17] 1984[10]). During the *tension-building phase* there is an escalation in tension around specific and intentional hurtful actions, but the woman may still believe that she can control the man's behavior and prevent the battering. During the *actual battering phase*, the batterer unleashes an overwhelming barrage of verbal and physical aggression. In the *final stage* the batterer may show kindness and remorse that is highly reinforcing to the woman. After the battering interaction has been well established, there may be no specific statements of kindness or remorse but simply a decline of tension and an end to the violence, which in itself may become reinforcing to the woman.

Some less prominent interpersonal theories explore threats to the victim's sense of self via issues of loyalty, control, and family ties. Ferraro (1984a[22]), Cohen (1984[23]), Dutton and Painter (1981[24]), and others have described the nature of traumatic bonding in which battered women, like POWs and hostages, form strong emotional attachments to their batterers under conditions of intermittent and continuous abuse.

Sociocultural theories examine legal, institutional, cultural, and political factors that are conducive to violence in intimate relationships and the victimization of women. Margolin et al. (1988,[1] pp. 98–99) and Straus (1977,[25] 1980[26]) cite the norms that are imparted when physical punishment of children is sanctioned: 1) those who love also have the right to hit, and 2) if something is really important, violence is justified. Patriarchal society's sanctions toward violence against women and male dominance have been cited as creating economic and legal conditions that maintain violence. Lower salaries, unequal distribution of labor and primary child care responsibilities, and lack of social support have made it difficult for many women to gather the necessary resources to leave their violent relationships. The legal system—which, as previously mentioned, permitted physical chastisement of wives until 1874—still impedes and discourages women during all steps of the legal process.

Gondolf and Fisher (1988[12]) have refuted the theory of learned helplessness by reviewing studies that document an increase, rather than a decrease, in help-seeking behavior as the abuse worsens in an assertive and persistent effort of the abused to survive. Gondolf and Fisher maintain that the women are stifled not by their learned helplessness but by unfavorable and ineffective responses from community systems of care and intervention. According to these theories, battering should decrease as families become more egalitarian and economic and resource opportunities are equalized. During the transition to this state, however, conflict may heighten as men's power is threatened.

Notes

1. Margolin G, Sibner LG, Gleberman L: Wife battering, in Handbook of Family Violence. Edited by Van Hasselt VB, Morrison RL, Bellack AS, et al. New York, Plenum, 1988, pp 89–117
2. Scott PD: Battered wives. Br J Psychiatry 125:433–441, 1974
3. Shainess N: Psychological aspects of wife battering, in Battered Women: A Psychosocial Study of Domestic Violence. Edited by Roy M. New York, Van Nostrand Reinhold, 1977, pp 111–118
4. Snell JE, Rosenwald J, Robey A: The wife-beaters wife. Arch Gen Psychiatry 11:107–112, 1964

5. Kuhl AF: Personality traits of abused women: masochism myth refuted. Victimology: An International Journal 9:450–463, 1984
6. Douglas MA, Der Ovanesian M: A comparative study of battered and not battered women in crisis. Paper presented at the 17th annual convention of the Association for the Advancement of Behavioral Therapy, Washington, DC, November 1983
7. Hughes HM, Rav TJ: Psychological adjustment of battered women in shelters. Paper presented at the American Psychological Association Meetings, Toronto, August 1984
8. Rosewater LB: The MMPI and battered women. Paper presented at the Second National Conference for Family Violence Researchers, Durham, NC, 1984
9. Telch CH, Lindquist CV: Violent vs nonviolent couples: a comparison of patterns. Psychotherapy 21:242–248, 1984
10. Walker LE: The Battered Woman Syndrome. New York, Springer, 1984
11. Hilberman E: Overview: the wife-beater's wife reconsidered. Am J Psychiatry 137:1336–1347, 1980 [Reprinted in The Gender Gap in Psychotherapy: Social Realities and Psychological Processes. Edited by Rieker PP, Hilberman E. New York, Plenum, 1984, pp 213–236]
12. Gondolf EW, Fisher ER: Battered Women as Survivors. Lexington, MA, Lexington Books, DC Heath, 1988
13. Gayford J: Wife battering: a preliminary survey of 100 cases. BMJ 1:195–197, 1975b
14. Rosenbaum A, O'Leary KD: Marital violence: characteristics of abusive couples. J Consult Clin Psychol 49:63–71, 1981
15. Roy M: A current survey of 150 cases, in Battered Women: A Psychosocial Study of Domestic Violence. Edited by Roy M. New York, Van Nostrand Reinhold, 1977, pp 25–44
16. Straus MA, Gelles RJ, Steinmetz SK: Behind Closed Doors: Violence in the American Family. New York, Anchor Press, 1980
17. Walker LE: The Battered Woman. New York, Harper & Row, 1979
18. Giles-Sims J: Wife Battering: A Systems Approach. New York, Guilford, 1983
19. Gelles RJ, Straus MA: Determinants of violence in the family: toward a theoretical integration, in Contemporary Theories About the Family, Vol 1. Edited by Burt WR, Hill R, Nye FI, et al. New York, Free Press, 1979, pp 549–581
20. Hornung CA, McCullough BC, Sugimoto T: Status relationships in marriage: risk factors in spouse abuse. Journal of Marriage and the Family 42:675–692, 1981

21. Traicoff ME: Family interventions from women's shelters, in Clinical Approaches to Family Violence. Edited by Hansen JC, et al. Rockville, MD, Aspen, 1982
22. Ferraro KJ: An existential approach to battering. Paper presented at the Second National Conference for Family Violence Researchers, Durham, NC, 1984a
23. Cohen P: Violence in the family: an act of loyalty. Psychotherapy 21:249–253, 1984
24. Dutton D, Painter SL: Traumatic bonding: the development of emotional attachments in battered women and other relationships of intermittent abuse. Victimology: An International Journal 6:139–155, 1981
25. Straus MA: A sociological perspective on the prevention and treatment of wife beating, in Battered Women: A Psychosociological Study of Domestic Violence. Edited by Roy M. New York, Van Nostrand Reinhold, 1977, pp 194–228
26. Straus MA: The marriage license as a hitting license: evidence from popular culture, law and social science, in The Social Causes of Husband-Wife Violence. Edited by Straus MA, Hotaling GT. Minneapolis, MN, University of Minneapolis Press, 1980, pp 39–50

Appendix N

Sexual Exploitation in Professional Relationships: Legal and Complaint Aspects of Treatment for Victims

From the onset of treatment, therapists must be sensitized to the fact that at some point in their recovery patients may need or wish to press charges against the offending professional via civil or criminal suits, or to lodge complaints with professional organizations or licensing boards. If legal action is taken, therapist and the therapy records may be subpoenaed for court proceedings. How patients and therapist will deal with the tension this creates regarding the confidentiality and the integrity of the therapy, especially if the therapist is harassed and the therapy devalued in the courtroom by opposing attorneys, needs to be honestly and directly addressed as early in the therapy as the patient's clinical status permits. Therapists and patients contemplating courtroom proceedings may wish to review *Sex in the Therapy Hour* (Bates and Brodsky 1989[1]), which provides a realistic and detailed account of the legal proceedings of a sexual exploitation case. In some instances it is possible to avoid many of these difficulties by utilizing a forensic psychiatrist who is retained to interview the patient, the therapist, and other relevant individuals, and to render an expert opinion regarding the psychiatric damages to the patient, as well as to provide testimony in court.

A second relevant legal issue involves the mandatory reporting required by some states regarding sexual exploitation by professionals. Therapists should be familiar with their state laws regarding the following issues:

- What types of professionals must be reported?
- To whom should they be reported?

- What steps will be taken by the agencies to which the incident is reported?
- How will these actions impact upon the patient?

Causing difficulties for an exploitative therapist who is still positively or ambivalently held can create an unnecessary burden of guilt for the patient. Additional trauma can also occur if a patient is prematurely drawn into a legal proceeding in an uncontrolled fashion at a time when she is vulnerable, unprepared, symptomatic, and lacking the perspective that working through the incident provides. If a therapist is unaware of the laws in this area and is confronted with an abuse victim who is entering treatment, time should be taken for the therapist to obtain the necessary information and discuss this freely, along with its implications, prior to encouraging the patient to fully disclose the identity of the offender. In this manner the patient may maintain control of the therapy boundaries and of any legal proceedings that may ensue. An extensive guide to current laws governing sexual exploitation and a wealth of additional legal resource information are available in a comprehensive textbook by Schoener et al. (1989[2]). Noel (1988[3]) and Gartrell et al. (1986b[4]) discuss issues that arise for therapists in reporting sexual misconduct by colleagues.

Lastly, the therapist working with patients who have been sexually exploited in other professional relationships should be familiar with the various ways in which patients attempt to address these issues with their offenders. This is necessary so that the therapist can assist the patients in assessing what impact various legal steps might have on their psychological well-being and sense of control and what form of redress is realistic and best suited to their needs. Milgrom (1989[5]) describes this process in great detail. She conceptualizes the variety of possible responses and combinations as a "wheel of options," including the following possibilities:

1. No action
2. Civil suit
3. Criminal complaint

4. Private damage compensation arrangement
5. Licensure complaint
6. Letter or call to the offender
7. Confrontation/processing meeting with the offender
8. Individual or group therapy for victim
9. Compensation from victims fund
10. Complaint to ethics committee or professional organization
11. Informing agency director or church official
12. Reporting to county or state authorities

To these we would add the corporate/institutional formal and informal complaint procedures summarized in Appendix J. These procedures can be helpful in student, mentoring, or work situations when the offending professional is an employee of an institution or corporation. These situations are subject to the civil rights laws governing employment, which make employers liable 1) if they do not take reasonable action when they have reason to know that improper sexual activity has taken place, and 2) if they refuse or fail to make inquiries of employees or from former employers about possible improper sexual contact when prior employment as a psychotherapist has occurred in the last 5 years. The former employers may also be liable for failure to disclose these facts upon inquiry. The pros and cons of the formal and informal complaint channels are summarized in Appendix J.

Therapists should be familiar with the advantages and disadvantages of all possible options, summarized briefly as follows. If the time commitment and trauma associated with the courtroom are contraindicated or if stopping the offender rather than obtaining financial reimbursement is the goal, a patient may wish to opt for reporting the therapist to a licensure board, professional organization ethics committee, agency, or church director. Impaired professionals' committees provide an option for many patients who wish to take action but are not comfortable with imposing sanctions on the offender or who wish more to encourage treatment for their offenders. Patients needing or wishing to face their abusers, enforce sanctions, and obtain financial reimbursement may opt to file suit, provided they can withstand the time, costs, and emotional rigor involved in a trial. Mediation or processing sessions that allow patients to confront and clarify issues directly with the offender in the presence of a third party may provide quicker, less stressful resolutions for patients. These sessions may also be helpful adjuncts to therapy. Models for this type of intervention are provided by Bouhoutsos and Brodsky (1985[6]) and Schoener and Milgrom (1989[7]).

Final relevant legal information involves therapists' understanding of the current trend toward criminalization of sexual exploitation. While current laws regarding statutory rape and sexual assault may be avenues for women who are minors or who are incompetent to give consent, there is also a current trend toward criminalization of sexual exploitation, particularly in the psychotherapy professions. We know of no states, however, that have devised laws to deal with the full spectrum of sexual exploitation in professional relationships. Several states have passed and several more are considering passing laws criminalizing sexual behavior within the psychotherapy relationship. What professional groups are covered, what constitutes sexual behavior, and what constitutes illegal behavior after the therapy has terminated and for what duration may vary from state to state. Therapists should also be aware that patients may not be able to recover financial reimbursement via malpractice suits, because insurers may not cover damages for sexual activities; specifically or generally they may refuse coverage on the basis that these practices are not ordinarily part of professional practice. Ironically, malpractice insurers may also be reluctant to provide legal defenses for those professionals falsely accused, again on the basis that this activity is not within the realm of normal practice and therefore not covered by malpractice. Thus, current insurance laws may protect the offenders by, in effect, making it impossible for their victims to obtain financial redress. Thus, as in the case of rape and battering, the legal system and other systems of redress may involve further traumatization for the victim and produce many secondary victims.

Notes

1. Bates CM, Brodsky AM: Sex in the Therapy Hour: A Case of Professional Incest. New York, Guilford, 1989
2. Schoener GT, Milgrom JH, Gonsiorek JC, et al (eds): Psychotherapists' Sexual Involvement With Clients: Intervention and Prevention. Minneapolis, MN, Walk-In Counseling Center, 1989
3. Noel MM: Reporting Colleagues Who Are Sexually Intimate With Clients: It's Time to Talk. New York, Haworth Press, 1988
4. Gartrell N, Herman J, Olarte S, et al: Report practices of psychiatrists who knew of sexual misconduct by colleagues. Am J Orthopsychiatry 57:287–295, 1986b
5. Milgrom JH: Advocacy: assisting sexually exploited clients through the complaint process, in Psychotherapists' Sexual Involvement With Clients: Intervention and Prevention. Edited by Schoener GT, Milgrom JH, Gonsiorek JC, et al. Minneapolis, MN, Walk-In Counseling Center, 1989, pp 305–312
6. Bouhoutsos JC, Brodsky AM: Mediation in therapist-client sex: a model. Psychotherapy 22:189–193, 1985
7. Schoener GR, Milgrom JH: Processing sessions, in Psychotherapists' Sexual Involvement With Clients: Intervention and Prevention. Edited by Schoener GT, Milgrom JH, Gonsiorek JC, et al. Minneapolis, MN, Walk-In Counseling Center, 1989, pp 345–358

Appendix O

Biology of Menopause

Any description of the psychodynamics of menopause must be accompanied by an understanding of its biology. Often, both biological and psychodynamic interventions are required. Sometimes, however, treatment of the hormonal fluctuations alone will correct the associated psychological problems.

A decline in ovarian sensitivity to gonadotropins, presumably due to a decreased number of oocytes, begins as early as 6 to 8 years prior to menopause, yielding a striking increase in follicle-stimulating hormone (FSH) levels throughout the menstrual cycle while luteinizing hormone (LH) levels remain normal. Serum estradiol and progesterone still reflect the cyclic fluctuation necessary for normal hypothalamic-pituitary interaction. Decreases in sex steroids, combined with anovulatory cycles, yield the changes in the menstrual cycle with regard to intermittent intervals, and the changes in quantity and duration of flow reported by women in this phase.

The reproductive hormones change gradually during the perimenopausal period, but, following the final menstrual period, serum FSH and LH are elevated. Twelve months later, when a menopause can be definitively identified, FSH levels are significantly higher than LH levels because of half-life and metabolic clearance differences. Hormonal replacement therapy may reduce these gonadotropin levels but not to premenopausal levels, perhaps because of the production of inhibin-like substances by the ovary, or perhaps because of decreased sensitivity by the hypothalamic-pituitary unit. These gonadotropin levels

---

The information in this appendix is adapted from Cumming DC: "Menarche, Menses and Menopause: A Brief Review." *Cleveland Clinic Journal of Medicine* 57:169–175, 1990; see pp. 172–174.

remain to some degree elevated for the remainder of life. With the end of the interactive relationship between pituitary, hypothalamic, and ovarian function comes the end of the cyclic fluctuation in gonadotropin levels and in circadian variations. Pulsative patterns are maintained and even exaggerated in frequency and amplitude, perhaps in response to elevated gonadotropin-releasing hormone production. Modulation of the frequency of pulsation activity by endogenous opiates no longer occurs, probably because of decreased sex steroid levels.

Estrogen administration reduces gonadotropin response to gonadotropin-releasing hormones. The hypothalamic-pituitary unit remains physiologically normal, and all the reported changes mentioned may not be due to decreases in the sex steroids. Ninety percent of postmenopausal women are hypoestrogenic, and 10% maintain estrogenic PAP smears. Circulatory estrogens change from premenopausal follicularly produced estradiol to the peripherally produced estrone, which is converted from androstenedione in adipose tissue. The ovary continues to manufacture androgenic and estrogenic steroids but produces androgens in far more significant amounts than estrogen.

Some clinical problems in the perimenstrual and postmenstrual periods are clearly linked to menopausal changes in sex steroids, but concomitant factors of aging, illness, and nutritional status may also play a role.

Appendix P

Biology of "Hot Flashes"

Current theories postulate the peripheral reaction of vasomotor instability, or *hot flashes*, as a compensatory mechanism to correct instability in the hypothalamic thermoregulatory mechanisms that result in a drop in the core body temperature. This instability is linked to an estrogen deficit, but the entire theory remains to be documented. The possibility of an additional endorphin-mediated mechanism has been postulated based on the positive response of some women to placebo, but this also has not yet been documented. The treatment of vasomotor episodes is with oral or transdermal estradiol patches. The addition of progesterone is indicated in women with an intact uterus to combat the risk of endometrial cancer due to unopposed estrogen. Estrogen replacement therapy should be carefully evaluated in women at risk for breast cancer. Medroxyprogesterone acetate, lofexidine, and clonidine have also been utilized with success, but their efficacy has not been well documented. Estrogen given above 150 to 200 pg/ml is contraindicated (because positive response has been documented at this level or below), unless there is the presence of an underlying problem such as hyperthyroidism, alcoholism, diabetes, or carcinoid syndrome.

The information in this appendix is adapted from Raunikar V: "Physiology and Treatment of Hot Flushes." *Obstetrics and Gynecology* 75:13–17, 1990

Appendix Q

Psychobiology of Midlife Depression

Recent studies (Guicheney et al. 1988[1]; Hankoff 1982[2]) show decreases in serotonin levels during the perimenopausal and menopausal period and have left some investigators to speculate on whether a temporary period of heightened susceptibility to suicide in vulnerable women who may already be depressed is a factor of menopause (Gitlin and Pasnau 1989[3]). Coulam (1981[4]), in reviewing several pathways by which estrogen interacts with catecholamines, views estrogen as a possible aggravator, rather than a cause, of midlife depressions and recommends estrogen replacement therapy (ERT) only when other conventional treatments have failed and estrogen deficiency is documented. At present there is no solid biochemical documentation of a link between depression and menopause physiology. Although contemporary analysts (Lax 1982[5]) continue to describe depressive reactions related to the psychodynamic meaning of menopause, recent epidemiological studies show that depressions are less common, rather than more common, in middle-age women (Myers et al. 1984[6]). As Gitlin and Pasnau (1989,[3] p. 1419) state, "The more recent research has seemingly put to rest the time honored concept of involutional depression first delineated by Kraepelin."

Notes

1. Guicheney P, Leger D, Barrat J, et al: Platelet serotonin content and plasma tryptophan in peri- and postmenopausal women: variations with plasma estrogen levels and depressive symptoms. Eur J Clin Invest 18:297–304, 1988
2. Hankoff CD: Suicide and attempted suicide, in Handbook of Affective Disorders. Edited by Paykel ES. New York, Guilford, 1982, pp 416–428

3. Gitlin MJ, Pasnau RO: Psychiatric syndromes linked to reproductive function in women: a review of current knowledge. Am J Psychiatry 146:1413–1422, 1989
4. Coulam CB: Age estrogens and the psyche. Clin Obstet Gynecol 24:219–229, 1981
5. Lax R: The expectable depressive climacteric reaction. Bull Menninger Clin 46:151–167, 1982
6. Myers JK, Weissman MM, Tischler GL: Six-month prevalence of psychiatric disorders in three communities. Arch Gen Psychiatry 41:959–967, 1984

Appendix R

Estrogen and Cardiovascular Disease

Estrogen decreases low-density lipoprotein (LDL) cholesterol and increases high-density lipoprotein (HDL) cholesterol levels by mechanisms that include possible induction of LDL receptors and the destruction of hepatic lipase, which degrades HDL cholesterol (Bush 1990[1]). In addition, estrogen also appears to have a direct beneficial effect on vessel wall physiology, perhaps increasing local prostacyclin production. Estrogen replacement therapy (ERT) is currently seen as a way to reverse some of these effects (Corson 1984[2]). The type of estrogen and the route of administration determine the positive and negative effects of estrogen on the cardiovascular system, with high-potency synthetic steroids contraindicated (Lobo 1990[3]). The addition of progesterones to mitigate against endometrial cancer is recommended but may cancel some of the beneficial cardiovascular effects. Low-dose nonandrogenic progesterones are advised if progesterone is indicated. The ways in which estrogen-related mechanisms interact with aging, stress, and lack of exercise in producing cardiovascular disease in women are not well known (Stampfer et al. 1990[4]; Sitruk-Ware and Iberra de Palacios 1989[5]).

Notes

1. Bush TL: The epidemiology of cardiovascular disease in postmenopausal women. Ann N Y Acad Sci 592:263–345, 1990
2. Corson SL: Impact of estrogen replacement therapy on cardiovascular risk. J Reprod Med 34:729–746, 1984
3. Lobo RA: Cardiovascular implications of estrogen replacement therapy. Obstet Gynecol 75:18S–35S, 1990
4. Stampfer MJ, Colditz GH, Willett WC: Menopause and heart disease. Ann N Y Acad Sci 592:193–262, 1990
5. Sitruk-Ware R, Iberra de Palacios P: Estrogen replacement therapy and cardiovascular disease in postmenopausal women: a review. Maturitas 11:259–274, 1989

Appendix S

Menopause and Sleep Disorders

Preliminary documentation of a relationship between sleep disorders and estrogen (Thompson 1976[1]; Thompson and Oswald 1977[2]), hot flushes (Erlik et al. 1981[3]), and progesterone and hormone-related changes in fat distribution (Block et al. 1980[4]; Fry 1987[5]) lend validation to the notion that at least some later-life sleep disturbances in women are related to hormonal changes of menopause and are therefore responsive to estrogen/progesterone replacement therapy. Readers are referred to a recent review by Fry (1987[5]) for more detail.

Notes

1. Thompson J: Double-blind study on the effect of estrogen on sleep, anxiety and depression in perimenopausal women: preliminary results. Royal Society of Medicine Proceedings 69:829–830, 1976
2. Thompson J, Oswald I: Effect of oestrogen on the sleep, mood, and anxiety of menopausal women. BMJ 2:1317–1319, 1977
3. Erlik Y, Tatryn IV, Meldrum DR, et al: Association of waking episodes with menopausal hot flushes. JAMA 245:1741–1744, 1981
4. Block AJ, Wynne JW, Boysen PG, et al: Sleep-disordered breathing and nocturnal oxygen desaturation in post-menopausal women. Am J Med 69:75–79, 1980
5. Fry JM: Sleep disorders. Med Clin North Am 71:95–111, 1987

Appendix T

Biology and Treatment of Osteoporosis

There is evidence that estrogen replacement used in minimum oral doses of 0.625 mg conjugated equine estrogen in the first 5 to 10 years after menopause significantly decreases postmenopausal rapid bone loss (Lindsay and Cosman 1990[1]) and is the treatment of choice for the prevention of osteoporosis. Risks for endometrial cancer can be minimized by the concomitant use of progesterone, but questions regarding a recent link of progesterone to breast cancer make it necessary to screen out patients who have a propensity or family history for breast cancer. Adequate intake of calcium and weight-bearing exercise are also important in the prevention of osteoporosis. Preliminary radiological screening of bone density by premenopausal women may be important in screening out women who should receive postmenopausal estrogen treatment (Sartoris et al. 1990[2]). Screening on the basis of blood chemistry and history risk indexes may soon be possible (Lee and Hoffman 1990[3]). Alternate drugs such as fluorides, vitamin A, anabolic steroids, and calcitonin have been utilized, but their efficacy is not yet well documented. Both estrogen and calcitonin have received Food and Drug Administration approval for treatment of established osteoporosis with bone fractures.

Notes

1. Lindsay R, Cosman F: Estrogen in prevention and treatment of osteoporosis. Ann N Y Acad Sci 592:326–333, 1990
2. Sartoris DJ, Moscona A, Resnick D: Progress in radiology: dual energy radiographic absorptiometry for bone densitometry. Ann N Y Acad Sci 592:307–325, 1990
3. Lee MJ, Hoffman R: Correlation of chemistry and history risk factors for osteoporosis. Ann N Y Acad Sci 592:441–442, 1990

Appendix U

Preparation for Widowhood

Numerous authors have documented adaptive coping in rehearsal for widowhood. Lopata (1973[2]), Cain (1974[3]), Scott and Kivelt (1985[4]), Remondet and Hansson (1987[5]), Carey (1979–1980[6]), and Neugarten (1968b[7]) have described subconscious monitoring of the husband's health and mental preparation for widowhood in middle-aged and older women. Cain (1974[3]), Gates (1990[8]), and Loewinsohn (1984[9]), authors of survival handbooks for widows, also allude to the importance of married couples planning for widowhood via the wife's familiarity with economic and household information. Cain, a widow herself, recommends a contingency day in which couples review wills, pertinent economic information, changes in living situations, and the use of professionals in the event of each other's deaths. This type of planning is of great help during the early stages of grief, which is accompanied by widespread disorganization. The planning provides a sense of ongoing love and support from the deceased that cushions the bereaved as well as protects the widow from poor and impulsive decisions. Unfortunately, only 39% of widows attempt to engage in this type of planning (Morgan 1986[10]). Others, perhaps in response to negative societal values, distance themselves, ignore or refuse to plan, or plan in isolation from the spouse.

The expansion and remodeling of social networks is another way in which prospective widows prepare for their loss. Hansson et al. (1986[11]) have documented the way in which loneliness and poor socialization correlate with maladaptive behaviors and the inability to restore social equilibrium after widowhood. Likewise, women accustomed to passive,

---

The information in this appendix is adapted from Heineman and Evans (1990[1]), pp. 142–168.

dependent roles in their marriage often lack the assertiveness to establish social networks (Lopata 1979[12]). In contrast, educated goal-setting women who are socialized to multidimensional roles and possess acquired resources stand a better chance of good adaptation (Lopata 1973[2]). Also figuring into the ultimate adjustment are poor health, limited levels of education, and economic difficulties, which correlate to social isolation after widowhood (Arens 1982[13]; Arling 1976b[14]). Ferraro et al. (1984[15]), in summarizing the literature on widowhood and social activity in later life, note that most widows are able to compensate for their losses by increasing certain aspects of social participation within a few years after the death of their spouses.

Notes

1. Heinemann GD, Evans PL: Widowhood: loss, change, and adaptation, in Family Relationships in Later Life, 2nd Edition. Edited by Brubaker TH. Newbury Park, CA, Sage, 1990, pp 142–168
2. Lopata HZ: Widowhood in an American City. Cambridge, MA, Schenkman, 1973
3. Cain L: Widow. New York, William Morrow, 1974
4. Scott JP, Kivelt VR: Differences in the morale of older, rural widows and widowers. Int J Aging Hum Dev 21:121–136, 1985
5. Remondet JH, Hansson RO: Assessing a widow's grief: a short index. Journal of Gerontological Nursing 13:30–34, 1987
6. Carey RG: Weathering widowhood: problems and adjustment of the widowed during the first year. Omega 10:163–174, 1979–1980
7. Neugarten BL: The awareness of middle age, in Middle Age and Aging. Edited by Neugarten BL. Chicago, IL, University of Chicago Press, 1968b, pp 93–98
8. Gates PA: Suddenly Alone: A Woman's Guide to Widowhood. New York, Harper & Row, 1990
9. Loewinsohn RJ: Survival Handbook for Widows. Glenview, IL, Scott, Foresman & Company, 1984
10. Morgan LA: The financial experience of widowed women: evidence from the LRHS. Gerontologist 26:663–668, 1986
11. Hansson RO, Jones WH, Carpenter BN, et al: Loneliness and adjustment to old age. Int J Aging Hum Dev 24:41–53, 1986

12. Lopata HZ: Women as Widows: Support Systems. New York, Elsevier, 1979
13. Arens DA: Widowhood and well-being: an examination of sex differences within a causal model. Int J Aging Hum Dev 15:27–40, 1982
14. Arling G: Resistance to isolation among elderly widows. Int J Aging Hum Dev 7:67–86, 1976b
15. Ferraro KF, Mutran E, Barresi CM: Widowhood, health and friendship support in later life. J Health Soc Behav 25:246–259, 1984

Appendix V

Review of the Psychoanalytic Literature on Mourning

In 1917 Freud[1] opened the problem of loss and mourning to future psychoanalytic psychodynamic study of grief with his classic paper "Mourning and Melancholia." Freud described grief and mourning as a profoundly painful dejection, a cessation of interest in the outside world, a loss of the capacity to love, and an inhibition of all activities. He described the work of mourning as a decathexis of the lost object, with energies reinvested in the formation of new relationships and readjustment to the environment in which whatever person was lost is missing. Freud differentiated mourning from melancholia in terms of the likelihood of a pronounced lowering of self-regard, sometimes to a delusional degree. He emphasized the importance of ambivalence toward the lost person in prolonged grief or melancholia, which he felt made it difficult, if not impossible, to decathect the lost object.

Other psychoanalytic theorists followed in Freud's footsteps. Abraham (1924/1953[2]) further explored the relationship between ambivalent feelings and the grieving process. He also elaborated the role of identification in the process of mourning and outlined the concept of introjection of the object and other aspects of object loss. Rank (1952[3]) emphasized the importance of separation in the formulation of character. Bonaparte (1928[4]) addressed various aspects of identification with the dead, while Deutsch (1937[5]) identified the problems that ensue in persons in whom there is a denial of grief. Peck (1939[6]) delineated a correlation between suicide attempts and reunion wishes toward a dead spouse. Klein's (1935,[7] 1940[8]) concept of infant mourning speaks to the concept of the reactivation of early development losses by the death of a loved object in later life.

Mahler has written of the developmental complexity of affect resulting from object loss. Bowlby has made important contributions to the area of loss, separation, and mourning despite current criticisms of his merging of child and adult mourning processes (Bowlby 1960,[9] 1961,[10] 1963,[11] 1973,[12] 1980[13]). More recently, Pollock (1961,[14] 1970,[15] 1971,[16] 1975,[17] 1978[18]) has made contributions connecting stages of mourning with specific affective states and outlining three possible outcomes to mourning: 1) successful completion, with a creative outcome; 2) arrest at various stages of the process; and 3) pathological or deviated processes related to melancholia. Krystal (1987[19]) has shed light on the importance of massive psychic trauma on the grieving process, and Volkan (1981[20]) has further clarified the issues of identification in grief, especially with regard to the notion of a linking object.

Various authors have focused on physical illness and somatic symptoms (Cobbs et al. 1939[21]; McDermott and Cobbs 1939[22]). Lindemann (1944[23]) and Horowitz et al. (1980[24]) introduced the notion of reactivation of latent self-images in pathological mourning. Wetmore (1963[25]) elaborated the role of grief in psychoanalysis. In focusing on depression and mourning, Bibring (1953[26]) emphasized the wish for a reunion with the lost love object and feelings of guilt at having not prevented the death. Dietrich and Shabad (1989[27]) have examined various adaptive and constructive reactions to losses from a psychoanalytic perspective.

In contrast to many of the psychoanalytic writers who have focused on the intrapsychic aspects of grief, stressing defenses and intrapsychic adaptations and etiologies of prolonged and aberrant grief reactions, other investigators have chosen to study the psychological aspects of grief in a more sequential and descriptive manner. Lindemann (1944[23]) was one of the earliest of these investigators. He described mourning as acute grief, with both psychological and somatic aspects, appearing immediately after death or delayed to a later point in time. He conceptualized grief as fairly uniform and phase-specific. Following a brief period of shock, numbness, and denial, a period of acute grief ensues, characterized by 1) physical and somatic distress such as choking, sighing, shortness of breath, exhaustion, malaise, digestive upset, anxiety symptoms, headaches, appetite disturbances, sleep disturbances; 2) preoccupation with the image of the lost person; 3) feelings of guilt; 4) hostile reactions; and 5) loss of patterned conduct. Lindemann joined Freud in outlining the task of grieving to include disinvestment of the lost object and reinvestment in new relationships and in acceptance of the world minus the deceased person. Lindemann's formulation included the use of denial and avoidance to ward off waves of anxiety. He postulated that this acute phase of chaos and disruption must be, by definition, self-limited, as the person could not remain indefinitely in such a state of disequilibrium. A resolution must be found, and the new balance may be healthy and growth-promoting or maladaptive and prolonged. He also defined roles for health workers and for family units in regard to promotion of adaptive coping. Lindemann's (1979[28]) work, along with Erikson's (1985[29]) model of developmental crisis occurring at transition points in the life cycle, formed the backbone of the crisis theory model of bereavement intervention.

Parkes, working with various associates, has also made many contributions to the understanding of grief and mourning and differed with Lindemann in noting a lack of differentiation and specific phases for grief (Parkes 1964,[30] 1970,[31] 1972,[32] 1991[33]; Parkes and Brown 1972[34]; Parkes and Weiss 1983[35]). Drawing on Bowlby's work on separation anxiety and attachment and loss, Parkes delineated undifferentiated 1) initial denial and avoidance of the loss; 2) alarm reactions such as anxiety, restlessness, and physiological complaints; 3) searching in an irrational manner to find the lost person; 4) anger and guilt reactions; 5) feelings of internal loss; 6) adoption of traits or mannerisms of the deceased; and 7) acceptance and resolution, including appropriate changes in identity. These phases, to some degree, resemble the sequences described for posttraumatic stress syndrome. Over a period of years, Parkes developed a concept of psychosocial transition to explain adaptation to bereavement and other stressful life changes. This model has important clinical implications for defining risk factors associated with pathological mourning as well as for the clarification of specific roles for significant others in clarifying and promoting the grieving process. From these primary models describing the sequential process of normal grief, models of pathological grief have evolved to explain the experiences of some widows who present for psychodynamic treatment.

Notes

1. Freud S: Mourning and melancholia (1917), in The Standard Edition of the Complete Psychological Works of Sigmund Freud, Vol 14. Translated and edited by Strachey J. London, Hogarth Press, 1961, pp 237–258
2. Abraham K: A short study of the development of the libido, viewed in the light of mental disorders (1924), in Selected Papers on Psycho-Analysis. New York, Basic Books, 1953, pp 418–501
3. Rank O: The Trauma of Birth. New York, Robert Brunner, 1952
4. Bonaparte M: L'identification d'une fille a sa mere morte. Revue Francaise Psychoanalytique 2:541–565, 1928
5. Deutsch H: Absence of grief. Psychoanal Q 6:12–22, 1937
6. Peck M: Notes on identification in a case of depression reactive to the death of a love object. Psychoanal Q 8:1–17, 1939
7. Klein M: A contribution to the psychogenesis of manic-depressive states. Int J Psychoanal 16:145–174, 1935
8. Klein M: Mourning and its relation to manic depressive states. Int J Psychoanal 21:125–153, 1940
9. Bowlby J: Grief and mourning in infancy and early childhood. Psychoanal Study Child 15:9–52, 1960
10. Bowlby J: Process of mourning. Int J Psychoanal 42:317–340, 1961
11. Bowlby J: Pathological mourning and childhood. J Am Psychoanal Assoc 11:500–541, 1963
12. Bowlby J: Attachment and Loss, Vol 2: Separation. New York, Basic Books, 1973
13. Bowlby J: Attachment and Loss, Vol 3: Loss, Sadness and Depression. New York, Basic Books, 1980
14. Pollock GH: Mourning and adaptation. Int J Psychoanal 42:341–361, 1961
15. Pollock GH: Anniversary reactions, trauma, and mourning. Psychoanal Q 39:347–371, 1970
16. Pollock GH: Temporal anniversary manifestations: hour, day, holiday. Psychoanal Q 40:123–131, 1971
17. Pollock GH: On mourning, immortality and utopia. J Am Psychoanal Assoc 23:334–362, 1975
18. Pollock GH: Process and affect: mourning and grief. Int J Psychoanal 59:255–276, 1978
19. Krystal H: The impact of massive psychic trauma and the capacity to grieve effectively, in Treating the Elderly With Psychotherapy. Edited by Sadavoy J, Leszcz M. Madison, CT, International Universities Press, 1987, pp 95–156

20. Volkan V: Linking Objects and Linking Phenomena: A Study of the Forms, Symptoms, Metapsychology and Therapy of Complicated Mourning. New York, International Universities Press, 1981
21. Cobbs S, Bauer W, Whiting I: Environmental factors in rheumatoid arthritis. JAMA 113:668–670, 1939
22. McDermott N, Cobbs S: A psychiatric survey of fifty cases of bronchial asthma. Psychosom Med 1:203–244, 1939
23. Lindemann E: Symptomatology and management of acute grief. Am J Psychiatry 101:141–148, 1944
24. Horowitz MJ, Wilner N, Marmar C, et al: Pathological grief and the activity of latent self-images. Am J Psychiatry 137:1157–1162, 1980
25. Wetmore R: The role of grief in psychoanalysis. Int J Psychoanal 44:97–103, 1963
26. Bibring E: The mechanism of depression, in Affective Disorders: Psychoanalytic Contribution to Their Study. Edited by Greenacre P. New York, International Universities Press, 1953, pp 13–48
27. Dietrich DR, Shabad PC: The Problem of Loss and Mourning: Psychoanalytic Perspectives. Madison, CT, International Universities Press, 1989
28. Lindemann E: Beyond Grief: Studies in Crisis Intervention. New York, Jason Aronson, 1979
29. Erikson EH: Childhood and Society, 2nd Edition. New York, WW Norton, 1985
30. Parkes CM: Recent bereavement as a cause of mental illness. Br J Psychiatry 110:198–204, 1964
31. Parkes CM: The first year of bereavement: a longitudinal study of the reaction of London widows to the death of their husbands. Psychiatry 33:444–467, 1970
32. Parkes CM: Bereavement: Studies in Grief in Adult Life. New York, International Universities Press, 1972
33. Parkes CM: Attachment, bonding and psychiatric problems after bereavement in adult life, in Attachment Across the Life Cycle. Edited by Parkes CM. London, Routledge Kegan Paul, 1991
34. Parkes CM, Brown RJ: Health after bereavement: a controlled study of young Boston widows and widowers. Psychosom Med 34:449–461, 1972
35. Parkes CM, Weiss RS: Recovery From Bereavement. New York, Basic Books, 1983

Bibliography

Abelin EL: The role of the father in the separation-individuation process, in Separation-Individuation: Essays in Honor of Margaret S. Mahler. Edited by McDevitt JB, Settlage CF. New York, International Universities Press, 1971, pp 229–252

Abraham G: Premenstrual tension, in Current Problems In Obstetrics and Gynecology. Chicago, IL, Year Book Medical, 1981, pp 1–39

Abraham K: Some remarks on the role of grandparents in the psychology of neurosis (1913), in Selected Papers of Karl Abraham, Vol 2: Clinical Papers on Psycho-Analysis. Edited by Abraham HC. New York, Basic Books, 1955, pp 44–48

Abraham K: A short study of the development of the libido, viewed in the light of mental disorders (1924), in Selected Papers on Psycho-Analysis. Edited by Abraham HC. New York, Basic Books, 1953, pp 418–501

Abraham K: The applicability of psychoanalytic treatment to patients at an advanced age, in Selected Papers of Karl Abraham, M.D. Edited by Abraham HC. London, Brunner/Mazel, 1927, pp 312–317

Adams M: The single woman in today's society: a reappraisal. Am J Orthopsychiatry 41:776–786, 1971

Adams-Tucker C: Proximate effects of sexual abuse in childhood. Am J Psychiatry 139:1252–1256, 1982

Adler NE: Emotional responses of women following therapeutic abortion. Am J Orthopsychiatry 45:446–454, 1975

Adler NE, David HP, Major BN, et al: Psychological responses after abortion. Science 248:41–44, 1990

Agras WS: Eating Disorders: Management of Obesity, Bulimia and Anorexia Nervosa. Elmsford, NY, Pergamon, 1987

Ahrons CR: The continuing coparental relationship between divorced spouses. Am J Orthopsychiatry 51:415–428, 1981

Aitken JM: Osteoporosis and its relation to estrogen deficiency, in The Management of the Menopause and Postmenopausal Years. Edited by Campbell S. Lancaster, MTP Press, 1976, pp 225–236

Aizenman M, Kelley G: The incidence of violence and acquaintance rape in dating relationships among college men and women. Journal of College Student Development 29:305–311, 1988

Akabas SH: Workers are parents too. Child Welfare 63:307–399, 1984

Akamatsu TJ: Intimate relationships with former clients: national survey of attitudes and behavior among practitioners. Professional Psychology: Research and Practice 19:454–458, 1988

Akiyama H, Holtzman JM, Britz WE: Pet ownership and health status during bereavement. Omega 17:187–193, 1986–1987

Alfonso DD, Domino G: Post partum depression: a review. Birth 11:231–235, 1984

Altshuler KZ, Weiner MF: Anorexia nervosa and depression: a dissenting view. Am J Psychiatry 142:328–332, 1985

American Association of Retired Persons: A Profile of Older Americans. Washington, DC, American Association of Retired Persons, 1987

American Psychiatric Association: Diagnostic and Statistical Manual of Mental Disorders (DSM-I). Washington, DC, American Psychiatric Association, 1952

American Psychiatric Association: Diagnostic and Statistical Manual of Mental Disorders, 3rd Edition, Revised. Washington, DC, American Psychiatric Association, 1987

Anda R, Williamson D, Escobed AL, et al: Depression and the dynamics of smoking. JAMA 264:1541–1545, 1990

Anderson TB: Widowhood as a life transition: its impact on kinship ties. Journal of Marriage and the Family 46:105–114, 1984

Andrews R: Adoption: the resolution of infertility. Fertil Steril 21:73–76, 1970

Anthony E, Benedek T (eds): Parenthood and Its Psychology. Boston, MA, Little, Brown, 1970

Apfel RJ, Simon B: Patient-therapist sexual contact: psychodynamic perspectives on the causes and the results. Psychother Psychosom 43:57–62, 1985a

Apfel RJ, Simon B: Patient-therapist sexual contact: problems of subsequent psychotherapy. Psychother Psychosom 43:63–68, 1985b

Applegarth A: Some observations on work inhibitions in women. J Am Psychoanal Assoc 24(suppl):251–268, 1976

Archer SL: Gender differences in identity development: issues of process domain and timing. J Adolesc 12:117–138, 1989

Arens DA: Widowhood and well-being: an examination of sex differences within a casual model. Int J Aging Hum Dev 15:27–40, 1982

Arling G: The elder widow, her family, neighbors and friends. Journal of Marriage and the Family 38:757–768, 1976a

Arling G: Resistance to isolation among elderly widows. Int J Aging Hum Dev 7:67–86, 1976b

Arlow JA, Freud A, Lampl–de Groot J, et al: Panel discussion. Int J Psychoanal 49:506–512, 1968

Arschault AM: Sources of support of elderly Acadian widows. Health Care of Women International 7:203–219, 1986

Asch S: Crib deaths; their possible relationship to post partum depression and infanticide. Journal of the Mount Sinai Hospital 35:214–220, 1968

Ashton J: The psychosocial outcome of induced abortion. Br J Obstet Gynaecol 87:1115–1122, 1980

Association of American Medical Colleges: Women and Minorities on U.S. Medical School Faculties. Washington, DC, Association of American Medical Colleges, 1988

Attorney General's Task Force on Domestic Violence: Domestic Violence. Washington, DC, U.S. Government Printing Office, 1984

Bachmann GA, Moeller T, Bennet J: Childhood and sexual abuse and the consequences in adult women. Obstet Gynecol 71:636–638, 1988

Bachmann GA: Sexual issues at menopause. Ann N Y Acad Sci 592:87–94, 1990

Bak RC: Being in love and object loss. Int J Psychoanal 54:1–8, 1973

Balint M: On genital love, in Primary Love and Psychoanalytic Technique. New York, Tavistock, 1948, pp 109–120

Ball JF: Widow's grief: the impact of age and mode of death. Omega 7:307–333, 1976–1977

Ballinger CB: Subjective sleep disturbance at the menopause. J Psychosom Res 20:509–513, 1976

Baltes PB, Reese HW, Lipsett LP: Life-span developmental psychology. Annu Rev Psychol 31:65–110, 1980

Bankoff EA: Effects of friendship support on the psychological well-being of widows. Research in the Interweave of Social Roles 2:109–113, 1981

Bankoff EA: Aged parents and their widowed daughters: a support relationship. J Gerontol 38:226–230, 1983a

Bankoff EA: Social support and adaptation to widowhood. Journal of Marriage and the Family 45:827–839, 1983b

Barnett R, Baruch G: Women in the middle years: a critique of research and theory. Psychology of Women Quarterly 3:187–197, 1978

Barnett RC, Baruch GK: Women's involvement in multiple roles, role strain and psychological distress. The Stone Center for Developmental Services and Studies, Work in Progress, Wellesley, MA, 1983, No 83-107

Barnhouse RT: Sex between patient and therapist. J Am Acad Psychoanal 6:533–546, 1978

Barraclough B, Bunch J, Nelson B, et al: A hundred cases of suicide: clinical aspects. Br J Psychiatry 125:355–373, 1974

Barrett CJ: Women in widowhood. Signs 2:856–868, 1977

Barrett CJ: Effectiveness of widows' groups in facilitating change. J Consult Clin Psychol 46:20–31, 1978

Barringer F: What are youth coming to? New York Times, August 19, 1990, pp 1, 5

Bart P, Grossman M: Menopause, in The Woman Patient VI: Medical and Psychological Interfaces. Edited by Notman M, Nadelson C. New York, Plenum, 1978, pp 337–354

Bass E, Davis L: The Courage to Heal: A Guide for Women Survivors of Child Sexual Abuse. New York, Harper & Row, 1988

Bates CM, Brodsky AM: Sex in the Therapy Hour: A Case of Professional Incest. New York, Guilford, 1989

Becker J: Level of post assault sexual function in post assault and incest victims. Arch Sex Behav 15:37–49, 1986

Beckwirth JB: The sudden infant death syndrome (DHEW Publ No HSA 75-5137). Washington, DC, U.S. Government Printing Office, 1975

Beeson W, McCollough E: Aesthetic Surgery of the Aging Face. St Louis, MO, CV Mosby, 1986

Begleiter ML, Burry VF, Harris DJ: Prevalence of divorce among parents of children with cystic fibrosis and other chronic diseases. Soc Biol 23:261–264, 1976

Bell R: Marriage and Family Interaction. Homewood, IL, Dorsey Press, 1971

Belsey EM, Greer HS, Lal S, et al: Predictive factors in emotional response to abortion: King's termination study IV. Soc Sci Med 11:71–82, 1977

Bender L, Blau A: The reaction of children to sexual relations with adults. Am J Orthopsychiatry 7:500–518, 1937

Benedek T: Climacterium: a developmental phase. Psychoanal Q 19:1–27, 1950

Benedek T: Infertility as a psychosomatic defense. Fertil Steril 3:527–541, 1952

Benedek T: Parenthood as a developmental phase: a contribution to the libido theory. J Am Psychoanal Assoc 7:389–417, 1959a

Benedek T: Sexual functions in women and their disturbances, in American Handbook of Psychiatry. Edited by Arieti S. New York, Basic Books, 1959b, pp 727–748

Benedek T: Motherhood and nurturing, in Parenthood: Its Psychology and Psychopathology. Edited by Anthony EJ, Benedek T. Boston, MA, Little, Brown, 1970a, pp 153–166

Benedek T: Parenthood during the life cycle, in Parenthood: Its Psychology and Psychopathology. Edited by Antony EJ, Benedek T. Boston, MA, Little, Brown, 1970b, pp 185–206

Benedek T: The psychobiology of pregnancy, in Parenthood: Its Psychology and Psychopathology. Edited by Antony EJ, Benedek T. Boston, Little, Brown, 1970c, pp 137–152

Bennett NM, Nickerson KG: Women families and academic medicine. N Y State J Med 90:284–285, 1990

Ben-Sita Z: Loss, stress and readjustment: the structure of coping with bereavement and disability. Soc Sci Med 17:1619–1632, 1983

Benzodiazepines: use, overuse, misuse, abuse (editorial). Lancet 1:1101–1102, 1978

Berger D: The role of the psychiatrist in a reproductive biology clinic. Fertil Steril 28:41, 1977

Bergler E: Divorce Won't Help. New York, Harper, 1970

Bergmann MV: The effect of role reversal on delayed marriage and maternity. Psychoanal Study Child 40:197–219, 1985

Bergmann MS: Psychoanalytic observations on the capacity to love, in Separation-Individuation. Edited by McDevitt JV, Settlage CF. New York, International Universities Press, 1971, pp 15–40

Berman EM, Lief HI: Marital therapy from a psychiatric perspective: an overview. Am J Psychiatry 132:583–592, 1975

Bernard J: No news but new ideas, in Divorce and After. Edited by Bohannan P. New York, Doubleday, 1970, pp 1–29

Bernard J: The Future of Marriage. New York, World, 1972

Bernardez-Bonesatti T: Women and anger: conflicts with aggression in contemporary women. J Am Med Wom Assoc 33:215–219, 1978

Bernardez-Bonesatti T: Women and anger: cultural prohibitions and the feminine ideal. The Stone Center for Developmental Services and Studies, Work in Progress, Wellesley, MA, 1988, No 88-31

Bernstein AE: A psychoanalytic contribution to the etiology of "back pain" and "spinal disc syndromes." J Am Acad Psychoanal 6:547–556, 1978

Bernstein AE: Analysis of two adult female patients who had been victims of incest in childhood. J Am Acad Psychoanal 17:207–221, 1989

Bernstein AE: The impact of incest trauma on ego development, in Adult Analysis and Childhood Sexual Abuse. Edited by Levine H. Hillsdale, NJ, Analytic Press, 1990, pp 65–93

Bernstein AE, Warner GM: Introduction to Contemporary Psychoanalysis. New York, Jason Aronson, 1981

Bernstein AE, Warner GM: Onset of anorexia nervosa after prolonged use of the Milwaukee brace. Psychosomatics 24:1033–1034, 1983

Bernstein AE, Warner GM: Female psychology and networking problems among female professionals. J Am Med Wom Assoc 39:156–158, 1984a

Bernstein AE, Warner GM: Women Treating Women. New York, International Universities Press, 1984b

Berny MD, Merry J: Alcoholism and eating disorders in women of fertile age. Br J Addict 81:685–687, 1986

Bibring E: The mechanism of depression, in Affective Disorders: Psychoanalytic Contribution to Their Study. Edited by Greenacre P. New York, International Universities Press, 1953, pp 13–48

Bibring GL: Some considerations of the psychological processes in pregnancy. Psychoanal Study Child 14:113–121, 1959

Bibring GL, Dwyer TF, Huntington DS, et al: A study of the psychological processes in pregnancy and of the earliest mother-child relationship. Psychoanal Study Child 16:9–72, 1961

Bidwell L, White P: The family context of marital rape. Journal of Family Violence 1:277–287, 1986

Bird C: The case against marriage, in The Future of the Family. Edited by Howe LK. New York, Simon & Schuster, 1972, pp 341–348

Black HC: Black's Law Dictionary, Revised 5th Edition. Edited by Nolan JR, Connolly MJ. St Paul, MN, West Publishing, 1979

Blackburn JA, Greenberg JS, Boss PG: Coping with normative stress from loss and change: a longitudinal study of rural widows. Journal of Gerontological Social Work 11:59–70, 1987

Blanchard CG, Blanchard EB, Becker JV: The young widow: depressive symptomatology throughout the grief process. Psychiatry 39:394–399, 1976

Blanck R, Blanck G: Marriage and Personal Development. New York, Columbia University Press, 1968

Blazer DG, Bachar JR, Marston KG: Suicide in late life: review and commentary. J Am Geriatr Soc 34:519–525, 1986

Block AJ, Wynne JW, Boysen PG, et al: Sleep-disordered breathing and nocturnal oxygen desaturation in post-menopausal women. Am J Med 69:75–79, 1980

Blood RO, Wolfe DM: Husbands and Wives: The Dynamics of Married Living. New York, Free Press, 1960

Blos P: On Adolescence. New York, Free Press, 1962

Blum EH: Youthful drug use, in Handbook on Drug Abuse. Edited by Dupont RI, Goldstein A, O'Donnell J. Washington, DC, U.S. Government Printing Office, 1979, pp 257–269

Blum H: Masochism, the ego ideal, and the psychology of women. J Am Psychoanal Assoc 24(suppl):157–191, 1976

Blumenthal SJ, Kupfer DJ: Suicide Over the Life Cycle: Risk Factors, Assessment, and Treatment of Suicidal Patients. Washington, DC, American Psychiatric Press, 1990

Blumstein P, Schwartz P: American Couples. New York, William Morrow, 1983

Bohannon P: Divorce and After. New York, Doubleday, 1970

Bohman M, Sigvardsson S, Cloninger CR: Maternal inheritance of alcohol abuse: cross-fostering analysis of adopted women. Arch Gen Psychiatry 38:965–969, 1981

Bonaparte M: L'identification d'une fille a sa mere morte. Revue Francaise Psychoanalytique 2:541–565, 1928

Bonaparte M: Passivity, masochism and frigidity. Int J Psychoanal 16:325–333, 1935

Bornstein H, Bornstein M: Marital Therapy: A Behavioral Communications Approach. New York, Pergamon, 1986

Borys DS, Pope KS: Dual relationships between therapist and client: a national study of psychologists, psychiatrists and social workers. Professional Psychology: Research and Practice 20:283–293, 1989

Bouhoutsos JC, Brodsky AM: Mediation in therapist-client sex: a model. Psychotherapy 22:189–193, 1985

Bouhoutsos JC, Holroyd J, Lerman H, et al: Sexual intimacy between psychotherapists and patients. Professional Psychology: Research and Practice 14:185–196, 1983

Bowlby J: Grief and mourning in infancy and early childhood. Psychoanal Study Child 15:9–52, 1960

Bowlby J: Process of mourning. Int J Psychoanal 42:317–340, 1961

Bowlby J: Pathological mourning and childhood. J Am Psychoanal Assoc 11:500–541, 1963

Bowlby J: Attachment and Loss, Vol 2: Separation. New York, Basic Books, 1973

Bowlby J: Attachment and Loss, Vol 3: Loss, Sadness, and Depression. New York, Basic Books, 1980

Bracken MB, Klerman LV, Bracken M: Coping with pregnancy resolution among never-married women. Am J Orthopsychiatry 48:320–334, 1978

Braithwaite J: The myth of social class and criminality reconsidered. American Sociological Review 46:36–57, 1981

Brazelton TB: Issues for working parents. Am J Orthopsychiatry 56:14–25, 1986

Brazelton TB: Stress for families today. Infant Mental Health Journal 9:65–71, 1988

Brazelton TB, Keefer CH: The early mother-child relationship: a developmental view of woman as mother, in The Woman Patient, Vol 2: Concepts of Femininity and the Life Cycle. Edited by Nadelson CC, Notman MT. New York, Plenum, 1982, pp 95–109

Breast cancer. P & S Journal, Fall 1989, p 9

Breckenridge JN, Gallagher D, Thompson LW, et al: Characteristic depressive symptoms of bereaved elders. J Gerontol 41:163–168, 1986

Bresnick E, Taymor M: The role of counseling. Fertil Steril 32:154, 1979

Breuer J, Freud S: Studies on hysteria (1892), in The Standard Edition of the Complete Psychological Works of Sigmund Freud, Vol 2. Translated and edited by Strachey J. London, Hogarth Press, 1966, pp 1–319

Briere J, Pruntz M: Suicidal thoughts and behaviors in former sexual abuse victims. Canadian Journal of Behavioural Sciences 18:413–423, 1986

Brinton LA: Menopause and the risk of breast cancer. Ann N Y Acad Sci 592:357–362, 1990

Brock AM, O'Sullivan P: From wife to widow: role transition in the elderly. J Psychosoc Nurs Ment Health Serv 23:6–12, 1985

Brodsky AM: Sex between patient and therapist: psychology's data and response, in Sexual Exploitation in Professional Relationships. Edited by Gabbard GO. Washington, DC, American Psychiatric Press, 1989, pp 15–25

Brody EM: Social, economic and environmental issues related to aging with some thoughts about "women in the middle." Aging: Research and Perspectives 3:37–45, 1979

Brody EM: Women in the middle and family help to older people. The Gerontologist 21:471–480, 1981

Brody EM, Schoonover CB: Patterns of parentcare when adult daughters work and when they do not. The Gerontologist 26:372–381, 1986

Bromberg EM: Mother/daughter relationships and later life: the effect of quality of relationship on mutual aid. Journal of Gerontological Social Work 6:75–92, 1983

Broverman IK, Broverman DM, Clarkson FE: Sex-role stereotypes and clinical judgments of mental health. J Consult Clin Psychol 34:1–7, 1970

Brown GL, Ebert MH, Goyer PF, et al: Aggression, suicide, and serotonin: relationships to CSF amine metabolites. Am J Psychiatry 139:741–746, 1982

Brownmiller S: Against Our Will: Men, Women & Rape, New York, Simon & Schuster, 1975

Bruce ML, Kim K, Leaf P, et al: Depressive episodes and dysphoria resulting from conjugal bereavement in a prospective community sample. Am J Psychiatry 147:608–611, 1990

Bruch H: Eating Disorders: Obesity, Anorexia Nervosa, and the Person Within. New York, Basic Books, 1973

Bruch H: The Golden Cage: The Enigma of Anorexia Nervosa. New York, Vintage Books, 1979

Brunswick K: The pre-oedipal phase of libido development. Psychoanal Q 9:293–319, 1940

Budoff PW: Zomepirac sodium in the treatment of primary dysmenorrhea. N Engl J Med 307:714–719, 1982

Buie DH: The abandoned therapist. International Journal of Psychoanalytic Psychotherapy 9:227–231, 1982–1983

Bumagin VE, Hirn KF: Observations on changing relationships for older married women. Am J Psychoanal 42:133–142, 1982

Bumiller E: May You Be the Mother of a Hundred Sons. New York, Random House, 1990

Bumpass L, Sweet L: Differentials in Marital Instability. American Sociological Review 37:754–766, 1972

Burch B: Psychotherapy and the dynamics of merger in lesbian couples, in Contemporary Perspectives on Psychotherapy With Lesbians and Gay Men. Edited by Stein TS, Cohen CJ. New York, Plenum, 1986, pp 57–71

Burgess AW, Holmstrom LL: Rape trauma syndrome. Am J Psychiatry 131:981–986, 1974a

Burgess AW, Holmstrom LL: Rape: Victims of Crisis. Bowie, MD, Robert J Brady Company, 1974b

Burgess AW, Holmstrom LL: Adaptive strategies and recovery from rape. Am J Psychiatry 136:1278–1282, 1979

Burr WR, Leigh GK, Day P, et al: Symbolic interaction and the family, in Contemporary Theories About the Family, Vol 2: General Theories and Theoretical Orientation. Edited by Burr WR, Hill R, et al. New York, Free Press, 1979, pp 42–111

Bush TL: The epidemiology of cardiovascular disease in postmenopausal women. Ann N Y Acad Sci 592:263–345, 1990

Bush TL, Cowan LD, Barrett-Connor E, et al: Estrogen use and all-cause mortality. JAMA 249:903–906, 1983

Busse EW: The myth, history and science of aging, in Geriatric Psychiatry. Edited by Busse EW, Blazer DG. Washington, DC, American Psychiatric Press, 1989, pp 3–34

Busse EW, Blazer DG: The theory and processes of aging, in Handbook of Geriatric Psychiatry. Edited by Busse EW, Blazer DG. New York, Van Nostrand Reinhold, 1980, pp 3–27

Busse EW, Blazer DG (eds): Geriatric Psychiatry. Washington, DC, American Psychiatric Press, 1989

Bydlowski M, Dagan-Lintzer M: A psychomedical approach to infertility: "suffering from sterility." Journal of Psychosomatic Obstetrics and Gynaecology 9:139–151, 1988

Byrne GJA: Studies on the Impact of Recent Spouse's Bereavement on Elderly Men. Herston Queensland, University of Queensland, 1989

Cain AC: The legacy of suicide; observations on the pathogenic impact of suicide upon marital partners. Psychiatry 29:406–411, 1966

Cain L: Widow. New York, William Morrow, 1974

Calhoun KS, Atkeson BM, Resick PA: A longitudinal examination of fear reactions in victims of rape. Journal of Counseling Psychology 29:655–661, 1982

Calogeras RC: Early object-relations conflicts in marital interaction. Psychoanal Rev 72:31–53, 1985

Cameron P: Masculinity/femininity of the generations: as self-reported as stereotypically appraised. Int J Aging Hum Dev 7:143–151, 1976

Campbell A: The American way of mating: marriages, children only maybe. Psychology Today, May 1975, pp 37–43

Campbell A, Converse P, Rodgers W: The Quality of American Life: Perceptions, Evaluations and Satisfactions. New York, Russell Sage, 1976

Carey RG: Weathering widowhood: problems and adjustment of the widowed during the first year. Omega 10:163–174, 1979–1980

Caron W, Doyle P: Contested custody intervention: an empirical assessment, in Child Custody: Literature Review and Alternative Approaches. Edited by Olsen D. Minneapolis, MN, University of Minnesota, Child Custody Research Project, 1979, pp 137–190

Carr M, Robinson GE: Fatal attraction: the ethical and clinical dilemma of patient-therapist sex. Can J Psychiatry 35:122–127, 1990

Carter H, Glick PC: Marriage and Divorce: A Social and Economic Study. Cambridge, MA, Harvard University Press, 1976

Casler L: Maternal deprivation: a critical review of the literature. Monogr Soc Res Child Dev, Vol 26, No 2, 1961

Cates W, Schulz KF, Grimes DA: The risks associated with teenage abortion. N Engl J Med 309:621–624, 1983

Cath S: Vicissitudes of grandfatherhood: a miracle of revitalization, in Father and Child. Edited by Cath SH, Gurwitt AR, Ross JM. Boston, MA, Little, Brown, 1982, pp 327–337

Chambers DL: Making Fathers Pay: The Enforcement of Child Support. Chicago, IL, University of Chicago Press, 1979

Chance S: Left for dead. Psychiatric Times, January 1991, pp 26–27

Charney DS, Heninger GR: Noradrenergic function and the mechanism of action of antianxiety treatment. Arch Gen Psychiatry 42:473–481, 1985

Cherland E, Matthews PC: Attempted murder of a newborn: a case history. Can J Psychiatry 34:337–339, 1989

Chernin K: The Obsession. New York, Harper & Row, 1981

Chilmon ES: Adolescent Sexuality in a Changing American Society: Social and Psychological Perspectives. Washington, DC, U.S. Government Printing Office, 1978

Chiriboga DA: The developmental psychology of middle age, in Modern Perspectives in the Psychiatry of Middle Age. Edited by Howell JG. New York, Brunner/Mazel, 1981, pp 3–25

Chodorow N: The Reproduction of Mothering: Psychoanalysis and the Sociology of Gender. Berkeley, CA, University of California Press, 1978

Christiansen C, Christiansen MS, Transbol I: Bone mass in postmenopausal women after withdrawal of oestrogen/gestagen replacement therapy. Lancet 1:459–461, 1981

Chused JF: Neutrality in the analysis of action-prone adolescents. J Am Psychoanal Assoc 38:679–704, 1990

Claman JM: Mirror hunger in the psychodynamics of sexually abusing therapists. Am J Psychoanal 47:35–40, 1987

Clark L, Lewis D: Rape: The Price of Coercive Sexuality. Toronto, Women's Press, 1977

Clark PG, Siviski RW, Weiner R: Coping strategies of widowers in the first year. Family Relations 35:425–430, 1986

Claven S: The impact of social class and social trends on the role of grandparent. The Family Coordinator 27:355–357, 1978

Clayton PJ: The clinical morbidity of the first year of bereavement: a review. Compr Psychiatry 14:151-157, 1973

Clayton PJ: Bereavement and its management, in Handbook of Affective Disorders. Edited by Paykel ES. New York, Guilford, 1982, pp 403–415

Clayton PJ, Desmarais L, Winokur G: A study of normal bereavement. Am J Psychiatry 125:168–178, 1968

Clayton PJ, Halikas JA, Maurice WL: The bereavement of the widowed. Diseases of the Nervous System 32:592–604, 1971

Clayton PJ, Halikas JA, Maurice WL: The depression of widowhood. Br J Psychiatry 120:71–78, 1972

Clayton PJ, Halikas J, Maurice W, et al: Anticipatory grief and widowhood. Br J Psychiatry 122:47–51, 1973

Clayton PJ, Herjanic M, Murphy G: Mourning and depression: their similarities and differences. Can J Psychiatry 19:309–312, 1974

Cleveland WP, Gianturco DT: Remarriage probability after widowhood; a retrospective method. J Gerontol 31:99–103, 1976

Cobbs S, Bauer W, Whiting I: Environmental factors in rheumatoid arthritis. JAMA 113:668–670, 1939

Cohen CJ, Stein TS: Reconceptualizing individual psychotherapy with gay men and lesbians, in Contemporary Perspectives on Psychotherapy With Lesbians and Gay Men. Edited by Stein TS, Cohen CJ. New York, Plenum, 1986, pp 27–54

Cohen P: Violence in the family: an act of loyalty. Psychotherapy 21:249–253, 1984

Cohen SI: Voodoo death, the stress response, and AIDS, in Psychological, Neuropsychiatric, and Substance Abuse Aspects of AIDS (Advances in Biochemical Psychopharmacology, Vol 44). Edited by Bridge TP, Mirsky AF, Goodwin FK. New York, Raven, 1988, pp 95–111

Cohler BJ, Greenbaum H: Mother, Grandmothers and Daughters. New York, Wiley, 1981

Cole C: A group design for adult female survivors of childhood incest. Woman and Therapy 4:71–82, 1985

Coleman WP: Dermatologic cosmetic surgery. J Dermatol Surg Oncol 16:170–176, 1990

Coley SM, Beckett JO: Black battered women: a review of empirical literature. Journal of Counseling and Development 6:266–270, 1988

Collins DT, Mebed AAK, Mortimer RL: Patient-therapist sex: consequences for subsequent treatment. McLean Hospital Journal 3:24–36, 1978

Coltrane S: Household labor and the routine production of gender. Social Problems 36:473–490, 1989

Conger JJ: Adolescent sexuality, in Adolescence and Youth: Psychological Development in a Changing World, 3rd Edition. Edited by Conger JJ, Peterson AC. New York, Harper & Row, 1984, p 277

Conger JJ, Petersen AF (eds): Adolescence and Youth: Psychological Development in a Changing World. New York, Harper & Row, 1984

Constantino RE: Bereavement crisis intervention for widows in grief and mourning. Nurs Res 30:351–353, 1981

Conte J, Schuerman J: Factor associated with an increased impact of child sexual abuse. Child Abuse Negl 11:201–211, 1987

Coolfront report: a PHS plan for prevention and control of AIDS and the AIDS virus. Public Health Rep 101:34–38, 1986

Coons P: Child abuse and multiple personality disorder: review of the literature and suggestions for treatment. Child Abuse Negl 10:455–462, 1986

Cord J, Wise L: Teenage mothers and teenage fathers: the impact of early childbearing on parents' personal and professional lives. Fam Plann Perspect 10:199–205, 1978

Corson SL: Impact of estrogen replacement therapy on cardiovascular risk. J Reprod Med 34:729–746, 1984

Coulam CB: Age estrogens and the psyche. Clin Obstet Gynecol 24:219–229, 1981

Courtois CA: Healing the Incest Wound: Adult Survivors in Therapy. New York, WW Norton, 1988

Cousins N: Anatomy of an Illness. New York, WW Norton, 1979

Cousins N: The Healing Heart. New York, WW Norton, 1983

Cox JL: Childbirth as a life event: sociocultural aspects of postnatal depression. Acta Psychiatr Scand Suppl 78 (suppl 344):75–83, 1988

Cox JL, Connor Y, Kendell RE: Prospective study of the psychiatric disorders of childbirth. Br J Psychiatry 140:111–117, 1982

Crull P: Stress effects of sexual harassment on the job: implications for counseling. Am J Orthopsychiatry 52:539–544, 1982

Cumming DC: Menarche, menses and menopause: a brief review. Cleve Clin J Med 57:169–175, 1990

Cutright P, Scanzoni J: Income supplements and the American family, in The Family Poverty and Welfare Programs: Factors Influencing Family Instability (Studies in Public Welfare No 12). Edited by Joint Economic Committee. Washington DC, U.S. Government Printing Office, 1973

Dacey J: Adolescents Today. Santa Monica, CA, Goodyear, 1979

Dahlberg CC: Sexual contact between patient and therapist. Contemporary Psychoanalysis 6:107–124, 1970

Daniluk J: Infertility: intrapersonal and interpersonal impact. Fertil Steril 49:982, 1988

Danto BL: Survivors of homicide, in The Human Side of Homicide. Edited by Danto BL, Bruhns J, Kutscher AH. New York, Columbia University Press, 1982, pp 85–97

Davis K: The American family in relation to demographic change: report of the U.S. Commission on Population Growth and the American future, in Demographic and Social Aspects of Population Growth, Vol 1. Edited by Westoff CCT, Raske R Jr. Washington, DC, U.S. Government Printing Office, 1972, pp 235–266

Dean C, Kendell RE: The symptomatology of puerperal illnesses. Br J Psychiatry 139:128–133, 1981

Debor L, Gallagher D, Lesher E: Group counseling with bereaving elderly. Clinical Gerontologist 1:81–90, 1983

Dege K, Gretzinger J: Attitudes of families towards menopause, in Changing Perspectives on Menopause. Edited by Voda AM, Dinnerstein M, O'Donnell SR. Austin, TX, University of Texas Press, 1982, pp 60–69

Denber H: Psychiatric aspects of infertility. J Reprod Med 20:23–29, 1978

Deutsch H: The psychology of women in relation to the functions of reproduction. Int J Psychoanal 6:405–418, 1925

Deutsch H: The significance of masochism in the mental life of women. Int J Psychoanal 11:40–60, 1930

Deutsch H: On female homosexuality. Psychoanal Q 1:484–510, 1932

Deutsch H: Homosexuality in women. Int J Psychoanal 14:34–56, 1933a

Deutsch H: Motherhood and sexuality. Psychoanal Q 2:476–488, 1933b

Deutsch H: Absence of grief. Psychoanal Q 6:12–22, 1937

Deutsch H: The Psychology of Women, A Psychoanalytic Interpretation, Vol 1. New York, Grune & Stratton, 1944

Deutsch H: The Psychology of Women, A Psychoanalytic Interpretation, Vol 2: Motherhood. New York, Grune & Stratton, 1945

Devlin MJ, Walsh BT: Eating disorders and depression. Psychiatric Annals 19:473–476, 1989

Deykin EY, Alpert JJ, McNamarra JJ: A pilot study of the effect of exposure to child abuse or neglect on adolescent suicidal behavior. Am J Psychiatry 142:1299–1303, 1985

Dicks HV: Object relations theory and marital studies. Br J Med Psychol 36:125–129, 1963

Dickstein LJ: The psychosocial effects of divorce on young adults, in Divorce as a Developmental Process. Edited by Gold JH. Washington, DC, American Psychiatric Press, 1988a, pp 1–26

Dickstein LJ: Spouse abuse and other domestic violence. Psychiatr Clin North Am 11:611–628, 1988b

Dietrich DR, Shabad PC: The Problem of Loss and Mourning: Psychoanalytic Perspectives. Madison, CT, International Universities Press, 1989

Dobash RE, Dobash RP: Violence Against Wives: A Case Against the Patriarchy. New York, Free Press, 1979

Dohrenwend BS: Social status and stressful life events. J Pers Soc Psychol 28:225–235, 1973

Doka KJ: Loss upon loss: the impact of death after divorce. Death Studies 10:441–449, 1986

Domash L: Motivations for motherhood and the nature of the self-object tie, in Critical Psychophysical Passages in the Life of a Woman: A Psychodynamic Perspective. Edited by Offerman-Zuckerman J. New York, Plenum, 1988, pp 93–102

Donaldson M, Gardner R: Diagnosis and treatment of post-traumatic stress among women after childhood incest, in Trauma and Its Wake: The Study and Treatment of Post Traumatic Stress Disorder. Edited by Figley CR. New York, Brunner/Mazel, 1985, pp 356–377

D'Orbán PT: Women who kill their children. Br J Psychiatry 134:560–571, 1979

Doty P, Sullivan E: Community involvement in combating abuse, neglect and maltreatment in nursing homes. Milbank Q 61:222–251, 1983

Douglas MA, Der Ovanesian M: A comparative study of battered and not battered women in crisis. Paper presented at the 17th annual convention of the Association for the Advancement of Behavioral Therapy, Washington, DC, November 1983

Downey J, Yingling M, McKinney M, et al: Mood disorders, psychiatric symptoms and distress in women presenting for infertility evaluation. Fertil Steril 52:425–432, 1989

Duke D: A study of the effects of bereavement. Unpublished thesis, Newcastle Polytechnic, Newcastle, UK, 1980

Duncan B, Duncan OD: Family stability and occupational success. Social Problems 16:271–306, 1969

Dutton D, Painter SL: Traumatic bonding: the development of emotional attachments in battered women and other relationships of intermittent abuse. Victimology: An International Journal 6:139–155, 1981

Dziech BW, Weiner L: The Lecherous Professor: Sexual Harassment on Campus. Boston, MA, Beacon Press, 1984

Eckert ED, Goldberg SC, Halmi KA, et al: Behaviour therapy in anorexia nervosa. Br J Psychiatry 134:55–59, 1979

Eck Menning B: The emotional needs of infertile couples. Fertil Steril 34:313–319, 1980

Egginton J: From Cradle to Grave: The Short Lives and Strange Deaths of Marybeth Tinning's Nine Children. New York, William Morrow, 1989

Elliot DS, Ageton SS: Reconciling of race and class differences in self-reported and official estimates of delinquency. American Sociological Review 45:95–110, 1980

Ellis EM: A review of empirical rape research: victim reactions and response to treatment. Clinical Psychology Review 3:473–490, 1983

Elman MR, Gilbert LA: Coping strategies for role conflict in married professional women with children. Family Relations 33:317–327, 1984

Emmore E: Lesbian Women and Society. London, Routledge & Kegan Paul, 1980

Enscobedo L, Anda R, Smith P, et al: Sociodemographic characteristics of cigarette smoking initiation in the United States. JAMA 264:1550–1555, 1990

Equal Employment Opportunities Commission, Federal Register 45(219):14–15, 1980

Erikson EH: Childhood and Society. New York, WW Norton, 1950

Erikson EH: The problem of ego identity. J Am Psychoanal Assoc 4:56–121, 1956

Erikson EH: Identity and the Life Cycle. New York, International Universities Press, 1959

Erikson EH: Identity, Youth, and Crisis. New York, WW Norton, 1968a

Erikson EH: Womanhood and the inner space, in Identity, Youth, and Crisis. New York, WW Norton, 1968b, pp 261–295

Erikson EH: Childhood and Society, 2nd Ed. New York, WW Norton, 1985

Erlik Y, Tatryn IV, Meldrum DR, et al: Association of waking episodes with menopausal hot flushes. JAMA 245:1741–1744, 1981

Erwin RJ, Mawhinney-Hee M, Gur RC, et al: Effects of task and gender on EEG indices of hemisphere activation: similarities to previous CBF findings. Neuropsychiatry Neuropsychology Behav Neurol 2:248–260, 1989

Estrich S: Real Rape. Cambridge, MA, Harvard University Press, 1987

Evans R, Henderson A, Hill P, et al: Smoking in children and adolescents: psychosocial determinants and prevention strategies, in Smoking and Health: A Report of the Surgeon General, Vol 17 (DHEW Publ No [PHS]-79-50066). Washington, DC, U.S. Department of Health, Education and Welfare (U.S. GPO No 017-000-00218-0), 1979, pp 1–30

Fairbairn WRD: An Object-Relations Theory of the Personality. New York, Basic Books, 1954

Farrell D, Wilner N: Mutual help groups for widows: a study of the process. Isr J Psychiatry Relat Sci 23:297–305, 1986

Fava M, Copeland PM, Schweiger V, et al: Neurochemical abnormalities of anorexia nervosa and bulimia nervosa. Am J Psychiatry 146:963–971, 1989

Federal Bureau of Investigation: Uniform Crime Reports. Washington, DC, U.S. Department of Justice, 1982

Feldman-Summers S, Jones G: Psychological impacts of sexual contact between therapists or other health care practitioners and their clients. J Consult Clin Psychol 52:1054–1061, 1984

Ferenczi S: Confusion of tongues between adults and children (1933), in Final Contribution to Psychoanalysis. New York, Basic Books, 1955, pp 156–174

Ferraro KF: An existential approach to battering. Paper presented at the Second National Conference for Family Violence Researchers, Durham, NC, 1984a

Ferraro KF: Widowhood and social participation in later life. Res Aging 6:451–468, 1984b

Ferraro KF: The effect of widowhood on the health status of older people. Int J Aging Hum Dev 21:9–25, 1985–1986

Ferraro KF, Mutran E, Barresi CM: Widowhood, health and friendship support in later life. J Health Soc Behav 25:246–259, 1984

Figley CR (ed): Trauma and Its Wake: The Study and Treatment of Post Traumatic Stress Disorder, New York, Brunner/Mazel, 1985

Figley CR (ed): Trauma and Its Wake, Volume 2: Traumatic Stress Theory, Research and Intervention. New York, Brunner/Mazel, 1986

Finell JS: Narcissistic problems in analysts. Int J Psychoanal 66:433–445, 1985

Finkelhor D, Hotaling GT: Sexual abuse in the national incidence study of child abuse and neglect: an appraisal. Child Abuse Negl 8:23–33, 1984

Finkelhor D, Yllo K: License to Rape: Sexual Abuse of Wives. New York, Free Press, 1985

Finkelstein L: Psychoanalysis, marital therapy, and object-relations theory. J Am Psychoanal Assoc 36:905–931, 1988

Fisch RZ, Tadmor O: Iatrogenic post-traumatic stress disorder. Lancet, December 9, no 8676, 1989, p 1397

Fish WC: Differences in grief intensity in bereaved parents, in Parental Loss of a Child. Edited by Rando TA. Champaign, IL, Research Press Co, 1986, pp 415–428

Fish WC, Whitney SM: Challenging conventional wisdom about parental bereavement. Forum for Death Education and Counsel Newsletter, No 6, 1983, p 4

Fleming JB: Stopping Wife Abuse. Garden City, NY, Anchor, 1979

Flint M: The menopause: reward or punishment. Psychosomatics 16:161–163, 1975

Flint M, Kronenberg F, Utian W (eds): Multidisciplinary Perspectives on Menopause. Annals of the New York Academy of Sciences, Vol 592. New York, New York Academy of Sciences, 1990

Fogarty TF: The role of romantic love in marriage, in Contemporary Marriage: Special Issues in Couples Therapy. Edited by Goldberg DC. Homewood, IL, Dorsey Press, 1985, pp 19–34

Folkman S, Lazarus RS: An analysis of coping in a middle age community sample. J Health Soc Behav 21:219–239, 1980

Ford C, Castelnuovo-Teddesco P, Long K: Abortion: is it a therapeutic procedure in psychiatry? JAMA 218:1173–1178, 1971

Foreman BD: Psychotherapy with rape victims. Psychotherapy: Theory, Research and Practice 17:304–311, 1980

Formanek R: Menopause: myth and reality, in Critical Psychophysical Passages in the Life of a Woman: A Psychodynamic Perspective. Edited by Offerman-Zuckerberg J. New York, Plenum, 1988, pp 199–214

Forrest JD, Sullivan E, Tietze C: Abortion in the United States. Fam Plann Perspect 11:329–341, 1979

Fourcroy J (chairperson): Presentation on the "female condom" at the annual meeting of the American Medical Women's Association, Philadelphia, PA, November 1990

Franco KN, Tamburrio MB, Campbell NS, et al: Psychological profile of dysphoric women post abortion. J Am Med Wom Assoc 44:113–119, 1989

Frank E, Anderson C, Rubinstein D: Frequency of sexual dysfunction in "normal" couples. N Engl J Med 299:111–115, 1978

Fraser S: My Father's House: A Memoir of Incest and of Healing. Toronto, Ticknor & Fields, 1987

Freedman AM, Blumenfield M: Recognizing the role of bereavement and reactive depression in modern psychiatry. Psychopathology 19:37–46, 1987

Freedman R: Beauty Bound. Lexington, MA, DC Heath, 1986

Freeman E, Rickels K, Huggins G, et al: Emotional disorder patterns among women having first or repeat abortions. Obstet Gynecol 55:630–636, 1980

Freud A: The ego and the mechanisms of defense (1936) (revised edition), in The Writings of Anna Freud, Vol 2. New York, International Universities Press, 1966

Freud S: Charçot (1893a), in Sigmund Freud, Collected Papers, Vol 1. Edited by Jones E. New York, Basic Books, 1953, pp 9–23

Freud S: Extracts from the Fliess papers: Draft B, the aetiology of the neuroses (1893b), in The Standard Edition of the Complete Psychological Works of Sigmund Freud, Vol 1. Translated and edited by Strachey J. London, Hogarth Press, 1966, pp 179–184

Freud S: Draft G, melancholia (1895), in The Standard Edition of the Complete Psychological Works of Sigmund Freud, Vol 1. Translated and edited by Strachey J. London, Hogarth Press, 1966, pp 200–206

Freud S: Heredity and the aetiology of the neuroses (1896), in The Standard Edition of the Complete Psychological Works of Sigmund Freud, Vol 3. Translated and edited by Strachey J. London, Hogarth Press, 1962, pp 141–156

Freud S: Sexuality in the aetiology of the neuroses (1898), in The Standard Edition of the Complete Psychological Works of Sigmund Freud, Vol 3. Translated and edited by Strachey J. London, Hogarth Press, 1962, pp 259–285

Freud S: Fragment of an anal analysis of a case of hysteria (1905a[1901]), in The Standard Edition of the Complete Psychological Works of Sigmund Freud, Vol. 7. Translated and edited by Strachey J. London, Hogarth Press, 1953, pp 1–122

Freud S: Three essays on the theory of sexuality (1905b), in The Standard Edition of the Complete Psychological Works of Sigmund Freud, Vol 7. Translated and edited by Strachey J. London, Hogarth Press, 1953, pp 123–245

Freud S: Analysis of a phobia in a five-year-old boy (1909a), in The Standard Edition of the Complete Psychological Works of Sigmund Freud, Vol 10. Translated and edited by Strachey J. London, Hogarth Press, 1955, pp 1–149

Freud S: Notes upon a case of obsessional neurosis (1909b), in The Standard Edition of the Complete Psychological Works of Sigmund Freud, Vol. 10. Translated and edited by Strachey J. London, Hogarth Press, 1955, pp 151–320

Freud S: A special type of choice of object made by men (contributions to the psychology of love I) (1910), in The Standard Edition of the Complete Psychological Works of Sigmund Freud, Vol 11. Translated and edited by Strachey J. London, Hogarth Press, 1957, pp 163–175

Freud S: On the universal tendency to debasement in the sphere of love (contributions to the psychology of love II) (1912a), in The Standard Edition of the Complete Psychological Works of Sigmund Freud, Vol 11. Translated and edited by Strachey J. London, Hogarth Press, 1957, pp 177–190

Freud S: Totem and taboo (1912b[1912–1913]), in The Standard Edition of the Complete Psychological Works of Sigmund Freud, Vol 13. Translated and edited by Strachey J. London, Hogarth Press, 1958, pp 1–162

Freud S: On narcissism: an introduction (1914a), in The Standard Edition of the Complete Psychological Works of Sigmund Freud, Vol 14. Translated and edited by Strachey J. London, Hogarth Press, 1957, pp 67–102

Freud S: Remembering, repeating and working-through (further recommendations on the technique of psycho-analysis II) (1914b), in The Standard Edition of the Complete Psychological Works of Sigmund Freud, Vol 12. Translated and edited by Strachey J. London, Hogarth Press, 1958, pp 145–156

Freud S: Observations on transference-love (further recommendations on the technique of psycho-analysis III) (1915[1914]), in The Standard Edition of the Complete Psychological Works of Sigmund Freud, Vol 12. Translated and edited by Strachey J. London, Hogarth Press, 1958, pp 157–173

Freud S: Introductory lectures on psycho-analysis, Parts I, II, and III (1916–1917[1915–1917]), in The Standard Edition of the Complete Psychological Works of Sigmund Freud, Vols 15 and 16. Translated and edited by Strachey J. London, Hogarth Press, 1961/1963

Freud S: Mourning and melancholia (1917), in The Standard Edition of the Complete Psychological Works of Sigmund Freud, Vol 14. Translated and edited by Strachey J. London, Hogarth Press, 1961, pp 237–258

Freud S: The taboo of virginity (contributions to the psychology of love III) (1918[1917]), in The Standard Edition of the Complete Psychological Works of Sigmund Freud, Vol 11. Translated and edited by Strachey J. London, Hogarth Press, 1957, pp 191–208

Freud S: Beyond the pleasure principle (1920a), in The Standard Edition of the Complete Psychological Works of Sigmund Freud, Vol 18. Translated and edited by Strachey J. London, Hogarth Press, 1955, pp 1–64

Freud S: The psychogenesis of a case of homosexuality in a woman (1920b), in The Standard Edition of the Complete Psychological Works of Sigmund Freud, Vol 18. Translated and edited by Strachey J. London, Hogarth Press, 1955, pp 145–172

Freud S: The ego and the id (1923a), in The Standard Edition of the Complete Psychological Works of Sigmund Freud, Vol. 19. Translated and edited by Strachey J. London, Hogarth Press, 1961, pp 1–66

Freud S: The infantile genital organization: an interpolation in the theory of sexuality (1923b), in The Standard Edition of the Complete Psychological Works of Sigmund Freud, Vol. 19. Translated and edited by Strachey J. London, Hogarth Press, 1961, pp 139–145

Freud S: The dissolution of the oedipus complex (1924a), in The Standard Edition of the Complete Psychological Works of Sigmund Freud, Vol. 19. Translated and edited by Strachey J. London, Hogarth Press, 1961, pp 171–179

Freud S: The economic problem of masochism (1924b), in The Standard Edition of the Complete Psychological Works of Sigmund Freud, Vol. 19. Translated and edited by Strachey J. London, Hogarth Press, 1961, pp 155–170

Freud S: Some psychical consequences of the anatomical distinction between the sexes (1925), in The Standard Edition of the Complete Psychological Works of Sigmund Freud, Vol 19. Translated and edited by Strachey J. London, Hogarth Press, 1961, pp 241–258

Freud S: Inhibitions, symptoms and anxiety (1926a), in The Standard Edition of the Complete Psychological Works of Sigmund Freud, Vol 20. Translated and edited by Strachey J. London, Hogarth Press, 1959, pp 75–175

Freud S: The question of lay analysis: conversations with an impartial person (1926b), in The Standard Edition of the Complete Psychological Works of Sigmund Freud, Vol 20. Translated and edited by Strachey J. London, Hogarth Press, 1959, pp 177–258

Freud S: Civilization and its discontents (1930[1929]), in The Standard Edition of the Complete Psychological Works of Sigmund Freud, Vol 21. Translated and edited by Strachey J. London, Hogarth Press, 1961, pp 57–145

Freud S: Female sexuality (1931) in The Standard Edition of the Complete Psychological Works of Sigmund Freud, Vol 21. Translated and edited by Strachey J. London, Hogarth Press, 1961, pp 221–243

Freud S: Femininity (1933a), in The Standard Edition of the Complete Psychological Works of Sigmund Freud, Vol 22. Translated and edited by Strachey J. London, Hogarth Press, 1964, pp 112–135

Freud S: New introductory lectures on psycho-analysis: femininity (1933b[1932]), in The Standard Edition of the Complete Psychological Works of Sigmund Freud, Vol 22. Translated and edited by Strachey J. London, Hogarth Press, 1964, pp 112–135

Freud S: Moses and monotheism (1939[1934–1938]), in The Standard Edition of the Complete Psychological Works of Sigmund Freud,

Vol 23. Translated and edited by Strachey J. London, Hogarth Press, 1964, pp 1–137

Freud S: Female sexuality, in Collected Papers. London, Hogarth Press, 1950, pp 225–243

Friday N: My Secret Garden: Women's Sexual Fantasies. New York, Pocket Books, 1973

Friday N: My Mother, My Self. New York, Dell, 1978

Friedl E: Women of Deh Koh: Lives in an Iranian Village. Washington, DC, Smithsonian Institute Press, 1988

Friedman AS, Bechner GM (eds): Treatment Services for Adolescent Substance Abusers (DHHS Publ No 87-1342). Rockville, MD, National Institute on Drug Abuse, 1985

Friedman CM, Greenspan R, Mittleman F: The decision-making process and the outcome of therapeutic abortion. Am J Psychiatry 131:1332–1337, 1974

Friedman RC: Male Homosexuality: A Contemporary Psychoanalytic Perspective. New Haven, CT, Yale University Press, 1988

Frieze IH: Investigating the causes and consequences of marital rape. Signs 8:532–553, 1983

Fry JM: Sleep disorders. Med Clin North Am 71:95–111, 1987

Fullilove MT, Fullilove RE: Intersecting epidemics: black crack use and sexually transmitted disease. J Am Med Wom Assoc 44:146–153, 1989

Fullilove MT, Fullilove RE, Haynes K, et al: Black women and AIDS prevention: a view towards understanding the gender roles. Journal of Sex Research 27:47–64, 1990

Fullilove RE, Fullilove MT, Bowser, et al: Risk of sexually transmitted disease among black adolescent crack users in Oakland and San Francisco, California. JAMA 263:851–856, 1991

Fulton R, Fulton JA: A psychosocial aspect of terminal care: anticipatory grief. Omega 2:91–99, 1971

Futterman EH, Hoffman I, Sabshin M: Parental anticipatory mourning, in Psychosocial Aspects of Terminal Care. Edited by Schoenberg B,

Carr AC, Peretz D, et al. New York, Columbia University Press, 1972, pp 243–272

Gabbard GO, Menninger RW: The psychology of the physician, in Medical Marriages. Edited by Gabbard GO, Menninger RW. Washington, DC, American Psychiatric Press, 1988, pp 23–38

Galenson E: A consideration of the nature of thought in childhood play, in Separation-Individuation; Essays in Honor of Margaret S. Mahler. Edited by McDevitt JB, Settlage CF. New York, International Universities Press, 1971, pp 41–59

Galenson E, Roiphe H: The impact of early sexual discovery on mood, defensive organization, and symbolization. Psychoanal Study Child 26:195–216, 1971

Galenson E, Roiphe H: Some suggested revisions concerning early female development. J Am Psychoanal Assoc 24(suppl):29–57, 1976

Galenson E, Blau S, Vogel S: Disturbance in sexual identity beginning at eighteen months of age. International Review of Psychoanalysis 2:389–393, 1975

Galenson E, Miller R, Roiphe H: The choice of symbols. Journal of the American Academy of Child Psychiatry 15:83–96, 1976

Ganzarain RC, Buchele BJ: Fugitives of Incest: A Perspective From Psychoanalysis and Groups. Madison, CT, International Universities Press, 1988

Gartrell N: Issues in psychotherapy with lesbian women. The Stone Center for Developmental Services and Studies, Work in Progress, Wellesley, MA, 1984, No 83-04:1–12

Gartrell N, Herman J, Olarte S, et al: Psychiatrist-patient sexual contact: results of a national survey, I: prevalence. Am J Psychiatry 143:1126–1131, 1986a

Gartrell N, Herman J, Olarte S, et al: Report practices of psychiatrists who knew of sexual misconduct by colleagues. Am J Orthopsychiatry 57:287–295, 1986b

Gartrell N, Herman J, Olarte S, et al: Psychiatric residents' sexual contact with educators and patients: results of a national survey. Am J Psychiatry 145:690–694, 1988

Gartrell N, Herman J, Olarte S, et al: Prevalence of psychiatrist-patient sexual contact, in Sexual Exploitation in Professional Relationships. Edited by Gabbard GO. Washington, DC, American Psychiatric Press, 1989, pp 3–13

Garvey MJ, Tollefson GD: Post partum depression. J Reprod Med 29:113–116, 1984

Gass KA: Coping strategies of widows. Journal of Gerontological Nursing 13:29–33, 1987

Gass KA, Chang AS: Appraisals of bereavement, coping, resources, and psychosocial health dysfunction in widows and widowers. Nurs Res 38:31–36, 1989

Gates PA: Suddenly Alone: A Woman's Guide to Widowhood. New York, Harper & Row, 1990

Gayford JJ: Battered wives. Med Sci Law 15:237–245, 1975a

Gayford J: Wife battering: a preliminary survey of 100 cases. BMJ 1:195–197, 1975b

Gechtman L: Sexual contact between social workers and their clients, in Sexual Exploitation in Professional Relationships. Edited by Gabbard GO. Washington, DC, American Psychiatric Press, 1989, pp 27–38

Gechtman L, Bouhoutsos JC: Social workers' attitudes and practices regarding erotic and nonerotic physical contact with their clients. Paper presented at the Annual Conference of the California Society for Clinical Social Work and The National Federation of Societies for Clinical Social Work, Universal City, CA, October 1985

Geller JA, Wasserman J: Conjoint therapy for the treatment of domestic violence, in Battered Women and Their Families. Edited by Roberts AR. New York, Springer, 1984, pp 33–48

Gelles RJ: The Violent Home: A Study of Physical Aggression Between Husbands and Wives. Beverly Hills, CA, Sage, 1972

Gelles RJ, Straus MA: Determinants of violence in the family: toward a theoretical integration, in Contemporary Theories About the Family, Vol 1. Edited by Burt WR, Hill R, Nye FI, et al. New York, Free Press, 1979, pp 549–581

Gentry M, Schulman A: Remarriage as a coping response for widowhood. Psychol Aging 3:191–196, 1988

Gentry M, Rosenman L, Schulman AD: Comparison of needs and support systems of remarried and non-remarried widows, in Widows, Vol 2: North America. Edited by Lopata HZ. Durham, NC, Duke University Press, 1987, pp 158–170

Geracioti TD, Liddle RA: Impaired cholecystokinin in bulimia nervosa. N Engl J Med 319:683–688, 1988

Gerber I, Rusalem W, Hannon N, et al: Anticipatory grief and aged widows and widowers. J Gerontol 30:225–229, 1975

Gerson MJ, Alpert JL, Richardson MS: Mothering: the view from psychological research. Signs 9:434–453, 1984

Getzel GS: Social work with family caregivers to the aged. Social Casework 62:201–210, 1981

Gilbert LA: Understanding dual-career families. Family Therapy Collections 10:57–81, 1984

Gilbert LA, Rachlin V: Mental health and psychological functioning of dual-career families. The Counseling Psychologist 15:7–49, 1987

Giles-Sims J: Wife Battering: A Systems Approach. New York, Guilford, 1983

Gilligan C: Women's place in the man's life cycle. Harvard University Review 49:431–446, 1979

Gilligan C: In a Different Voice. Cambridge, MA, Harvard University Press, 1982

Gilligan C: Making Connections: The Relational Worlds of Adolescent Girls at Emma Willard School. Cambridge, MA, Harvard University Press, 1990

Gilson E, Kane S: Unnecessary Choices: The Hidden Life of the Executive Woman. New York, William Morrow, 1987

Gise LH, Paddison P: Rape, sexual abuse, and its victims. Psychiatr Clin North Am 11:629–648, 1988

Gitlin MJ, Pasnau RO: Psychiatric syndromes linked to reproductive function in women. Am J Psychiatry 146:1413–1422, 1989

Glaser RD, Thorpe JS: Unethical intimacy: a survey of sexual contact and advances between psychology educators and female graduate students. Am Psychol 41:43–51, 1986

Glassman A, Helzer J, Coveny L, et al: Smoking, smoking cessation and major depression. JAMA 264:1546–1549, 1990

Glick ID: Marital and Family Therapy. New York, Grune & Stratton, 1980

Glick IO, Weiss RS, Parkes CM: The First Year of Bereavement. New York, Wiley, 1974

Glick PC: A demographer looks at American families. Journal of Marriage and the Family 37:15–26, 1975

Glick PC: How American Families Are Changing. American Demography 6:20–27, 1984

Glick PC, Norton AJ: Perspectives on the recent upturn in divorce and remarriage. Demography 10:301–314, 1973

Gold JH: Divorce as a Developmental Process. Washington, DC, American Psychiatric Press, 1988

Gold PW, Kaye WH, Robertson RL, et al: Abnormalities in plasma and cerebrospinal fluid arginine vasopressin in patients with anorexia nervosa. N Engl J Med 308:1117–1123, 1983

Goldberg GS, Kantrow R, Kremen E, et al: Spouseless, childless elderly women and their social supports. Social Work 31:104–112, 1986

Goldberg M: The dynamics of marital interaction and marital conflict. Psychiatr Clin North Am 5:449–467, 1982

Goldberg MC: Women's friendships—women's groups. Psychiatric Annals 20:398–401, 1990

Goldstein MZ: Aspects of gender and ethnic identity in menopause: two Italian-American women. J Am Acad Psychoanal 15:383–394, 1987

Gomes-Schwartz B, Horowitz JM, Sauzier M: Severity of emotional distress among sexually abused preschool, school-age, and adolescent children. Hosp Community Psychiatry 36:503–508, 1985

Gondolf EW, Fisher ER: Battered Women as Survivors. Lexington, MA, DC Heath, 1988

Good WJ: After Divorce. New York, Free Press, 1956

Gooden W, Toye R: Occupational dream, relation to parents and depression in the early adult transition. J Clin Psychol 40:945–954, 1984

Goodman MJ: Age at menopause in relation to reproductive history in Japanese, Caucasian, Chinese and Hawaiian women living in Hawaii. J Gerontol 33:688–694, 1978

Goodman MJ: Patterns of menopause: a study of certain medical and physiological variables among Caucasian and Japanese women living in Hawaii. J Gerontol 32:291–298, 1977

Goodwin DW, Guze SB: Psychiatric Diagnosis, 2nd Edition. New York, Oxford University Press, 1979

Goodwin J: Evaluation and treatment of incest victims and their families: a problem-oriented approach, in Modern Perspectives in Psychosocial Pathology. Edited by Howells J. New York, Brunner/Mazel, 1988, pp 43–57

Gorer G: Death, Grief and Mourning. New York, Doubleday, 1965

Gorman JM, Levy GF, Liebowitz MR, et al: Effect of acute ß-adrenergic blockade on lactate-induced panic. Arch Gen Psychiatry 40:1079–1082, 1983

Gorman JM, Askanazi J, Liebowitz MR, et al: Response to hyperventilation in a group of patients with panic disorder. Am J Psychiatry 141:857–861, 1984

Gottman JM, Krokoff LJ: Marital interaction and satisfaction: a longitudinal view. J Consult Clin Psychol 57:47–52, 1989

Gould MS, Shaffer D: The impact of suicide in television movies: evidence of imitation. N Engl J Med 315:690–694, 1986

Gove WR: Sex, marital status and mortality. American Journal of Sociology 79:45–67, 1973

Gray LA, Christopherson WM, Hoover RN: Estrogens and endometrial carcinoma. Obstet Gynecol 49:385–389, 1977

Green BL: A Clinical Approach to Marital Problems: Evaluation and Management. Springfield, IL, Charles C Thomas, 1970

Green JW, Keown M: Depression and suicide in children and adolescents. Compr Ther 12:38–43, 1986

Green R: Human sexuality: research and treatment frontiers, in American Handbook of Psychiatry, Vol 1. Edited by Arieti S. New York, Basic Books, 1976, pp 665–691

Green R, Dalton R: Premenstrual syndrome. BMJ 1:1007–1014, 1953

Greenacre P: Human sexuality: research and treatment frontiers, in American Handbook of Psychiatry. Edited by Arieti S. New York, Basic Books, 1948, pp 665–691

Greenacre P: Anatomical structure and superego development (1948), in Trauma, Growth, and Personality. New York, International Universities Press, 1952a, pp 149–164

Greenacre P: Some factors producing different types of genital and pregenital organization, in Trauma, Growth, and Personality. New York, International Universities Press, 1952b, pp 293–302

Greenacre P: Certain relationships between fetishism and the faulty development of the body image (1953a), in Emotional Growth: Psychoanalytic Studies of the Gifted and a Great Variety of Other Individuals, Vol 1. New York, International Universities Press, 1971, pp 9–30

Greenacre P: Penis awe and its relation to penis envy (1953b), in Emotional Growth: Psychoanalytic Studies of the Gifted and a Great Variety of Other Individuals, Vol 1. New York, International Universities Press, 1971b, pp 31–49

Greenbaum E: Unfolding of identifications: repetition and change in identity formation. J Am Acad Psychoanal 1:125–143, 1973

Greenbaum H: On the nature of marriage and marriage therapy. J Am Acad Psychoanal 11:284–297, 1983

Greenblatt DJ, Shader R: Benzodiazepines in Clinical Practice. New York, Raven, 1974

Greene JG, Cook DJ: Life stress and symptoms at the climacterium. Br J Psychiatry 136:486–491, 1980

Greganti MA, Fletcher SW: House staff pregnancy in internal medicine residencies. Ann Intern Med 102:123–125, 1985

Guicheney P, Leger D, Barrat J, et al: Platelet serotonin content and plasma tryptophan in peri- and postmenopausal women: variations with plasma estrogen levels and depressive symptoms. Eur J Clin Invest 18:297–304, 1988

Guinan ME, Hardy A: Epidemiology of AIDS in women in the United States, 1981–1986. JAMA 261:2039–2042, 1987

Gunther J: Death Be Not Proud. New York, Harper & Row, 1949

Gur RC, Gur RE, Obrist WD, et al: Sex and handedness differences in cerebral blood flow during rest and cognitive activity. Science 217:256–261, 1982

Gur RC, Erwin RJ, Gur RE: Neurobehavioral probes for physiological neuroimaging studies. Arch Gen Psychiatry 49:409–414, 1992

Gurdus L: The Death Train. New York, National Council on Art in Jewish Life, 1978

Gutek BA: Sex and the Workplace: The Impact of Sexual Behavior and Harassment on Women, Men, and Organizations. San Francisco, CA, Jossey-Bass, 1985

Guttman HA: Autonomy and motherhood. Psychiatry 46:230–235, 1983

Haglund RMJ, Schuckit MA: The epidemiology of alcoholism, in Alcoholism: Development, Consequences and Interventions. Edited by Estes N, Heinemann E. St Louis, MO, CV Mosby, 1982, pp 32–48

Hall E: The gynaecologist and artificial reproduction. Journal of Psychosomatic Obstetrics and Gynaecology 4:317–320, 1985

Hamilton JA, Alagna SW, King LS, et al: The emotional consequences of gender-based abuse in the workplace: new counseling programs for sex discrimination, in Women, Power, and Therapy: Issues for Women. Edited by Braude M. New York, Haworth Press, 1988, pp 155–182

Hankoff CD: Suicide and attempted suicide, in Handbook of Affective Disorders. Edited by Paykel ES. New York, Guilford, 1982, pp 416–428

Hanneke CR, Shields NM, McCall GJ: Assessing the prevalence of marital rape. Journal of Interpersonal Violence 1:350–361, 1986

Hansson RO, Remondet JH: Old age and widowhood: issues of personal control and independence. Journal of Social Issues 44:159, 1988

Hansson RO, Jones WH, Carpenter BN, et al: Loneliness and adjustment to old age. Int J Aging Hum Dev 24:41–53, 1986

Harding JJ: Post partum psychiatric disorders: a review. Compr Psychiatry 30:109–112, 1989

Hardy JB: Premature sexual activity, pregnancy, and sexually transmitted diseases: the pediatrician's role as counselor. Pediatr Rev 10:69–76, 1988

Harlow HF, Harlow MK: The effect of rearing conditions on behavior. Bull Menninger Clin 26:213–224, 1962

Harlow HF, Harlow MK: Learning to love. American Scientist 54:244–247, 1966

Harmsworth HC, Minnis M: Non-statutory causes of divorce: the lawyers' point of view. Marriage and Family Living 17:316–321, 1955

Harvey M, Koss MP: The Rape Victim: Clinical and Community Approaches to Treatment. Lexington, MA, Greene Press, 1987

Havighurst RJ: Developmental Tasks and Education. New York, Longmans Green, 1948

Heinemann GD, Evans PL: Widowhood: loss, change, and adaptation, in Family Relationships in Later Life, 2nd Edition. Edited by Brubaker TH. Newbury Park, CA, Sage, 1990, pp 142–168

Heiss J: On the transmission of marital instability in black families. American Sociological Review 37:82–92, 1972

Hennig M, Jardim A: The Managerial Woman. New York, Anchor Press/Doubleday, 1977

Henshaw S, O'Reilly R: Characteristics of abortion patients in the United States, 1979–80. Fam Plann Perspect 15:5–16, 1983

Herman J, Russell D, Trocki K: Long-term effects of incestuous abuse in childhood. Am J Psychiatry 143:1293–1296, 1986

Herman JL (with Hirschman L): Father-Daughter Incest. Cambridge, MA, Harvard University Press, 1981

Heyman DK, Gianturco DT: Long-term adaptation by the elderly to bereavement. J Gerontol 28:359–363, 1973

Hilberman [Carmen] EH: The Rape Victim. Washington, DC, American Psychiatric Association, 1976

Hilberman E: Overview: the "Wife-Beater's Wife" reconsidered. Am J Psychiatry 137:1336–1347, 1980 [Reprinted in The Gender Gap in Psychotherapy: Social Realities and Psychological Processes. Edited by Rieker PP, Carmen EH. New York, Plenum, 1984, pp 213–236]

Hilberman E, Munson K: Sixty battered women. Victimology: An International Journal 2:460–471, 1977–1978

Hochschild A (with Machung A): The Second Shift. New York, Avon Books, 1989

Hoefel BG, Liebowitz SF: Brain monoamines in the modulation of self stimulation, feeding, and body weight. Res Publ Assoc Res Nerv Ment Dis 59:103–147, 1981

Hofferth SL: Teenage pregnancy and its resolution, in Risking the Future. Edited by Hofferth SL, Hayes CD. Washington, DC, National Academy Press, 1987, pp 78–92

Hoffman, Dustin. New York Times, December 21, 1983, pp 6–11

Hollander E, Liebowitz MR, Gorman JM: Anxiety disorders, in American Psychiatric Press Textbook of Psychiatry. Edited by Talbott JA, Hales RE, Yudofsky SC. Washington, DC, American Psychiatric Press, 1987, pp 443–491

Holmes TH, Rahe RH: The social readjustment rating scale. J Psychosom Res 11:213–218, 1967–1968

Holroyd JC, Brodsky AM: Psychologists' attitudes and practices regarding erotic and non-erotic physical contact with patients. Am Psychol 32:843–849, 1977

Holroyd JC, Brodsky AM: Does touching patients lead to sexual intercourse? Professional Psychology: Research and Practice 11:807–811, 1980

Hopkins J, Marcus N, Campbell S: Post partum depression: a critical review. Psychol Bull 95:498–515, 1984

Horner MS: Toward an understanding of achievement-related conflicts in women. Journal of Social Issues 28:157–175, 1972

Horney K: The flight from womanhood: the masculinity-complex in women as viewed by men and women. Int J Psychoanal 7:324–339, 1926 [Reprinted in Miller JB: Psychoanalysis and Women: Contributions to New Theory and Therapy. New York, Brunner/Mazel, 1973, pp 3–16]

Horney K: The dread of woman: observations on a specific difference in the dread felt by men and by women respectively for the opposite sex. Int J Psychoanal 13:348–360, 1932

Horney K: The denial of the vagina: a contribution to the problem of the genital anxieties specific to women (1933a), in Horney K: Feminine Psychology. Edited by Kelman H. New York, WW Norton, 1967, pp 147–161

Horney K: The problem of feminine masochism (1933b), in Horney K: Feminine Psychology. Edited by Kelman H. New York, WW Norton, 1967, pp 214–233

Horney K: Feminine Psychology. Edited by Kelman H. New York, WW Norton, 1967

Hornig M: The impact of welfare payment levels on family stability, in The Family Poverty and Welfare Programs: Factors Influencing Family Instability (Studies in Public Welfare 12). Edited by Joint Economic Committee. Washington, DC, U.S. Government Printing Office, 1973

Hornung CA, McCullough BC, Sugimoto T: Status relationships in marriage: risk factors in spouse abuse. Journal of Marriage and the Family 43:675–692, 1981

Horowitz MJ: Stress Response Syndromes. New York, Jason Aronson, 1976

Horowitz MJ: A model of mourning: change in schemas of self and other. J Am Psychoanal Assoc 38:297–324, 1990

Horowitz MJ, Wilner N, Marmar C, et al: Pathological grief and the activity of latent self-images. Am J Psychiatry 137:1157–1162, 1980

Hott JR: The telephone rape: crisis intervention for an obscene phone call. Issues in Health Care of Women 4:107–113, 1983

Hotta M, Shibasaki T, Masuda A, et al: The responses of plasma adrenocorticotropin and cortisol to corticotropin-releasing hormone and cerebrospinal immunoreactive CRH in anorexia nervosa patients. J Clin Endocrinol Metab 62:319–324, 1986

Hoyt JR: The telephone rape: crisis intervention for an obscene phone call. Issues in Health Care of Women 4:107–113, 1984

Hudson JI, Pope HG Jr: Depression and eating disorders, in Presentations of Depression: Depression in Medical and Other Psychiatric Disorders. Edited by Cameron OG. New York, Wiley, 1987, pp 33–66

Hughes HM, Rav TJ: Psychological adjustment of battered women in shelters. Paper presented at the American Psychological Association Meetings, Toronto, August 1984

Hughes JO, Sandler BR: In Case of Sexual Harassment: A Guide for Women Students. Washington, DC, Project on the Status and Education of Women, Association of American Colleges, 1986

Hunt JG, Hunt LL: The dualities of careers and families: new integrations or new polarizations? Social Problems 29:499–510, 1982

Hunt M, Hunt B: The Divorce Experience, New York, McGraw-Hill, 1977

Hyman DA: Aesthetics and ethics: the implications of cosmetic surgery. Perspect Biol Med 33:190–202, 1990

Iddenden DA: Sexuality during the menopause. Med Clin North Am 71:87–94, 1987

Idiculla AA, Goldberg G: Physical fitness for the mature woman. Med Clin North Am 71:135–143, 1987

Imboden JP, Urbaitis JC: Practical Psychiatry in Medicine. New York, Appleton-Century-Crofts, 1978

Inciardi JA: Over-the-counter drugs: epidemiology, adverse reactions, overdose deaths, and mass media promotion. International Journal of Addictive Diseases 3:253–272, 1977

Inglis A, Greenglass ER: Motivation for marriage among women and men. Psychol Rep 65:1035–1042, 1989

Isay RA: Being Homosexual: Gay Men and Their Development. New York, Farrar, Straus & Giroux, 1989

Isselbacher KJ, Adams RD, Braunwald E, et al (eds): Harrison's Principles of Internal Medicine, 9th Edition, Vol 1. New York, McGraw-Hill, 1980

Jacobs SC, Kim K: Psychiatric complications of bereavement. Psychiatric Annals 20:314–317, 1990

Jacobs SC, Nelson JC, Zisook S: Treating depressions of bereavement with antidepressants; a pilot study. Psychiatr Clin North Am 10:501–511, 1987

Jacobson E: Development of the wish for a child in boys. Psychoanal Study Child 5:139–152, 1950

Jacobson E: The Self and the Object World. New York, International Universities Press, 1964

Jacobson GF: The Multiple Crises of Marital Separation and Divorce. New York, Grune & Stratton, 1983

Jacobson NS, Bussod N: Marital and family therapy, in The Clinical Psychology Handbook. Edited by Hersen M, Kazdin AE, Bellard AK. New York, Pergamon, 1983, pp 611–630

Jaffe JH: Drug addiction and drug abuse, in The Pharmacological Basis of Therapeutics. Edited by Goodman LS, Gilman A. New York, Macmillan, 1980, pp 535–584

Jamison KR, Wellisch D, Pasnau RO, et al: Psychosocial aspects of mastectomy, I: the woman's perspective. Am J Psychiatry 135:432–436, 1978

Jaszmann L, Van Lith WP, Zaat JLA: The perimenopausal symptoms; the statistical analysis of a survey. Med Gynaecol Sociol 4:268, 1969

Jehu D: Beyond Sexual Abuse: Therapy With Women Who Were Childhood Victims. Chichester, UK, Wiley, 1988

Jehu D, Gazan M, Klassen C: Therapy With Women Who Were Sexually Abused in Childhood, Part 8: Stress Disorders. Winnipeg, University of Manitoba, Psychological Services Center, 1987

Jessner L, Welgern E, Farg J: The development of parental attitudes during pregnancy, in Parenthood. Edited by Anthony EJ, Benedek T. Boston, MA, Little, Brown, 1986, pp 209–245

Johnson CL: Dyadic family relationships and social support. The Gerontologist 23:377–383, 1983

Johnson CL, Johnson FA: Parenthood, marriage and careers: situational constraints and role strain, in Dual-Career Couples. Edited by Pepitone-Rockwell F. Beverly Hills, CA, Sage, 1980

Johnston GD, Bachman JF, O'Malley PM: Highlights from student drug use in America, 1975–78 (DHHS Publ No ADM-82-1208). Rockville, MD, National Institute on Drug Abuse, 1979

Johnstone EC, Cunningham Owens DG, Frith CD, et al: Neurotic illness and its response to anxiolytic and antidepressant treatment. Psychol Med 10:321–328, 1980

Jolleys JV: Reported prevalence of urinary incontinence in women in a general practice. BMJ 296:1300–1302, 1988

Jones E: Early development of female sexuality. Int J Psychoanal 8:459–472, 1927

Jones E: Early female sexuality. Int J Psychoanal 16:263–273, 1935

Jones E: The Life and Work of Sigmund Freud, Vol 1–3. New York, Basic Books, 1955

Jordan JV: The meaning of mutuality. The Stone Center for Developmental Services and Studies, Work in Progress, Wellesley, MA, 1986, No 86, p 23

Jordan J, Surrey J, Kaplan A: Women and empathy: implications for psychological development and psychotherapy. The Stone Center for Developmental Services and Studies, Work in Progress, Wellesley, MA, 1983, No 82

Josselyn IM: The capacity to love: a possible reformulation. Journal of the American Academy of Child Psychiatry 10:6–22, 1971

Kahn RJ, McNair DM, Lipman RS, et al: Imipramine and chlordiazepoxide in depression and anxiety disorders, II: efficacy in anxious outpatients. Arch Gen Psychiatry 43:79–85, 1986

Kalogerakis MG: The Emotionally Troubled Adolescent and the Family Physician. Springfield, IL, Charles C Thomas, 1973

Kansky J: Sexuality of widows: a study of the sexual practices of widows during the first fourteen months of bereavement. J Sex Marital Ther 12:307–321, 1986

Kaplan EH: Career change in early adulthood: developmental considerations. Adolesc Psychiatry 16:259–277, 1989

Kaplan HI, Sadock BJ: Synopsis of Psychiatry: Behavioral Sciences, Clinical Psychiatry, 5th Edition. Baltimore, MD, Williams & Wilkins, 1988

Kaplan HI, Freedman A, Sadock BJ: Comprehensive Textbook of Psychiatry/V, 5th Edition. Baltimore, MD, Williams & Wilkins, 1985

Kaplan HS: Disorders of Sexual Desire. New York, Brunner/Mazel, 1979

Karahanasoglu A, Barglow P, Grow G: Psychological aspects of infertility. J Reprod Med 9:241–247, 1972

Kardener SH, Fuller M, Mensh IN: A survey of physicians' attitudes and practices regarding erotic and nonerotic contact with patients. Am J Psychiatry 130:1077–1081, 1973

Karme L: A clinical report of penis envy: its multiple meanings and defensive function. J Am Psychoanal Assoc 29:427–446, 1981

Katan A: Children who were raped. Psychoanal Study Child 28:208–224, 1973

Kaufert P: Myth and the menopause. Sociology of Health and Illness 4:141–166, 1982

Kaufert PA, Gilbert P: Women, menopause and medicalization. Cult Med Psychiatry 10:7–21, 1986

Kaye WH, Gwirtsman HE, George DT, et al: Elevated cerebrospinal fluid levels of immunoreactive corticotropin-releasing hormone in anorexia nervosa: relation to state of nutrition, adrenal function, and intensity of depression. J Clin Endocrinol Metab 64:203–208, 1987

Kaye WH, Gwirtsman HE, Breweston FD, et al: Binging behavior and plasma amino acids: a possible involvement of brain serotonin in bulimia nervosa. Psychiatry Res 23:31–43, 1988

Keiser S: Female sexuality. J Am Psychoanal Assoc 4:563–574, 1956

Kelly EE: Marital compatibility as related to personality traits of husbands and wives as rated by self and spouse. J Soc Psychol 13:193–198, 1941

Kendell RE: Emotional and physical factors in the genesis of puerperal mental disorders. J Psychosom Res 29:3–11, 1985

Kerchoff AC: The social context of interpersonal attraction, in Foundation of Interpersonal Attractions. Edited by Huston TL. New York, Academic, 1974, pp 61–78

Kernberg OF: Barriers to falling and remaining in love. J Am Psychoanal Assoc 22:486–511, 1974a

Kernberg OF: Mature love: prerequisites and characteristics. J Am Psychoanal Assoc 22:743–768, 1974b

Kertzner R: The psychiatric aspects of AIDS and HIV infection. Unpublished manuscript, Psychiatric Medicine, Columbia University College of Physicians and Surgeons, January 1989

Kestenberg JS: On the development of maternal feelings in early childhood: observations and reflections. Psychoanal Study Child 11:275–291, 1956a

Kestenberg JS: Vicissitudes of female sexuality. J Am Psychoanal Assoc 4:453–576, 1956b

Kestenberg JS: Outside and inside, male and female. J Am Psychoanal Assoc 16:457–520, 1968

Kestenberg JS: Children and Parents: Psychoanalytic Studies in Development. New York, Jason Aronson, 1975

Kestenberg JS: Psychoanalytic Studies in Development. New York, Jason Aronson, 1978

Keye WR, Hammond DC, Strong C: Medical and psychologic characteristics of women presenting with menstrual symptoms. Obstet Gynecol 68:634–637, 1986

Keys A, Brozek J, Henshel A, et al: The Biology of Human Starvation. Minneapolis, MN, Minnesota University Press, 1950

Kilpatrick DG, Veronen LJ, Resick PA: The aftermath of rape: recent empirical findings. Am J Orthopsychiatry 49:658–669, 1979

Kilpatrick DG, Veronen LJ, Resick PA: Effects of a rape experience: a longitudinal study. Journal of Social Issues 37:(4)105–122, 1981

Kilpatrick DG, Best CL, Veronen LJ, et al: Mental health correlates of criminal victimization: a random community survey. J Consult Clin Psychol 53:866–873, 1985

Kipper D, Zigler-Shani Z, Sern D: Psychogenic infertility, neuroticism and the female role: a methodological inquiry. J Psychosomat Res 221:353–358, 1977

Kirkpatrick C: Community of interest and the measurement of adjustment in marriage. The Family 18:133–137, 1937

Kirkpatrick M: Some clinical perception of middle-aged divorcing women, in Divorce as a Developmental Process. Edited by Gold JH. Washington, DC, American Psychiatric Press, 1988, pp 79–99

Kitson GC, Zyzanski SJ: Grief in widowhood and divorce. Psychiatr Clin North Am 10:369–386, 1987

Klaus MH, Kennell JH: Maternal-Infant Bonding: The Impact of Early Separation or Loss on Family Development. St Louis, MO, CV Mosby, 1976

Kleber H: Cocaine abuse: historical, epidemiological, and psychological perspectives. J Clin Psychiatry 49:3–7, 1988

Kleber RJ: A double-blind comparative study of desipramine hydrochloride and diazepam in the control of mixed anxiety/depression symptomatology. J Clin Psychiatry 40:165–170, 1979

Kleeman J: The establishment of core gender identity in normal girls, introduction: development of ego capacity to differentiate. Arch Sex Behav 1:117–129, 1971

Kleeman J: Genital self-stimulation in infant and toddler girls, in From Infancy to Senescence. Edited by Marcus I, Francis JJ. New York, International Universities Press, 1975, pp 97–106

Klein DF: Delineation of two drug-responsive anxiety syndromes. Psychopharmacologia 5:397–408, 1964

Klein DF: Anxiety reconceptualized, in Anxiety: New Research and Changing Concepts. Edited by Klein DF, Rabkin JG. New York, Raven, 1981, pp 235–265

Klein F: Sexual harassment in federal employment: factors affecting its incidence, severity, duration and relationship to productivity. Doctoral dissertation, Brandeis University, Waltham, MA, 1984

Klein F: The 1988 Working Women Sexual Harassment Report. Executive Report, Klein Associates, Cambridge, MA, 1988

Klein F: Sexual Harassment in Massachusetts trial courts and the legal profession: implications from the gender bias study. Boston Bar Journal, July/August 1989a, pp 17–19

Klein F: Unpublished survey of sexual harassment in a university system. Cambridge, MA, Klein Associates, 1989b

Klein M: Early stages of the oedipus conflict. Int J Psychoanal 9:167–180, 1928

Klein M: The Psychoanalysis of Children. London, Hogarth Press, 1932

Klein M: A contribution to the psychogenesis of manic-depressive states. Int J Psychoanal 16:145–174, 1935

Klein M: Mourning and its relation to manic depressive states. Int J Psychoanal 21:125–153, 1940

Klein M (with Joan Reviere): Love, Hate and Reparation. London, Hogarth Press, 1953

Kleinberg L: Coming home to self, going home to parents: lesbian identity disclosure. The Stone Center for Developmental Services and Studies, Work in Progress, Wellesley, MA, 1986, No 86-24:1–16

Klingbeil KS, Boyd VD: Emergency room intervention: detection, assessment, and treatment, in Battered Women and Their Families: Intervention Strategies and Treatment Programs. Edited by Roberts AR. New York, Springer, 1984, pp 7–32

Kluft RP: Childhood Antecedents of Multiple Personality. Washington, DC, American Psychiatric Press, 1985

Kluft RP: Treating the patient who has been sexually exploited by a previous therapist. Psychiatr Clin North Am 12:483-500, 1989

Kluft RP, Braun B, Sachs R: Multiple personality intrafamilial abuse and family psychiatry. Int J Fam Psychiatry 5:283–301, 1985

Kohlberg L: A cognitive-developmental analysis of children's sex role concepts and attitudes, in The Development of Sex Differences. Edited by Maccoby E. Stanford, CA, Stanford University Press, 1966, pp 82–173

Kohut H: The Analysis of the Self: A Systematic Approach to the Psychoanalytic Treatment of Narcissistic Personality Disorders. New York, International Universities Press, 1971

Kohut H: The Restoration of the Self. New York, International Universities Press, 1977

Korner AF: Sex differences in newborns with special reference to differences in the organization of oral behavior. J Child Psychol Psychiatry 14:19–29, 1973

Korsten MA, Matsuzaki S, Feinman L, et al: High blood acetaldehyde levels after ethanol administration: difference between alcoholic and non-alcoholic subjects. N Engl J Med 292:386–389, 1975

Koss MP: The hidden rape victim: personality, attitudinal and situational characteristics. Psychology of Women Quarterly 9(2):193–212, 1985

Koss MP, Leonard KE: Sexually aggressive men: a review of empirical findings, in Pornography and Sexual Aggression. Edited by Malamuth NM, Donnerstein E. Orlando, FL, Academic, 1984, pp 213–232

Koss MP, Oros CJ: Sexual Experiences Survey: a research instrument investigating sexual aggression and victimization. J Consult Clin Psychol 50:455–457, 1982

Koss MP, Gidycz CA, Wisniewski N: The scope of rape: incidence and prevalence of sexual aggression and victimization in a national sample of higher education students. J Consult Clin Psychol 55:162–170, 1987

Kraft AD, Palombo J, Mitchell D, et al: The psychological dimensions of infertility. Am J Orthopsychiatry 50:618–628, 1980

Krausz SL: Sex roles within marriage. Social Work 31:457–464, 1986

Kressel K: The Process of Divorce: How Professionals and Couples Negotiate Settlements. New York, Basic Books, 1985

Krugman S: Trauma in the family: perspectives on the intergenerational transmission of violence, in Psychological Trauma. Edited by van der Kolk BA. Washington, DC, American Psychiatric Press, 1987, pp 127–151

Krystal H: The impact of massive psychic trauma and the capacity to grieve effectively, in Treating the Elderly With Psychotherapy. Edited by Sadavoy J, Leszcz M. Madison, CT, International Universities Press, 1987, pp 95–156

Krystal H: Integration and Self-Healing: Affect, Trauma, Alexithymia. Hillsdale, NJ, Analytic Press, 1988

Kuchan A: Survey of incidence of psychotherapists' sexual contact with clients in Wisconsin, in Psychotherapists' Sexual Involvement With Clients: Intervention and Prevention. Edited by Schoener GR, Milgrom JH, Gonsiorek JC, et al. Minneapolis, MN, Walk-In Counseling Center, 1989, pp 51–64

Kuhl AF: Personality traits of abused women: masochism myth refuted. Victimology: An International Journal 9:450–463, 1984

Kumar R, Robson KM: A prospective study of emotional disorders in childbearing women. Br J Psychiatry 144:35–47, 1984

LaFarge L: Emptiness as defense in severe regressive states. J Am Psychoanal Assoc 37:965–995, 1989

Lalos A, Lalos O, Jacobson L, et al: A psychosocial characterization of infertile couples before surgical treatment of the female. Journal of Psychosomatic Obstetrics and Gynaecology 4:83–93, 1985

Lampl de Groot A: The evolution of the oedipus conflict in women. Int J Psychoanal 9:332–345, 1928

Lampl de Groot J: On the process of mourning. Psychoanal Study Child 38:9–13, 1983

Lansky SB: Childhood leukemia: the child psychiatrist as a member of the oncology team. Journal of the American Academy of Child Psychiatry 13:499–508, 1974

Law Enforcement Assistance Administration: Criminal Victimization Surveys in 13 American Cities. Washington DC, U.S. Government Printing Office, 1975

Laws JL: The psychology of tokenism: an analysis. Sex Roles 1:51–67, 1975

Lax R: The expectable depressive climacteric reaction. Bull Menninger Clin 46:151–167, 1982

Lazare C: The adoptive parents experience, in Infertility: Medical, Emotional, and Social Considerations. Edited by Mazor M, Simons H. New York, Human Sciences Press, 1984, p 108

Lebe DM: Female ego ideal conflicts in adulthood. Am J Psychoanal 46:22–32, 1986

Lee MJ, Hoffman R: Correlation of chemistry and history risk factors for osteoporosis. Ann N Y Acad Sci 592:441–442, 1990

Lenhart SA, Klein F, Falcao P, et al: Gender bias against and sexual harassment of AMWA members in Massachusetts. J Am Med Wom Assoc 46:121–125, 1991

Lennon MC: The psychological consequences of menopause: the importance of timing of a strange life event. J Health Soc Behav 23:353–366, 1982

Lerner HE: Early origins of envy and devaluation of women: implications for sex role stereotypes. Bull Menninger Clin 38:538–553, 1974a

Lerner HE: The hysterical personality: a "woman's" disease. Compr Psychiatry 15:157–164, 1974b

Lerner HE: Internal prohibitions against female anger. Am J Psychoanal 40:137–148, 1980

Lerner HE: Female dependency in context: some theoretical and technical considerations. Am J Orthopsychiatry 53:697–705, 1983

Lerner HE: The Dance of Anger. New York, Harper & Row, 1985

Lerner HG: Work and success inhibitions in women: family systems level interventions in psychodynamic treatment. Bull Menninger Clin 51:338–360, 1987

Lester EP, Notman MT: Pregnancy, developmental crisis and object relations: psychoanalytic considerations. Int J Psychoanal 67:357–366, 1986

Lester EP, Notman MT: Pregnancy and object relations: clinical considerations. Psychoanalytic Inquiry 8:196–221, 1988

Levan I: Mortality and psychopathology following the death of an adult child: an epidemiologic review. Isr J Psychiatry Relat Sci 119:23–38, 1982

Levenkron S: The Best Little Girl in the World. New York, Warner Books, 1978

Levinger G: Marital cohesiveness and dissolution: an integrative review. Journal of Marriage and the Family 27:19–28, 1965

Lewis SNC, Cooper CL: The transition to parenthood in dual-earner couples. Psychol Med 18:477–486, 1988

Lewittes HJ: Just being friendly means a lot—women, friendship and aging, in Women in the Later Years. Edited by Gray L. New York, Haworth Press, 1989, pp 139–159

Lieberman MA, Videka-Sherman L: The impact of self-help groups on the mental health of widows and widowers. Am J Orthopsychiatry 56:435–449, 1986

Lindberg F, Distad L: Post-traumatic stress disorder in women who experienced childhood incest. Child Abuse Negl 9:329–334, 1985

Lindemann E: Symptomatology and management of acute grief. Am J Psychiatry 101:141–148, 1944

Lindemann E: Beyond Grief: Studies in Crisis Intervention. New York, Jason Aronson, 1979

Lindsay R, Cosman F: Estrogen in prevention and treatment of osteoporosis. Ann N Y Acad Sci 592:326–333, 1990

Lindsay R, Hart DM, MacLean A, et al: Bone response to termination of oestrogen treatment. Lancet 1:1325–1327, 1978

Livingston R: Sexually and physically abused children. Journal of the American Academy of Child Psychiatry 26:413–415, 1987

Lobo RA: Cardiovascular implications of estrogen replacement therapy. Obstet Gynecol 75:18S–35S, 1990

Lock M: Models and practice in medicine: menopause as syndrome or life transition. Cult Med Psychiatry 7:261–280, 1982

Locke HJ: Predicting Adjustment in Marriage: A Comparison of a Divorced and Happily Married Group. New York, Henry Holt, 1951

Loebuck JB, Kessler RG: The Etiology of Alcoholism. Springfield, IL, Charles C Thomas, 1971

Loewinsohn RJ: Survival Handbook for Widows. Glenview, IL, Scott, Foresman & Company, 1984

London RS, Murphy L, Ktlowski KE, et al: Efficacy of alpha-tocopherol in the treatment of premenstrual syndrome. J Reprod Med 32:400–404, 1987

Loombs M: By food possessed. Women's Sports, February 1982, pp 12–18

Lopata HZ: Widowhood in an American City. Cambridge, MA, Schenkman, 1973

Lopata HZ: Women as Widows: Support Systems. New York, Elsevier, 1979

Lopata HZ: Widows: North America, in Widows, Vol 2: North America. Edited by Lopata HZ. Durham, NC, Duke University Press, 1987, pp 3–31

Lopata HZ: Support systems of American urban widowhood. Journal of Social Issues 44:113–128, 1988

Luepker ET: Clinical assessment of clients who have been sexually exploited by their therapists and development of differential treatment plans, in Psychotherapists' Sexual Involvement With Clients: Intervention and Prevention. Edited by Schoener GR, Milgrom JH, Gonsiorek JC, et al. Minneapolis, MN, Walk-In Counseling Center, 1989a, pp 159–176

Luepker ET: Time-limited treatment/support groups for clients who have been sexually exploited by therapists: a nine-year perspective, in Psychotherapists' Sexual Involvement With Clients: Intervention and Prevention. Edited by Schoener GR, Milgrom JH, Gonsiorek JC, et al. Minneapolis, MN, Walk-In Counseling Center, 1989b, pp 181–194

Lynn DB: Intellectual development of women, in Dual-Career Couples. Edited by Pepitone-Rockwell F. Beverly Hills, CA, Sage, 1980, pp 55–71

Maccoby E, Jacklin C: The Psychology of Sex Differences. Stanford, CA, Stanford University Press, 1974

Mack TM, Pike MC, Henderson BE, et al: Estrogens and endometrial cancer in a retirement community. N Engl J Med 294:1262–1267, 1976

Maddison D, Viola A: The health of widows in the year following bereavement. J Psychosom Res 12:297–306, 1968

Maddison D, Walker WL: Factors affecting the outcome of conjugal bereavement. Br J Psychiatry 113:1057–1067, 1967

Mahler MS: Thoughts about development and individuation. Psychoanal Study Child 18:307–324, 1963

Mahler MS: On human symbiosis and the vicissitudes of individualism. J Am Psychoanal Assoc 15:740–763, 1967

Mahler MS, Furer M: Certain aspects of the separation-individuation phase. Psychoanal Q 32:1–14, 1963

Mahler MS, La Perriere K: Mother-child interaction during separation-individuation. Psychoanal Q 34:483–498, 1965

Mahler MS, Pine F, Bergman A: The Psychological Birth of the Human Infant: Symbiosis and Individuation. London, Hutchinson and Company, 1975

Mahlstedt P: The psychological component of infertility. Fertil Steril 43:335–346, 1985

Mai FM, Munday RN, Rump EE: Psychiatric interview comparisons between infertile and fertile couples. Psychosom Med 34:431–440, 1972

Main TF: Mutual projection in a marriage. Compr Psychiatry 7:432–449, 1966

Major B, Mueller P, Hildebrandt K: Attributions, expectations, and coping with abortion. J Pers Soc Psychol 48:585–599, 1985

Malatesta UJ, Chambless DL, Pollack M, et al: Widowhood, sexuality and aging: a life span analysis. J Sex Marital Ther 14:49–62, 1988

Margolin G, Sibner LG, Gleberman L: Wife battering, in Handbook of Family Violence. Edited by Van Hasselt VB, Morrison RL, Bellack AS, et al. New York, Plenum, 1988, pp 89–117

Margolis M: A preliminary report of a case of consummated mother/son incest. Annual of Psychoanalysis 5:276–294, 1977

Margolis M: A case of mother-adolescent son incest: a follow-up study. Psychoanal Q 53:355–385, 1984

Marks I, Lader M: Anxiety states (anxiety neurosis): a review. J Nerv Ment Dis 156:3–18, 1973

Marks J: The Benzodiazepines: Use, Overuse, Misuse, and Abuse. Lancaster, UK, MT-P Press, 1978

Marks SR: Multiple roles and role strain. American Sociological Review 42:921–936, 1977

Marmar CR, Horowitz MJ, Weiss DS, et al: A controlled trial of brief psychotherapy and mutual help group treatment of conjugal bereavement. Am J Psychiatry 145:203–209, 1988

Martin CA, Warfield MC, Braen GR: Psychotherapy of rape. Current Psychiatric Therapies 23:65–73, 1986

Martin D: Battered Wives. San Francisco, CA, Glide, 1976

Martin PA: A Marital Therapy Manual. New York, Brunner/Mazel, 1976

Masotti M, Guidotti A, Costa E: Characterization of benzodiazepine and gamma-aminobutyric acid recognition sites and their hydrogenous modulators. J Neurosci 1:409–418, 1981

Masters W, Johnson V: Human Sexual Response. Boston, Little, Brown, 1966

Masters WH, Johnson JE: Human Sexual Inadequacy. Boston, MA, Little, Brown, 1970

May R: Love and Will. New York, WW Norton, 1969

Mayer EL: "Everybody must be just like me": observations on female castration anxiety. Int J Psychoanal 66:331–347, 1985

McAnarney R, McAnarney MD, Hendee WR: Adolescent pregnancy and its consequences. JAMA July 7, 1988, p 76

McCombie SL (ed): The Rape Crisis Intervention Handbook: A Guide for Victim Care. New York, Plenum, 1980

McCormick MC, Shapiro S, Starfield B: High risk mothers: infant mortality and morbidity in four areas in the United States, 1973–78. Am J Public Health 79:18–23, 1984

McCrae RR, Costa Jr PT: Psychological resilience among widowed men and women: a 10-year follow-up of a national sample. Journal of Social Issues 44:129–142, 1988

McDermott N, Cobbs S: A psychiatric survey of fifty cases of bronchial asthma. Psychosom Med 1:203–244, 1939

McDonald TW, Annegers JF, O'Fallon WM: Exogenous estrogen and endometrial carcinoma; case control and incidence study. Am J Obstet Gynecol 127:572–580, 1977

McFarlane AC, McFarlane CM, Gilchrist PN: Posttraumatic bulimia and anorexia nervosa. International Journal of Eating Disorders 7:705–708, 1988

McGuire D: Psychological management of infertile women. Postgrad Med 57:173, 1975

McIntire MS, Angle CK: Evaluation of suicidal risk in adolescents. J Fam Pract 2:339–341, 1975

McIntosh P: Feeling like a fraud. The Stone Center for Developmental Services and Studies, Work in Progress, Wellesley, MA, 1985, No 85-03:1–11

McKenny P, Tishler C, Keeley C: Adolescent suicide: a comparison of attempters and non-attempters in an emergency room population. Clin Pediatr (Phila) 21:266–270, 1982

McKinlay S, Jefferys M: The menopausal syndrome. British Journal of Preventive and Social Medicine 28:108–115, 1974

McKinlay S, McKinlay J: Selected studies on the menopause. J Biosoc Sci 5:533–555, 1973

McKinlay S, Jeffrey SM, Thompson B: An investigation of the age at menopause. J Biosoc Sci 4:161–173, 1972

McLeer SV: Psychoanalytic perspectives on family violence, in Handbook of Family Violence. Edited by Van Hasselt VB, Morrison RL, Bellack AS, et al. New York, Plenum, 1988, pp 11–30

McPherson K: Menopause as disease: the social construction of a metaphor. ANS 3:95–113, 1980–1981

Mead M: Male and Female: A Study of the Sexes in a Changing World. New York, Dell, 1968

Meade M: Anomalies in American post-divorce relationships, in Divorce and After. Edited by Tew BJ, Payne H, Lawrence KM. New York, Doubleday, 1970

Mednick MT: Single mothers: a review and critique of current research. Applied Sociology and Psychology Annals 7:184–201, 1987

Mellinger GD, Balter MB, Manheimer DI, et al: Psychic distress, life crisis, and use of psychotherapeutic medications: National Household

Survey data. Arch Gen Psychiatry 35:1045–1052, 1978

Melton LJ: Epidemiology of osteoporosis; predicting who is at risk. Ann N Y Acad Sci 592:295–306, 1990

Meltzer ES, Kumar R: Puerperal mental illness, clinical features and classification: a study of 142 mother-and-baby admissions. Br J Psychiatry 147:647–654, 1985

Mendell D: A study of menopausal women in analytic treatment, in Critical Psychophysical Passages in the Life of a Woman: A Psychodynamic Perspective. Edited by Offerman-Zuckerberg J. New York, Plenum, 1988, pp 183–197

Menning BE: Infertility: A Guide for Childless Couples. Englewood Cliffs, NJ, Prentice-Hall, 1977

Menninger KA: Emotional factors in organic gynecological conditions. Bull Menninger Clin 7:47–55, 1943

Michels R: Adulthood, in The Course of Life: Psychoanalytic Contributions Toward Understanding Personality Development, Vol 3: Adulthood and the Aging Process (DHHS Publ No [ADM] 81-1000). Edited by Greenspan SI, Pollock GH. Washington, DC, National Institute of Mental Health, 1980, pp 25–34

Middleton W: Studies in the Phenomenology of Grief. Herston Queensland, University of Queensland, 1989

Milgrom JH: Advocacy: assisting sexually exploited clients through the complaint process, in Psychotherapists' Sexual Involvement With Clients: Intervention and Prevention. Edited by Schoener GT, Milgrom JH, Gonsiorek JC, et al. Minneapolis, MN, Walk-In Counseling Center, 1989, pp 305–312

Miller JB: Toward a New Psychology of Women. Boston, MA, Beacon Press, 1976

Miller JB: The construction of anger in women and men. The Stone Center for Developmental Services and Studies, Work in Progress, Wellesley, MA, 1983, No 83-01:1–7

Miller JB: Date rape: time for a new look at prevention. Journal of College Student Development 29:553–555, 1988

Mittelmann B: The concurrent analysis of married couples. Psychoanal Q 17:182–197, 1948

Money J: Androgyne becomes bisexual in sexological theory: Plato to Freud and neuroscience. J Am Acad Psychoanal 18:392–413, 1990

Money J, Erhardt A: Man and Woman, Boy and Girl. Baltimore, MD, Johns Hopkins University Press, 1972

Monge RH: Structure of the self-concept from adolescence through old age. Exp Aging Res 1:281–291, 1975

Moore K, Spain D, Bianchi S: Working wives and mothers. Marriage and Family Review 7:77–98, 1984

Morgan LA: The financial experience of widowed women: evidence from the LRHS. The Gerontologist 26:663–668, 1986

Morokoff PJ: Sexuality in perimenopausal and postmenopausal women. Psychology of Women Quarterly 12:489–511, 1988

Morton R: Phthisiologia: On a Treatise of Consumption. London, S Smith and B Walford, 1689

Moseley DT, Follingstad DR, Harley H, et al: Psychological factors that predict reaction to abortion. J Clin Psychol 37:276–279, 1981

Moss MS, Moss SZ: Some aspects of the elder widow(er)'s persistent tie with the deceased spouse. Omega 15:195–206, 1984

Moss-Kanter RM: Men and Women of the Corporation. New York, Basic Books, 1977a

Moss-Kanter RM: Some effects of proportions on group life: skewed sex ratios and responses to token women. American Journal of Sociology 82:965-990, 1977b [Reprinted in Rieker PP, Carmen EH (eds): The Gender Gap in Psychotherapy: Social Realities and Psychological Processes. New York, Plenum, 1984, pp 53–78]

Moss-Kanter RM: Some effects of proportions on group life: skewed sex ratios and responses to token women, in The Gender Gap in Psychotherapy: Social Realities and Psychological Processes. Edited by Rieker PP, Carmen EH. New York, Plenum, 1984, pp 53–78

Most youth who attempt suicide go unidentified, unhelped. Psychiatric News, Vol 26, May 18, 1990

Mueller P, Major B: Self-blame, self-efficacy, and adjustment to abortion. J Pers Soc Psychol 57:1059–1068, 1989

Murphy L: The Widening Circle of Childhood. New York, Basic Books, 1962

Murray AD: Maternal employment reconsidered: effects on infants. Am J Orthopsychiatry 45:773–790, 1975

Musa K, Roach M: Adolescent appearance and self concept. Adolescence 8:385–394, 1973

Myers JK, Weissman MM, Tischler GL: Six-month prevalence of psychiatric disorders in three communities. Arch Gen Psychiatry 41:959–967, 1984

Myers WA: Dreams of mourning and separation in older individuals, in The Interpretations of Dreams in Clinical Work. Edited by Rothstein A (Workshop Monograph 3). New York, American Psychoanalytic Association, 1987, pp 125–144

Myers WA: I can't play ball anymore. J Geriatr Psychiatry 21:121–139, 1989

Nadelson CC: Marital therapy from a psychoanalytic perspective, in Marriage and Marital Therapy: Psychoanalytic, Behavioral, and Systems Theory Perspectives. Edited by Paolino TJ Jr, McCrady BS. New York, Brunner/Mazel, 1978, pp 89–164

Nadelson CC, Notman MT, Bennett MB: Success or failure: psychotherapeutic considerations for women in conflict. Am J Psychiatry 135:1092–1096, 1978

Nadelson CC, Notman MT: To marry or not to marry: a choice. Am J Psychiatry 138:1352–1356, 1981

Nadelson CC, Notman MT, Zackson H, et al: A follow-up study of rape victims. Am J Psychiatry 139:1266–1270, 1982

Napolion A, Lewis CM: Psychological considerations in lipoplasty: the problematic or "special care" patient. Ann Plast Surg 23:430–432, 1989

Napolion A, Lewis CM: Psychological considerations in the elderly cosmetic surgery candidates. Ann Plast Surg 24:165–169, 1990

National Center for Health Statistics: Monthly Vital Statistics Report, Vol 29. U.S. Department of Health and Human Services, Public Health Service, Office of Health Research Statistics and Technology, 1981, p 13

National Council on Alcoholism, Criteria Committee: Criteria for the diagnosis of alcoholism. Am J Psychiatry 129:127–135, 1972

National Prescription Audit (NPA): The top 20 drugs. Pharmacy Times, April 1972–1984

Neidig PH, Friedman DH: Spouse Abuse: A Treatment Program for Couples. Champaign, IL, Research Press Company, 1984

Nemiroff RA, Colarusso CA: The Race Against Time: Psychotherapy and Psychoanalysis in the Second Half of Life. New York, Plenum, 1985

Neugarten BL: Adult personality: toward a psychology of the life cycle, in Middle Age & Aging. Chicago, IL, University of Chicago Press, 1968a, pp 137–147

Neugarten BL: The awareness of middle age, in Middle Age and Aging. Edited by Neugarten BL. Chicago, IL, University of Chicago Press, 1968b, pp 93–98

Neugarten BL, Kraines RJ: "Menopausal symptoms" in women of various ages. Psychosom Med 27:266–273, 1965

Neugarten BL, Weinstein K: The changing American grandparent. Journal of Marriage and the Family 26:204, 1964

Neugarten BL, Wood V, Kraines RJ, et al: Women's attitudes towards the menopause. Vita Humana 6:140–151, 1963

Neugarten DA, Shafritz JM (eds): Sexuality in Organizations: Romantic and Coercive Behaviors at Work. Oak Park, IL, Moore Publishing, 1980

Nicholi AM Jr: The adolescent, in The Harvard Guide to Modern Psychiatry. Edited by Nicholi AM Jr. Cambridge, MA, Belknap Press/Harvard University Press, 1978, pp 519–540

Niemela P, Lechtinen P, Rauramo L, et al: The first abortion and the last: a study of the personality factors underlying repeated failure of contraception. Int J Gynaecol Obstet 19:193–200, 1981

Niswander K, Patterson R: Psychologic response to therapeutic abortion: subjective patient response. Obstet Gynecol 29:702–706, 1967

Noel MM: Reporting Colleagues Who Are Sexually Intimate With Clients: It's Time to Talk. New York, Haworth Press, 1988

Notelovitz M: Exercise and health maintenance in menopausal women, in Multidisciplinary Perspectives on Menopause. Edited by Flint M, Kronenberg F, Utian W. Annals of the New York Academy of Sciences, Vol 592. New York, New York Academy of Sciences, 1990, pp 204–262

Notman MT: Women and midlife: a different perspective. Psychiatric Opinion 15:15–25, 1978

Notman MT: Midlife concerns of women: implications of the menopause. Am J Psychiatry 136:1270–1274, 1979

Notman MT: Psychiatric disorder of menopause. Psychiatric Annals 14:448–453, 1984

Notman MT: The menopause, in The Psychiatric Implications of Menstruation. Edited by Gold JH. Washington, DC, American Psychiatric Press, 1985, pp 87–102

Notman MT: Menopause and adult development. Ann N Y Acad Sci 592:151, 1990

Notman MT, Nadelson CC: The rape victim: psychodynamic considerations. Am J Psychiatry 133:408–413, 1976

Notman MT, Nadelson CC: Psychodynamic and life-stage considerations in the response to rape, in The Rape Crisis Intervention Handbook: A Guide for Victim Care. Edited by McCombie SL. New York, Plenum, 1980, pp 131–142

Notman MT, Nadelson CC: Changing views of the relationship between femininity and reproduction, in The Woman Patient, Vol 2: Concepts of Femininity and the Life Cycle. Edited by Nadelson CC, Notman MT. New York, Plenum, 1982a, pp 31–42

Notman MT, Nadelson CC: Maternal work and children, in The Woman Patient, Vol 2: Concepts of Femininity and the Life Cycle. Edited by Nadelson CC, Notman MT. New York, Plenum, 1982b, pp 121–134

Oates MR: The treatment of psychiatric disorders in pregnancy and the puerperium. Clin Obstet Gynecol 13:385–395, 1986

O'Brien JD: The effects of incest on female adolescent development. J Am Acad Psychoanal 15:83–92, 1987

O'Bryant SL: Neighbors' support of older widows who live alone in their own homes. The Gerontologist 25:305–310, 1985

Ochberg FM (ed): Post-Traumatic Therapy and Victims of Violence. New York, Brunner/Mazel, 1988

Offer D: The Psychological World of the Teenager: A Study of Normal Adolescent Boys. New York, Basic Books, 1969

Offer D, Offer JL: Profiles of normal adolescent girls. Arch Gen Psychiatry 19:513–522, 1968

Offer D, Marcus D, Offer JL: A longitudinal study of normal adolescent boys. Am J Psychiatry 126:914–924, 1970

O'Hara MW: Social support, life events, and depression during pregnancy and the puerperium. Arch Gen Psychiatry 43:569–573, 1986

O'Neill JM, Fishman DM, Kinsella-Shaw M: Dual career couples' career transitions and normative dilemmas: a preliminary assessment model. Counseling Psychologist 15:50–96, 1987

Osborn M: Depression at the menopause. Br J Hosp Med 32:128–129, 1984

Osterweiss M, Solomon F, Green M (eds): Bereavement: Reaction, Consequences, and Care. Report by the Committee for the Study of Health Consequences of the Others of Bereavement, Institute of Medicine, National Academy of Sciences. Washington, DC, National Academy Press, 1988

Parens H: A contribution of separation-individuation to the development of psychic structure, in Separation-Individuation; Essays in Honor of Margaret S. Mahler. Edited by McDevitt JB, Settlage CF. New York, International Universities Press, 1971, pp 100–112

Parkes CM: Recent bereavement as a cause of mental illness. Br J Psychiatry 110:198–204, 1964

Parkes CM: Bereavement and mental illness. Br J Med Psychol 38:1–26, 1965

Parkes CM: The first year of bereavement: a longitudinal study of the reaction of London widows to the death of their husbands. Psychiatry 33:444–467, 1970

Parkes CM: Bereavement: Studies in Grief in Adult Life. New York, International Universities Press, 1972

Parkes CM: Determinants of outcome following bereavement. Omega 6:303–323, 1975

Parkes CM: Risk factors in bereavement: implications for the prevention and treatment of pathologic grief. Psychiatric Annals 20:308–313, 1990

Parkes CM: Attachment, bonding and psychiatric problems after bereavement in adult life, in Attachment Across the Life Cycle. Edited by Parkes CM. London, Routledge Kegan Paul, 1991

Parkes CM, Brown RJ: Health after bereavement: a controlled study of young Boston widows and widowers. Psychosom Med 34:449–461, 1972

Parkes CM, Weiss RS: Recovery From Bereavement. New York, Basic Books, 1983

Parlee MB: Social factors in the psychology of menstruation, birth and menopause. Prim Care 3:477–490, 1976

Parlee MB: Integrating biological and social science research on menopause. Ann N Y Acad Sci 592:379–389, 1990

Pascarelli EF: Methaqualone: the quiet epidemic, in Drug Use in America: Problem in Perspective, Second Report of the National Commission on Marijuana and Drug Abuse, Vol 1. Edited by Shafer RP. Washington, DC, U.S. Government Printing Office, No 5266-00004, 1973, pp 102–105

Patt SL, Rappaport RG, Barglow P: Follow-up of therapeutic abortion. Arch Gen Psychiatry 20:408–414, 1969

Paykel ES, Emms EM, Fletcher J, et al: Life events and social support in puerperal depression. Br J Psychiatry 136:339–346, 1980

Payne EC, Kravitz AR, Notman MT, et al: Outcome following therapeutic abortion. Arch Gen Psychiatry 33:725–733, 1976

Peck M: Notes on identification in a case of depression reactive to the death of a love object. Psychoanal Q 8:1–17, 1939

Pelham AO, Clark WF: Widowhood among low income racial and ethnic groups in California, in Widows, Vol 2: North America. Edited by Lopata HZ. Durham, NC, Duke University Press, 1987, pp 191–222

Pennington G, Atlay R: Some surprising results in the investigation of the infertile woman. Journal of Obstetrics and Gynaecology of the British Commonwealth 79:651–653, 1972

Perlmutter J: A gynecological approach to menopause, in The Woman Patient VI: Medical and Psychological Interfaces. Edited by Notman M, Nadelson C. New York, Plenum, 1978, pp 323–336

Perosa SL, Perosa LM: The mid-career crisis in relation to Super's career and Erikson's adult developmental theory. International Journal of Aging and Human Development 20:53–68, 1984–1985

Person ES: Women working: fears of failure, deviance and success. J Am Acad Psychoanal 10:67–84, 1982

Person ES: Dreams of Love and Fateful Encounters: The Power of Romantic Passion. New York, WW Norton, 1989

Persons J, Burns D: Mechanisms of action of cognitive therapy: the relative contribution of technical and interpersonal interventions. Cognitive Therapy and Research 9:539–551, 1985

Peterson RC, Stillman RC: Phencyclidine (PCP) Abuse: An Appraisal (GPO 017-024-00785-04). Washington, DC, U.S. Government Printing Office, 1979, p 231

Pfeffer CR: The Suicidal Child. New York, Guilford, 1986

Pfeffer CR, Plutchik R, Mizruchi MS: Suicidal and assaultive behavior in children: classification, measurement, and interrelations. Am J Psychiatry 140:154–157, 1983

Pfeffer CR, Zuckerman S, Plutchik R, et al: Suicidal behavior in normal school children: a comparison with child psychiatric inpatients. Journal of the American Academy of Child Psychiatry 23:416–423, 1984

Phillips DP, Carstensen LL: Clustering of teenage suicides after television news stories about suicide. N Engl J Med 315:685–689, 1986

Pillay M, Crisp AH: The impact of social skills training within an established in-patient treatment programme for anorexia nervosa. Br J Psychiatry 139:533–539, 1981

Pillemer K: The dangers of dependency: new findings on domestic violence against the elderly. Social Problems 33:146–158, 1985

Pillemer K: Maltreatment of patients in nursing homes: overview and research agenda. J Health Soc Behav 29:227–238, 1988

Pillemer K, Finkelhor D: Causes of elder abuse: caregiver stress versus problem relatives. Am J Orthopsychiatry 59:179–187, 1989

Pines D: Pregnancy and motherhood: interaction between fantasy and reality. Br J Med Psychol 45:333–343, 1972

Pines D: The relevance of early psychic development to pregnancy and abortion. Int J Psychoanal 63:311–319, 1982

Pirog-Good MA, Stets JE: Violence in Dating Relationships: Emerging Social Issues. New York, Praeger, 1989

Pitt B: "Atypical" depression following childbirth. Br J Psychiatry 114:1325–1335, 1968

Pitt B: "Maternity blues." Br J Psychiatry 122:431–433, 1973

Pitts FN, McClune JN: Lactate metabolism in anxiety neurosis. N Engl J Med 277:1329–1336, 1967

Planned Parenthood Foundation: Eleven million teenagers: what can be done about the epidemic of adolescent pregnancies in the United States? New York, Planned Parenthood Foundation of America, 1976

Platt J, Ficher I, Silver M: Infertile couples: personality traits and self-ideal concept discrepancies. Fertil Steril 24:972–976, 1973

Polit DF, LaRocco SA: Social and psychological correlates of menopausal symptoms. Psychosom Med 42:335–345, 1980

Polivka J: Cartoon humor as an aid in therapy. Clinical Gerontologist 7:63–67, 1987

Pollock GH: Mourning and adaptation. Int J Psychoanal 42:341–361, 1961

Pollock GH: Anniversary reactions, trauma, and mourning. Psychoanal Q 39:347–371, 1970

Pollock GH: Temporal anniversary manifestations: hour, day, holiday. Psychoanal Q 40:123–131, 1971

Pollock GH: On mourning, immortality and utopia. J Am Psychoanal Assoc 23:334–362, 1975

Pollock GH: The mourning process and creative organizational change. J Am Psychoanal Assoc 25:3–34, 1977

Pollock GH: Process and affect: mourning and grief. Int J Psychoanal 59:255–276, 1978

Pollock GH: Aging or aged: development or pathology, in The Course of Life: Psychoanalytic Contributions Toward Understanding Personality Development, Vol 3. Edited by Greenspan SI, Pollock GH. Washington, DC, National Institute of Mental Health, 1981, pp 549–585

Poloma MM: Role conflict and the married professional woman, in Toward a Sociology of Women. Edited by Safilios-Rothschild C. Lexington, MA, Xerox College Publications, 1972, pp 187–198

Pope H, Mueller C: The intergeneration transmission of marital instability: comparisons by race and sex, in Divorce and Separation: Context, Causes and Consequences. Edited by Levinger G, Mole O. New York, Basic Books, 1977, pp 89–113

Pope KS: How clients are harmed by sexual contact with mental health professionals: the syndrome and its prevalence. Journal of Counseling and Development 67:222–226, 1988

Pope KS, Bouhoutsos JC: Sexual Intimacy Between Therapists and Patients. New York, Praeger, 1986

Pope KS, Levenson H, Schover LR: Sexual intimacy in psychology training: results and implications of a national survey. Am Psychol 34:682–689, 1979

Pope KS, Keith-Spiegel P, Tabachnick BG: Sexual attraction to clients: the human therapist and the (sometimes) inhuman training system. Am Psychol 41:147–158, 1986

Pope KS, Tabachnick BG, Keith-Spiegel P: Ethics of practice: the beliefs and behaviors of psychologists as therapists. Am Psychol 42:993–1006, 1987

Posner J: It's all in your head: feminist and medical models of menopause (strange bedfellows). Sex Roles 5:179–191, 1976

Post SG: History, infanticide and imperiled newborns. Hastings Cent Rep 18:14–17, 1988

Price LH, Charney DS, Robin AL, et al: Alpha$_2$ adrenergic receptor function in depression. Arch Gen Psychiatry 43:849–858, 1986

Prior J: Conditioning exercise and premenstrual symptoms. J Reprod Med 32:423–427, 1987

Pugliesi K: Employment characteristics, social support and the well-being of women. Women Health 14:35–58, 1988

Quadrio C: Analysis and system: a marriage. Aust N Z J Psychiatry 20:219–224, 1986

Ramu GN, Tavuchis N: The valuation of children and parenthood among the voluntary childless and parental couples in Canada. Journal of Comparative Family Studies 17:99–116, 1986

Rando RA: An investigation of grief and adaptation in parents whose children have died from cancer. J Ped Psychol 8:3–20, 1983

Rando TA: Grief, Dying and Death: Clinical Interventions for Caregivers. Champaign, IL, Research Press Company, 1984

Ranier JD: Genetic factors in depression and suicide. Am J Psychother 38:329–340, 1984

Rank O: The Trauma of Birth. New York, Robert Brunner, 1952

Rapaport D: The theory of ego autonomy, in Collected Papers. Edited by Gill MM. New York, Basic Books, 1967, pp 722–744

Rapoport R, Rapoport RN: Dual-Career Families. London, Penguin, 1971

Raphael B: Preventive intervention with the recently bereaved. Arch Gen Psychiatry 34:1450–1454, 1977

Raphael B: Mourning and the prevention of melancholia. Br J Med Psychol 51:303–310, 1978

Raphael B: The Anatomy of Bereavement. New York, Basic Books, 1983

Raphael B, Middleton W: What is pathologic grief? Psychiatric Annals 6:304–308, 1990

Raphael-Leff J: Psychotherapeutic needs of mothers-to-be. Journal of Child Psychotherapy 8:3–13, 1982

Rascovsky MW de, Rascovsky A: On consummated incest. Int J Psychoanal 31:42–47, 1950

Rassieur CL: The Problem Clergymen Don't Talk About. Philadelphia, PA, Westminster Press, 1976

Raunikar V: Physiology and treatment of hot flushes. Obstet Gynecol 75:13–17, 1990

Read NO, Elliot MR, Escobar MD, et al: The effects of marital status and motherhood on the career concerns of reentry women. Career Development Quarterly 37:47–55, 1988

Recker RR, Saville PD, Heany RP: Effect of estrogen and calcium carbonate on bone loss in postmenopausal women. Ann Intern Med 87:649–655, 1977

Redburn DE, Juretich M: Some considerations for using widowed self-help group leaders. Gerontology and Geriatrics Education 9(3):89–98, 1989

Reich A: Narcissistic object choices in women. J Am Psychoanal Assoc 1:22–44, 1953

Reich A: Pathologic forms of self-esteem regulation. Psychoanal Study Child 15:215–232, 1960

Reid RL, Yen SS: Premenstrual syndrome. Am J Obstet Gynecol 139:85–104, 1981

Reinhardt JP, Fisher CB: Kinship versus friendship: social adaptation in married and widowed elderly women. Doctoral dissertation, Fordham University, Bronx, NY (New York, Haworth Press), 1989

Remer R, Elliot JE: Characteristics of secondary victims of sexual assault. International Journal of Family Psychiatry 9:373–387, 1988

Remnet VL: How adult children respond to role transitions in the lives of their aging parents. Educational Gerontology 13:341–355, 1987

Remondet JH, Hansson RO: Assessing a widow's grief: a short index. Journal of Gerontological Nursing 13:30–34, 1987

Renshaw DC: Treatment of sexual exploitation: rape and incest. Psychiatr Clin North Am 12:257–277, 1989

Resnick PJ: Murder of the newborn: a psychiatric review of neonaticide. Am J Psychiatry 126:1414–1420, 1970

Rhoades FP: Minimizing the menopause. J Am Geriatr Soc 15:346–354, 1967

Rickels K, Csanalosi I, Chung HR, et al: Amitriptyline in anxious-depressed outpatients: a controlled study. Am J Psychiatry 131:25–30, 1974

Ritvo S: Late adolescence: developmental and clinical considerations. Psychoanal Study Child 26:241–263, 1971

Ritvo S: Adolescent to woman, in Female Psychology: Contemporary Psychoanalytic Views. Edited by Blum HP. New York, International Universities Press, 1977, pp 127–137

Roark ML: Preventing violence on college campuses. Journal of Counseling and Development 65:367–371, 1987

Roberto KA, Scott JP: Confronting widowhood: the influence of informal support. American Behavioral Scientist 29:497–511, 1986

Robins E, Gassner S, Kayes J, et al: The communication of suicidal intent: a study of 134 consecutive cases of successful (completed) suicide. Am J Psychiatry 115:724–733, 1959

Robinson GE, Stewart DE: Motivation for motherhood and the experience of pregnancy. Can J Psychiatry 34:861–865, 1989

Robinson GE, Perrotta M, Burne S: Autonomy in mothers with careers. Can J Psychiatry 27:270–274, 1982

Robinson LH: Grandparenting: intergenerational love and hate. J Am Acad Psychoanal 17:483–491, 1989

Rohsenow DJ, Corbett R, Devine D: Molested as children: a hidden contribution to substance abuse? J Subst Abuse Treat 5:13–18, 1988

Roiphe H: On an early genital phase, with an addendum on Genesis. Psychoanal Study Child 23:348–365, 1968

Roiphe H, Galenson E: Early genital activity and the castration complex. Psychoanal Q 41:334–347, 1972

Roiphe H, Galenson E: Object loss and early sexual development. Psychoanal Q 42:73–90, 1973

Rose DS: "Worse than death": psychodynamics of rape victims and the need for psychotherapy. Am J Psychiatry 143:817–824, 1986

Rose R: Review of Tannen D: You Just Don't Understand: Women and Men in Conversation. New York Times Book Review, Aug 26, 1990, p 27

Rosenbaum A, O'Leary KD: Marital violence: characteristics of abusive couples. J Consult Clin Psychol 49:63–71, 1981

Rosenblatt PC: Bitter, Bitter Tears: Nineteenth-Century Diarists and Twentieth-Century Grief Theorists. Minneapolis, MN, University of Minnesota Press, 1983

Rosenfeld AA, Nadelson CC, Krieger M, et al: Incest and sexual abuse of children. Journal of the American Academy of Child Psychiatry 16:327–339, 1977

Rosenwald GC, Wiersma J: Women, career changes, and the new self: an analysis of rhetoric. Psychiatry 46:213–229, 1983

Rosewater LB: The MMPI and battered women. Paper presented at the Second National Conference for Family Violence Researchers, Durham, NC, 1984

Ross ED, Mesulam M-M: Dominant langauage functions of

Ross HL, Sawhill IV: Time of Transition: The Growth of Families Headed by Women. Washington, DC, The Urban Institute, 1975

Rossi A: Transition to parenthood. Journal of Marriage and the Family 38:26–39, 1968

Rowe MP: Dealing with sexual harassment. Harvard Business Review, May/June 1981, pp 42–48

Rowe MP: Barriers to equality: the power of subtle discrimination to maintain unequal opportunity. Employee Responsibilities and Rights Journal 3:153–163, 1990

Roy M: A current survey of 100 cases, in Battered Women: A Psychosocial Study of Domestic Violence. Edited by Roy M. New York, Van Nostrand Reinhold, 1977, pp 25–44

Roy P: Sex in the factory: informal heterosexual relations between supervisors and work groups, in Deviant Behavior: Occupational and Organizational Bases. Edited by Bryant C. Chicago, IL, Rand-McNally, 1974, pp 44–67

Roy A, Markku L, Jimerson DC, et al: Pre-menopausal and post-menopausal depressed women. Aust N Z J Psychiatry 20:464–469, 1986

Rubenstein B: An emotional factor in infertility. Fertil Steril 2:80–86, 1951

Rubinstein RL: Singular Paths: Old Men Living Alone. New York, Columbia University Press, 1986

Rush F: The Best Kept Secret: Sexual Abuse of Children. Englewood Cliffs, NJ, Prentice-Hall, 1980

Russell DEH: Rape in Marriage. New York, Macmillan, 1982

Russell DEH: The incidence and prevalence of intrafamilial and extrafamilial sexual abuse of female children. Child Abuse Negl 7:133–146, 1983

Russell DEH: Sexual Exploitation: Rape, Child Sexual Abuse, and Workplace Harassment. Beverly Hills, CA, Sage, 1984

Russell DEH: The Secret Trauma: Incest in the Lives of Girls and Women. New York, Basic Books, 1986

Russell DEH, Van de Ven L: Crimes Against Women: Proceedings of the International Tribunal. Millbrae, CA, Les Femmes, 1976

Russell GFM, Szmukler GI, Dare C, et al: An evaluation of family therapy in anorexia nervosa and bulimia nervosa. Arch Gen Psychiatry 44:1047–1056, 1987

Rutter M: The Qualities of Mothering: Maternal Deprivation Reassessed. New York, Jason Aronson, 1974

Rutter P: Sex in the Forbidden Zone. Los Angeles, CA, Jeremy Tarcher, 1989

Rynearson EK: Pathologic grief: the queen's croquet ground. Psychiatric Annals 20:295–304, 1990

Sack L, Sturner W, Lipsitt L, et al: Relationship of maternal and perinatal conditions to eventual adolescent suicide. Lancet 1:624–627, 1985

Sager CJ: Marriage Contracts and Couple Therapy: Hidden Forces in Intimate Relationships. New York, Brunner/Mazel, 1976

Sales E, Baum M, Shore B: Victim readjustment following assault. Journal of Social Issues 37:5–27, 1984

Sanders CM: Risk factors in bereavement outcome. Journal of Social Issues 44:97–111, 1988

Sanders HS: A comparison of adult bereavement in the death of a spouse, child and parent. Omega 10:303–322, 1979–1980

Sandler B: Infertility of emotional origin. Journal of Obstetrics and Gynaecology of the British Commonwealth 68:809–815, 1961

Sandroff R: Sexual harassment in the Fortune 500. Working Women Magazine, December 1988

Sanford L, Donovan M: Women and Self-Esteem. Garden City, NY, Anchor Press/Doubleday, 1984

Sanford W (ed): Fighting Sexual Harassment: An Advocacy Handbook. Boston, MA, Allyson Publication/The Alliance Against Sexual Coercion, 1981

Sarrel PM: Sexuality in the middle years. Obstet Gynecol Clin North Am 14:49–62, 1987

Sarrel PM: Sexuality and menopause. Obstet Gynecol 75:26S-30S, 1990

Sarrel PM, DeCherney M: Psychotherapeutic intervention for treatment of couples with secondary infertility. Fertil Steril 43:897–903, 1985

Sartoris DJ, Moscona A, Resnick D: Progress in radiology: dual energy radiographic absorptiometry for bone densitometry. Ann N Y Acad Sci 592:307–325, 1990

Sayres M, Wyshak G, Denterlein G, et al: Pregnancy during residency. N Engl J Med 314:418–423, 1986

Schachere K: Attachment between working mothers and their infants: the influence of family processes. Am J Orthopsychiatry 60:19–34, 1990

Schafer R: Problems in Freud's psychology of women. J Am Psychoanal Assoc 22:459–485, 1974

Schiff H: The Bereaved Parent. New York, Crown Publishers, 1977

Schindler B: The psychiatric disorders of midlife. Med Clin North Am 71:71–85, 1987

Schlesinger B: Lasting marriages in the 1980s. Conciliation Courts Review 20:43–49, 1982

Schoener GR, Milgrom JH: Processing sessions, in Psychotherapists' Sexual Involvement With Clients: Intervention and Prevention. Edited by Schoener GT, Milgrom JH, Gonsiorek JC, et al. Minneapolis, MN, Walk-In Counseling Center, 1989, pp 345–358

Schoener GR, Milgrom JH, Gonsiorek J: Sexual exploitation of clients by therapists. Women and Therapy 3(3–4):63–69, 1984

Schoener GR, Milgrom JH, Gonsiorek JC, et al (eds): Psychotherapists' Sexual Involvement With Clients: Intervention and Prevention. Minneapolis, MN, Walk-In Counseling Center, 1989

Schoonover CB, Brody EM, Hoffman C, et al: Parent care and geographically distant children. Research on Aging 10:472–492, 1988

Schreiner-Engel P: Differential diagnosis of hypoactive sexual desire: reported to the American Society of Psychosomatics in Obstetrics and Gynecology. Clinical Psychiatry News, No 18, 1990, p 30

Schuchter SSR, Zisook S: Widowhood: the continuing relationship with the dead spouse. Bull Menninger Clin 52:269–279, 1988

Schuchter SSR, Zisook S: Hovering over the bereaved. Psychiatric Annals 20:327–333, 1990

Schuckit MA: Alcoholism and sociopathy—diagnostic confusion. Quarterly Journal of Studies on Alcohol 34:157–164, 1973

Schuckit MA: Current therapeutic options in the management of typical anxiety. J Clin Psychiatry 42(no 11, sec 2):15–26, 1981

Schuckit MA: A study of alcoholism with secondary depression. Am J Psychiatry 140:711–714, 1983

Schuckit MA, Haglund RMJ: Etiological theories on alcoholism, in Alcoholism: Development, Consequences and Interventions. Edited by Estes N, Heinemann E. St Louis, MO, CV Mosby, 1982, pp 16–31

Schuckit MA, Rayser V: Ethanol ingestion: differences in blood acetaldehyde concentrations in relatives of alcoholics and controls. Science 203:54–55, 1979

Schuckit MA, Winbeur R: A short-term follow-up of women alcoholics. Diseases of the Nervous System 33:672–678, 1972

Schwab JJ, Chalmers J, Conroy S, et al: Studies in grief: a preliminary report, in Bereavement: Its Psychosocial Aspects. Edited by Schoenberg B, Gerber I, Wiener A, et al. New York, Columbia University Press, 1975, pp 78–91

Schwab JJ, Farris PB, Conroy SJ, et al: Funeral behavior and unresolved grief, in Acute Grief and the Funeral. Edited by Pine VR, Kutscher A, Peretz D, et al. Springfield, IL, Charles C Thomas, 1976, pp 241–249

Schwartz AM: Comments in section on "The Parents," in Understanding Bereavement and Grief. Edited by Linzer N. New York, Yeshiva University Press, 1977, pp 193–196

Schwartzman LC, Leiblum SR: Changing perspectives on the menopause. Journal of Psychosomatic Obstetrics and Gynecology 6:11–24, 1987

Scott JP, Kivelt VR: Differences in the morale of older rural widows and widowers. Int J Aging Hum Dev 21:121–136, 1985

Scott PD: Parents who kill their children. Medicine, Science and the Law 13:120–126, 1973

Scott PD: Battered wives. Br J Psychiatry 125:433–441, 1974

Searles HF: Countertransference and Related Subjects: Selected Papers. New York, International Universities Press, 1979

Seelback WC: Correlates of aged person's filial responsibility, expectation and realizations. Family Coordinator 27:341–350, 1978

Sefton MS: Dual-career families and the family life cycle. Australian Journal of Sex, Marriage and Family 8:118–123, 1987

Seibel M, Taymor M: Emotional aspects of infertility. Fertil Steril 37:137–141, 1982

Severino K, Teusink J, Pender V, et al: Overview: the psychology of grandparenthood. J Geriatr Psychiatry 19:13–17, 1986

Severne L: Psychosocial aspects of the menopause, in Changing Perspectives on Menopause. Edited by Voda AM, Dinnerstein M, O'Donnell SR. Austin, TX, University of Texas Press, 1982, pp 239–247

Shaffer D: Suicide in children and early adolescence. J Child Psychol Psychiatry 15:275–291, 1974

Shainess N: Psychological aspects of wife battering, in Battered Women: A Psychosocial Study of Domestic Violence. Edited by Roy M. New York, Van Nostrand Reinhold, 1977, pp 111–118

Shammas E: Controlled comparison of bromazepam, amitriptyline, and placebo in anxiety-depressive neurosis. Diseases of the Nervous System 38:201–207, 1977

Shanas E: Older people and their families: the new pioneers. Journal of Marriage and the Family 42:9–15, 1980

Shanfield SB, Benjamin GAH, Swain BJ: Parents' reactions to the death of an adult child from cancer. Am J Psychiatry 141:1092–1094, 1984

Shanfield SB, Swain BJ: Death of adult children in traffic accidents. J Nerv Ment Dis 172:533–538, 1984

Shengold L: Child abuse and deprivation: soul murder. J Am Psychoanal Assoc 27:553–559, 1979

Shengold L: Some reflections on a case of mother/adolescent son incest. Int J Psychoanal 61:461–475, 1980

Shengold L: Soul Murder: The Effects of Childhood Abuse and Deprivation. New Haven, CT, Yale University Press, 1989

Sherfy M: The evolution and nature of female sexuality in relation to psychoanalytic theory. J Am Psychoanal Assoc 14:28–128, 1966

Sherfy M: The Nature and Evolution of Female Sexuality. New York, Random/Village, 1973

Sherkow S: Consequences of childhood sexual abuse on the development of ego structure: a comparison of child and adult abuse cases, in Adult Analysis and Childhood Sexual Abuse. Edited by Levine H. Hillsdale, NJ, Analytic Press, 1990a, pp 93–116

Sherkow SP: Evaluation and diagnosis of sexual abuse of little girls. J Am Psychoanal Assoc 38:347–369, 1990b

Shusterman LR: Predicting the psychological consequences of abortion. Soc Sci Med 13A:683–689, 1979

Sieber SD: Towards a theory of role accumulation. American Sociological Review 39:567–578, 1974

Siegel B: A Death in White Bear Lake. New York, Bantam Books, 1990

Silverman DC, Apfel RJ: Caring for victims of rape, in Treatment Interventions in Human Sexuality. Edited by Nadelson CC, Marcotte DB. New York, Plenum, 1983, pp 195–213

Simmel G: The Sociology of Georg Simmel. Translated by Wolff KH. Glencoe, IL, Free Press, 1950

Simon NM, Senturia AG, Rothman D: Psychiatric illness following therapeutic abortion. Am J Psychiatry 124:59–65 [97–103], 1967

Singh HB, Raphael B: Post-disaster morbidity of the bereaved: a possible role for preventive psychiatry. J Nerv Ment Dis 169:203–212, 1981

Sitruk-Ware R, Iberra de Palacios P: Oestrogen replacement therapy and cardiovascular disease in postmenopausal women: a review. Maturitas 11:259–274, 1989

Skinner DA: Dual-career family stress and coping. Family Relations 29:473–481, 1980

Skolnick P, Paul SM: Benzodiazepine receptors in the central nervous system. Int Rev Neurobiol 23:103–140, 1982

Smith DC, Prentice R, Thompson DJ, et al: Association of exogenous estrogen and endometrial carcinoma. N Engl J Med 293:1164–1167, 1975

Smith S: The seduction of the female patient, in Sexual Exploitation in Professional Relationships. Edited by Gabbard GO. Washington, DC, American Psychiatric Press, 1989, pp 57–69

Snell JE, Rosenwald J, Robey A: The wife-beaters wife. Arch Gen Psychiatry 11:107–112, 1964

Socarides CW: Theoretical and clinical aspects of overt female homosexuality. J Am Psychoanal Assoc 10:579–592, 1962

Socarides CW: The historical development of theoretical and clinical concepts of overt female homosexuality. J Am Psychoanal Assoc 11:386–414, 1963

Sontag S: The double standard of aging. Saturday Review of the Society, September 1972, pp 29–38

Sours JA: Starving to Death in a Sea of Objects: The Anorexia Nervosa Syndrome. New York, Jason Aronson, 1980

Spanier FR, Casto RF: Adjustment in separation and divorce, in Divorce and Separation: Context, Causes and Consequences. Edited by Levinger G, Moles O. New York, Basic Books, 1979, pp 211–227

Spanier GB, Glick PC: Paths to remarriage. Journal of Divorce 3:283–298, 1980

Spiegel D: Multiple personality as a post-traumatic stress disorder. Psychiatr Clin North Am 7:101–110, 1984

Spitz RA, Wolf KM: Anaclitic depression: an inquiry into the genesis of psychiatric conditions in early childhood, II. Psychoanal Study Child 2:313–342, 1946a

Spitz RA, Wolf KM: The smiling response: a contribution to the ontogenesis of social relations. Genetic Psychology Monographs 34:57–125, 1946b

Stampfer MJ, Colditz GH, Willett WC: Menopause and heart disease. Ann N Y Acad Sci 592:193–263, 1990

Stanley EJ, Barter J: Adolescent suicidal behavior. Am J Orthopsychiatry 83:180–185, 1978

Stannard V: The mask of beauty, in Women in a Sexist Society. Edited by Gornick V, Moran B. New York, Basic Books, 1971, pp 118–130

Steele D: Child abuse, in The Reconstruction of Trauma. Edited by Rothstein A (Workshop Series of the American Psychoanalytic Association). NJ, American Psychoanalytic Press, 1986, pp 59–72

Steketee G, Foa EB: Rape victims: post traumatic stress responses and their treatment: a review of the literature. Journal of Anxiety Disorders 1:69–86, 1987

Stern P: Mother and infant at play: the dyadic interaction involving facial, vocal, and gaze behavior, in The Effect of the Infant on Its Caregiver. Edited by Lewis M, Rosenblum M. New York, Wiley, 1974, pp 187–215

Stiver I: Work inhibitions in women. The Stone Center for Developmental Services and Studies, Work in Progress, Wellesley, MA, 1983, No 82-03:1–11

Stiver I: The meaning of "dependency" in female-male relationships. The Stone Center for Developmental Services and Studies, Working Papers, Wellesley, MA, 1984, No 83-07:1–12

Stoller K: A contribution to the study of gender identity. Int J Psychoanal 45:220–226, 1964

Stoller RJ: The sense of maleness. Psychoanal Q 34:207–218, 1965

Stoller RJ: The sense of femaleness. Psychoanal Q 37:42–55, 1968

Stoller RJ: Primary femininity. J Am Psychoanal Assoc 24(suppl):59–78, 1976

Stoller RJ: Observing the Erotic Imagination. New Haven, CT, Yale University Press, 1985

Stone AB: Report at the Annual Meeting of the American Psychiatric Association. Clinical Psychiatry News, No 18, 1990, p 16

Straus MA: A sociological perspective on the prevention and treatment of wife beating, in Battered Women: A Psychosociological Study of Domestic Violence. Edited by Roy M. New York, Van Nostrand Reinhold, 1977, pp 194–228

Straus MA: The marriage license as a hitting license: evidence from popular culture, law and social science, in The Social Causes of Husband-Wife Violence. Edited by Straus MA, Hotaling GT. Minneapolis, MN, University of Minneapolis Press, 1980, pp 39–50

Straus MA, Gelles RJ, Steinmetz SK: Behind Closed Doors: Violence in the American Family. Garden City, NY, Anchor Books, 1980

Streib GF, Beck RW: Older families: a decade review. Journal of Marriage and the Family 42:937–956, 1980

Strober M, Katz IL: Depression in the eating disorders: a review and analysis of descriptive, family, and biological findings, in Diagnostic Issues in Anorexia Nervosa and Bulimia Nervosa. Edited by Garner DM, Garfinkel PE. New York, Brunner/Mazel, 1988, pp 80–111

Stroebe W, Stroebe MS: Bereavement and Health: The Psychological and Physical Consequences of Partner Loss. London, UK, Cambridge University Press, 1987

Stromberg AH, Harkess S: Women Working: Theories and Facts in Perspective. Palo Alto, CA, Mayfield, 1978

Strugnell C: Who the widow-to-widow program served, in Helping Each Other in Widowhood. Edited by Silverman P, MacKenzie MP, Wilson E. New York, Health Sciences Publishing, 1974, pp 31–56

Studd JW, Thom MH, Paterson MEL, et al: The prevention and treatment of endometrial pathology in postmenopausal women receiving exogenous estrogens, in The Menopause and Postmenopause. Edited by Pasetto R, Paoletti R, Ambrus JL. Lancaster, UK, MTP Press, 1980, pp 127–139

Surrey JL: Self in relation: a theory of women's development. The Stone Center for Developmental Services and Studies, Working Paper, Wellesley, MA, 1983, No 83-13

Surrey JL: Eating problems as a reflection of women's development. The Stone Center for Developmental Services and Studies, Working Papers, Wellesley, MA, 1985, No 83-06:1–7

Sutherland S, Scherl DJ: Patterns of response among victims of rape. Am J Orthopsychiatry 40:503–511, 1970

Sutton JJ, Pillemer K: Explaining conflict when adult children and elderly parents live together. Journal of Marriage and the Family 50:1037–1047, 1988

Swift WJ, Andrews D, Barklage NE: The relationship between affective disorder and eating disorders: a review of the literature. Am J Psychiatry 143:290–299, 1986

Symonds A: The dynamics of depression in functioning women—sexism in the family. J Am Acad Psychoanal 14:395–406, 1986

Tallman JF, Paul SM, Skolnick P, et al: Receptors for the age of anxiety: pharmacology of the benzodiazepines. Science 207:274–281, 1980

Task Panel on Mental Health and American Families: Report of the Sub-Task Panel on General Issues and Adult Years, President's Commission on Mental Health. Washington, DC, U.S. Government Printing Office, 1978

Taylor J, Defrain J, Ernst L: Sudden infant death syndrome, in Parental Loss of a Child. Edited by Rando RA. Champaign, IL, Research Press Co, 1986, pp 159–180

Telch CH, Lindquist CV: Violent vs nonviolent couples: a comparison of patterns. Psychotherapy 21:242–248, 1984

Terman LM, Oden MH: Genetic Studies of Genius V5: The Gifted Group at Midlife. Stanford, CA, Stanford University Press, 1959

Tew BJ, Payne H, Laurence KM: Must a family with a handicapped child be a handicapped family? Medical and Childhood Neurology 16 (suppl 32):95–98, 1974

Tew BJ, Laurence KM, Payne H, et al: Marital stability following the birth of a child with spina bifida. Br J Psychiatry 131:79–82, 1977

Thiebault J, Kelly H: The Social Psychology of Groups. New York, Wiley, 1959

Thoits PA: Multiple identities and psychological well-being. American Sociological Review 48:174–187, 1983

Thomas CB: The relationship of smoking and habits of nervous tension, in Smoking Behavior: Motives and Incentives. Edited by Dunn WL Jr. Washington, DC, Winston, 1973, pp 157–170

Thomas LE, DiGiulio RC, Sheehan WW: Identity loss and psychological crisis in widowhood: a re-evaluation. Int J Aging Hum Dev 26:225–239, 1988

Thompson C: Cultural pressures in the psychology of women. Psychiatry 5:331–339, 1942

Thompson C: Some effects of the derogatory attitude towards female sexuality. Psychiatry 13:349–354, 1950 [Reprinted in Miller JB: Psychoanalysis and Women: Contributions to New Theory and Therapy. New York, Brunner/Mazel, 1973, pp 65–74]

Thompson J: Double-blind study on the effect of estrogen on sleep, anxiety and depression in perimenopausal women: preliminary results. Royal Society of Medicine Proceedings 69:829–830, 1976

Thompson J, Oswald I: Effect of oestrogen on the sleep, mood, and anxiety of menopausal women. BMJ 2:1317-1319, 1977

Touyz SW, Beumont PJV, Glaun D, et al: A comparison of lenient and strict operant conditioning programmes in refeeding patients with anorexia nervosa. Br J Psychiatry 144:517–520, 1984

Towns K, Gentzler R: Empowering re-entry women: an organizational case study, in The Dynamics of Feminist Therapy. New York, Haworth Press, 1986, pp 159–166

Traicoff ME: Family interventions from women's shelters, in Clinical Approaches to Family Violence. Edited by Hansen JC, et al. Rockville, MD, Aspen, 1982, pp 105–115

Tucker S: The role of psychiatry: evaluation and treatment of altered mental status in persons with AIDS, in What to Do About AIDS: Physicians and Health Professionals Discuss the Issues. Edited by McKusichl S. Berkeley, CA, University of California Press, 1986, pp 45–50

Twemlow SW, Gabbard GO: The lovesick therapist, in Sexual Exploitation in Professional Relationships. Edited by Gabbard GO. Washington, DC, American Psychiatric Press, 1989, pp 71–87

Uhlenhuth EH, Balter MB, Mellinger GD, et al: Symptom checklist syndrome in the general population. Arch Gen Psychiatry 40:1167–1173, 1983

Ulman RB, Brothers D: The Shattered Self: A Psychoanalytic Study of Trauma. Hillsdale, NJ, Analytic Press, 1988

U.S. Bureau of the Census: Current Population Reports, Series P-20:31C: Marriage, Divorce, Widowhood and Remarriage by Family Characteristics, June 1975. Washington, DC, U.S. Government Printing Office, 1977

U.S. Merit Systems Protection Board: Sexual Harassment in the Federal Workplace: Is It a Problem? Washington, DC, U.S. Government Printing Office, 1987

Utian WH: The menopause in perspective: from potions to patches. Ann N Y Acad Sci 592:1–8, 1990

Vachon MLS, Rogers J, Lyall WA, et al: Predictors and correlates of adaptation to conjugal bereavement. Am J Psychiatry 139:998–1002, 1982a

Vachon MLS, Sheldon AR, Lanacee WJ, et al: Correlates of enduring distress patterns following bereavement: social network, life situation and personality. Psychol Med 12:783–788, 1982b

Vaillant G: Dangers of psychotherapy in the treatment of alcoholism, in Dynamic Approaches to Understanding and Treatment of Alcoholism. Edited by Bean HH, Zisberg NE. New York, Free Press, 1981, pp 36–55

Vaillant G, Sobowale N, McArthur C: Some psychologic vulnerabilities of physicians. N Engl J Med 287:372–375, 1972

Van der Hart O, Goossens FA: Leavetaking rituals in mourning therapy. Isr J Psychiatry Relat Sci 24:87–98, 1987

Van der Kolk BA: Psychological Trauma. Washington, DC, American Psychiatric Press, 1987

Van Keep PA, Kellerhals JM: The impact of socio-cultural factors on symptom formation: some results of a study on ageing women in Switzerland. Psychother Psychosom 23:251–263, 1974

Van Praag HM: Depression, suicide and serotonin metabolism, in The Neuro-Biology of Manic Depressive Illness. Edited by Post IM, Ballinger JC. Baltimore, MD, Williams & Wilkins, 1984, pp 601–618

Van Rooijen L: Widows' bereavement stress and depression after one and a half years. Paper presented at the Advanced Study Institute in Environmental Stress, Cambridge, UK, 1978

Veevers JE: Voluntary childlessness; a review of issues and evidence. Marriage and Family Review 2:1–261, 1979

Veevers JE: Childless by Choice. Toronto, Butterworths, 1980

Viederman M: Personality change through life experience (I): a model. Psychiatry 49:204–217, 1986

Volkan V: Typical findings in pathological grief. Psychiatr Q 44:231–250, 1970

Volkan V: Linking Objects and Linking Phenomena: A Study of the Forms, Symptoms, Metapsychology and Therapy of Complicated Mourning. New York, International Universities Press, 1981

Voydanoff P: Work and Family Life. Newbury Park, CA, Sage, 1987

Wahl CW: The psychodynamics of consummated maternal incest: a report of two cases. Arch Gen Psychiatry 3:96–101 [188–219], 1960

Waldhera A, Nair C: Legal abortions among teenagers in Canada, 1974 through 1978. Can Med Assoc J 122:1386–1388, 1980

Walker HE: Sexual problems and infertility. Psychosomatics 19:477–484, 1978

Walker K, McBride A, Vachon M: Social support and the crisis of bereavement. Soc Sci Med 11:34-41, 1977

Walker LE: The Battered Woman. New York, Harper & Row, 1979

Walker LE: The Battered Woman Syndrome. New York, Springer, 1984

Walling M, Anderson BL, Johnson SR: Hormonal replacement therapy for postmenopausal women: a review of sexual outcomes and related gynecologic effects. Arch Sex Behav 2:119–137, 1990

Wambach JA: The grief process as a social construct. Omega 16:201–211, 1985–1986

Warner SL: A comparative study of widows' and widowers' perceived social support during the first year of bereavement. Arch Psychiatr Nurs 1:241–250, 1987

Warshaw R: I Never Called It Rape. New York, Harper & Row, 1988

Wasser S, Isembert D: Reproductive failure among women: pathology or adaptation? Journal of Psychosomatic Obstetrics and Gynaecology 5:153–176, 1986

Weingourt R: Wife rape: barriers to identification and treatment. Am J Psychother 39:187–192, 1985

Weissman MM: The myth of involutional melancholia. JAMA 42:742–744, 1979

Weissman MM: The epidemiology of anxiety disorders: rates, risks, familial patterns. Paper presented at the National Institute of Mental Health Conference on Anxiety and Anxiety Disorders, Sterling Forest Conference Center, Tuxedo, NY, September 1983

Weissman MM, Klerman GL: Sex differences and the epidemiology of depression. Arch Gen Psychiatry 34:98–111, 1977

Wengle HP: The psychology of cosmetic surgery: a critical overview of the literature, 1960–62, Part 1. Ann Plast Surg 16:435–443, 1986

Wetmore R: The role of grief in psychoanalysis. Int J Psychoanal 44:97–103, 1963

Wetzel JR: American Youth: A Statistical Snapshot. New York, William T Grand Foundation, 1987, pp 11–13

Whanger AD, Myers AC (eds): Mental Health Assessment and Therapeutic Intervention With Older Adults. Rockville, MD, Aspen, 1984

Whitehead MI, Townsend PT, Pryse-Davies J, et al: Effects of estrogens and progestins on the biochemistry and morphology of the postmenopausal endometrium. N Engl J Med 305:1599–1605, 1981

Whittington HG: Evaluation of therapeutic abortion as an element of preventive psychiatry. Am J Psychiatry 126:1224–1229, 1970

Wilkins AJ: Attempted infanticide. Br J Psychiatry 146:206–208, 1985

Wilson RA: Feminine Forever. New York, Evans, 1966

Wilson RA, Wilson TA: The fate of the nontreated postmenopausal woman. J Am Geriatr Soc 11:347–362, 1963

Windholz MJ, Marmar CR, Horowitz MJ: A review of research on conjugal bereavement: impact on health and efficacy of intervention. Compr Psychiatry 26:433–447, 1985

Winnicott DW: The theory of the parent-infant relationship. Int J Psychoanal 41:585–595, 1960

Winnicott DW: Transitional Objects and Transitional Phenomena in Playing and Reality. New York, Penguin, 1980

Winokur G: Depression in the menopause. Am J Psychiatry 130:92–93, 1973

Wisnack S, Wisnack R, Kassan A, et al: Drinking and drinking problems among women in a U.S. National Survey. Alcohol Health and Research World 9:3–13, 1985

Wolfman BR: Women and their many roles. The Stone Center for Developmental Services and Studies, Work in Progress, Wellesley, MA, 1984, No 83-03

Woods N: Menopausal distress: a model for epidemiological investigation, in Changing Perspectives on Menopause. Edited by Voda AM, Dinnerstein M, O'Donnell SR. Austin, TX, University of Texas Press, 1982, pp 220–238

Woolf V: A Room of One's Own. New York, Harcourt, Brace, 1919, pp 35–36

Worden JW: Grief Counseling and Grief Therapy: A Handbook for the Mental Health Practitioner. New York, Springer, 1982

Working Group on HIV Testing of Pregnant Women and the Newborn. JAMA 264:2416–2420, 1990

World Health Organization: Ninth Revision of the International Classification of Diseases—Clinical Modification (ICD-9-CM). Geneva, World Health Organization, 1977

Wurthman J: Report presented to the American Society for Psychosomatics in Obstetrics and Gynecology. Clinical Psychiatry News, No 18, 1990, p 16

Wurthman RS: Nutrients that modify brain function. Sci Am 246:50–59, 1982

Yalom ID, Lunde DT, Moos RH, et al: "Postpartum blues" syndrome: a description and related variables. Arch Gen Psychiatry 18:16–27, 1968

Yandow V: Alcoholism in women. Psychiatric Annals 19:243–247, 1989

Yankauskas E: Primary female syndromes: an update. N Y State J Med 90:105–301, 1990

Ylikor Kala O, Dawood MY: New concepts in dysmenorrhea. Am J Obstet Gynecol 130:833–847, 1978

Yogev S, Vierra A: The state of motherhood among professional women. Sex Roles 9:391–396, 1983

Young DD: Some misconceptions concerning the menopause. Obstet Gynecol 75:881–883, 1990

Ziel HK, Finkle WD: Increased risk of endometrial carcinoma among users of conjugated estrogens. N Engl J Med 293:1167-1170, 1975

Zinberg NE: Psychoanalytic consideration of aging. J Am Psychoanal Assoc 12:151–159, 1964

Zuckerman BS, Amaro H, Beardstein W: Mental health of adolescent mothers: the implications of depression and drug use. J Dev Behav Pediatr 8:111–116, 1987

Supplemental Readings

Anath J: Hysterectomy and depression. Obstet Gynecol 52:724–730, 1978

Backstrom T: Estrogen and progesterone in plasma in relation to premenstrual tension. J Steroid Biochem 5:257–260, 1974

Barker MG: Psychiatric illness after hysterectomy. BMJ 2:91–95, 1968

Beaumont PJ, Richards DH, Gelden MG: A study of minor psychiatric and physical symptoms during the menstrual cycle. Br J Psychiatry 126:431–434, 1975

Bernstein AE: Psychological meaning of mastectomy after surgical removal of the inner reproductive organs. J Am Med Wom Assoc 40:178–180, 1985

Blackstrom CT, Boyle H, Baird DT: Persistence of symptoms of premenstrual tension in hysterectomized women. Br J Obstet Gynaecol 88:530–536, 1981

Chuong CJ, Coulan CB, Bergsbach ER, et al: Clinical trials of naltrexone in premenstrual syndrome. Obstet Gynecol 72:332–336, 1978

Clare AW: Hormones, behavior, and the menstrual cycle. J Psychosom Res 29:225–233, 1985

DePirro R: Insulin receptors during the menstrual cycle in normal women. J Clin Endocrinol Metab 47:1387–1391, 1978

Drellich MB, Dieber I: Psychological importance of the uterus and its functions. J Nerv Ment Dis 126:322, 1958

Elsner CW, Buster JE, Schindler KA, et al: Bromocriptine in the treatment of premenstrual tension syndrome. Obstet Gynecol 56:723–726, 1980

Gath DH: Psychiatric aspects of hysterectomy, in The Social Consequences of Psychiatric Illness. Edited by Robin L, Clayton TJ, Wing JW. New York, Brunner/Mazel, 1980, pp 33–46

Gath DH, Cooper P, Bond A, et al: Hysterectomy and psychiatric disorder, II: demographic, psychiatric, and physical factors in relation to psychiatric outcome. Br J Psychiatry 140:343–350, 1982

Gath DH, Cooper P, Day A, et al: Hysterectomy and psychiatric disorder, I: levels of psychiatric morbidity before and after hysterectomy. Br J Psychiatry 140:335–342, 1982

Lindemann E: Observations on psychiatric sequelae to surgical operations in women. Am J Psychiatry 98:132–137, 1941

Maguire RP, Lu EG, Beungton PJ, et al: Psychiatric problems in the first year after mastectomy. BMJ 118:963–965, 1978

Martin RL, Roberts WV, Clayton PJ, et al: Psychiatric illness and noncancer hysterectomy. Diseases of the Nervous System 38:974–980, 1977

Martin RL, Roberts WV, Clayton PJ, et al: Psychiatric status after hysterectomy. JAMA 144:350–353, 1980

Pfefferbaum B: A comprehensive program of psychosocial care for mastectomy patients. International Journal of Medicine 1:63–72, 1977

Polivy J: Psychological reactions to hysterectomy: a critical review. Am J Obstet Gynecol 118:417–426, 1974

Rasuch JL: Hormonal and neurotransmitter hypothesis of premenstrual tension. Psychopharmacol Bull 18:26–34, 1982

Richards D: Depression after hysterectomy (letter). Lancet 2:652–673, 1973

Richards DH: A post-hysterectomy syndrome. Lancet 2:983–985, 1974

Roy-Byrne PP, Rubinow DR, Hoban MC, et al: TSH and prolactin responses to TRH in patients with premenstrual syndrome. Am J Psychiatry 144:480–484, 1987

Rubinow DR, Roy-Byrne PP: Premenstrual syndromes: an overview from a methodological perspective. Am J Psychiatry 141:113–142, 1984

Sloan D: The emotional and psychosexual aspects of hysterectomy. Am J Obstet Gynecol 131:598–605, 1978

Stewart A: Clinical and biochemical effects of nutritional supplementation. J Reprod Med 32:405–422, 1987

Witkin MH: Sex after mastectomy. Med Aspects Hum Sex 16:50–59, 1982

Zussman L, Zussman S, Sunley R, et al: Sexual response after hysterectomy-oophorectomy: recent studies and reconsideration of psychogenesis. Am J Obstet Gynecol 140:725–729, 1981

Index

Page numbers printed in **boldface type** *refer to case studies.*